Snapshots in
GASTROENTEROLOGY

Snapshots in
GASTROENTEROLOGY

S Devaji Rao
MS MNAMS FICS

Teaching Faculty
National Board of Examinations

Senior Consultant in General Surgery
Department of Surgical Gastroenterology and
Surgical Oncology
St Isabel's Hospital
Chennai Meenakshi Multispeciality Hospital Ltd
and
Kauvery Hospital
Chennai, Tamil Nadu, India

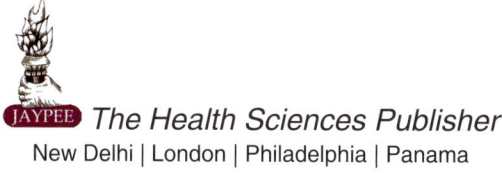

JAYPEE The Health Sciences Publisher
New Delhi | London | Philadelphia | Panama

Jaypee Brothers Medical Publishers (P) Ltd

Headquarters
Jaypee Brothers Medical Publishers (P) Ltd
4838/24, Ansari Road, Daryaganj
New Delhi 110 002, India
Phone: +91-11-43574357
Fax: +91-11-43574314
Email: jaypee@jaypeebrothers.com

Overseas Offices

J.P. Medical Ltd
83 Victoria Street, London
SW1H 0HW (UK)
Phone: +44 20 3170 8910
Fax: +44 (0)20 3008 6180
Email: info@jpmedpub.com

Jaypee Medical Inc.
The Bourse
111 South Independence Mall East
Suite 835, Philadelphia, PA 19106, USA
Phone: +1 267-519-9789
Email: jpmed.us@gmail.com

Jaypee Brothers Medical Publishers (P) Ltd
Bhotahity, Kathmandu, Nepal
Phone: +977-9741283608
Email: kathmandu@jaypeebrothers.com

Jaypee-Highlights Medical Publishers Inc.
City of Knowledge, Bld. 237, Clayton
Panama City, Panama
Phone: +1 507-301-0496
Fax: +1 507-301-0499
Email: cservice@jphmedical.com

Jaypee Brothers Medical Publishers (P) Ltd
17/1-B Babar Road, Block-B, Shaymali
Mohammadpur, Dhaka-1207
Bangladesh
Mobile: +08801912003485
Email: jaypeedhaka@gmail.com

Website: www.jaypeebrothers.com
Website: www.jaypeedigital.com

© 2016, Jaypee Brothers Medical Publishers

The views and opinions expressed in this book are solely those of the original contributor(s)/author(s) and do not necessarily represent those of editor(s) of the book.

All rights reserved. No part of this publication may be reproduced, stored or transmitted in any form or by any means, electronic, mechanical, photocopying, recording or otherwise, without the prior permission in writing of the publishers.

All brand names and product names used in this book are trade names, service marks, trademarks or registered trademarks of their respective owners. The publisher is not associated with any product or vendor mentioned in this book.

Medical knowledge and practice change constantly. This book is designed to provide accurate, authoritative information about the subject matter in question. However, readers are advised to check the most current information available on procedures included and check information from the manufacturer of each product to be administered, to verify the recommended dose, formula, method and duration of administration, adverse effects and contraindications. It is the responsibility of the practitioner to take all appropriate safety precautions. Neither the publisher nor the author(s)/editor(s) assume any liability for any injury and/or damage to persons or property arising from or related to use of material in this book.

This book is sold on the understanding that the publisher is not engaged in providing professional medical services. If such advice or services are required, the services of a competent medical professional should be sought.

Every effort has been made where necessary to contact holders of copyright to obtain permission to reproduce copyright material. If any have been inadvertently overlooked, the publisher will be pleased to make the necessary arrangements at the first opportunity.

Inquiries for bulk sales may be solicited at: jaypee@jaypeebrothers.com

Snapshots in Gastroenterology

First Edition: **2016**

ISBN: 978-93-5152-881-4

Printed at Sanat Printers

Dedicated to

My teachers

My parents
Uma Bai and Siva Rao

My daughters and their husbands
Bhavna and Dhananjai
Kirthana and Rakesh

My beloved wife
Kalpana

Preface

Gastroenterology is a large subdivision of medicine and has been the major attraction for many students in medicine. The explosion of technology and knowledge has changed the diagnostic and therapeutic concepts in this field. The books on gastroenterology have become voluminous for this reason.

The book *Snapshots in Gastroenterology* published by M/s Jaypee Brothers Medical Publishers (P) Ltd, New Delhi, India, is designed to collate all the details in a bulleted and understandable form.

The book is aimed at a well read and sophisticated audience, and has a wealth of information essential and necessary for those interested in gastroenterology. Thoughtfully, it covers both the medical and surgical aspects of gastroenterology, making the presentation complete, but concise.

The photographs and the figures add the color and quality to this prized manual, which I hope will fulfill the needs of those practitioners of medicine, more so the students of medical schools.

S Devaji Rao

Acknowledgments

My first thanks goes to Shri Jitendar P Vij (Group Chairman), Mr Ankit Vij (Group President) and Mr Tarun Duneja (Director-Publishing) of M/s Jaypee Brothers Medical publishers (P) Ltd. New Delhi, India, for choosing me to author this book on gastroenterology belonging to the series, Snapshots.

My special thanks to my friends Dr Mani Veeraraghavan for the endoscopy photographs and Dr V Ganesan for the ultrasound photographs. Most of the CT and MRI pictures were procured from Bharat Scans, Chennai, and I sincerely thank Dr R Emmanuel for providing them.

My very special thanks goes to my wife Kalpana for the tolerance during the preparation of this manual.

Detailed chapter corrections were done by my daughter Dr Bhavna Rao, and above all I express my very sincere thanks to my daughter Dr Kirthana Rao for patiently drawing the computer-aided illustrations.

I am grateful to all those working for M/s Jaypee Brothers Medical Publishers (P) Ltd, New Delhi, India, for their expertise in shaping this edition.

Contents

Chapter 1: Acute Abdominal Pain — 1
- Acute Upper Abdominal Pain   3
- Acute Lower Abdominal Pain   9
- Colic   14

Chapter 2: Chronic Abdominal Pain — 19
- Etiology   19
- Diagnosis   19
- Management   30

Chapter 3: Dysphagia — 31
- Surgical Anatomy of Esophagus   31
- Physiology of Swallowing   31
- Dysphagia   32

Chapter 4: Diarrhea — 38
- Definition   38
- Types of Diarrhea   38
- Acute Diarrhea   38
- Dysentery   39
- Traveler's Diarrhea   42
- Chronic Diarrhea   43

Chapter 5: Constipation and Fecal Incontinence 50

- Anatomy of Anorectum 50
- Physiology of Defecation 50
- Constipation 51
- Fecal Incontinence 58

Chapter 6: Nausea and Vomiting 61

- Causes of Nausea and Vomiting 61
- Pathogenesis 61
- Diagnosis 63

Chapter 7: Gaseousness 65

- Belching 65
- Bloating 66
- Flatulence 67

Chapter 8: Jaundice 69

- Bilirubin Metabolism 69
- Anatomy of Biliary System 69
- Disorders of Bilirubin Metabolism 72
- Gilbert's Syndrome (GS) 73
- Crigler–Najjar Syndrome 76
- Dubin–Johnson Syndrome (DJS) 79
- Rotor Syndrome 81
- Lucey–Driscoll Syndrome 82
- Obstructive Jaundice 82

Contents

Chapter 9: Gastrointestinal Hemorrhage 88
- Upper Gastrointestinal Bleed 88
- Management (Step By Step) 93
- Lower Gastrointestinal Bleed 99
- Obscure Gastrointestinal Bleed 112

Chapter 10: Esophagus 116
- Anatomy and Physiology 116
- Approach to a Patient with Esophageal Pathology 118
- Atresia of Esophagus 119
- Achalasia Cardia (Cardiospasm) 122
- Esophageal Webs 127
- Schatzki's Ring 129
- Diverticula of the Esophagus 131
- Hiatus Hernia 134
- Reflux Esophagitis (Gastroesophageal Reflux Disease—GERD) 137
- Transthoracic Belsey Mark IV Operation 148
- Transthoracic Nissen Fundoplication 151
- Nissen's Fundoplication (Open Procedure) 152
- Modified Hill Repair 155
- Collis Gastroplasty 158
- Endoscopic Treatment of GERD 160
- Barrett's Esophagus 165
- Strictures of Esophagus 169
- Esophageal Injury 172
- Infections of Esophagus 173

- Diffuse Esophageal Spasm 175
- Foreign Bodies of Esophagus 176
- Esophageal Varices 179
- Mallory–Weiss Tear of Esophagus 181
- Benign Tumors 182
- Esophageal Malignancy 184
- Esophageal Resections 191
- Transhiatal Esophagectomy 193
- Postesophagectomy Complications 195

Chapter 11: Stomach and Duodenum 197

- Surgical Anatomy 197
- Approach to a Patient with Upper Gastrointestinal Pathology 204
- Gastric Volvulus 205
- Gastritis 209
- Acid Peptic Disease 214
- Zollinger–Ellison Syndrome (ZES) 228
- Gastroparesis 230
- Gastric Polyps 232
- Gastric Malignancy 236
- Congenital Pyloric Stenosis 251
- Injuries of Duodenum 255
- Bezoars 256
- Dieulafoy's Ulcer 258
- Menetrier's Disease 260
- Bariatric Surgery 261

- Surgeries of Stomach and Duodenum 265
- Partial/Subtotal Gastrectomy 268
- Complications of Gastric Surgery and Management 281
- Long-term Complications of Gastric Surgery 306

Chapter 12: Small Intestine 347

- Anatomy 347
- Physiology 349
- Approach to the Patient with Small Bowel Disease 350
- Small Bowel Atresia 352
- Volvulus of Midgut 354
- Injuries of Small Intestine 357
- Intussusception 359
- Abdominal Tuberculosis 365
- Crohn's Disease 369
- Whipple's Disease 377
- Celiac Disease 379
- Irritable Bowel Syndrome 380
- Strictures 383
- Paralytic Ileus 385
- Ischemic Enteritis/Mesenteric Vascular Obstruction 386
- Intestinal Obstruction 389
- Diverticulitis of Small Bowel 393

xvi Snapshots in Gastroenterology

- Angiodysplasia   400
- Benign Tumors   401
- Malignant Tumors   402
- Surgery of Small Bowel   410
- Postoperative complications   419

Chapter 13: Vermiform Appendix   435

- Surgical Anatomy   435
- Congenital Anomalies   437
- Acute Appendicitis   438
- Recurrent Appendicitis   452
- Neoplasms of Appendix   453
- Surgery of Appendix   460
- Complications of Appendicectomy   469

Chapter 14: Large Intestine   477

- Anatomy   477
- Physiology   479
- Volvulus   479
- Injuries of Large Intestine   489
- Ulcerative Colitis   490
- Pseuodmembranous Colitis   497
- Radiation Colitis   500
- Ischemic Colitis   502
- Ogilvie's Syndrome   506
- Diverticulitis   511
- Cecal Diverticulitis   520

Contents xvii

- Colorectal Polyps 522
- Polyposis Syndromes 534
- Colonic Malignancy 537
- Hereditary Non-polyposis Colorectal Cancer (HNPCC) 550
- Surgeries of Colon 551
- Ileorectal/Ileoanal Anastomosis 561
- Ileal Pouch–Anal Anastomosis 561
- Complications of Colonic Surgery 562

Chapter 15: Rectum and Anal Canal 569

- Anatomy 569
- Physiology 571
- Approach to the Patient with Anorectal Disease 571
- Hirschsprung's Disease 572
- Anorectal Malformations 575
- Injuries of Rectum 579
- Hemorrhoids 580
- Perianal Hematoma 611
- Anal Fissures 612
- Anorectal Abscesses 617
- Fistula in Ano 621
- Amebic Proctitis and Ulcers 634
- Rectal Polyps 635
- Rectal Malignancy 636
- Anal Malignancy 649

- Rectal Prolapse 653
- Solitary Rectal Ulcer 661

Chapter 16: Intestinal Stomas 663

- Input Stomas 663
- Jejunostomy 672
- Complications of Input Stomas 679
- Output Stomas 680
- Ileostomy 683
- Colostomy 685
- Appliances 696
- Problems 705
- Complications of Ostomy 707
- Continent Ileostomy 716
- Complications 717

Chapter 17: Liver 720

- Surgical Anatomy 720
- Physiology 724
- Approach to the Patient with Liver Disease 726
- Hepatomegaly 737
- Injuries of Liver 739
- Viral Hepatitis 743
- Autoimmune Hepatitis 755
- Alcoholic Liver Disease (ALD) 759
- Alcohol Withdrawal Syndrome 764

Contents xix

- Non-alcoholic Fatty Liver Disease (NAFLD)   766
- Drug-induced Liver Disease (DILD)   768
- Metabolic Liver Diseases   772
- Cirrhosis   780
- Primary Biliary Cirrhosis   785
- Portal Vein Thrombosis   787
- Budd–Chiari Syndrome   790
- Portal Hypertension   793
- Ascites   799
- Hepatic Encephalopathy   805
- Hepatorenal Syndrome   808
- Focal Liver Masses   809
- Liver Abscess   814
- Cystic Liver Diseases   822
- Congenital Liver Cysts   824
- Hydatid Cyst of Liver   828
- Neoplastic Liver Cysts   832
- Benign Liver Tumors   833
- Hepatoblastoma   840
- Primary Liver Malignancy   841
- Hepatocellular Carcinoma   842
- Metastatic Liver Disease   849
- Surgical Procedures: Shunt Procedures   852
- Hepatectomy   856
- Liver Transplantation   862

Chapter 18: Gallbladder and Bile Ducts   869

- Anatomy 869
- Physiology 871
- Anomalies 871
- Biliary Atresia 872
- Choledochal Cysts 874
- Gallstones (Cholelithiasis) 881
- Chronic Cholecystitis 885
- Acute Cholecystitis 890
- Acalculous Cholecystitis 900
- Emphysematous Cholecystitis 902
- Choledocholithiasis 904
- Gallstone Ileus 914
- Injuries to the Biliary Tract 915
- Bile Duct Strictures 924
- Primary Sclerosing Cholangitis (PSC) 928
- Sphincter of Oddi Dysfunction 932
- Gallbladder Polyps 934
- Carcinoma of Gallbladder 937
- Cholangiocarcinoma 943
- Operative Procedures 951
- Management of Choledocholithiasis 973

Chapter 19: Pancreas   983

- Anatomy and Physiology 983
- Approach to a Patient with Pancreatic Disease 987
- Acute Pancreatitis (AP) 992

- Chronic Pancreatitis (CP) 1008
- Pancreatic Pseudocyst 1023
- Ampullary and Periampullary Carcinoma 1026
- Pancreatic Malignancy 1030
- Cystic Neoplasms of Pancreas 1037
- Islet Cell Tumors of Pancreas 1041
- Surgery of Pancreas: Pancreatic Resections 1043
- Complications of Pancreatic Surgery 1045

Index　　　　　　　　　　　　　　　　　　　　　　　　　　　　*1053*

Abbreviations

5HIAA	:	5 Hydroxy indole acetic acid
ACTH	:	Adrenocorticotrophic hormone
ADH	:	Antidiuretic hormone
AIDS	:	Acquired immunodeficiency syndrome
APC gene	:	Adenomatous polyposis coli gene
APUD	:	Amine precursor uptake and decarboxylation
ARDS	:	Acute respiratory distress syndrome
ASA	:	Acetyl salicylic acid
BMI	:	Body mass index
BE	:	Barrett's esophagus
CBD	:	Common bile duct
CCK	:	Cholecystokinin
CEA	:	Carcinoembryonic antigen
CECT	:	Contrast-enhanced computed tomography
CHD	:	Common hepatic duct
CRP	:	C-reactive protein
CT	:	Computerized tomography
CUSA	:	Cavitron ultrasonic surgical aspirator
DNA	:	Deoxyribonucleic acid
EG junction	:	Esophagogastric junction
ELISA	:	Enzyme-linked immunosorbent assay
ERCP	:	Endoscopic retrograde cholangiopancreatography

ESR	:	Erythrocyte sedimentation rate
EUS	:	Endoscopic ultrasound
FNA	:	Fine needle aspiration
GE junction	:	Gastroesophageal junction
GERD	:	Gastroesophageal reflux disease
GIT	:	Gastrointestinal tract
H. pylori	:	*Helicobacter pylori*
HCV	:	Hepatitis C virus
HDV	:	Hepatitis D virus
HEV	:	Hepatitis E virus
HIDA	:	Hydroxy iminodiacetic acid
IBD	:	Inflammatory bowel disease
IL	:	Interleukin
INR	:	International normalized ratio
LFT	:	Liver function tests
LHA	:	Left hepatic artery
MALT	:	Mucosa-associated lymphoid tissue
MDCT	:	Multi-detector computed tomography
MEN	:	Multiple endocrine neoplasia
MODS	:	Multiorgan dysfunction syndrome
MPR	:	Multiplanar reformation
MRCP	:	Magnetic resonance cholangiopancreatography
MRI	:	Magnetic resonance imaging
NBM	:	Nil by mouth
NBT-PABA	:	N-benzoyl-tyrosyl-para-aminobenzoic acid
NG tube	:	Nasogastric tube
NSAID	:	Nonsteroidal anti-inflammatory drug

PAS	:	Para-aminosalicylic acid
PCR	:	Polymerase chain reaction
PEG	:	Polyethylene glycol
PET	:	Positron emission tomography
PJ	:	Pancreatojejunostomy
PPI	:	Proton-pump inhibitor
PTBD	:	Percutaneous transhepatic biliary drainage
PTFE	:	Polytetrafluoroethylene
PTC	:	Percutaneous transhepatic cholangiography
RHA	:	Right hepatic artery
RIBA	:	Recombinant immunoblot assay
RNA	:	Ribonucleic acid
SIRS	:	Systemic inflammatory response syndrome
SLE	:	Systemic lupus erythematosus
TAUS	:	Transabdominal ultrasonography
TEF	:	Tracheoesophageal fistula
TNF	:	Tumor necrosis factor
TSH	:	Thyroid stimulating hormone
UDCA	:	Ursodeoxycholic acid
US	:	Ultrasonography
VIP	:	Vasoactive intestinal polypeptide

Chapter 1

Acute Abdominal Pain

INTRODUCTION

Abdominal pain is the most common symptom of the pathologies of the gastrointestinal tract. The pain can occur in any part of the abdomen, but for convenience, it can be divided into upper abdominal and lower abdominal.

The main visceral pain receptors in the abdomen respond to mechanical and chemical stimuli.

- **Mechanical stimuli:** Stretch, distension, contraction, compression and torsion.
- **Chemical stimuli:** Bradykinin, substance P, serotonin and prostaglandins. These receptors are located on the serosal surfaces, within the mesentery and within the walls of hollow viscera.
- Gut related visceral pain is usually perceived in the midline because it is a midline structure in an embryo and has bilateral symmetric innervations, except for pains originating from the gallbladder and the ascending and descending colon. Pain from other intra-abdominal organs tends to be unilateral.
    a. **Pain at epigastrium—Diseases of the foregut** (abdominal esophagus, stomach and proximal half of second part of duodenum and their offshoots like liver, gallbladder, pancreas and spleen) (e.g. gastric and duodenal ulcers).
    b. **Pain at the umbilical region—Diseases of midgut** (distal half of second part of duodenum, small bowel, colon up to the proximal 2/3 of transverse colon) (e.g. intestinal tuberculosis).

Snapshots in Gastroenterology

c. **Pain at the hypogastrium—Diseases of hindgut** (distal 1/3 of transverse colon to the anorectal junction) (e.g. colorectal pathologies).

- The perception of visceral pain corresponds to the spinal segments where the visceral afferent nerve fibers enter the spinal cord. **Table 1.1** shows some common spinal segments where visceral pain is perceived.
- The abdominal pain has particular pattern and has regional localization. The abdomen is divided into ten arbitrary regions for convenience of understanding and localization **(Fig. 1.1)**.

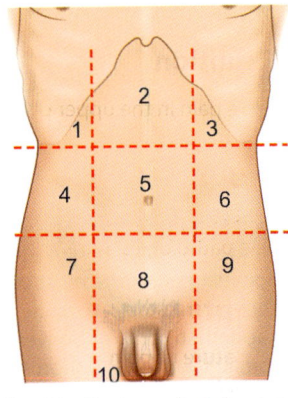

Fig. 1.1: Regions of abdomen: 1. Right hypochondrium, 2. Epigastrium, 3. Left hypochondrium, 4. Right lumbar, 5. Umbilical, 6. Left lumbar, 7. Right iliac fossa, 8. Hypogastrium, 9. Left iliac fossa, 10. External genitalia

Table 1.1: Visceral pain and dermatomal perceptions

Organ of pathology	Site of pain	Dermatome
Stomach	Epigastrium	T5–T10
Small bowel	Umbilicus	T9–T10
Large bowel proximal to splenic flexure	Umbilicus	T11–L1
Large bowel distal to splenic flexure	Hypogastrium	L1–L2
Gallbladder	Epigastrium, right scapular region	T7–T9
Pancreas	Epigastrium	T6–T10

ACUTE UPPER ABDOMINAL PAIN

Definition

Severe pain in the upper part of the abdomen.

Diagnosis

While evaluating the upper abdominal pain, it is necessary to keep some pathologies in mind (**Table 1.2**).

Symptoms

1. **Nature of pain**
   - Continuous (e.g. acute pancreatitis)
   - Episodic (e.g. acute hyperacidity)
   - Colicky (e.g. biliary colic).
2. **Location of pain**
   - Epigastric pain (e.g. acute hyperacidity, acute pancreatitis)
   - Left hypochondrial pain (e.g. acute hyperacidity, left renal colic)
   - Right hypochondrial pain (e.g. acute cholecystitis, acute hepatitis).

Table 1.2: Acute upper abdominal pain and related pathologies

Right upper quadrant pain	Epigastric pain	Left upper quadrant pain
Acute cholecystitis	Acute hyperacidity	Acute pancreatitis
Acute cholangitis	Acute pancreatitis	Acute hyperacidity
Acute hepatitis	Perforated duodenal ulcer	Splenic infarct
Acute hyperacidity	Acute hepatitis (left lobe)	
Perforated duodenal ulcer		

3. **Association of vomiting**
   – Presence of vomiting is not a very reliable symptom to narrow down the diagnosis, as it can be present with any severe painful pathology in the upper abdomen.
4. **Association of fever**
   – Fever indicates infective pathology (e.g. acute cholecystitis, acute pancreatitis, acute colitis, perforated duodenal ulcer).
5. **Association of jaundice**
   – Jaundice may be present with acute cholangitis, acute hepatitis or acute cholecystitis.
6. **Association of loose stools**
   Association of loose stools may indicate colitis or rarely acute pancreatitis.
7. **Radiation**
   Radiation to right scapula or shoulder is common with acute cholecystitis, perforated duodenal ulcer due to irritation of diaphragm.
8. **Aggravating factors**
   – Food—in acute hyperacidity
   – Lying supine—in acute pancreatitis
   – Deep breathing—in acute cholecystitis.
9. **Relieving factors**
   – Leaning forward while sitting—acute pancreatitis.
10. **Referred pain**
    In some pathologies, the pathology and the area of the pain are different, since both of them share the same nerve supply. **(Fig. 1.2) (Table 1.1)**.

Past History

- History of pain (e.g. acute on chronic cholecystitis)

Acute Abdominal Pain

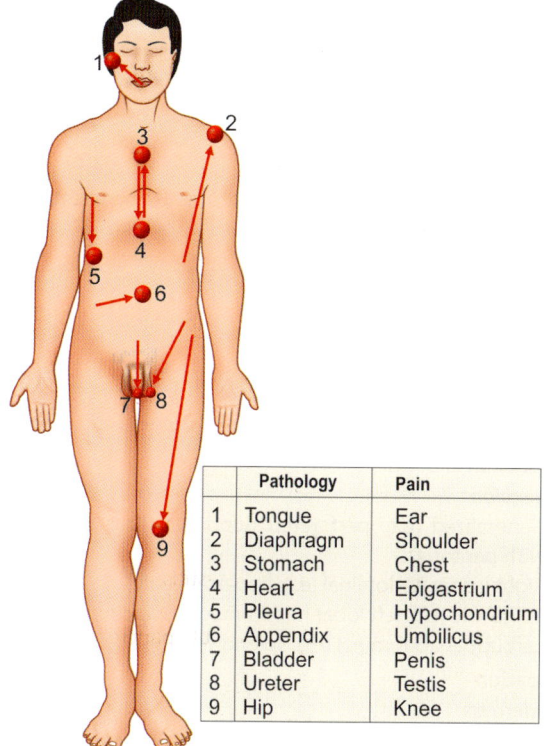

Fig. 1.2: Referred pain

- Previous surgery (e.g. cholecystectomy will rule out cholecystitis from consideration).

Family History

- Gallstones.

Signs

General

- Breath for fetor (e.g. alcoholic hepatitis, acute pancreatitis)
- Conjunctiva for anemia, jaundice
- Tongue for anemia
- Neck for lymphadenopathy
- Hands for signs of liver failure (e.g. clubbing, palmar erythema, liver flap, etc.).

Abdomen

- **Inspection**
  Distension
  - Generalized (e.g. perforated duodenal ulcer or gallbladder with peritonitis)
  - Right upper abdominal (e.g. hepatomegaly)
  - Epigastric (e.g. left lobar hepatomegaly, carcinoma stomach)
  - Left upper abdominal (e.g. splenomegaly).
- **Palpation**
  Tenderness
  - All quadrants—generalized peritonitis
  - Right upper quadrant (e.g. acute hepatitis, acute cholecystitis, acute hyperacidity)
  - Epigastric (e.g. acute gastritis, acute hepatitis)
  - Left upper quadrant (e.g. acute gastritis, acute pancreatitis).

Lump
- Right upper quadrant (e.g. hepatomegaly, distended gall-bladder)
- Epigastric (e.g. carcinoma stomach, left lobar hepatomegaly)
- Left upper quadrant (e.g. carcinoma stomach, splenomegaly).

- **Percussion**

  Percuss the liver for:
  - Its enlargement (e.g. acute hepatitis)
  - Obliteration of liver dullness (e.g. perforated duodenal ulcer).
- **Auscultation**
  - Absence of bowel sounds indicates paralytic ileus (e.g. perforated peritonitis).
  - Normal bowel sounds indicate that there is no gross infection of the peritoneum.

Differential Diagnosis of Acute Upper Abdominal Pain of GI Etiologies

- *Right hypochondrial pain*
  - *Without fever and but local tenderness* (e.g. acute cholecystitis, acute hepatitis, acute hyperacidity).
  - *With fever and local tenderness*
    - *± distension* (e.g. acute cholecystitis)
    - *Obliteration of liver dullness* (e.g. perforated duodenal ulcer)
    - *± hepatomegaly* (e.g. acute liver abscess).
  - *With vomiting and*
    - *Local tenderness* (e.g. acute cholecystitis, acute hyperacidity)
    - *Local tenderness with obliteration of liver dullness* (e.g. perforated duodenal ulcer).

- With diarrhea and local tenderness (e.g. acute colitis).
- With jaundice and
  - *Local tenderness ± hepatomegaly* (e.g. acute hepatitis, acute cholecystitis, choledocholithiasis, cholangitis, acute liver abscess)
  - *Local tenderness, fever, +/- abdominal lump* (e.g. mucocele gallbladder, choledochal cyst)
- *Colicky in nature +/- local tenderness* (e.g. biliary colic).
- *Epigastric pain*
  - *Without fever but with local tenderness* (e.g. acute hyperacidity, acute pancreatitis, acute hepatitis—left lobe)
  - *With fever and local tenderness ± distension* (e.g. acute pancreatitis, perforated duodenal or gastric ulcer).
  - *With vomiting and*
    - *Local tenderness* (e.g. acute hyperacidity, acute pancreatitis)
    - *Local tenderness and obliteration of liver dullness* (e.g. perforated ulcer).
  - *With diarrhea and local tenderness* (e.g. acute colitis).
  - *With jaundice*
    - *± tender hepatomegaly* (e.g. left lobar hepatitis, left lobar liver abscess)
    - *Non-tender hepatomegaly* (e.g. metastatic liver).
- *Left hypochondrial pain*
  - *Without fever but with local tenderness* (e.g. acute gastritis, acute pancreatitis)
  - *With fever and local tenderness +/- splenomegaly* (e.g. acute pancreatitis, splenic infarct)
  - *With diarrhea and local tenderness* (e.g. acute colitis).

Investigations

Blood tests

- **Leukocytosis** in infective pathologies (e.g. acute cholecystitis, perforated duodenal ulcer, perforated cholecystitis, acute pancreatitis)
- **Raised ESR** in all infective pathologies.

Radiology

- **Plain X-ray abdomen**—gas under the diaphragm (e.g. perforated hollow viscus). Radiopaque shadows in the right upper abdomen (e.g. renal stones, gallstones)
- **Ultrasonography**—renal stones, gallstones.

Management

- **Non-perforated pathologies**—medical management.
- **Perforated pathologies**—early surgical management.
- **Diagnosis not clear and not responding to medical management**—exploratory laparotomy.

Clinical Pearl

- Acute nephritis and renal colic can cause upper abdominal pain in their respective sides.

ACUTE LOWER ABDOMINAL PAIN

Definition

Severe pain in the lower part of the abdomen.

Diagnosis

While evaluating lower abdominal pain, it is necessary to keep some pathologies in mind **(Table 1.3)**.

Symptoms

1. **Nature of pain**
   - Continuous (e.g. acute appendicitis)
   - Colicky (e.g. appendicular colic).
2. **Location of pain**
   - Right lower abdomen (e.g. acute appendicitis, right ureteric colic)
   - Hypogastrium (e.g. acute colorectal pathologies)
   - Left lower abdomen (e.g. acute diverticulitis, left ureteric colic).
3. **Association of nausea and vomiting**
   Presence of vomiting is not a very reliable symptom to narrow down the diagnosis, as it can be present with any severe painful pathology in the lower abdomen. Nausea is a predominant symptom of acute appendicitis.

Table 1.3: Acute lower abdominal pain and GI pathologies

Right lower quadrant pain	Hypogastric pain	Left lower quadrant pain
Acute appendicitis	Acute cystitis	Acute diverticulitis
Acute Meckel's diverticulitis	Acute congestive dysmenorrhea	
Perforated appendicitis	Meckel's diverticulitis	
Acute mesenteric adenitis		
Ureteric colic		
Acute cecal diverticulitis		

Note: Diabetic ketoacidosis is one of the important metabolic causes of acute lower abdominal pain.

4. **Association of fever**
   Fever indicates infective pathology (e.g. acute appendicitis, acute colitis).
5. **Association of loose stools**
   Association of loose stools may indicate colitis, acute diverticulitis.

Past History

- History of pain (e.g. acute on chronic appendicitis)
- Previous surgery (e.g. appendicectomy will rule out appendicitis from consideration).

Family History

- Diverticulosis
- Colonic malignancy.

Signs

General

- Conjunctiva for anemia (e.g. GI malignancy)
- Tongue for anemia (e.g. GI malignancy).

Abdomen

- **Inspection**
  Distension
  – Generalized (e.g. perforated appendicitis with generalized peritonitis)
  – Right lower abdominal (e.g. ruptured appendicitis).

- **Palpation**
  Tenderness
  – All quadrants—generalized peritonitis
  – Right lower quadrant (e.g. acute appendicitis, acute mesenteric adenitis)
  – Left lower quadrant (e.g. acute colitis, acute diverticulitis).
  Lump
  – Right lower quadrant (e.g. acute appendicitis mesenteric adenitis, right ovarian cyst)
  – Left lower quadrant (e.g. carcinoma colon).
- **Percussion**
  Percuss the liver for:
  – Its enlargement (e.g. associated metastases liver)
  – Obliteration of liver dullness (e.g. perforated appendicitis and diverticulitis).
- **Auscultation**
  – Absence of bowel sounds indicates paralytic ileus (e.g. perforation and peritonitis)
  – Exaggerated bowel sounds may indicate obstruction of small bowel (e.g. intestinal colic)
  – Normal bowel sounds indicate that there is no gross infection of the peritoneum.

Differential Diagnosis of Acute Lower Abdominal Pain of GI Etiologies

- *Pain in the right iliac fossa with*
  – ***Nausea/vomiting and fever and local tenderness*** (e.g. acute catarrhal/perforated appendicitis, acute typhlitis, acute Meckel's diverticulitis, acute mesenteric adenitis).

Acute Abdominal Pain

  - *Vomiting and*
    - *± local tenderness* (colicky pain, e.g. appendicular colic)
    - ***Abdominal lump*** (e.g. ileocecal tuberculosis, Crohn's disease, cecal malignancy).
  - *Diarrhea or dysentery and local tenderness* (e.g. acute amebic typhlitis, cecal diverticulitis).
- *Pain in the left iliac fossa with vomiting*
  - *± local tenderness* (e.g. left ureteric colic)
  - *Abdominal lump* (e.g. colonic malignancy)
  - *Diarrhea or dysentery with or without local tenderness* (e.g. acute colitis, acute diverticulitis).
- *Hypogastric pain with*
  - *Constipation (*e.g. rectal pathology).
- *Acute lower abdominal pain (any or all quadrants of lower abdomen) with*
  - *Vague symptoms and signs* (e.g. Metabolic causes- diabetes mellitus).

Investigations

Blood Tests

- *Reduced hematocrit* (e.g. colonic malignancy)
- *Leukocytosis* in infective pathologies (e.g. acute appendicitis, perforated appendicitis, and diverticulitis)
- *Raised ESR* in all infective pathologies.

Radiology

- Plain X-ray abdomen
  - Gas under the diaphragm (e.g. perforated appendicitis and diverticulitis)

- Opaque abdomen (e.g. peritonitis)
- Radiopaque shadows (e.g. ureteric stone).
- *Ultrasonography*
  - Cystic swelling (e.g. appendicular abscess, paracolic abscess).

Management

- *Non-perforated pathologies*—medical management (except acute appendicitis)
- *Perforated pathologies*—early surgical management
- *Diagnosis not clear and not responding to medical management*—exploratory laparotomy or diagnostic laparoscopy.

Clinical Pearls

- Obstetric conditions like ruptured ectopic gestation should be thought of in a woman of reproductive age
- Gynecologic conditions like torsion of ovarian cyst should be considered in acute lower abdominal pain
- Urologic conditions like acute cystitis should be considered in patients with acute lower abdominal pain with urinary symptoms
- Ureteric colic should be considered in patients with acute pain in the iliac fossae
- Complicated hernia should be considered in patients with acute lower abdominal pain.

COLIC

Definition

Colic is defined as a sudden squeezing or griping pain lasting for about 3–5 minutes with pain free intervals.

Acute Abdominal Pain

- Nausea, vomiting and retching are common accompaniments
- The cause of a colic is partial obstruction of a tubular structure due to varied causes.

Diagnosis

While evaluating abdominal colic, the following GI pathologies should be kept in mind (**Table 1.4**).

Clinical Features

The clinical features of various colics of GI pathologies are given in **Table 1.5**.

Table 1.4: Colic related to GI pathologies

Right hypochondrium	Umbilical region	Right iliac fossa
Biliary colic	Intestinal colic	Appendicular colic

Table 1.5: Clinical features of various colics

Clinical feature	Biliary colic	Intestinal colic	Appendicular colic
Incidence	Fat, fertile, flatulent, female of fifty	Any age	Any age
Etiology	Gallstones	Parasitic infestations (younger age), strictures (middle age), malignancy (old age)	Fecaliths, Worms
Nature of pain	Right hypochondrial pain, referred to right scapula or shoulder	Colicky pain in the umbilical region	Colicky pain in the right iliac fossa
Associated symptom	Dyspepsia	Constipation or diarrhea	Repeated attacks of dull pain in right iliac fossa

Eliciting History

1. **Nature of pain**
   - Severe griping pain with pain free intervals.
2. **Location of pain**
   - Location almost gives the clue.
3. **Association of vomiting**

   Presence of vomiting is not a very reliable symptom to narrow down the diagnosis, as it can be present with any colic.
4. **Association of fever**
   - Fever indicates associated infections (e.g. cholangitis in biliary colic).
5. **Association of jaundice**
   - Jaundice may be present with biliary colic (e.g. acute cholangitis, acute hepatitis or acute cholecystitis).
6. **Association of loose stools**
   - Association of loose stools may indicate colitis.
7. **Radiation**
   - Radiation to right scapula or shoulder is common with biliary colic (e.g. acute cholecystitis).

Past History

- History of pain (e.g. colics can be recurrent)
- Previous surgery (e.g. intestinal colic can occur in adhesive obstruction of small bowel).

Family History

- Gallstones.

Differential Diagnosis by Clinical History

Depends mostly on:
- Location of pain
- Associated jaundice (e.g. cholangitis).

Clinical Examination

General
- May not be contributory.

Abdomen

- **Inspection**

  Distension
  - Generalized (e.g. intestinal colic of intestinal obstruction)
  - Localized (e.g. intussusception).
- **Palpation**

  Tenderness
  - Elicitable in infective pathologies.

  Lump
  - Right upper quadrant (e.g. distended gallbladder)
  - Umbilical (e.g. post operative adhesions)
- **Percussion**
  - Not a very useful method.
- **Auscultation**
  - Exaggerated bowel sounds may indicate obstruction of small bowel (e.g. intestinal colic)
  - Normal bowel sounds does not rule out any pathology.

Investigations

Hematology

- *Leukocytosis* in infective pathologies (e.g. acute cholecystitis)
- *Raised ESR* in all infective pathologies.

Radiology

- *Plain X-ray abdomen*—gas filled loops of bowel (e.g. acute intussusceptions, acute intestinal obstruction)
- *Ultrasonography*—intussusception.

Management

- Medical management will suffice in most instances
- Obstructive pathologies may require surgery to relieve the cause of obstruction
- Repeated attacks of colic will require evaluation and management.

Chapter 2

Chronic Abdominal Pain

INTRODUCTION

Abdominal pain lasting for more than 6 months is referred to as chronic abdominal pain.

ETIOLOGY

While evaluating chronic abdominal pain of GI etiology, the pathologies listed in **Table 2.1** should be kept in mind.

DIAGNOSIS

Symptoms

1. **Nature of pain**
    - Severe and continuous (e.g. chronic pancreatitis)
    - Dull and continuous (e.g. chronic appendicitis)
    - Episodic (e.g. chronic hyperacidity)
    - Burning pain (e.g. acid peptic disease).
2. **Aggravating factors**
    - Physical movements like jolting (e.g. infections, abdominal malignancies)
    - Deep inspiration (e.g. hepatic malignancy)
    - Intake of fatty food (e.g. chronic cholecystitis)

Table 2.1: Chronic abdominal pain and various pathologies

Right hypochondrium	Epigastrium	Left hypochondrium
• Chronic cholecystitis • Gallbladder malignancy • Chronic hepatitis • Space occupying lesions of liver • Malignant hepatic disease (Primary and secondary) • Acid peptic disease • Gastric malignancy	• Acid peptic disease • Gastric malignancy • Chronic pancreatitis • Pancreatic head malignancy • Lesions of liver (left lobe)	• Chronic pancreatitis • Acid peptic disease • Splenic infarct
Right lumbar region	**Umbilical region**	**Left lumbar region**
• Carcinoma of ascending colon	• Gastric/pancreatic malignancy • Malignancy of transverse colon • Dissection of abdominal aorta	• Carcinoma of descending colon
Right iliac fossa	**Hypogastrium**	**Left iliac fossa**
• Chronic appendicitis • Amebic typhlitis • Ileocecal tuberculosis • Crohn's disease • Malignancy of cecum	• Rectal inflammation • Rectal malignancy	• Ulcerative colitis • Diverticulitis • Malignancy of colorectum

   – Intake of spicy food, alcohol (e.g. acid peptic disease)
   – Lying supine (e.g. chronic pancreatitis)
   – Drugs—analgesics (e.g. acid peptic disease).
3. **Relieving factors**
   – Vomiting (e.g. acid peptic disease)
   – Intake of bland food (e.g. acid peptic disease)

Chronic Abdominal Pain

- Leaning forward (e.g. chronic pancreatitis)
- Drugs—antacids, H_2 blockers (e.g. acid peptic disease)

4. **Association of vomiting**

   Presence of vomiting is a reliable symptom to narrow down the diagnosis, as it can represent an obstructive pathology or an acute exacerbation, but the following is to be considered:
   - Character of vomiting
     - ***Projectile*** (e.g. high intestinal obstruction)
     - ***Regurgitative*** (e.g. low intestinal obstruction).
   - Frequency of vomiting
     - ***Constant*** (e.g. gastric outlet obstruction)
     - ***Periodical*** (e.g. intestinal obstruction).
   - Nature of vomitus
     - ***Brownish to dark brown*** (coffee ground color) (e.g. chronic duodenal ulcer, gastritis, carcinoma of stomach)
     - ***Greenish*** due to the presence of bile (e.g. high intestinal obstruction)
     - ***White or colorless*** due to the absence of bile (e.g. gastric outlet obstruction and pyloric or antral growth which prevent the bile reflux)
     - ***Reddish*** (e.g. frank blood due to bleeding esophageal varices)
     - ***Yellowish or yellowish green (foul smelling)*** (e.g. gastrojejunocolic fistula).
   - Quantity of vomitus
     - ***Large quantities*** indicate distal bowel obstruction
     - ***Small quantities*** indicate gastric outlet obstruction.
   - Relationship with pain
     - Pain preceding vomiting (e.g. gastric outlet obstruction)
     - Pain and vomiting occurring together (e.g. high intestinal obstruction)

- Vomiting occurs much later than the pain (e.g. low intestinal obstruction)
- Vomiting as a late feature or absent (e.g. large intestinal obstruction).

5. **Association of dyspepsia**
   - *Dyspepsia and flatulence* (e.g. chronic cholecystitis)
   - *Dyspepsia and early satiety* (e.g. duodenal stenosis and gastric outlet obstruction, gastric carcinoma)
   - *Feeling of fullness* (e.g. chronic pancreatitis, obstructive jaundice).

6. **Association of fever**
   - Fever indicates infective pathology (e.g. ileocecal tuberculosis), rarely malignancies (e.g. malignancy).

7. **Association of jaundice**
   Jaundice may be present with chronic pancreatitis, malignancy of liver.

8. **Change in bowel habits**
   - *Constipation* (e.g. obstructive colonic malignancy, strictures of intestinal tuberculosis)
   - *Diarrhea* (e.g. ulcerative colitis, intestinal tuberculosis)
   - *Alternating diarrhea and constipation* (e.g. left sided colonic tumors)
   - *Spurious diarrhea* (e.g. left sided obstructing colonic tumors).

9. **Color of stools**
   - *Blood stained hard stools* (e.g. left sided colonic malignancy)
   - *Blood stained mucoid loose stools* (e.g. Crohn's disease, ulcerative colitis, colorectal malignancy)
   - *Black colored stools* (e.g. upper gastrointestinal bleed proximal to DJ flexure)

- *White clay colored stools* (e.g. obstructive jaundice)
- *Large, fatty, offensive frothy stools* (e.g. chronic pancreatitis).

10. **Radiation**

    Radiation to right scapula or shoulder is common with chronic cholecystitis.

11. **Appetite and weight loss**

    Appetite loss is a common feature and an early sign of gastrointestinal malignancy.

Past History

- History of treatment (e.g. recurrent appendicitis, tuberculosis)
- Previous surgery (e.g. cholecystectomy will rule out cholecystitis from consideration, consider recurrence of intra-abdominal malignancy).

Family History

- Gallstones
- Pancreatitis
- Colonic malignancy.

Personal History

- *Alcohol* (e.g. chronic duodenal ulcer)
- *Tobacco* (e.g. chronic duodenal ulcer, pancreatitis)
- *Drugs like NSAIDs*, *steroids* (e.g. chronic duodenal ulcer).

Menstrual History

- Metrorrhagia (e.g. uterine malignancies).

Clinical Examination

General

- Breath for fetor (e.g. chronic hepatitis)
- Conjunctiva for anemia (e.g. malignancies), jaundice (e.g. obstructive jaundice)
- Tongue for anemia (e.g. malignancies)
- Neck for lymphadenopathy (e.g. GI malignancies)
- Hands—clubbing, palmar erythema, liver flap etc. (e.g. signs of liver failure).

Abdomen

- **Inspection**
  Distension
  - Generalized (e.g. ascites, large cysts)
  - Right upper abdominal (e.g. hepatomegaly)
  - Epigastric (e.g. left lobar hepatomegaly, carcinoma stomach)
  - Left upper abdominal (e.g. splenomegaly)

Scars, Swellings and Sinuses

- **Palpation**
  Tenderness
  - Right upper quadrant (e.g. hepatitis)
  - Epigastric (e.g. hepatitis, acid peptic disease)
  - Left upper quadrant (e.g. acid peptic disease)
  - Lumbar (e.g. colonic infections)
  - Right iliac fossa (e.g. chronic appendicitis)
  - Hypogastrium (e.g. chronic cystitis)
  - Left iliac fossa (e.g. chronic ulcerative colitis, diverticulitis).

Lump
- Right upper quadrant (e.g. hepatomegaly, carcinoma gallbladder, distended gallbladder)
- Epigastric (e.g. left lobar hepatomegaly, carcinoma stomach)
- Left upper quadrant (e.g. left lobar hepatomegaly, carcinoma stomach)
- Lumbar (e.g. renal/colonic mass)
- Right iliac fossa (e.g. ileocecal tuberculosis, carcinoma cecum)
- Hypogastrium (e.g. uterine fibroid)
- Left iliac fossa (e.g. carcinoma colon).

- **Percussion**
  Percuss the liver for:
  - Its enlargement (e.g. chronic hepatitis, metastatic liver).
- **Auscultation**
  - Bowel sounds are usually normal in patients with chronic abdominal pain
  - Exaggerated bowel sounds may indicate obstruction of terminal ileum (e.g. ileocecal tuberculosis).

Differential Diagnosis of Chronic Abdominal Pain of GI Etiologies

- *Chronic abdominal pain with no clinical findings* (e.g. any chronic intra-abdominal pathology)
- *Chronic abdominal pain with distension*
  - *Generalized*
    - *Without previous surgery scars and positive fluid thrill* (e.g. ascites)
    - *With previous surgery scars* (e.g. incisional hernia).

- *Localized*
    - Right upper abdominal (e.g. hepatomegaly)
    - Epigastric (e.g. left lobar hepatomegaly, carcinoma stomach)
    - Left upper abdominal (e.g. splenomegaly)
    - Central abdominal (e.g. intestinal tuberculosis)
    - Flanks (e.g. distal colonic obstruction).
- *Chronic abdominal pain with*
    - *Fever ± local tenderness, ± lump* (e.g. intestinal tuberculosis, Crohn's disease, lymphoma of GIT).
    - *Nausea and*
        - *Epigastric tenderness* (e.g. acid peptic disease)
        - *Right iliac fossa tenderness* (e.g. chronic appendicitis).
    - *Vomiting ± fever ± local tenderness* (e.g. malignancy of gastrointestinal tract, obstructing lesions of GIT).
    - *Jaundice*
        - *No clinical findings* (e.g. CBD stones)
        - *Enlarged gallbladder* (e.g. pancreatic head malignancy)
        - *Hepatomegaly* (e.g. metastatic liver).
    - *Diarrhea and local tenderness* (e.g. inflammatory bowel disease, diverticulitis).
    - *Constipation ± palpable lump in the line of colon* (e.g. obstructing lesions of colon).
    - *Constipation and diarrhea alternating*
        - *± abdominal lump* (e.g. intestinal tuberculosis—in young, obstructing malignancy—in old).
- *Colicky pain with local tenderness*
    - *Right upper abdomen* (e.g. cholelithiasis)
    - *Right lower abdomen* (e.g. appendicular colic)
    - *Urinary symptoms* (e.g. urolithiasis).

Chronic Abdominal Pain

Investigations

Blood Tests

- **Leukocytosis** in infective pathologies (e.g. intestinal tuberculosis)
- **Raised ESR** (e.g. intestinal tuberculosis, Crohn's disease, GI malignancies).

Radiology

- **Plain X-ray abdomen (Table 2.2).**
- **Intestinal contrast studies are shown in Table 2.3.**
- **Biliary contrast studies**
  - **Magnetic resonance cholangiopancreatography (MRCP)**—a noninvasive procedure to delineate the anatomy of biliary tree
  - **Endoscopic retrograde cholangio pancreatography (ERCP)**—to delineate the biliary tree, and for nasobiliary decompression, basketing of stones, and stenting of biliary tree in unresectable tumors.
  - **Percutaneous transhepatic cholangiography (PTC)**—to delineate the biliary tree proximal to the obstruction and for decompression in impassable strictures.
- **Computed radiology**
  - **CT and MRI of abdomen**: These non-invasive investigations have revolutionized in the diagnosis of abdominal pathologies.

Table 2.2: Plain X-ray findings in chronic abdominal pain

Plain X-ray abdomen		
Findings		**Pathology**
Radiopaque shadows	Single or multiple faceted shadows in the gallbladder area	Gallstones
	Radiopaque gallbladder shadow	Porcelain gallbladder
	Radiopaque shadows in the pancreatic region	Pancreatic calculi

Table 2.3: Contrast studies and chronic abdominal pain

Intestinal contrast studies		
Procedure	**Findings**	**Pathology**
Barium meal series	Niche in the lesser curvature	Gastric ulcer
	Filling defect in the stomach	Growth
	Convergence of gastric rugae towards the ulcer	Benign ulcer
	Divergence of gastric rugae from the ulcer	Malignant ulcer
	Dilated stomach	Gastric outlet obstruction
	Deformed duodenal cap "Trifoiling"	Chronic duodenal ulcer with cicatrization
	Contracted narrowed stomach	Linitis plastica
	Pad sign of duodenum	Carcinoma head of pancreas
	Inverted 3 appearance	Periampullary carcinoma
	Displacement of stomach	Pancreatic pseudocyst
Hypotonic duodenography	Flattening of medial margin of duodenum	Early stages of chronic pancreatitis
	Inverted 3 appearance	Late stages of chronic pancreatitis
	Filling defects	Carcinoma head of pancreas, polyps, diverticulum, periampullary carcinoma
Barium meal followthrough	Pulled up cecum	Ileocecal tuberculosis
	String sign of Kantor	Crohn's disease
	Filling defect of cecum or ascending colon	Malignant growths
Barium enema	Claw or pincer shape	Chronic intussusception
	Segmental spasm or saw tooth appearance	Diverticulitis
	Linear ulcers, transverse sinuses and clefts—cobble stone appearance	Crohn's disease
	Filling defects in the colon and rectum	Malignant growth

Oral and intravenous contrast enhancements give excellent information.

- **US of the abdomen:** Used to diagnose the lesions of the abdominal cavity, especially of the liver, gallbladder, pancreas and hepatopancreaticobiliary anatomy and many others.

Vascular Studies

- *Angiography* is useful in diagnosing vascular abnormalities (during acute bleed) and also malignant tumors
- *CT or MR angiography* are useful adjuncts to this evaluation.

Endoscopy

- *Upper GI endoscopy* is required in conditions, which cause confusion in diagnosis (e.g. acute gastritis and acute pancreatitis)
- *Lower GI endoscopy* is required in conditions like ulcerative colitis, and intussusception or growths
- *Capsule endoscopy* is useful in diagnosing small bowel lesions.

Radionuclide Imaging

This is useful in cases of hepatobiliary disorders, and diagnoses Meckel's diverticulitis.

Laparoscopy

Extremely useful in diagnosing intra-abdominal pathologies (e.g. adhesions) and also used for therapy at the same time (e.g. adhesion release).

Exploratory Laparotomy

Laparotomy as a diagnostic mode is very rarely used today, due to the advent of diagnostic laparoscopy.

MANAGEMENT

- *Non-perforated pathologies*—medical management
- *Perforated pathologies*—early surgical management
- *Diagnosis not clear and not responding to medical management*—exploratory laparotomy.

Clinical Pearls

- Chronic renal pain occurs in the lumbar regions and renal angles, and may be caused by hydronephrosis or renal malignancy
- Chronic hypogastric pain may be caused by uterine malignancy, urinary bladder pathology
- Chronic ovarian pathology can give rise to pain in the iliac fossae, mimicking many gastrointestinal pathologies.

Chapter 3

Dysphagia

SURGICAL ANATOMY OF ESOPHAGUS

Esophagus is a muscular tube connecting the pharynx and the stomach, guarded by sphincters at both ends. It is lined by squamous epithelium, excepting in its lower part and the esophagogastric junction, where it is lined by columnar epithelium. It lies anterior to the cervical vertebrae and lies in the posterior mediastinum, and enters the abdomen through a hiatus 'esophageal hiatus' of the diaphragm. The esophagus is devoid of serosal layer. The lower sphineter and the acute gastroesophageal angle prevent gastroesophageal reflux, and the esophagus normally remains empty.

PHYSIOLOGY OF SWALLOWING

Before the act of actual swallowing, preparation takes place (preparatory phase) in which chewing, sizing, shaping and positioning of the bolus on tongue take place. Then the actual act of swallowing starts.

Normal swallowing is a very complex mechanism consisting of coordination of four elements. They are:
1. Voluntary muscular contractions of oropharynx.
2. Protection of the larynx and respiratory passages by its striated muscles.

3. Relaxation of esophageal sphincters.
4. Peristaltic wave.

Dysphagia may occur due to the derangement of one or more of the above four elements, or narrowing of the lumen by stricture or tumor or extraneous causes.

DYSPHAGIA

Introduction

Dysphagia is defined as difficulty in swallowing.

It is a very reliable symptom and should never be dismissed as psychological, unless proved otherwise.

For clinical purposes, dysphagia is divided into two varieties:
1. Oropharyngeal
2. Esophageal

Patients with dysphagia complain of the sensation of food sticking somewhere in its passage to the stomach, usually at the level of obstruction, but many times point at the suprasternal notch, even though the level of obstruction is far below.

Globus sensation is defined as the feeling of a lump in the throat. This is present as a continuous sensation and not related to dysphagia. The common causes of globus sensation are:
- Gastroesophageal reflux disease (GERD)
- Early malignancy of hypopharynx
- Anxiety disorder
- Goiter.

Pain can accompany dysphagia (Odynophagia), if there is associated esophageal spasm. Very severe pain may occur, which may be radiating to the base of neck, angles of jaw, arms, epigastrium and back. *Esophageal pain may mimic cardiac pain.*

Heartburn is a retrosternal sensation of burning and discomfort, which occurs due to regurgitation of stomach contents into the normally empty esophagus, which may reach even the pharynx if the quantity is large *(Water brash).*

Causes of Dysphagia

Oropharyngeal Dysphagia

Etiology

It has many causes. They are:
- Propulsive
- Structural
- Iatrogenic

Propulsive causes of oropharyngeal dysphagia are many but they are mainly neurological. They are given in **Table 3.1**.

Structural causes of oropharyngeal dysphagia are given in **Table 3.2**.

Iatrogenic causes of oropharyngeal dysphagia include the following:

Drug-induced

- Mucosal inflammation following chemotherapy
- Steroid myopathy.

Radiation-induced

- Xerostomia
- Oral ulcers.

Prosthesis-induced

- Ill-fitting dental prosthesis.

Table 3.1: Propulsive causes of oropharyngeal dysphagia

Neurologic	Degenerative	Muscular	Metabolic	Inflammatory	Infectious
Cerebrovascular accidents	Alzheimer's disease	Muscular dystrophy	Hyperthyroidism with myxedema	Systemic lupus erythematosus (SLE)	Acquired immunodeficiency syndrome (AIDS)
Parkinson's disease	Huntington's chorea	Myasthenia gravis		Amyloidosis	Syphilis
Multiple sclerosis	Recurrent laryngeal nerve palsy	Myositis		Sarcoidosis	Botulism
	Cranial nerve palsies				Rabies
					Diphtheria
					Meningitis

Table 3.2: Structural causes of dysphagia

Etiology	Oral cavity	Pharynx	Larynx	Esophagus
Congenital	Macroglossia	Pharyngeal pouch	Subglottic stenosis, laryngomalacia	Atresia
Traumatic	Injuries of oral cavity	Impacted foreign bodies (coin, tooth, dentures)	Injuries to larynx/laryngopharynx, Impacted foreign bodies	Postoperative and corrosive strictures, foreign bodies, radiotherapy
Inflammatory	Stomatitis, tonsillitis, peritonsillar abscess	Acute pharyngitis, retropharyngeal abscess, cervical lymphadenopathy	Acute epiglottitis, tuberculous laryngitis	Reflux esophagitis, post-chemotherapy fungal infections
Neoplastic benign	Benign tumors	Benign tumors	Benign tumors	Benign tumors

Contd...

Contd...

Etiology	Oral cavity	Pharynx	Larynx	Esophagus
Neoplastic malignant	Carcinoma tongue, cancers of oral cavity	Carcinoma hypopharynx	Carcinoma larynx	Esophageal malignancy
Miscellaneous	Paralysis of soft palate (bulbar palsy)	Paterson-Kelly syndrome	Vocal cord palsy, neuroasthenia	Scleroderma, diffuse esophageal spasm, achalasia, paterson-Kelly syndrome, diverticula of the esophagus, para-esophageal hiatus hernia, pressure from extrinsic pathologies

Post-surgery

- Resections of oropharynx.

Esophageal dysphagia is almost always caused by diseases in and adjacent to the esophagus and rarely by the lesions in the pharynx or stomach. Esophageal narrowing causes dysphagia when the lumen is not able to expand beyond a diameter of about 10 mm. Chronic obstructions of esophagus like achalasia cardia, allow the patients to compensate and present at a very late date, but by this time, there is marked weight loss and severe undernutrition.

Diagnosis

Symptoms and Signs

Oropharyngeal Dysphagia
- Inability to initiate the act of swallowing
- Sticky feeling of food in the throat
- Cough or choking sensation during swallowing
- Nasopharyngeal regurgitation
- Voice change
- Visual disturbances.

Esophageal Dysphagia
- Regurgitation
- Water brash
- Chest pain.

Complication

- Aspiration pneumonia.

Management

- Treatment of primary pathology
- Swallow therapy
    - Softening of food, optimizing food bolus volume, rate of bolus consumption
    - Tongue exercises
    - Psychotherapy.

Clinical Pearls

- Patients with oropharyngeal dysphagia usually point to the level of obstruction as the oropharynx, but majority of patients with esophageal dysphagia are not able to recognize the level of obstruction, and point it proximal to the level of obstruction.
- Oropharyngeal and esophageal dysphagia do not coexist as anatomically these areas are different in respect to musculature, nerve supply and neural regulation.

Chapter 4

Diarrhea

DEFINITION

Diarrhea is defined as passing increased number of stools of less than normal consistency and form.

TYPES OF DIARRHEA

- *Acute diarrhea:* This refers to acute onset of symptoms of less than 14 to 30 days duration.
- *Chronic diarrhea:* This refers to persistence of diarrhea for over 1 month.

ACUTE DIARRHEA

This can be classified into three forms
- *Mild:* Not associated with any change in daily activities.
- *Moderate:* Associated with changes in daily activities but patient is able to function.
- *Severe:* Patient is disabled by symptoms.

Etiology and Pathogenesis

The common organisms being
- Viruses (e.g. caliciviruses—norovirus, rotavirus, coronavirus)

- Bacteria (e.g. *Shigella, Salmonella, E. coli, Campylobacter*)
- Parasites (e.g. *Entamoebae*).

The organisms are obtained by oral consumption of infected raw or undercooked food, or animal product such as chicken, beef and eggs.

The organisms produce toxins, which cause watery diarrhea. There are two varieties of toxins. They are:
1. Cytotonic
2. Cytotoxic

Cytotonic toxins activate the intracellular enzymes, which cause fluid secretion into the intestinal lumen (e.g. *V. cholerae*).

Cytotoxic toxins cause injury to the intestinal mucosal structure, which in turn causes inflammation and mucosal bleeding (e.g., enterohemorrhagic *E. coli*).

Management

- Most cases resolve spontaneously and require no treatment
- Evaluation and treatment is reserved for those who have toxic symptoms (fever, dehydration, bloody diarrhea, severe abdominal pain, elderly and immunocompromised patients).

DYSENTERY

Definition

Dysentery is defined as a disease process characterized by loose stools containing blood and polymorphonuclear cells.

Causes of Dysentery

- Infectious dysentery (e.g. parasitic infections, bacterial infection)
- Inflammatory bowel disease
- Ischemic bowel disease.

Pathogenesis

Dysentery results due to the inflammatory reaction caused by:
1. Direct invasion of ileal/colonic epithelium.
2. Producing a toxin that causes cellular death and tissue damage.

Diagnosis

Symptoms and Signs

- Loose stools containing blood and mucus
- Abdominal pain and cramping
- Tenesmus (painful urge to pass stool)
- Fever
- Dehydration.

Investigations

Stool Tests

- *Bacterial infections*
  - Fecal leukocyte test—microscopic/immunoassay (presence of leukocytes in stool indicates infection).
- *Amebic infections*
  - Microscopy yields in only 50% of amebic dysentery.
  - Monoclonal antibody-based EIA stool assay for *E. histolytica* has a sensitivity of about 95%.

- Circulating antibodies to *E. histolytica* antigens by indirect hemagglutination test—sensitivity of 90%.

Complications

Complications of Amebic Dysentery

- Liver abscess
- Toxic megacolon
- Intestinal perforation
- Peritonitis
- Intussusception
- Ameboma.

Management

- *Fluids*—plenty of oral fluids
- *Diet*—bland diet.

Bacterial Infections
- *Drugs*
  - *Antibiotics:* Ciprofloxacin or Norfloxacin for 5 days
  - *Antimotility drugs:* Loperamide.

Amebic Infections
- *Metronidazole* 500 mg thrice daily for 7–10 days followed by iodoquinol 650 mg thrice daily for 20 days (intraluminal cysticide).

Clinical Pearls

- Normally, leukocytes are not found in the stool
- Complete cooking of food will kill the bacteria, and raw vegetables are common sources of infection causing diarrhea

- Typhoid fever is a clinical syndrome of marked fever, persistent bacteremia, hepatosplenomegaly and abdominal pain, due to intestinal infection caused by *S. typhi*.
- *Giardia*, *Cryptosporidium* and *Cyclospora* species cause self limiting non-bloody diarrhea
- Antimotility agents like loperamide will reduce the pathogen clearance and are not indicated in viral diarrhea
- Travellers diarrhea occurs due to infections contracted from infected areas
- Cholera is a severe diarrheal disorder caused by gram-negative, comma-shaped bacteria, *Vibrio cholera*.
- Fluid replacement (oral/IV) is the mainstay of therapy for cholera or any diarrhea with heavy fluid loss
- Apart from infections, the causes of acute diarrhea include food poisoning, drugs, ischemic colitis, bacterial overgrowth, fecal impaction and partial bowel obstruction
- Patients with mild illness do not require elaborate evaluation, but in those with high fever, bloody diarrhea, and invasion with a powerful pathogen, it is reasonable to culture the stools for appropriate treatment.

TRAVELER'S DIARRHEA

Introduction

Acute loose stools following a travel to an endemic area or high-risk areas, commonly by the infestation of *E. coli* organisms.

Management

- Quinolone (ciprofloxacin) 500 mg bid for 3 days.

Prevention

- ***Dietary precautions*** (consumption of heated food, safe drinking water, carbonated bottled beverages, hot beverages, fruits)
- *A single dose of quinolone daily is useful when traveling in high-risk areas*
- *Azithromycin or rifaximin is also useful.*

CHRONIC DIARRHEA

Definition

Chronic diarrhea is defined as diarrhea persisting for over one month.

Pathogenesis

Diarrhea occurs due to incomplete absorption of fluid from the intestinal contents. Normally, stools contain 75% water and 25% solids. Some solutes in the solids prevent water absorption, and this process results in osmotic diarrhea (e.g. lactose malabsorption).

When water absorption is reduced and more water and electrolytes are secreted into the lumen, it is called secretory diarrhea (e.g. mucosal inflammation).

Classifications

Epidemiological Classification

- *Epidemic diarrhea*
  - Viral infections
  - Bacterial infections
  - Protozoal infections.

- *Travelers' diarrhea*
  - Bacterial infections
  - Protozoal infections
  - Tropical sprue.

Classification Based on Stool Characteristics

- *Watery diarrhea*—watery stools without blood, pus or fat.
  - *Secretory diarrhea (stool with excessive electrolytes)— IBD, Bacterial toxins.*
  - *Osmotic diarrhea (stool with reduced electrolytes)—osmotic laxatives.*
- *Inflammatory diarrhea* (stool with pus and or blood)—IBD, infections.
- *Fatty diarrhea (stool with excessive fat)—(malabsorption syndromes—celiac disease, maldigestion—pancreatic exocrine insufficiency).*

The causes of chronic diarrhea are given in **Table 4.1**.

Table 4.1: Causes of chronic diarrhea

Secretory watery diarrhea	Osmotic watery diarrhea	Inflammatory diarrhea	Fatty diarrhea
Infections	Osmotic laxatives	Inflammatory bowel disease	Pancreatic exocrine deficiency
Inflammatory bowel disease	Carbohydrate malabsorption	Intestinal tuberculosis	Bile acid deficiency
Drugs		Infectious diseases	Mucosal diseases (celiac disease)
Stimulant laxatives		Ischemic colitis	Bacterial overgrowth
Endocrine diseases		Radiation colitis	Small bowel fistulae
Tumors		Neoplasms	Short bowel syndrome
Idiopathic			

Systemic Diseases Associated with Chronic Diarrhea

Endocrine Diseases

- Hyperthyroidism
- Addison's disease
- Hypopituitarism
- Diabetes mellitus.

Hematologic Diseases

- Leukemia
- Lymphoma
- Multiple myeloma.

Endocrine Syndromes

- MEN 1 (Wermer syndrome—hyperparathyroidism, pancreatic endocrine tumors, pituitary tumors)
- MEN 2a (Sipple syndrome—medullary thyroid cancer, pheochromocytoma, hyperparathyroidism)
- MEN 2b (Sipple syndrome features + neuromas + Marfanoid phenotype).

Immune System Disorders

- AIDS
- Amyloidosis.

Diagnosis

Symptoms

- ***Criteria for diagnosis of chronic diarrhea***

1. >2 stools/day
2. Unformed stools
3. Increased stool weight (>240 g/day for men, >180 g/day for women).

- ***Association of pain:*** IBD, IBS, ischemic bowel disease.
- ***Weight loss:*** Malabsorption, malignancy.
- ***Aggravating factors:*** Diet, stress.
- ***Relieving factors:*** Diet, drugs.
- ***Iatrogenic causes:*** Drugs, radiation, surgery (short bowel syndrome).
- ***Systemic diseases:*** Hyperthyroidism, diabetes mellitus, neoplastic syndromes.

Signs

- Features of water and electrolyte imbalance
- Features of malnutrition
- ***Skin:*** Flushing, rashes, dermographism
- ***Neck:*** Thyromegaly
- ***Chest:*** Rhonchi
- ***Abdomen:*** Hepatomegaly, mass, ascites, local tenderness
- ***Rectum:*** Anal sphincter laxity.

Investigations

Blood Tests

- ***Complete blood count:*** Low hematocrit, leukocytosis, raised ESR
- ***Serum electrolytes:*** Electrolyte disturbances
- ***Serum proteins:*** Hypoalbuminemia.

Stool Tests

- *Stool weight*
- *Fecal fat content by Sudan staining and quantitative analysis* (high fat content in fatty diarrhea)
- *Fecal electrolytes:* (low electrolyte content in osmotic diarrhea and high content in secretory diarrhea)
- *Fecal osmotic gap determination:* This represents the osmotic activity in stool water not due to electrolytes. Sum of concentration of sodium and potassium in stool water is multiplied by 2 which accounts for the anions that are present in the stool, which is subtracted from 290 mOsm/kg. Fecal osmotic gap of <50 mOsm/kg indicates secretory diarrhea and >50 mOsm/kg may indicate osmotic diarrhea.
- *Fecal pH:* Low pH <5 is due to carbohydrate malabsorption
- *Fecal occult blood:* Seen in inflammatory and neoplastic conditions
- *Fecal leukocytes:* Increased in infective conditions.

Investigations Related to Causes of Secretory Diarrhea

- *Stool examination:* Infections (identify pathogens)
- *Colonoscopy biopsy:* Local pathologies
- *CT abdomen with oral contrast:* Structural changes in GIT, mass, neoplasm
- *Capsule endoscopy/Sonde enteroscopy:* Local pathologies in small bowel
- *Other tests*
  - *Plasma peptides* (gastrin, calcitonin, somatostatin, VIP)
  - *Urinalysis* (5HIAA, histamine, metanephrine)
  - *Tests related to systemic diseases* (TSH, ACTH stimulation, serum protein electrophoresis).

Investigations Related to Causes of Fatty Diarrhea

- *Secretin test* (pancreatic exocrine insufficiency)
- *Stool examination*
  - Chymotrypsin activity (pancreatic exocrine insufficiency)
  - Fat content (increased in pancreatic exocrine insufficiency)
- *CT abdomen with oral contrast:* Structural changes in GIT, mass, neoplasm
- *Capsule endoscopy/Sonde enteroscopy:* Local pathologies in small bowel, celiac disease
- *Other tests*
  - *IgA antibodies against tissue transglutaminase (tTG):* To rule out celiac disease

Investigations Related to Causes of Inflammatory Diarrhea

- Stool test to identify the pathogens
- *Colonoscopy biopsy:* Local pathologies
- *CT abdomen with oral contrast:* Structural changes in GIT, mass, neoplasm

Capsule endoscopy/Sonde enteroscopy: Local pathologies in small bowel.

Careful history taking, clinical examination and investigations should help in differentiating the type of diarrhea into watery (secretory/osmotic), inflammatory or fatty diarrhea.

Management

- Management of cause if found
- Since the evaluation itself takes several weeks, the patient needs therapy, which may be nonspecific
- Opiates are the most effective (**Table 4.2**)
- When no cause is found in about 25% of cases, opiate administration becomes a longstanding and specific therapy.

Table 4.2: Nonspecific opiates used in the treatment of chronic diarrhea

µ opiate receptor selective	δ opiate receptor selective
Diphenoxylate—2.5–5 mg QID	Racecadotril—1.5 mg/kg TID
Loperamide—2–4 mg QID	Clonidine (adrenergic agonist)—0.1–0.3 mg TID
Codeine—15–60 mg QID	Octreotide (Somatostatin analogue)—50–250 µg TID
Morphine—2–20 mg QID	Cholestyramine (Bile acid binding resin)—4 g QID

Clinical Pearls

- Neuroendocrine tumors are very uncommon causes of chronic diarrhea, and investigations related to them should be done only when common causes are ruled out
- In a quarter of patients, no cause can be found for chronic diarrhea in spite of all the investigations
- Once a thorough evaluation has been done, symptomatic treatment is the only option
- Small bowel mucosal biopsy is the definitive test for celiac disease
- Most common cause of iatrogenic diarrhea is drugs (antibiotics, chemotherapeutic drugs, anti-inflammatory drugs, anti-hypertensives, herbal drugs).

Chapter 5

Constipation and Fecal Incontinence

ANATOMY OF ANORECTUM

Continence is maintained by the pelvic floor muscles, which include the internal, external anal sphincters, and puborectalis muscle.

- *Internal anal sphincter (IAS)* is controlled by the autonomic nervous system via the enteric nervous system, is contracted tonically to contribute to the majority of anal resting pressure (80%).
- *External anal sphincter (EAS)* is controlled by the pudendal nerve, and is partially contracted at rest periods. This contraction is stimulated by external factors like coughing, etc.
- *Puborectalis muscle* is like a U-shaped sling around the anorectal junction and creates an angle of 90° between the rectum and anal canal. Contraction of this muscle further creates an acute angle, which physically obstructs the stools from moving down the rectum involuntarily. Contraction of puborectalis sling is a voluntary physical act.

PHYSIOLOGY OF DEFECATION

When stool mass reaches and distends the rectum, the reflex relaxation of IAS occurs (called sampling reflex). At this stage, the presence of stools is felt by the anal mucosa, EAS contracts to prevent soiling. Defecation occurs by coordinated movements of these muscles, and simultaneously, the puborectalis relaxes to open the anorectal angle to about 130°. Stretch receptors in the rectum which sense the presence of fecal matter causes a spinal reflex to relax the IAS (rectoanal inhibitory reflex). Further to this, sitting or squatting position, stretches the anal canal anteroposteriorly, causing the relaxation of EAS, which facilitates the smooth passage of stools. The ultimate expulsion of fecal matter is aided by diaphragmatic and abdominal muscle contractions.

CONSTIPATION

Introduction

Constipation means different things to different people
- Straining to pass stool
- Sense of incomplete evacuation
- Passing stools of hard consistency
- Diminished frequency of bowel movements.

Constipation is defined as frequency of bowel movements of three or less in a week with the need to strain at quarter or more of all bowel movements.

However, Rome III committee developed the criteria for constipation (**Table 5.1**).

Constipation depends on various factors also. They are given in **Table 5.2**.

The patients with constipation are divided into two categories:
- Patients with normal colon
- Patients with organic pathology.

Table 5.1: Criteria for constipation

Chronic constipation*	
It must include ≥2 of the following:	
In at least 25% of defecations	Straining
In at least 25% of defecations	Lumpy or hard stools
In at least 25% of defecations	Sensation of incomplete evacuation
In at least 25% of defecations	Sensation of anorectal obstruction/blockage
In at least 25% of defecations	Manual maneuvers to facilitate
And the following criteria must be met	
Loose stools are rarely present (excluding the use of laxatives)	
Insufficient criteria to establish a diagnosis of irritable bowel syndrome	
Functional defecation disorders	
At least two of the following must be present during repeated attempts to defecate: • Impaired evacuation (based on balloon expulsion test or imaging test) • Inappropriate contraction of the pelvic floor muscles or less than 20% relaxation of the basal resting anal sphincter pressure as seen on manometry, imaging or EMG • Inadequate propulsive forces as determined by manometry or imaging	

* Criteria fulfilled for 3 or more months with onset of symptoms at least 6 months prior to diagnosis.

Table 5.2: Causes of constipation

Factor	Pathologies
Psychosocial	Lack of childhood toilet training
	Depression
Physiologic	Delayed colonic transit (colonic or hindgut inertia)
	Impaired rectal motor function
	Reduced rectal filling
	Outlet obstruction
	Absent gastrocolic reflex
	Idiopathic megacolon and megarectum
	Irritable bowel syndrome

Etiology of Constipation

Constipation is classified into primary and secondary.
- *Primary constipation* (with no external known cause or physical abnormality, but may be due to gastrointestinal function disorder). The common causes are:
  - Impaired colonic transit
  - Constipation predominant IBS
  - Pelvic floor dysfunction.
- *Secondary constipation* (with recognizable cause).

Organic Causes

Patients with organic pathologies in and around the colorectum, present with constipation. They are listed in **Table 5.3**.

In patients with megacolon and megarectum, the causes are:
- Hirschsprung's disease (congenital megacolon)
- Chagas' disease
- Neurological diseases
- Endocrine and metabolic diseases
- Acquired megacolon.

In patients with normal colon, constipation is caused by various factors. They are listed in **Table 5.4**.

Table 5.3: Causes of constipation in patients with organic local pathologies

Intraluminal	Intramural	Extramural
Fecal impaction	Colorectal malignancies	Uterine tumors
Polyps	Anorectal infections	Prostatic enlargement
Foreign bodies	Strictures	Pelvic metastases
		Post-anal dermoid
		Pessaries

Snapshots in Gastroenterology

Table 5.4: Causes of constipation in patients with normal colon

Cause	Conditions
Endocrine	Hypothyroidism, hyperparathyroidism, hypercalcemia, hyperglucagonemia, pheochromocytoma
Metabolic	Diabetes mellitus
Nervous system disorders	Autonomic neuropathies, high spinal cord transection, cauda equina syndrome, multiple sclerosis, Parkinson's disease
Muscular disorders	Myotonic dystrophy
Collagen vascular disorders	Scleroderma, amyloidosis, dermatomyositis
Medications	Anticholinergics, antidepressants, opiates, anticonvulsants, calcium channel blockers
Functional disorders	Anorexia nervosa, dementia
General causes	Old age, bedridden patient

Functional Causes

When no obvious organic pathology is found, constipation is said to be functional or primary, which occurs due to two mechanisms. They are:

1. *Slow transit:* The fecal matter travels slowly from the cecum to rectum due to decreased contractions and uncoordinated contractions of the left colon.
2. *Pelvic dysfunction:* Feces get stored in the rectum for a longer period due to lack of coordinated rectal emptying.

Diagnosis

Symptoms

- Thorough careful eliciting of history (including blood per rectum, weight loss, risk factors, systemic illnesses)
- The presenting symptom is constipation (number of bowel movements less than three per week)

Constipation and Fecal Incontinence

- Abdominal discomfort, pain, distension, nausea are frequent accompaniments
- Rectal bleeding may be associated with lesions like, colorectal cancers, solitary rectal ulcers and hemorrhoids.

Signs

- ***Abdominal examination*** may show
  - Palpable fecal masses in the sigmoid colon
  - Palpable malignant growths of colon.
- ***Rectal examination*** may show
  - Fecal soiling of perineum, due to overflow incontinence around a hard fecal mass in the rectum, decreased tone of anal sphincter
  - Palpable growth in the rectum.

Investigations

Blood Tests

- ***Hemoglobin*** (e.g. anemia)
- ***Serum calcium*** to evaluate hypercalcemia
- ***Thyroid function test*** for evaluation of hypothyroidism.

Radiology

- ***Plain X-rays: Chest*** (e.g. lung metastases of colorectal malignancies), ***abdomen*** (e.g. air fluid levels, foreign bodies)
- ***Contrast study (Barium enema):*** Administration of barium contrast in the colon is diagnostic (e.g. malignancies) but histopathological confirmation can only be had from endoscopy
- ***CT or MRI scan of abdomen*** (e.g. to assess malignant lymph node deposits of colorectal malignancies, pelvic tumors presenting with constipation)

- *Ultrasonography of abdomen* may be useful in assessing the liver parenchyma (e.g. malignant deposits, pelvic tumors and prostatic enlargement presenting with constipation)
- *Virtual colonoscopy* is useful in localizing obstructing colorectal lesions in patients who are very old and not willing to undergo colonoscopy.

Endoscopy

- *Lower gastrointestinal endoscopy (Total colonoscopy)* is the most important investigation to identify the cause (e.g. malignancies). It has the advantage of obtaining tissues for histopathology.
- *Histopathology: Biopsy* through colonoscopy is confirmative.

Colonic Function Tests

- *Colonic transit time*
- *Defecography*
- *Anorectal manometry.*

Management

- Dietary and lifestyle modifications:
  - Consumption of dietary fiber of about 20–35 g/day
  - Consumption of 2.5 liters of water daily
- Avoidance of constipating drugs
- Medical therapy is to be initiated (**Table 5.5**).

Refractory Constipation

The constipation, which is not responding to medical management, is called refractory constipation, and this needs work up. The studies, which are required at this point, are:
- *Colon marker study*: Patient is given 24 radiopaque plastic rings. Number and distribution of rings are evaluated using plain

Constipation and Fecal Incontinence

Table 5.5: Medical therapy of chronic constipation

Medication	Mechanism of action	Examples
Bulk forming laxatives	Increase stool weight, accelerate transit	Wheat bran, methylcellulose
Stool softeners	Creates soft stool by interacting with stool	Docusate
Osmotic laxatives	Cause water retention in the lumen	Lactulose 15 mL thrice daily, Polyethylene glycol 3350—17 g daily, Sorbitol 1–2 tsp twice daily, Magnesium hydroxide 3 tsp daily
Stimulant laxatives	Promotes intestinal contractions by stimulating nerve endings, may have inhibitory effect on absorption of water	Bisacodyl 5 mg daily, Senna 2 tabs daily
Suppositories, enema	Stimulate rectum	Glycerin, bisacodyl, sodium phosphate enemas

abdominal radiographs after 5 days, and if 5 or lesser markers are seen, transit is said to be normal.
- *Scintigraphy:* Patient is given radiolabeled material and transit time is evaluated after 3–5 days
- *Anorectal manometry:* Pressure recording with a balloon catheter in the rectum
- *Electromyography:* EMG of pelvic muscles to assess the anorectal muscle strength
- *Balloon expulsion study:* Water filled balloon is inserted into the rectum and asked to expel the balloon, which can be done in a minute's time. Delay indicates dyssynergia
- *Defecography (MR defecography):* Contrast is kept in the rectum. Assessment of expulsion determined by videoradiography before and after expulsion
- *Colon manometry:* Probes kept in the colon at various levels and pressure recordings done after meals, sleep, etc.

Surgical Therapy of Functional Bowel Disorders
- **Slow colonic transit constipation:** Total abdominal colectomy with ileorectal anastomosis.

Clinical Pearls

- Constipation dating back to childhood is habitual and needs no special investigation, whereas constipation of recent onset or short duration, and a change in the pattern of chronic constipation needs special attention, especially in the elderly.
- Coexistence of constipation and weight loss suggests colorectal malignancy
- In patients with combined slow transit constipation and pelvic floor dysfunction, pelvic floor training should always be given before surgical therapy
- Slow small bowel transit and gastroparesis are absolute contra-indications for surgical therapy for slow large bowel transit
- Segmental colectomy gives effective result when compared to total colectomy.

FECAL INCONTINENCE

Introduction

- Fecal incontinence is more common in women
- Highest incidence in the elderly.

Etiology and Pathogenesis

- The etiology is multifactorial
- Irritable bowel syndrome is the commonest cause

> **Box 5.1**
>
> *Congenital*
> - Congenital anomalies of anus and rectum
>
> *Acquired*
> - Autonomic neuropathy (internal sphincter defect of diabetes/alcohol consumption)
> - Pelvic floor injuries (external sphincter defects of multiparity, perineal tears)
> - Spurious diarrhea
> - Irritable bowel syndrome
> - Inflammatory bowel disease
> - Rectal prolapse
> - Fistula in ano
> - Traumatic injuries of anorectum
> - Pelvic floor neuropathy

- Obstetric anal sphincter injuries are common iatrogenic causes of incontinence
- There are some acquired causes of incontinence (**Box 5.1**).

Diagnosis

Investigations
- ***Colonoscopy*** to rule out neoplastic conditions (adenoma, carcinoma), inflammatory bowel disease
- ***Anorectal physiology studies***
- ***Evacuating proctography***
- ***Anorectal ultrasound*** to determine the integrity of the anal sphincters
- ***MRI*** to define the anorectal anatomy.

Management

Treatment depends on the clinical assessment.

Medical

- Reassurance
- Antidiarrheal agents
- Bowel washouts for those with spurious diarrhea
- Management of irritable bowel syndrome.

Surgical

- Internal anal sphincter repair—internal sphincterotomy, hemorrhoidectomy
- External anal sphincter repair—scar excision and overlap repair
- Post-anal repair (plication of pelvic floor muscles)
- Surgery for rectal prolapse
- Stoma creation for refractory fecal incontinence
- Artificial bowel sphincters
- Dynamic gracilis muscle transposition
- Sacral nerve stimulation.

Clinical Pearls

Sacral nerve stimulation is the most promising treatment available for fecal incontinence today, but long-term follow-up is necessary.

Chapter 6

Nausea and Vomiting

INTRODUCTION

- *Nausea* is defined as a feeling of the imminent desire to vomit.
- *Vomiting* is defined as the forceful expulsion of gastric contents through mouth.
- *Retching* denotes the labored rhythmic respiratory activity that frequently precedes vomiting.

Nausea and vomiting may occur independently but nausea precedes or accompanies vomiting. Nausea is usually associated with diminished activity of stomach and duodenum for a period of time. When a severe episode of nausea occurs, there is some altered autonomic activity. They are: skin pallor, increased perspiration, salivation, occasionally hypotension and bradycardia.

CAUSES OF NAUSEA AND VOMITING

Nausea is a very nonspecific symptom of a variety of conditions. Nausea and vomiting can be acute or chronic. The causes are tabulated in **Table 6.1**.

PATHOGENESIS

The act of vomiting is controlled by two distinct medullary centers, vomiting center and chemoreceptor trigger zone, which lie close

Table 6.1: Causes of nausea and vomiting

Nausea and vomiting	Acute	Chronic
Gastrointestinal	• Infectious gastroenteritis • Acute gastritis • Food poisoning • Acute abdominal conditions	• Malignant gastric outlet obstruction • Intestinal obstruction • Gastroparesis
Drugs	• Cancer chemotherapy • NSAIDs • Antibiotics	• Cancer chemotherapy
Metabolic abnormalities	• Fluid and electrolyte disturbances • Addison's disease • Acute renal failure	• Chronic renal failure • Chronic hyponatremia
Neuropsychiatric	• Migraine • Increased intracranial tension	• Psychiatric disorders
Otologic	• Acute labyrinthitis • Acute otitis media	• Chronic disorders
Postoperative	• Electrolyte disturbances • Mechanical obstruction	• Adhesions • Recurrence of obstructive disease
Others	• Systemic infection	

to each other near the centers which regulate the vasomotor and autonomic responses in the brainstem. The vomiting center receives afferent stimuli from the intestines and also from the chemoreceptor trigger zone. The efferent pathways are the phrenic nerves (to the diaphragm) and spinal nerves (to the abdominal musculature). The activation of vomiting center causes the act of vomiting. The chemoreceptor trigger zone is activated by many stimuli, including drugs.

The muscles of the abdomen provide the major ejection force by forceful contraction, which increases the intra-abdominal pressure with concomitant relaxation of the gastric fundus and the gastroesophageal sphincter and annular contraction of pylorus push the gastric contents into the esophagus. Increased intrathoracic pressure along with reverse peristalsis of esophagus causes forceful expulsion of esophageal contents into the mouth. Elevation of soft palate prevents the contents to regurgitate into the nasopharynx, and reflex closure of glottis prevents pulmonary aspiration.

Prolonged and recurrent acts of vomiting can lead to dehydration and loss of gastric secretions lead to metabolic alkalosis with hypokalemia.

DIAGNOSIS

Diagnosis of the disorder related to nausea and vomiting requires:
- Eliciting history*
- Physical examination**
- Judicious use of laboratory investigations
- Quantity (large–proximal intestinal obstruction, moderate–distal small bowel obstruction)
- Nature–gastric contents (gastric outlet obstruction), bilious (proximal intestinal obstruction), feculent (distal small bowel/proximal large bowel obstruction).

Management

- Management depends on the diagnosis
- When exact diagnosis is not possible, treatment is empiric
- Antiemetics and prokinetics.

---

* Vomiting immediately after food intake indicates gastritis or pylorospasm, but vomiting 4–6 hours after food intake indicates gastric stasis (e.g. gastroparesis, gastric outlet obstruction).
** Character of vomiting

Clinical Pearls

- Psychogenic vomiting is defined as the act of vomiting associated with psychiatric disturbances or emotional upset
- Alcoholic gastritis can give rise to early morning vomiting called 'dry heaves'
- Vomiting is not a characteristic feature of distal colonic obstruction.

Chapter 7

Gaseousness

Gaseousness is defined as the sensation of gas filling up the abdomen, which may give a tight feeling of the abdomen. This so-called gas has to find its way through the mouth as a belch or escape through the anus, for the patient to get the relief.

BELCHING

Introduction

Belching is defined as an involuntary expulsion of air from the stomach and esophagus. Usually, this regurgitation is the swallowed air in the stomach as a normal physiological event.

Etiology

Though belching is a physiological event, it can be caused by a variety of organic conditions. The conditions include
- Those which interfere with the integrity of the esophagogastric junction:
  - GERD
  - Hiatus hernia
  - Achalasia cardia.
- Those which interfere with gastric emptying:
  - Gastroparesis
  - Gastric outlet obstruction.

Persons who swallow excessive air present with belching, a condition called *'aerophagia'* is associated with anxiety, asthma, COPD.

Diagnosis

If the clinical history and examination suggest an organic pathology, further investigations may be justified.

Management

- Physiological belching can be left alone
- Discomforting or embarrassing episodes of belching may be treated empirically with PPIs
- Patients with aerophagia may need counseling and convinced that it is not due to an organic illness, or gas produced in the stomach.

BLOATING

Introduction

Bloating is defined as a distended feeling of the abdomen.

Etiology

Unlike belching, bloating is not a physiological event. Though an obvious cause may not be documented in many cases, chronic upper abdominal dyspepsia and hyperacidity are associated with bloating. Many causes are associated with bloating. They are:
- **General**
  - Diet (legumes, beans, starches)
  - Constipation

    - Malabsorption
    - Dyspepsia (biliary and appendicular)
    - Irritable bowel syndrome.
- **Organic causes**
    - GERD
    - Gastroparesis
    - Acid peptic disease
    - Diverticular disease
    - Intra-abdominal malignancy.
- **Systemic causes**
    - Diabetes mellitus (gastroparesis)
    - Neuromuscular disorders (muscular dystrophy)
    - Endocrine disorders (hypothyroidism).
- **Drugs**
    - Narcotics
    - Analgesics
    - Calcium channel blockers.

FLATULENCE

Introduction

Flatulence is production of flatus in the intestine, which passes rectally. Normally, 2,500 mL of flatus is produced in a day, which is passed out rectally about 20–25 times a day, and some movements are not felt by the individual.

Etiology

The gas or flatus is a combination of swallowed air and gas produced in the colon by bacteria. The swallowed air is rich in oxygen, whereas the colonic gas consists of hydrogen, methane, malodorous sulfur. Some conditions are known to produce increased quantities of gas. They are:

- Malabsorptive diseases (pancreatic diseases, bacterial overgrowth, celiac disease)
- Lactose intolerance
- Fructose containing foods
- Starchy foods.

Diagnosis

- Diagnosis depends on careful history taking (including dietary history) and examination
- Rectal examination and manometry may document the sphincter tone.

Management

- Gas without bad odor may be due to swallowing of air, and this habit may be curtailed by counseling
- Gas adsorbents like charcoal may be useful
- Avoidance of food which is expected to produce excessive flatulence.

Chapter 8

Jaundice

Jaundice is defined as yellowish discoloration of body tissues due to excess of circulating bilirubin.
- Normal serum bilirubin levels range from 0.5 to 1.0 mg%
- Jaundice is detected clinically when serum bilirubin levels go above 2.0 mg%
- The discoloration is most evident in tissues abundant in elastic collagen tissue, such as bulbar conjunctiva over the sclera, skin, oral cavity and undersurface of tongue.

BILIRUBIN METABOLISM

Bilirubin metabolism (**Fig. 8.1**), and its defects and diseases are given in **Table 8.1**.

ANATOMY OF BILIARY SYSTEM

Bile canaliculi form a network surrounding the hepatocytes, and unite to form intralobular and interlobular ductules. These ductules converge to form the left and right hepatic ducts. The hepatic ducts unite to form the common hepatic duct. Cystic duct joins the common hepatic duct to form the common bile duct. The common bile duct lies most anterior in the lesser omentum and travels down through the posterior substance of the pancreas and is joined by the

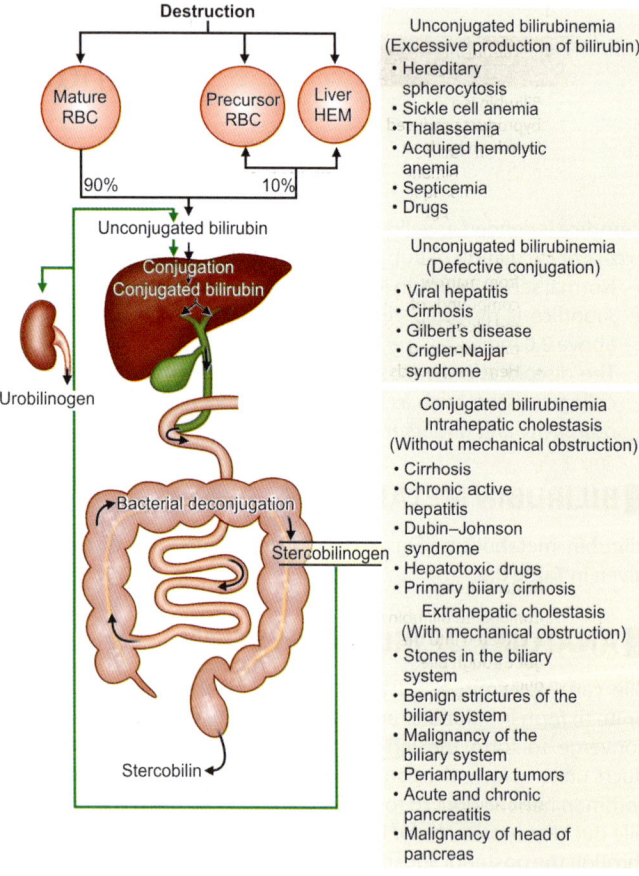

Fig. 8.1: Bilirubin metabolism

Table 8.1: Bilirubin metabolism and its defects and its diseases

Step	Metabolism	Defect in metabolism	Diseases
1.	Bilirubin is a byproduct produced from hem by three routes: • 90% is derived from mature red blood cells • 7% is derived from marrow compounds of red blood cell precursors and • Hem compounds in the liver	Increased production of bilirubin produces excessive *unconjugated* bilirubin	• Hereditary spherocytosis • Sickle cell anemia • Thalassemia • Acquired hemolytic anemia • Septicemia • Drugs
2.	Unconjugated bile (lipid soluble) reaches liver transported by plasma proteins	Defective conjugation produces excessive *unconjugated* bilirubin	• Viral hepatitis • Cirrhosis • Gilbert's disease • Crigler-Najjar syndrome
3.	In the liver, it is conjugated into bilirubin glucuronide (water soluble)		
4.	Conjugated bilirubin is excreted into the gut through bile ducts	Defective excretion produces excessive *conjugated* bilirubin	**Intrahepatic cholestasis (without mechanical obstruction)** • Cirrhosis • Chronic active hepatitis • Dubin-Johnson syndrome • Hepatotoxic drugs • Primary biliary cirrhosis
5.	Conjugated bilirubin undergoes bacterial deconjugation in colon to stercobilinogen	Non-conjugation of bilirubin produces absent stercobilinogen and stercobilin excretion produces 'putty' stools	

Contd...

Step	Metabolism	Defect in metabolism	Diseases
			Extrahepatic cholestasis (with mechanical obstruction)
6.	Stercobilinogen is partly reabsorbed to be excreted through urine as urobilinogen, and partly excreted in the feces as stercobilin	Non-absorption of stercobilinogen produces absent urobilinogen	• Stones in the biliary system • Benign strictures of the biliary system • Acute and chronic pancreatitis • Malignancy of head of pancreas • Malignancy of the biliary system • Periampullary tumors

pancreatic duct. The confluence is flask shaped and is called ampulla of Vater. The duct ultimately opens in the posteromedial part of the duodenum. This opening is surrounded by circular muscle, sphincter of Oddi **(Fig. 8.2)**.

DISORDERS OF BILIRUBIN METABOLISM

Gilbert's syndrome, Crigler–Najjar syndrome (types I and II), Dubin–Johnson syndrome, and Rotor syndrome, make up the five known hereditary defects in bilirubin metabolism. Unlike Gilbert's syndrome, only a few hundred cases of Criger–Najjar syndrome are known.

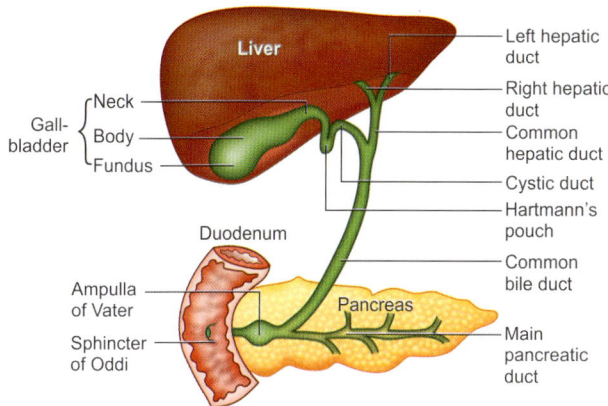

Fig. 8.2: Anatomy of biliary system

GILBERT'S SYNDROME (GS)

Introduction

Gilbert's syndrome, also called Gilbert-Meulengracht syndrome, is the most common hereditary cause of increased bilirubin and is found in up to 5% of the population. It is a phenotypic effect. A major characteristic is jaundice, caused by unconjugated hyperbilirubinemia.

Etiology and Pathogenesis

The reduced activity of the enzyme uridine-diphosphate-glucuronosyl transferase isoform 1A1 (UDP-glucuronosyl transferase 1A1) or glucuronyltransferase, which conjugates bilirubin causes hyperbilirubinemia. There is a considerable reduction of UGT1A1 in this disorder. The UGT1A1 gene is associated with a TATA box promoter region; this region most commonly contains the genetic sequence A (TA6) TAA; this variant accounts for about 50% of alleles in many populations. There are however several allelic polymorphic variants of this region, the most common adding another dinucleotide repeat TA to the promoter region, so that it is thus referred to as A (TA7) TAA, also called UGT1A1*28; this common variant accounts for about 40% of alleles in some populations, but is seen less often, approximately 3% of alleles, in Southeast and East Asian people and Pacific Islanders.

In most populations, Gilbert's syndrome is most commonly associated with homozygous A (TA7) TAA alleles. In 95% of GS cases, two other glucuronosyltransferase enzymes, UGT1A6 (rendered 50% inactive) and UGT1A7 (rendered 83% ineffective), are also affected.

However, Gilbert's syndrome can arise without TATA box promoter polymorphic mutations; in some populations, particularly in healthy Southeast and East Asians, Gilbert's syndrome is more often a consequence of heterozygote missense mutations (such as Gly71Arg also known as UGT1A1*6, Tyr486Asp also known as UGT1A1*7, Pro364Leu also known as UGT1A1*73) in the actual gene coding region, which may be associated with significantly higher bilirubin levels.

Because of its effects on drug and bilirubin breakdown and because of its genetic inheritance, Gilbert's syndrome can be classed as a minor inborn error of metabolism.

Diagnosis

Symptoms and Signs

Mild jaundice may appear under conditions of exertion, stress, fasting, and infections, but the condition is otherwise usually asymptomatic. It has been reported that GS may contribute to an accelerated onset of neonatal jaundice, especially in the presence of increased hemolysis due to diseases like G6PD deficiency. This situation can be especially dangerous if not quickly treated as the high bilirubin causes irreversible neurological disability in the form of kernicterus.

Nonspecific symptoms: Fatigue, difficulty in maintaining concentration, loss of appetite, abdominal pain, loss of weight and others, but scientific studies found no clear pattern of adverse symptoms related to the elevated levels of unconjugated bilirubin in adults.

Investigations

- Unconjugated hyperbilirubinemia at moderate levels
- Liver enzymes and albumin levels remain normal.

Complications

Detoxification of Certain Drugs

While paracetamol is not metabolized by UGT1A1, it is metabolized by one of the other enzymes also deficient in some people with GS. A subset of people with GS may have an increased risk of paracetamol toxicity.

Differential Diagnosis

- *Hemolysis* should be excluded by blood count, haptoglobin, LDH levels and absence of reticulocytosis (feature of hemolytic anemia)
- *Viral hepatitis* by antigens and antibody levels of viruses
- *Cholestasis* should be excluded by increased levels of alkaline phosphatase, and ultrasound screening
- *Crigler–Najjar syndrome (types I and II)* should be excluded.

Clinical Pearls

- There is consequently a debate about whether GS should be classified as a disease
- Gilbert's syndrome was first described by French gastroenterologist Augustin Nicolas Gilbert et al. in 1901. In German literature, it is commonly associated with Jens Einar Meulengracht.

CRIGLER–NAJJAR SYNDROME

Introduction

The condition is named after John Fielding Crigler (1919), an American pediatrician and Victor Assad Najjar (1914), a Lebanese-American pediatrician. Crigler–Najjar Syndrome or CNS is a rare disorder affecting the bilirubin metabolism. The disorder results in an inherited form of nonhemolytic jaundice, which results in high levels of unconjugated bilirubin and often leads to brain damage in infants. There are two types:
- **Type I**
- **Type II** (also called Arias syndrome).

Crigler–Najjar Syndrome, Type I

- Very rare disease (estimated at 0.6–1.0 per million live births), and consanguinity increases the risk of this condition (other rare diseases may be present)
- Inheritance is autosomal recessive
- Most patients (type IA) have a mutation in one of the common exons (2–5), and have difficulties conjugating several additional substrates (several drugs and xenobiotics)
- A smaller percentage of patients (type IB) have mutations limited to the bilirubin-specific A1 exon; their conjugation defect is mostly restricted to bilirubin itself.

Diagnosis

Symptoms and Signs

Intense jaundice appears in the first days of life and persists thereafter.

Investigations

Type 1 is characterized by a serum bilirubin usually above 345 µmol/L (310–755) (whereas the reference range for total bilirubin is 2–14 µmol/L).

Management

Before the availability of phototherapy, these children died of kernicterus (bilirubin encephalopathy) or survived until early adulthood with clear neurological impairment. Today, therapy includes:
- Exchange transfusions in the immediate neonatal period
- 12 hours/day phototherapy
- Heme oxygenase inhibitors to reduce transient worsening of hyperbilirubinemia (although the effect decreases over time)

- Oral calcium phosphate and carbonate to form complexes with bilirubin in the gut
- Liver transplantation before the onset of brain damage and before phototherapy becomes ineffective at later age.

Crigler–Najjar Syndrome, Type II

Type II differs from type I in several aspects:
- Bilirubin levels are generally below 345 µmol/L (100–430; thus, there is overlap), and some cases are only detected later in life.
- Because of lower serum bilirubin, kernicterus is rare in type II.
- Bile is pigmented, instead of pale in type I or dark as normal, and monoconjugates constitute the largest fraction of bile conjugates.
- UGT1A1 is present at reduced but detectable levels (typically <10% of normal), because of single base pair mutations.
- The inheritance pattern of Crigler–Najjar syndrome type II has been difficult to determine but is generally considered to be autosomal recessive.

Hyperbilirubinemia of the unconjugated type may be caused by:
- Increased production
  - Hemolysis (e.g. hemolytic disease of the newborn, hereditary spherocytosis, sickle cell disease)
  - Ineffective erythropoiesis
  - Massive tissue necrosis or large hematomas.
- Decreased clearance
  - Drug-induced
  - Physiological neonatal jaundice and prematurity
  - Liver diseases such as advanced hepatitis or cirrhosis
  - Breast milk jaundice and Lucey–Driscoll syndrome
  - Crigler–Najjar syndrome and Gilbert syndrome.

Investigations

In Crigler–Najjar syndrome and Gilbert syndrome, routine liver function tests are normal, and hepatic histology usually is, too. There is no evidence for hemolysis.

Differential Diagnosis

Neonatal jaundice may develop in the presence of sepsis, hypoxia, hypoglycemia, hypothyroidism, hypertrophic pyloric stenosis, galactosemia, fructosemia, etc.
- Drug-induced *hepatitis* typically regresses after discontinuation of the substance.
- *Physiological neonatal jaundice* may peak at 85–170 µmol/L and decline to normal adult concentrations within 2 weeks.
- *Prematurity* results in higher levels.

Management

Treatment with phenobarbital is effective, generally with a decrease of at least 25% in serum bilirubin.

Clinical Pearl
- Treatment with phenobarbital can be used, along with these other factors, to differentiate type I and II.

DUBIN–JOHNSON SYNDROME (DJS)

Introduction

It is an autosomal recessive disorder that causes an increase of conjugated bilirubin in the serum without elevation of liver enzymes (ALT, AST). This condition is associated with a defect in the ability of hepatocytes to secrete conjugated bilirubin into the bile, and is similar to Rotor syndrome. It is usually asymptomatic but may be diagnosed in early infancy based on laboratory tests.

Pathophysiology

- The conjugated hyperbilirubinemia is a result of ***defective endogenous and exogenous transfer of anionic conjugates from hepatocytes into the bile***.
- Impaired biliary excretion of bilirubin glucuronides is due to a mutation in the canalicular multidrug resistance protein 2 (MRP2).
- Pigment deposition in lysosomes causes the liver to turn black.

Diagnosis

A hallmark of DJS is the unusual ratio between the byproducts of heme biosynthesis.

- Normal subjects have a coproporphyrin III to coproporphyrin I ratio of approximately 3–4:1. In patients with DJS, this ratio is reversed with coproporphyrin I being 3–4 times higher than coproporphyrin III. Analysis of urine porphyrins show a normal level of coproporphyrin but the I isomer accounts for 80% of the total (normally 25%).
- In postmortem autopsy, the liver will have a dark pink or black appearance due to pigment accumulation. There is plenty of canalicular multidrug resistant protein that causes bilirubin transfer to bile canaliculi. An isoform of this protein is localized to the apical hepatocyte membrane, allowing transport of glucuronide and glutathione conjugates back into the blood. High levels of gamma-glutamyl transferase (GGT) help in diagnosing pathologies involving biliary obstruction.
- DJS is due to a defect in the multispecific anion transporter (cMOAT) gene (ABC transporter superfamily). It is an autosomal recessive disease and is likely due to a loss of function mutation, since the mutation affects the cytoplasmic/binding domain.

Prognosis

Prognosis is good, and treatment of this syndrome is usually unnecessary. Most patients are asymptomatic and have normal life spans. Some neonates will present with cholestasis.

ROTOR SYNDROME

Introduction

- **Rotor syndrome**, also called **Rotor type hyperbilirubinemia**
- It is named after the Filipino internist, Arturo Belleza Rotor.
- It is a rare, relatively benign autosomal recessive bilirubin disorder of unknown origin.
- It is a distinct disorder, yet similar to Dubin–Johnson syndrome—both diseases cause an increase in conjugated bilirubin.
- Rotor syndrome has many things in common with Dubin-Johnson syndrome, an exception being that the liver cells are not pigmented. The main symptom is a non-itching jaundice. It can be differentiated from Dubin–Johnson syndrome in the following ways (**Table 8.2**).

Table 8.2: Differentiating features of Rotor and Dubin–Johnson syndromes

	Rotor syndrome	Dubin Johnson syndrome
Appearance of liver	Normal histology and appearance	Liver has black pigmentation
Gallbladder visualization	Gallbladder can be visualized by oral cholecystogram	Gallbladder cannot be visualized
Total urine coproporphyrin content	High with <70% being isomer 1	Normal with >80% being isomer 1 (normal urine contains more of isomer 3 than isomer 1)

LUCEY–DRISCOLL SYNDROME

Lucey–Driscoll syndrome is an autosomal recessive metabolic disorder affecting enzymes involved in bilirubin metabolism. It is one of several disorders classified as a transient familial neonatal unconjugated hyperbilirubinemia.

Etiology

The common cause is congenital, but it can also be caused by maternal steroids passed on through breast milk to the newborn. It is different from breast milk jaundice (breast-fed infants have higher bilirubin levels than formula-fed ones). A defect in the UGT1A1-gene, also linked to Crigler–Najjar syndrome and Gilbert's syndrome, is responsible for the congenital form of Lucey–Driscoll syndrome.

OBSTRUCTIVE JAUNDICE

Extrahepatic obstruction producing cholestasis and jaundice, is otherwise called **surgical or obstructive cholestatic jaundice**.

Causes

The causes of obstruction (**Fig. 8.3**) are mechanical and are given in **Table 8.3**.

The surgeon is concerned with surgical jaundice, as it requires surgical intervention to remove the cause and or relieve the obstruction.

Causes of obstructive jaundice can be classified based on its etiology (**Table 8.4**).

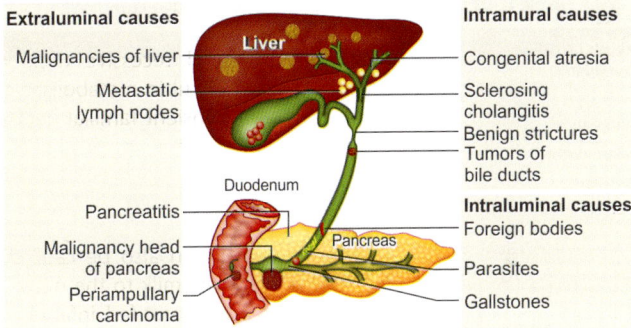

Fig. 8.3: Causes of mechanical obstruction of biliary system

Table 8.3: Causes of mechanical obstruction of biliary system

Location of obstruction	Nature of obstruction
Inside the biliary ducts (intraluminal)	• Gallstones • Foreign bodies (e.g. broken T tube) • Parasites (e.g. hydatid, roundworm, flukes)
In the duct wall (intramural)	• Congenital atresia • Benign strictures • Sclerosing cholangitis • Tumors of the bile ducts
Outside the biliary ducts (extraluminal)	• Pancreatitis • Metastatic lymph nodes • Malignancies of liver • Malignancy of head of pancreas • Periampullary carcinoma

Table 8.4: Etiological classification of obstructive jaundice

Etiology	Pathology
Congenital	• Biliary atresia • Choledochal cyst
Traumatic	• Traumatic strictures
Inflammatory	• Sclerosing cholangitis
Neoplastic	• Hepatocellular carcinoma • Cholangiocarcinoma • Periampullary carcinoma • Carcinoma head of pancreas • Metastatic liver disease • Metastatic lymph nodes
Metabolic and miscellaneous	• Gallstones • Parasitic diseases

Investigations

1. **Urine examination**
   - ***Bile salts*** presence in the urine indicate bilirubinuria
   - ***Urobilinogen***—absence indicates obstructive jaundice and excess indicates hemolytic jaundice.
2. **Stool examination**
   - ***Bile pigment***—absence indicates obstructive jaundice, and excess amount indicates hemolytic jaundice
   - ***Positive occult blood*** suggests gastrointestinal malignancy, bleeding esophageal varices
3. **Hematology**
   - ***Hemoglobin*** for anemia
   - ***Total and differential leukocyte count,*** e.g. infections
   - ***ESR*** may be raised in infections and malignancies.

4. **Liver function tests**
   - *Raised bilirubin levels* indicate jaundice
   - *Raised levels of serum alkaline phosphatase* indicate biliary obstruction
   - *Albumin globulin levels* get reversed in hepatocellular damage
   - *Transaminase levels* are raised in hepatocellular damage.
5. **Coagulation profile**
   - Prolonged prothrombin time is an accompaniment of deranged liver function tests.
6. **Radiology**
   - *US of abdomen* may be useful in assessing the liver parenchyma (e.g. malignant deposits, cirrhosis) and biliary system (e.g. nature and level of obstruction of biliary tree)
   - *CT or MRI scan* (e.g. nature and level of obstruction of biliary tree)
   - *Contrast studies*
     - *MRCP* has the advantage of being noninvasive with high sensitivity
     - *ERCP*—Administration of radiopaque dye into the biliary tree by ERCP may identify the underlying cause (e.g. CBD stones, ductal malignancies) but used only when therapy is planned
     - *PTC* is ideal for demonstrating an extrahepatic impassable obstruction and also for stenting to relieve jaundice.
7. **Radionuclide studies (HIDA):** Bile duct visualization helpful in fistulas, but anatomical details are poorly displayed.
8. **Endoscopy**
   - *Upper gastrointestinal endoscopy* is important to identify the upper GI causes (e.g. esophageal varices, malignancies)

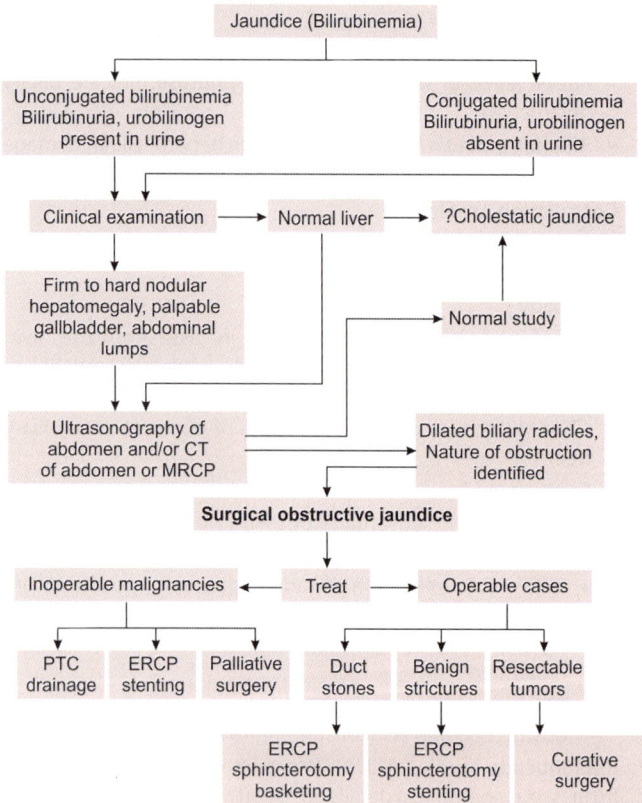

Fig. 8.4: Flowchart for evaluation and management of obstructive jaundice

- *Total colonoscopy* may be needed to eliminate primary colorectal cancer
- *Proctoscopy* is an inherent part of rectal examination, and is a mandatory investigation to make a clinical diagnosis
- *Laparoscopy* as diagnostic tool and for obtaining biopsies (e.g. cirrhosis of liver)
- *Spyglass cholangiography* to directly visualize and treat the cause.

9. **Histopathology**
   - **Biopsy** (percutaneous) of the liver is needed to have a final diagnosis. Ultrasound or CT guided biopsies have reduced the incidence of laparoscopy and laparotomy aided biopsies

The evaluation and management process of patient with obstructive jaundice is shown in **Figure 8.4**.

Chapter 9

Gastrointestinal Hemorrhage

Gastrointestinal hemorrhages, when they are in large quantities, called major hemorrhages present either as vomiting of blood or passage of blood per rectum.

The blood loss due to gastrointestinal hemorrhage is divided into three types:
1. *Mild*—less than 500 mL
2. *Moderate*—500–1500 mL
3. *Severe*—more than 1500 mL

Mild hemorrhages are rarely associated with systemic signs. When the blood loss approaches about 40% of the blood volume, shock ensues. Actual loss of 1,000 mL will produce orthostatic changes of 10–20 mm Hg in systolic blood pressure and a pulse raise of 20 beats/minute, and loss of more than 2,000 mL will produce shock.

UPPER GASTROINTESTINAL BLEED

Introduction

- Any bleeding from the gastrointestinal tract from a source proximal to the ligament of Treitz is called upper gastrointestinal bleed (UGIB).
- It is five to six times more common than lower gastrointestinal bleed (LGIB).

- It presents as vomiting of blood, called **hematemesis,** which may be fresh or partly altered. Altered blood is dark in color (contact of blood with hydrochloric acid produces acid hematin), and has the typical appearance of 'coffee grounds'. Some blood passes down the alimentary tract, and is subjected to digestion, to pass per rectum as altered blood called **'melena'**.
- The blood should remain in the gut for approximately 8 hours to produce melena, but when the bleeding from the upper gastrointestinal tract is large and rapid, and when the gastrointestinal transit time is prolonged, bleeding from small bowel and even ascending colon can pass rectally as black stools, as melena.
- Approximately about 60 mL of blood is required to produce a single black stool; loss more than this amount can cause melena for more than 3 days.
- Even after the color of the stools returns to normal, the test for occult blood in the stool may remain positive for a week or longer.
- Hematemesis and melena usually coexist.
- UGIB can also present with melena as the sole clinical symptom.

Etiology

The causes of upper GI bleed are tabulated in **Table 9.1** and shown in **Figure 9.1**.

Risk Factors

- Smoking
- Alcohol
- NSAIDs
- Prior GI bleed
- UGI symptoms.

Table 9.1: Causes of upper GI bleed

Parts of upper GIT	Pathology	Clinical presentation
Esophagus	• Reflux esophagitis • Esophageal varices • Mallory–Weiss tears	Hematemesis and/or melena
Stomach and duodenum	• Acid peptic disease • Gastric polyps • Gastric lymphoma • Carcinoma stomach	

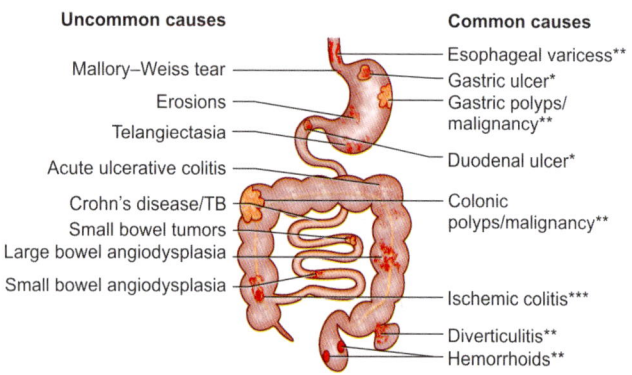

Fig. 9.1: Causes of gastrointestinal bleeding
Note: * Very common, ** Common, *** Fairly common

Diagnosis

Clinical Presentation

Vomiting
- *Color*
  - Bright red color (e.g. pathologies of esophagus)
  - Blackish color (e.g. pathologies of stomach).
- *Duration*
  - Long history (e.g. bleeding acid peptic disease, esophageal varices)
  - Short history (e.g. bleeding acid peptic disease, esophageal varices, malignancy).
- *Volume of bleed*
  - Small to moderate quantities (e.g. any upper GI pathology)
  - Large bleeds (e.g. esophageal varices, bleeding ulcer).
- *Abdominal pain*
  - Presence of pain (e.g. acid peptic disease)
  - Absence of pain (e.g. esophageal varices, malignancy).
- *Retching*
  - Associated with retching (e.g. Mallory Weiss tears).

Signs
- Positive gastric aspirate, black stool per rectum (melena)
- *Tenderness*
  - Epigastric tenderness (e.g. acid peptic disease)
  - No area of tenderness (e.g. esophageal varices, gastric polyps, esophageal/gastric malignancy).
- *Quantity of bleed:* Large bleeds (e.g. esophageal varices)

Clinical diagnosis towards the cause of UGIB can be done using **Table 9.2**.

Table 9.2: Differential diagnosis of UGIB by clinical history and examination

GI hemorrhage	Associated symptoms	Clinical diagnosis after eliciting history	Clinical findings	Clinical diagnosis after examination
Hematemsis and melena	Upper abdominal pain	Bleeding duodenal/gastric ulcer	Epigastric tenderness	Bleeding duodenal/gastric ulcer
	No abdominal pain	Esophageal varices, vascular malformations, upper GI malignancy	No clinical finding	Varices, vascular malformations, upper GI malignancy
			Abdominal lump	Upper GI malignancy
	Painless increasing jaundice	Upper GI malignancy with liver metastases	Abdominal lump, ± hepatomegaly	Upper GI malignancy + liver metastases
	Painless fluctuating jaundice	Periampullary carcinoma, liver metastases	Palpable GB, ± hepatomegaly	Periampullary carcinoma, ± liver metastases
Melena	Abdominal pain	Bleeding duodenal ulcer, Inflammatory bowel disease, duodenal diverticulitis	Epigastric tenderness	Bleeding duodenal/gastric ulcer, duodenal diverticulitis
			Umbilical tenderness	Inflammatory bowel disease
			Palpable lump	Upper GI malignancy
	Painless	Esophageal varices, vascular malformations, upper GI malignancy	No clinical finding	Varices, vascular malformations, upper GI malignancy
			Abdominal lump	Upper GI malignancy

Gastrointestinal Hemorrhage

Investigations

Investigations are done as a part of management schedule.

MANAGEMENT (STEP BY STEP)

1. Quick evaluation of hemodynamic status.
2. Quick intravenous access with large bore catheters and fluid replacement (crystalloids—normal saline/lactated Ringer's solution).
3. Blood tests (hematocrit, platelet count, prothrombin time, partial thromboplastin time) from the blood taken during the intravenous access.
4. If there is no recovery of vitals, vasopressors are to be administered.
5. Insertion of nasogastric tube to confirm and assess the quantity of bleed.
6. Unstable patients should be transferred to intensive care unit.
7. Clearing of stomach of all blood with water wash, and prepare for a quick endoscopy to identify the source (**Figs 9.2 to 9.8**) and briskness of bleed.
8. Management based on endoscopy findings (Forrest classification) (**Table 9.3**).

Table 9.3: Forrest classification for bleeding peptic ulcer

Description	Class
Spurting active bleeding	IA
Nonspurting active bleeding	IB
Nonbleeding 'visible vessel'	IIA
Nonbleeding ulcer with overlying clot	IIB
Nonbleeding ulcer with hematin covered base	IIC
Clean ulcer base with no signs of bleeding	III

- *Forrest Grade IA, IB and II A*—high risk
    - Endoscopic hemostasis
    - Intensive care
    - Intravenous PPI (80 mg bolus + continuous infusion (8 mg/hr) for 72 hours

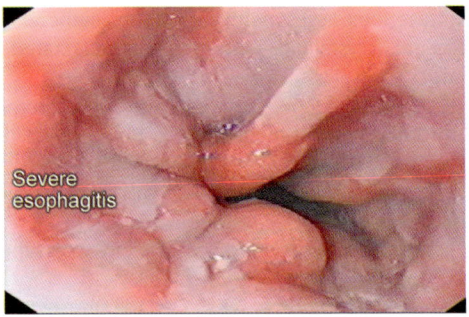

Fig. 9.2: Esophagoscopy—Bleeding esophagitis

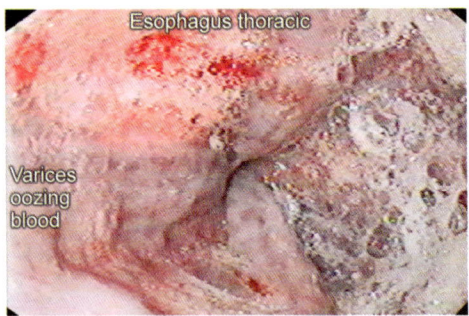

Fig. 9.3: Esophagoscopy—Bleeding esophageal varices

Gastrointestinal Hemorrhage

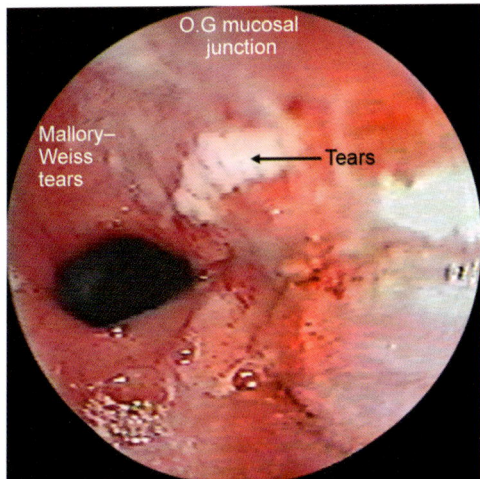

Fig. 9.4: Esophagoscopy—Bleeding from Mallory–Weiss tear

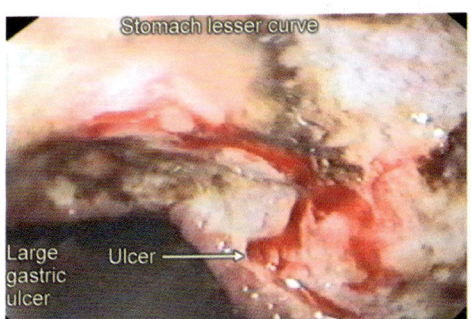

Fig. 9.5: Gastroscopy—Bleeding gastric ulcer

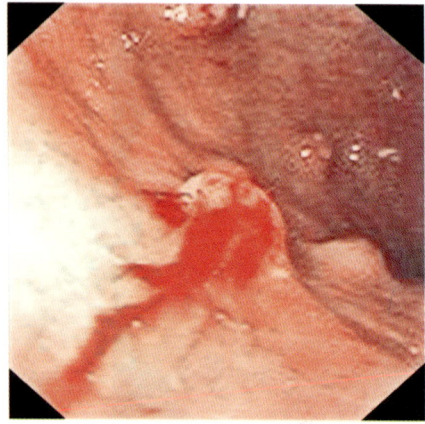

Fig. 9.6: Gastroscopy—Bleeding from polyp of stomach

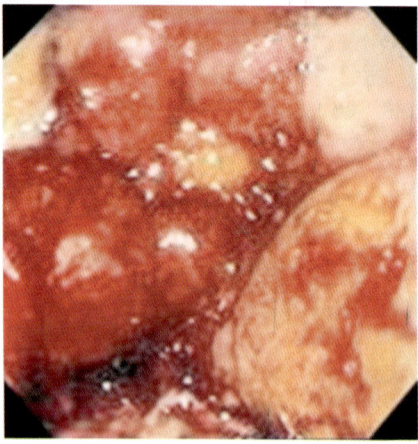

Fig. 9.7: Gastroscopy—Bleeding gastric lymphoma

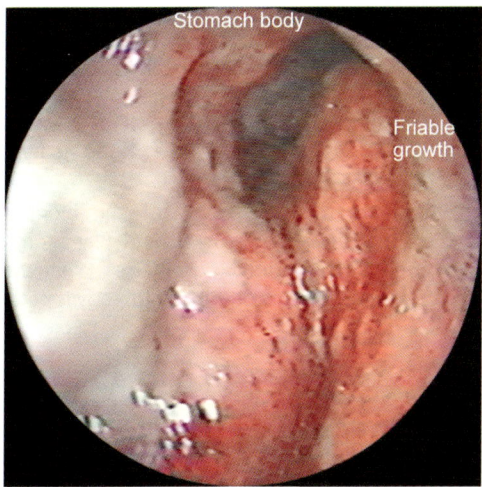

Fig. 9.8: Gastroscopy—Bleeding from gastric malignancy

  - Clear liquid diet after 6 hours
  - Oral PPI after 72 hours
  - Test for *H. pylori* and treat if positive.
- ***Forrest Grade IIB and IIC***—high risk
  - Endoscopic hemostasis only if bleeding vessel is seen below clot
  - Treatment as Grade IA.
- ***Forrest Grade III***—low risk
  - No need for hemostasis
  - Oral PPI
  - Regular diet after 6 hours of endoscopy
  - Test for *H. pylori* and treat if positive.

Clinical Pearls

- Absence of risk factors may indicate malignancy of upper GIT
- The volume of blood loss either by vomiting or through rectum, is not a very reliable measure, as large amounts stay in the bowel. Whatever be the external visible loss, signs of hypovolemia should be watched for
- Though there are methods to assess the blood loss and predict the seriousness (e.g. Rockall and Blatchford scores—**Tables 9.4 and 9.5**), it is better to hospitalize the patient of upper GI bleed at least for 24 hours or until endoscopy is performed.

Table 9.4: Rockall score

Variable	Score 0	Score 1	Score 2	Score 3
Age	<60	60–79	>80	
Shock	No shock	Pulse >100	SBP <100	
Comorbidity	Nil major	All other diagnoses	CHF, IHD, major morbidity	Renal failure, liver failure, metastatic cancer
Diagnosis		Mallory-Weiss	GI malignancy	
Evidence of bleeding		None	Blood, adherent clot, spurting vessel	

It attempts to identify patients at risk of adverse outcome following acute upper gastrointestinal bleeding. The scoring system uses clinical criteria (increasing age, comorbidity, shock) as well as endoscopic finding (diagnosis, stigmata of acute bleeding).

Interpretation: Total score is calculated by simple addition. A score less than 3 carries good prognosis but total score of more than 8 carries high risk of mortality.

Table 9.5: Blatchford admission risk markers

Admission risk marker	Score component value
Blood urea (mMol/L)	
6.5–8.0	2
8.0–10.0	3

Contd...

Contd...

Admission risk marker	Score component value
10.0–25.0	4
>25	6
Hemoglobin (g/L) for men	
120–130	1
100–120	3
<100	6
Hemoglobin (g/L) for women	
100–120	1
<100	6
Systolic blood pressure (mm Hg)	
100–109	1
90–99	2
<90	3
Other markers	
Pulse >100 per min	1
Presentation with melena	1
Presentation with syncope	2
Hepatic disease	2
Cardiac failure	2

Interpretation: Total score is calculated by simple addition. A score less than 3 carries good prognosis but total score of more than 8 carries high risk of mortality.

LOWER GASTROINTESTINAL BLEED

Introduction

- Any bleeding from the gastrointestinal tract from a source distal to the ligament of Treitz is called lower gastrointestinal bleed (LGIB)
- It is one fifth to one sixth as common as UGIB
- This presents as bleeding per rectum and it is bright red in color. This is called **hematochezia**.

Etiology

The causes of lower GI bleed are tabulated in **Table 9.6**.

Table 9.6: Causes of lower GI bleeding

Part of GIT		Pathology	Clinical presentation
Lower	Small bowel	Angiodysplasia	Melena
		Diverticulitis	
		Radiation enteritis	
		Infections and inflammations	
		Ischemic disease	
		Intussusception	
		Richter's hernia	
		Benign tumors	
		Malignant tumors	
	Large bowel	Angiodysplasia	Fresh rectal bleed (diarrhea/constipation as per etiology)
		Diverticulitis	
		Radiation colitis	
		Infections and inflammations	
		Ischemic disease	
		Ulcerative colitis	
		Benign polyps	
		Malignant tumors	
	Rectum and anus	Polyps	Fresh rectal bleed (constipation)
		Malignant tumors	
		Hemorrhoids fissures	

Note: Lower gastrointestinal hemorrhages do not present with hematemesis, but hematochezia results from UGIB in about 10% of cases, and when in doubt, nasogastric lavage should be done to confirm or exclude its source.

Risk Factors
- Smoking
- Alcohol
- NSAID
- Prior GI bleed
- UGI symptoms.

Diagnosis

Clinical Presentation

Bleeding Per Rectum
- *Color*
  - Bright red color (e.g. pathologies in the lower GI tract)
  - Blackish color (e.g. pathologies in the upper GI tract).
- *Duration*
  - Long history (e.g. benign conditions like ulcerative colitis, hemorrhoids)
  - Short history (e.g. malignancy).
- *Bowel habits*
  - Recent onset constipation (e.g. malignancy)
  - Habitual constipation (e.g. hemorrhoids)
  - Diarrhea (e.g. inflammatory bowel disease).
- *Volume of bleed*
  - Small to moderate quantities (e.g. hemorrhoids)
  - Large bleeds (e.g. angiodysplasia).
- *Abdominal pain*
  - Presence of pain (e.g. inflammatory bowel disease, infection)
  - Absence of pain (e.g. hemorrhoids, malignancy).

- *Anal pain*
  - Presence of pain (e.g. complicated hemorrhoids, anal malignancy, radiation proctitis)
  - Absence of pain (e.g. hemorrhoids, rectal malignancy).

Clinical Examination

- Vital signs.

Abdomen

- Tenderness
  - Presence of tenderness (e.g. inflammatory bowel disease)
  - Absence of tenderness (e.g. polyps, angiodysplasia, malignancy).

Rectum

- **Digital examination** (e.g. malignant growths)
- **Proctoscopy** (e.g. hemorrhoids, polyps, ulcers).

Clinical diagnosis towards the cause of LGIB can be done using **Table 9.7**.

Investigations

- Complete blood count
- Coagulation profile
- Electrolytes
- Colonoscopy
- Nuclear scintigraphy
- Capsule endoscopy
- Selective mesenteric angiography (useful in acute bleeds occurring at a rate of 0.5–1 mL/min, and has the advantage of therapeutic intervention).

Table 9.7: Differential diagnosis of LGIB by clinical history and examination

GI hemorrhage	Associated symptoms	Clinical diagnosis after eliciting history	Clinical findings	Clinical diagnosis after examination
Hematochezia	Pain during defecation	Acute fissure in ano	Positive inspection findings	Acute fissure in ano
	Painless	Hemorrhoids, colorectal pathologies	Positive proctoscopy findings	Hemorrhoids, rectal pathology
			Negative proctoscopy findings	Colonic pathologies
	Abdominal pain and fever	Inflammatory bowel disease, diverticulitis	Local tenderness	Inflammatory bowel disease, diverticulitis
	Colicky pain	Colonic obstruction	Abdominal lump	Colonic malignancy
	Jaundice (Painless) ± abdominal pain	Obstructive jaundice	± abdominal lyump, ± hepatomegaly	Colonic malignancy with liver metastases

Management

1. Quick evaluation of hemodynamic status.
2. Resuscitation: Quick intravenous access with large bore catheters and fluid replacement (crystalloids—normal saline/lactated Ringer's solution).
3. Blood tests (hematocrit, platelet count, prothrombin time, partial thromboplastin time) from the blood taken during the intravenous access.
4. If there is no recovery of vitals, blood transfusions are needed and vasopressors are to be administered.
5. Insertion of nasogastric tube to confirm and assess the quantity of bleed (only for patients having melena).

104 Snapshots in Gastroenterology

6. Unstable patients (patients requiring 2 units of blood or has had a drop of 6% hematocrit) should be transferred to intensive care unit.
7. A quick colonoscopy to identify the source **(Figs 9.9 to 9.17)** and briskness of bleed is as fallows:
   - Management based on endoscopy findings
   - Endoscopic contact electrocautery and argon plasma coagulation are used for bleeding vascular lesions and polyps
   - Bleeding pedunculated polyps can be snared during colonoscopy.

The management approach to lower GI bleeding is given in **Figure 9.18**.

Clinical Pearls

- Large majority of patients with LGIB resolve without therapeutic intervention

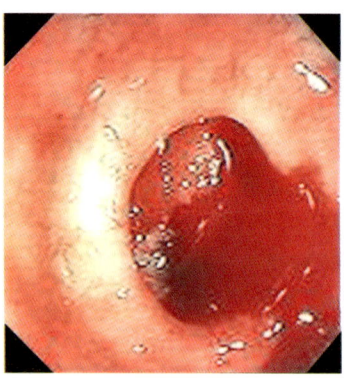

Fig. 9.9: Colonoscopy—Bleeding from colonic diverticulitis

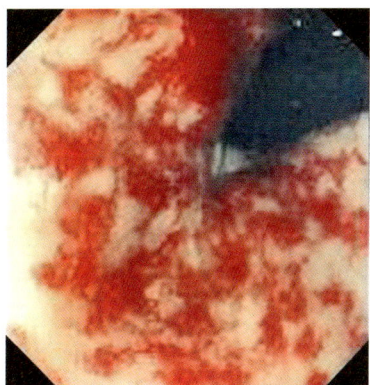

Fig. 9.10: Colonoscopy—Radiation colitis

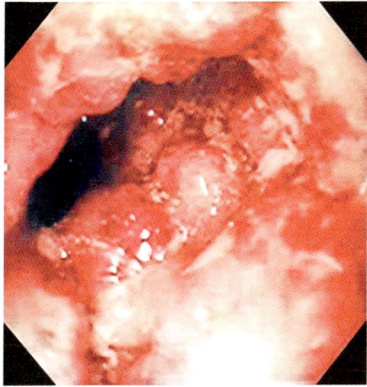

Fig. 9.11: Colonoscopy—Bleeding from Crohn's disease of colon

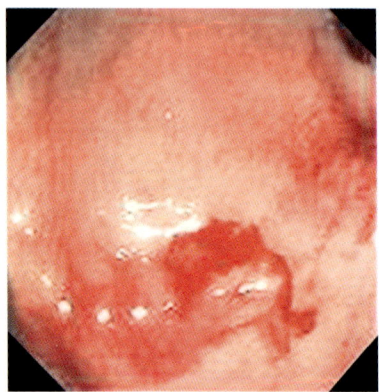

Fig. 9.12: Colonoscopy—Bleeding angiodysplasia of large bowel

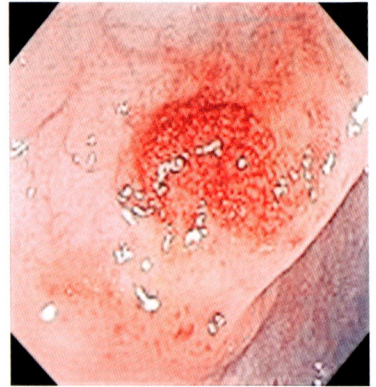

Fig. 9.13: Colonoscopy—Hemangioma of rectum

Gastrointestinal Hemorrhage

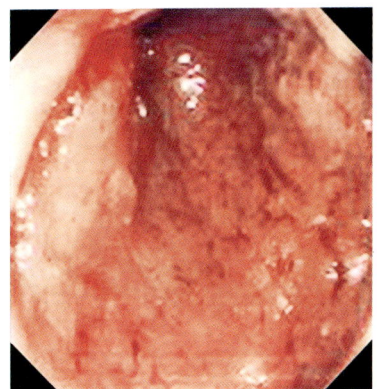

Fig. 9.14: Colonoscopy—Bleeding ulcerative colitis

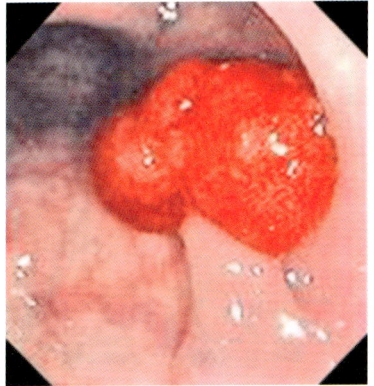

Fig. 9.15: Colonoscopy—Bleeding colonic polyp

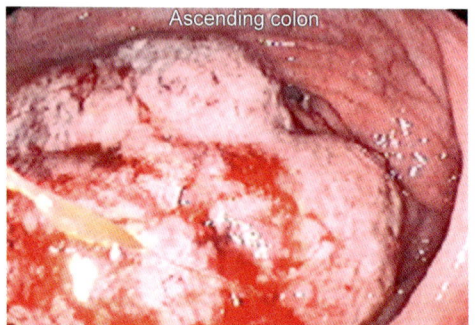

Fig. 9.16: Colonoscopy—Bleeding from carcinoma of cecum

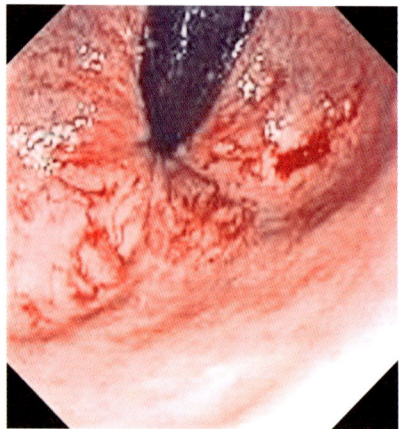

Fig. 9.17: Colonoscopy—Bleeding hemorrhoids

Gastrointestinal Hemorrhage

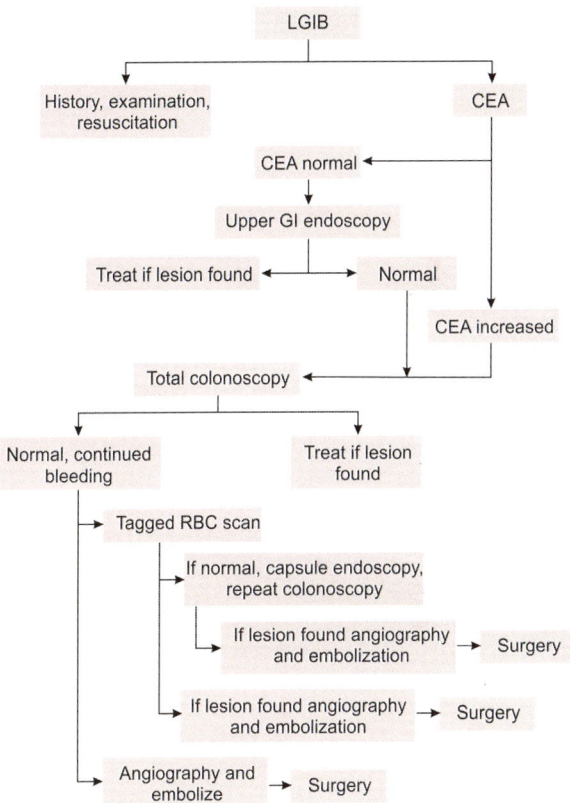

Fig. 9.18: The management approach to lower GI bleeding

- Majority of sites of LGIB originate in the colon or rectum, and a small but substantial percentage come from the small intestine
- It is difficult to assess whether the LGIB is continuous or not, and patient's hematocrit is the only possible indicator of continued bleeding
- A common cause of massive LGIB occurs from the mucosal erosion of a colonic diverticulum adjacent to perforating vessels
- NSAIDs are associated with LGIB due to colonic diverticulosis, NSAIDs can exacerbate IBD
- Unstable patients in the presence of adequate volume substitution should make one suspect continued bleeding
- During acute LGIB, colon can be screened by colonoscopy, but small bowel screening is not possible and technetium^{99} labeled red cell scintigraphy and selective angiography may be useful
- Small bowel screening is done only when the colon is normal
- Chronic small bowel pathology bleeding can be diagnosed by capsule endoscopy (**Figs 9.19 and 9.20**)
- Capsule endoscopy, though noninvasive, has the disadvantages like not able to take a biopsy, when compared to double balloon enteroscopy, which has better resolution and camera control and biopsies can be obtained
- Angiography is most useful in LGIB of diverticulosis, as such bleeding is arterial and massive compared to other pathologies
- About 10% of patients do have a localized pathology before surgery, which operation to perform is a dilemma
- In patients with no palpable or visual abnormality during laparotomy, intraoperative enteroscopy (insertion of colonoscopy through an enterotomy) may be of benefit
- In patients with no demonstrable pathology, and bleed recurrently, total abdominal colectomy may be necessary
- The mortality associated with lower GI bleeding is very low, and is rarely a direct cause of death.

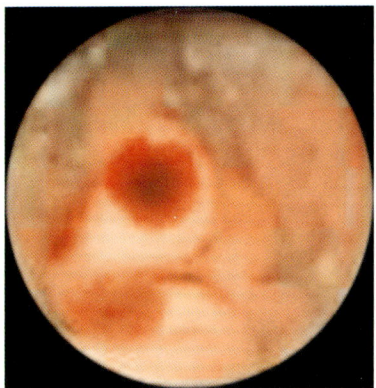

Fig. 9.19: Capsule endoscopy—Angiodysplasia of stomach

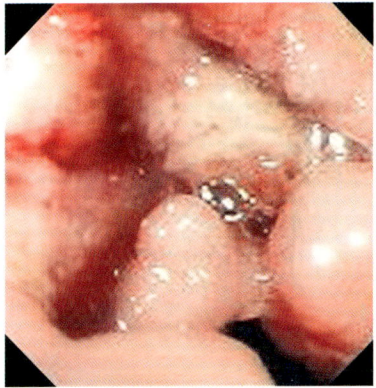

Fig. 9.20: Capsule endoscopy—Bleeding from small bowel lymphoma

OBSCURE GASTROINTESTINAL BLEED

Introduction

Obscure GI bleeding is defined as bleeding that persists or recurs without a demonstrable etiology after a thorough workup including all endoscopies. They are divided into:
- **Obscure occult bleeding:** Bleeding that is not visible (not frank blood loss) to the naked eye but its presence is manifested by occult blood test.
- **Obscure overt bleeding:** Clinically observable frank bleeding with negative endoscopic examinations.

Etiology

The etiologies which can cause overt GI bleeding are given in **Box 9.1**.

Box 9.1: Etiologic factors of overt GI bleeding

Common
- AV malformation (telangiectasia)
- Neoplasms (GIST, adenocarcinoma, carcinoid)
- Small bowel lesions (NSAID-related ulcers or erosions)

Uncommon
- Lipoma
- Dieulafoy's lesion
- Cameron's erosion

Rare
- Nevus
- Kaposi's sarcoma
- Tuberculosis
- Hemobilia
- Foreign body
- Crohn's disease
- Celiac sprue
- Aortoenteric fistula
- Watermelon stomach (gastric antral vascular ectasia)

Associated Factors

- Oral or facial telangiectasia associated with gut telangiectasia (Osler–Weber–Rendu syndrome)
- Acanthosis nigricans in the axilla suggests GI malignancy
- Perioral hyperpigmentation suggests Peutz-Jeghers syndrome
- Purpura may suggest a possible bleeding disorder.

Diagnosis

Symptoms

- Usually patients are asymptomatic and identification of GI bleed is only by fecal occult blood test
- Rarely, some patients with anemia with chronic blood loss, show signs of cardiac failure, general weakness.

Signs

- Cheilosis, glossitis and koilonychias (signs of iron deficiency anemia).

Investigations

Stool Test

Occult blood is tested in the stool. There are two methods:
1. Guaiac fecal occult blood test.
2. Immunochemical method.

Tumor Markers

- CEA determination is useful (elevated in colonic adenocarcinoma).

Endoscopy

- If the occult blood test is positive, and CEA values are high, colon should be evaluated with colonoscopy, if found normal, followed by upper GI endoscopy. When upper GI scopy is also normal, random biopsies should be taken from the 2nd and 3rd part of duodenum to look for tropical sprue. When CEA values are normal, upper GI endoscopy is done first as it is a simpler procedure with no formal preparation, followed by total colonoscopy
- If duodenal biopsy is negative for sprue, small bowel endoscopy (Sonde enteroscopy/Capsule endoscopy) should be performed and appropriate biopsies should be taken
- Intraoperative endoscopy is very sensitive and yields best results.

Radiology

- Barium meal follow through may be useful
- CT enteroclysis is more informative.

Scintigraphy and Angiography

- Tagged red cell scan can demonstrate bleeding with a rate of >0.1 mL/min
- Angiography demonstrates bleeding source if the bleeding rate is 0.5–1 mL/min.

Management

Management Depends on the Cause

- Angiodysplasia—endoscopic cautery (laser, bipolar, heater probe, argon plasma coagulation)
- Benign lesion—local excision
- Polyp—endoscopic removal
- Malignancy—radical excision.

Clinical Pearls

- Patients with obscure GI bleeding pose a challenge to surgeons, especially when the bleeding is intermittent, variable in amount and not accessible by routine localization techniques
- About 2 mL of blood in the GIT is enough to produce a positive fecal occult blood test
- Foods like red meat, raw broccoli, cauliflower, radish and turnip consumption cause false positive fecal occult blood test due to the pseudoperoxidase content
- Patient should avoid aspirin and NSAIDs and the vegetables mentioned above for 3 days prior to the fecal sample collection for occult blood test
- A sizable proportion of gastroduodenal and colonic lesions are not appreciated on initial endoscopy, and when bleeding persists or recurs, repeat endoscopy is warranted. Such missed lesions are usually, Cameron's erosions, Dieulafoy lesion, angiodysplasia and gastric antral vascular ectasia.

Chapter 10

Esophagus

ANATOMY AND PHYSIOLOGY

The esophagus is a long muscular tube starting at the lower border of pharynx (at the lower border of 6th cervical vertebra) and ends at the GE junction, the cardia. It is fixed at two places, one to the cricoid cartilage above and the other to the diaphragm below. It is in the midline, with a deviation to the left in the lower portion of neck and upper portion of the thorax, but returns to the midline in the midthorax. It deviates again to the left and anteriorly to pass through the esophageal hiatus in the diaphragm.

There are three narrowings in the esophagus. They are caused by:
1. Cricopharyngeus muscle (at about 15 cm from the incisor tooth).
2. Left main bronchus and arch of aorta (at about 25 cm from the incisor tooth).
3. Diaphragmatic crux at the hiatus (at about 40 cm from the incisor tooth).

The esophagus is divided into three parts:
- *Cervical esophagus* (approximately 5 cm long extending from the 6th cervical vertebra to the 2nd thoracic vertebra corresponding to the suprasternal notch)
- *Thoracic esophagus* (approximately 20 cm long extending from the thoracic inlet to the diaphragmatic hiatus)
- *Abdominal part of esophagus* (approximately 2 cm extending from the diaphragmatic hiatus to the GE junction).

Musculature

It can be divided into:
- Outer longitudinal muscle
- Inner circular muscle.

Arterial Supply

- Cervical esophagus—inferior thyroid artery
- Thoracic esophagus—bronchial arteries, branches from aorta
- Abdominal esophagus—left gastric artery.

Venous Drainage (Through Submucosal Plexus)

- Cervical esophagus—inferior thyroid vein
- Thoracic esophagus—bronchial veins, azygos and hemiazygos veins
- Abdominal esophagus—coronary vein.

Nerve Supply

- Entire esophagus—vagus nerves.

Lymphatics (Through Submucosal Plexus)

- *Upper third*—travel upwards (paratracheal and deep cervical nodes)
- *Middle third*—paratracheal nodes
- *Lower third*—travel downward (subcarinal, inferior pulmonary and superior gastric nodes).

Physiology

Swallowing is the act by which food is taken from the mouth to the stomach. The first phase is called the oropharyngeal phase, which consists of:
- Elevation and posterior movement of tongue (pushes the bolus into the posterior oropharynx)
- Elevation of soft palate (closes the passage between the oropharynx and nasopharynx)
- Elevation of hyoid and larynx (opens the retrolaryngeal space)
- Tilting of epiglottis (covers the opening of the larynx and prevents aspiration).

The entire act takes about 1.5 seconds.

Pressure gradient, propels the food from the hypopharynx into the esophagus and further by the peristaltic contraction of posterior pharyngeal constrictors. The food bolus then travels down the esophagus into the stomach. The LES prevents the reflux of bolus, which enters the stomach.

APPROACH TO A PATIENT WITH ESOPHAGEAL PATHOLOGY

Signs and Symptoms

The most common symptoms of esophageal disease are:
- Dysphagia
- Odynophagia
- Weight loss
- Early satiety
- Anorexia
- Anemia

- Regurgitation
- Cough.

Signs of esophageal diseases are:
- Direct—nil
- Indirect—cervical lumps, respiratory signs, hepatomegaly.

Investigations

- Tests to detect structural abnormalities
  - Radiologic tests (Barium swallow, CT scan and MRI, chest X–ray)
  - Endoscopic evaluation (esophagoscopy).
- Tests to detect functional abnormalities
  - Stationary manometry
  - High resolution manometry
  - Esophageal impedance
  - Esophageal transit scintigraphy
  - Video and cine radiography.
- Tests to detect exposure to gastric juice
  - 24-hour ambulatory pH monitoring
  - Radiographic detection of reflux.
- Tests of duodenogastric function.

ATRESIA OF ESOPHAGUS

Introduction

- Congenital anomaly in which there is interruption of elongation and partitioning of esophageal and tracheal tubes
- Occurs in 1 in 4,000 births
- Occurs when embryonic foregut fails to recanalize to form an esophagus, and the exact reason is not known.

Classification

- Esophageal atresia (**Figs 10.1A and B**) is classified as follows:
  - *Type A*—Pure esophageal atresia (8%)
  - *Type B*—Esophageal atresia with upper pouch fistula to the trachea (1%)

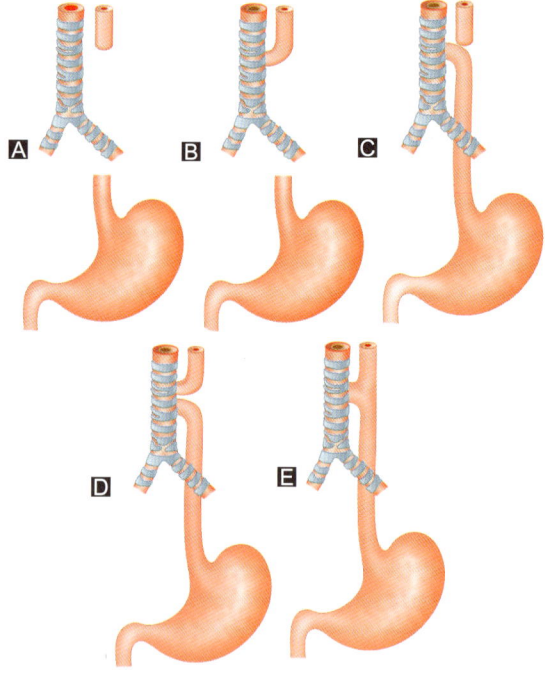

Fig. 10.1A: Esophageal atresia

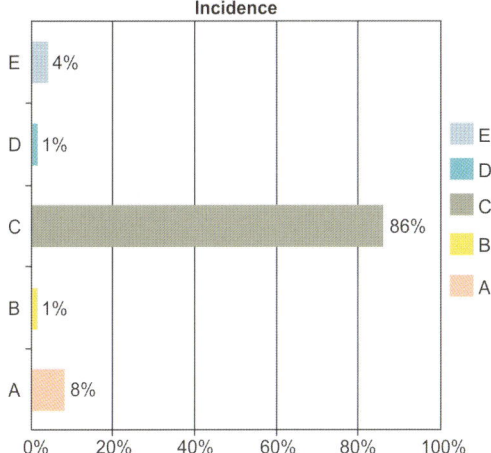

Fig. 10.1B: Incidence of varieties of esophageal atresia

- *Type C*—Esophageal atresia with lower pouch fistula to the trachea (86%)
- *Type D*—Esophageal atresia with upper and lower fistulae (1%)
- *Type E*—Fistula without atresia (4%).
- Associated congenital anomalies occur in 20% patients.

Diagnosis

Symptoms and Signs

- Child presents with inability to retain the food intake resulting in vomiting, aspiration, choking, cyanosis and respiratory distress
- The abdomen progressively distends due to the air entry through the fistula.

Investigations

- Passing the nasogastric tube is impossible
- *Administration of contrast through the tube will clinch the diagnosis (Fig. 10.2).*

Management

- *Medical:* Head up position, intravenous fluids, antibiotics
- *Surgical: Transthoracic approach: Transpleural or extrapleural*
  - *Excision of fistula with end to end anastomosis*
  - *Esophageal replacement using stomach, colon or jejunum may be required to fill long gaps*
  - *Feeding gastrostomy may be necessary, if surgery is delayed.*

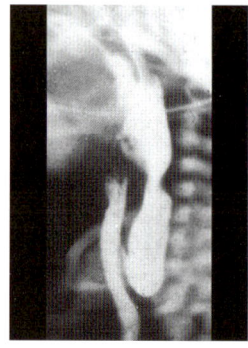

Fig. 10.2: Barium swallow—Esophageal atresia with tracheoesophageal fistula

ACHALASIA CARDIA (CARDIOSPASM)

Introduction

- An uncommon motility disorder of the esophagus with a peristalsis and failure of lower esophageal sphincter relaxation while swallowing
- Occurs due to degeneration of ganglion cells of myenteric plexus resulting in the non-relaxation of the lower esophageal sphincter during deglutition, and the bolus is retained in the lower esophagus for some time.

Associated Pathologies

- Alacrimation and Addison's disease *(Triple A syndrome)*
- **Loss of inhibitory nerves in the stomach and duodenum**
- **Sphincter of Oddi dysfunction**
- Infection with *Trypanosoma cruzi* may produce a similar syndrome, which is common in South America.

Association with Malignancy

Esophageal cancer may develop in cases of achalasia cardia but seems to occur in the dilated mid-esophagus and is usually of squamous variety. The incidence is about 3% and increases after 15 years of achalasia. Though this is considered a premalignant condition, the risk of cancer in most patients adequately treated is very small. The question of periodic endoscopic surveillance remains unanswered by insufficient data.

Diagnosis

Symptoms and Signs

- Progressive dysphagia to liquids and solids
- Regurgitation of food several hours after intake, probably due to the dilated esophagus acting as a reservoir and eject its contents when the intra-esophageal pressure reaches its maximum
- Retrosternal pain (caused by fermentation of food)
- Weight loss is common.

Investigations

Radiology

- ***X-ray chest*** is usually normal, but when the disease progresses, it shows a widened mediastinum with air fluid level in the atonic and dilated esophagus.

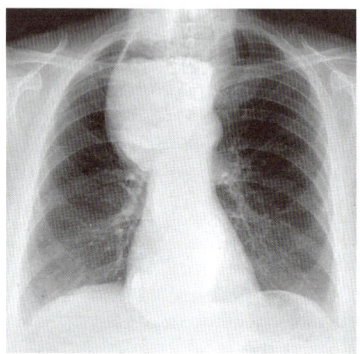

Fig. 10.3: Barium swallow—Achalasia

- *Barium swallow* (**Fig. 10.3**) shows a smooth tapering of distal esophagus *(Bird's beak appearance)* and allows very small quantity of contrast to pass through. *Sigmoid esophagus* is an elongated and dilated esophagus in longstanding achalasia.

Endoscopy

- *Esophagoscopy* (**Fig. 10.4**) shows disproportionate amount of food residue at the esophagogastric junction and is essential to differentiate it from malignant disease, especially in older patients. A tight or an elastic feel while passing through the GE junction is characteristic of achalasia.

Pressure Studies

- *Manometry* is diagnostic of achalasia, when it shows lack of peristalsis in the body of the esophagus with abnormal or absent lower esophageal sphincter (LES) relaxation in response to swallowing.

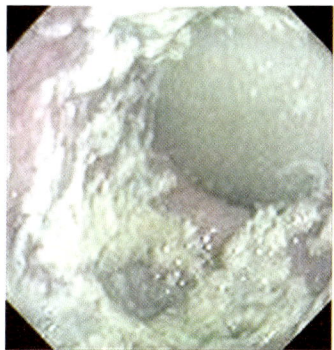

Fig. 10.4: Esophagoscopy—Achalasia showing retained fluid

Blood Test
- *Blood smear* may show *T. cruzi*.

Differential Diagnosis

- Pseudoachalasia
- Chagas' disease
- Motility disorders
- Esophageal stricture.

Complications

- Squamous cell carcinoma of esophagus.

Management

Medical

- Smooth muscle relaxants
- Botulinum toxin injection
- **Balloon dilatation** of esophagogastric junction resolves majority of lesions. Though the overall immediate response is good, more than half will require one or more dilatations over a 5-year period, and eventually require surgery. Perforation is a dreaded complication of dilatation, but majority of them are very small and conservative management will suffice.

Surgical

- ***Cardiomyotomy (Heller's operation)—longitudinal myotomy of the distal esophagus and GE junction down to the level of the mucosa*** is the treatment of choice and it is curative in majority of cases
- ***Antireflux procedures*** may be needed in some cases.

Clinical Pearls

- Patients with achalasia carry a higher risk of malignancy, and they develop at about 10 years younger than the general population, with a poor prognosis due to late diagnosis
- Use of drugs like nitrates and calcium channel blockers are useful in some cases, but most patients require surgical management
- Though intrathoracic myotomy is logical, transabdominal laparoscopic myotomies are widely practiced today with good long-term results

- Perforation is the commonest complication of cardiomyotomy, which needs to be repaired if recognized. Unrecognized perforation presents with fever, tachycardia and pleural effusion, which may require reoperation, if conservative management fails
- Previous medical management like dilatation and botulinum injections increase the difficulty during myotomy
- Heller myotomy should be offered to young patients as early as possible for best results.

ESOPHAGEAL WEBS

Introduction

- Esophageal webs can be associated with iron deficiency anemia. This is called *Plummer–Vinson syndrome*
- When additional features like angular cheilitis and glossitis are found, it is referred to as *Brown Paterson Kelly syndrome*
- A complex described by Paterson and Kelly in 1919, and Plummer and Vinson's name got associated later
- Esophageal webs are associated with squamous cell carcinoma of the hypopharynx and upper esophagus, though the exact link is not defined.

Diagnosis

Symptoms

Intermittent dysphagia for solids is the hallmark.

Signs

Atrophic oral mucosa, spoon-shaped fingers with brittle nails, and a longstanding anemia (iron deficiency).

Investigations

Blood Test

- *Hematocrit and peripheral smear* for anemia.

Radiology

- *Barium swallow* **(Fig. 10.5A)** demonstrates a fibrous web obstructing the lumen in an eccentric fashion just below the cricopharyngeus muscle
- *Videofluoroscopy with lateral views* is the best method to visualize the web.

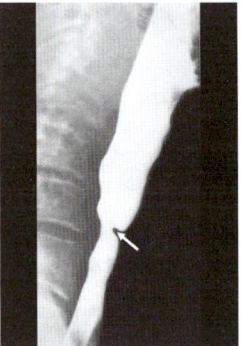

Fig. 10.5A: Barium swallow—Esophageal web

Endoscopy

- *Esophagoscopy* **(Fig. 10.5B)** is diagnostic.

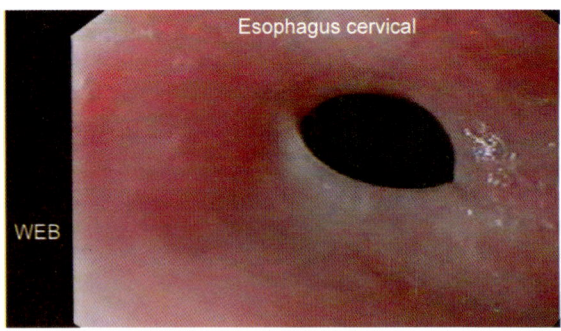

Fig. 10.5B: Esophagoscopy—Esophageal web

Complications

- Food impaction.

Management

- *Correction of anemia*
- *Dilatation of esophagus* (dilators or balloons).

Clinical Pearls

Dysphagia manifests only when the inner diameter is less than 13 mm.

SCHATZKI'S RING

Introduction

There are two types of esophageal rings. They are named as A and B.
- *The A ring* occurs about 2 cm proximal to the GE junction, is muscular in origin and asymptomatic
- *The B ring* also known as *Schatzki's ring*, is mucosal and occurs at the squamocolumnar junction.

The precise cause of esophageal rings is not known. It is suggested that it may be associated with esophageal dysmotility, and the B rings are thought to be reflux related or congenital in nature.

Diagnosis

Symptoms and Signs

- Majority remain asymptomatic

- Dysphagia (intermittent dyspagia to solids induced by hurrying or anxiety) is a common symptom when the diameter is less than 13 mm
- Foreign body impaction is common.

Investigations

Radiology

- *Barium swallow* can demonstrate the ring.

Endoscopy

- *Esophagoscopy* **(Fig. 10.6)** is diagnostic.

Management

- *Endoscopic dilatations* are useful, though repeated dilatations may be required.

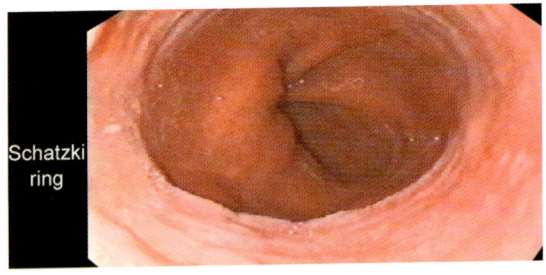

Fig. 10.6: Esophagoscopy—Schatzki's ring

DIVERTICULA OF THE ESOPHAGUS

Introduction

The esophageal diverticula are of acquired variety and are protrusions of epithelial lined mucosal pouches. They are of three varieties:
1. *Pharyngoesophageal pouch (Pharyngeal pouch/Zenker's [hypopharyngeal] diverticulum)*—located in the midline, protruding between the oblique fibers of inferior pharyngeal constrictor and the transverse fibers of cricopharyngeus in the proximal esophagus (Killian's dehiscence).
2. *Parabronchial pouch*—occurs at the mid-esophageal level due to traction by the lymph nodes of tuberculosis or histoplasmosis of subcarinal region
3. *Epiphrenic diverticulum*—a pulsion diverticulum usually occurs in the distal esophagus–typically within 10 cm of the cardia. Hernial sac consists of mucosa and submucosa covered by thin bands of attenuated esophageal musculature.

Diagnosis

Symptoms and Signs

- *Pharyngeal pouch:* Sensation of high cervical obstruction is the most common symptom. Regurgitation of recently consumed food with offensive odor is a characteristic symptom. A mass may be felt in the neck.
- *Parabronchial pouch*: Usually asymptomatic, unless complicated. They rarely cause dysphagia.
- *Epiphrenic diverticulum*: Many are asymptomatic, but dysphagia, regurgitation and retrosternal pain are the com-mon symptoms.

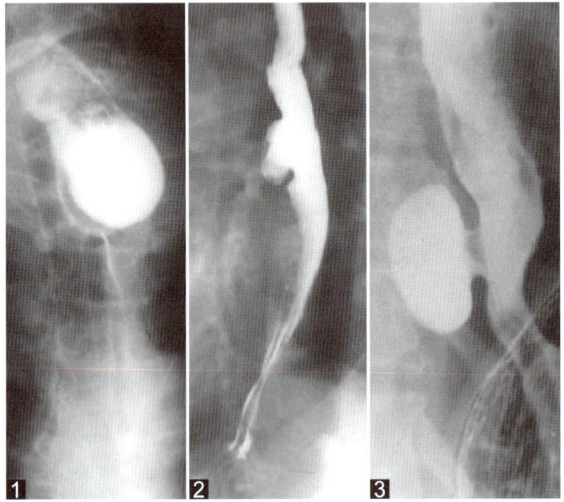

Fig. 10.7A: Barium swallow—esophageal diverticula. (1) Zenker's diverticulum; (2) Parabronchial pouch; (3) Epiphrenic diverticulum

Investigations

Radiology
- ***Barium swallow* (Fig. 10.7A)** is diagnostic.

Endoscopy
- ***Esophagoscopy* (Fig. 10.7B)** is confirmatory.

Pressure Studies
- ***Esophageal manometry*** is diagnostic.

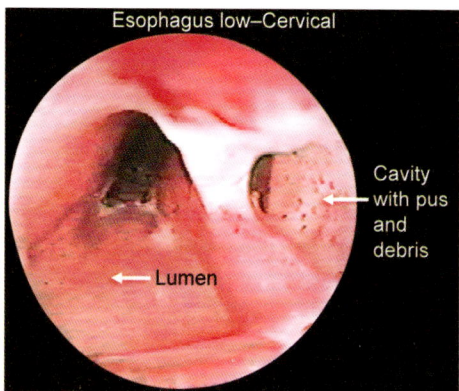

Fig. 10.7B: Endoscopy—Esophageal diverticulum. Pus and debris oozing from opening

Management

- *Pharyngeal pouch*
  - *Cricopharyngeal myotomy* is effective for small diverticula
  - *Excision* is for large diverticula (Open or endoscopic)
- *Parabronchial pouch*: Large diverticula need excision
- *Epiphrenic diverticulum*: Excision is curative.

Clinical Pearls

- Severely symptomatic diverticula of any region of esophagus need excision.

HIATUS HERNIA

Introduction

This is a herniation of the stomach along the esophagus through the esophageal hiatus into the chest.

Classification

Hiatus hernia is of four types (**Fig. 10.8**) (**Table 10.1**)
- *Type I—Sliding or esophagogastric* (most common)
- *Type II—Rolling or paraesophageal*
- *Type III—Mixed*
- *Type IV—Mixed with herniation of other intra-abdominal contents.*

Diagnosis

Symptoms and Signs
- Usually asymptomatic
- Postprandial fullness of stomach, vomiting and dysphagia if the hernial sac is very big.

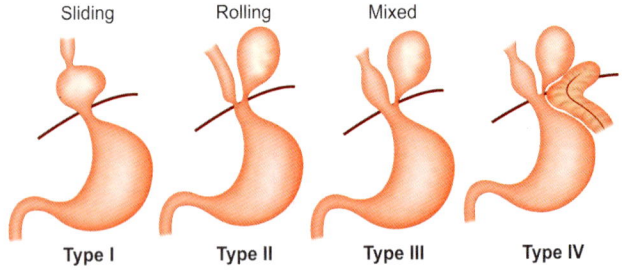

Fig. 10.8: Hiatus hernia types

Table 10.1: Hiatus hernia and their characteristics

Type of hiatus hernia	Location of GE junction	Contents of hernia	Reducibility	Rotation
Type I	Intrathoracic	Gastric fundus	Reducible	None
Type II	Intra-abdominal	Gastric fundus + body	Usually not reducible	None or organoaxial
Type III	Intrathoracic	Gastric fundus + body	Not reducible	Organoaxial or mesentericoaxial
Type IV	Intrathoracic	Gastric fundus + body + other organ	Not reducible	Organoaxial or mesentericoaxial

Investigations

- *X-ray chest* **(Fig. 10.9A)** shows retrocardiac air bubble with or without an air-fluid level on the lateral view
- *Barium contrast studies and CT* are diagnostic
- *Esophagoscopy (Fig. 10.9B)* is confirmatory.

Management

Severely symptomatic patients require surgical correction (reduction of herniated stomach, narrowing of the hiatus, re-establishment of the esophagogastric angle and an anti-reflux procedure—fundoplication) by open surgery (thoracotomy/ laparotomy) or laparoscopic surgery.

Clinical Pearls

- A paraesophageal hiatus hernia is to be suspected when retrocardiac gas shadow is seen in an incidental chest X-ray (lateral view)
- If dysphagia is present, esophageal manometry should be performed to rule out achalasia.

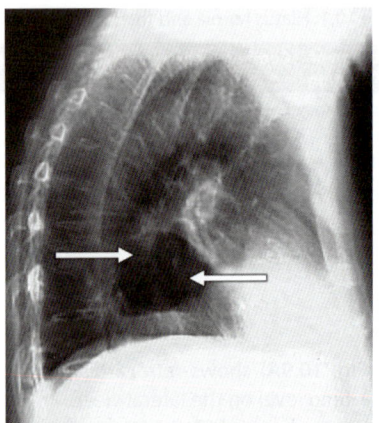

Fig. 10.9A: X-ray—Paraesophageal hernia

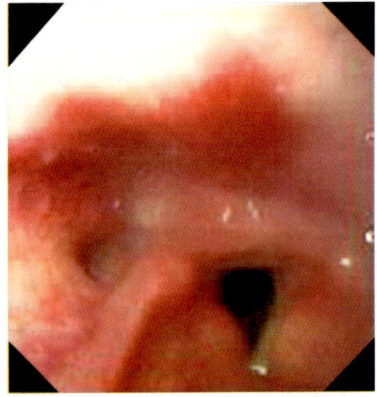

Fig. 10.9B: Esophagoscopy—Paraesophageal hernia

REFLUX ESOPHAGITIS (GASTROESOPHAGEAL REFLUX DISEASE—GERD)

Introduction

GERD is defined as a complex of symptoms with or without mucosal injury due to abnormal reflux of gastric contents into the esophagus.

Etiology and Pathogenesis

- Incompetence of the esophagogastric junction, which allows the acidic gastric contents into the lower esophagus, causes esophagitis
- The relaxation of the lower esophageal sphincter is transient and occurs commonly in normal individuals, but acid reflux occurs in patients with GERD
- GERD is closely associated with hiatus hernia. Hiatus hernia augments lower esophageal pressure and interferes with the integrity of the right crus of the diaphragm, contributing to acid reflux.

Risk Factors

- Hiatus hernia
- Delayed gastric emptying
- Scleroderma (due to impaired esophageal clearance of hypotonic esophagus)
- Emotional stress
- Tobacco smoking
- Obesity
- *H. pylori* infection.

Diagnosis

Symptoms

- *Typical symptoms:* Retrosternal burning (Heartburn) with choking sensation, usually in the immediate postprandial period, especially on lying down
- *Atypical symptoms:* Asthma, lingual or dental erosion, chest pain, cough, recurrent otitis in children, hiccups, hoarseness, episodes of sleep apnea.

Heartburn

Heartburn is a retrosternal sensation of burning and discomfort, which occurs due to regurgitation of stomach contents into the normally empty esophagus, which may reach even the pharynx if the quantity is large.

Investigations

Radiology

- *Barium meal of the stomach* (Fig. 10.10) may show reflux in Trendelenburg position, but in about quarter of patients only.

Pressure Studies

- *Acid perfusion test (Bernstein test)*: Measurement of intraesophageal pH after instilling 0.1 N HCl (300 mL) into the stomach. If the sphincter is competent, the intraesophageal pH will remain above 5 or 6

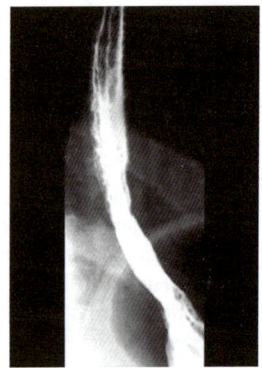

Fig. 10.10: Barium meal— Reflux esophagitis

and if there is reflux, it will fall down to 1.5 or 2, at least intermittently.
- *Esophageal manometry* is useful. Recording the pressure in the esophagus for a period of 12 hours is more informative.
- *Ambulatory esophageal pH monitoring:* A soft gel capsule called Bravo capsule is placed just above the squamo- columnar junction with the help of an endoscope and stapled. This capsule helps in intraesophageal monitoring, continuously.

Isotope Studies
- *Radioisotope scan* may demonstrate the ingested ^{99m}Tc in water, and this procedure needs no intubation.

Endoscopy
- *Esophagoscopy* is diagnostic to see the reflux (**Fig. 10.11A**), and also for Barrett's esophagus (**Fig. 10.11B**).

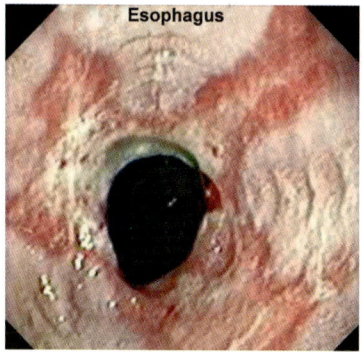

Fig. 10.11A: Esophagoscopy—Severe esophagitis

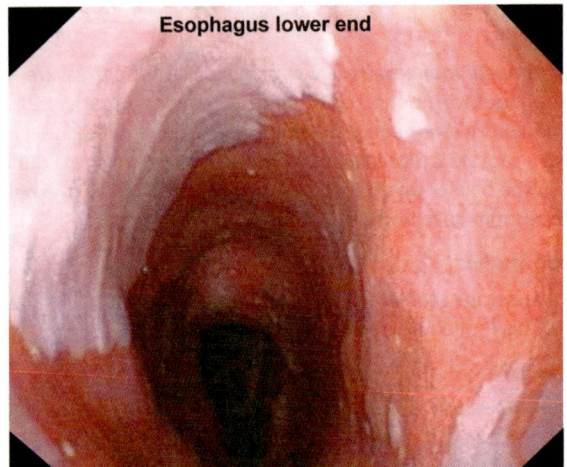

Fig. 10.11B: Esophagoscopy—Barrett's esophagus

Tissue Diagnosis
- *Histopathology* confirms esophagitis and intestinal metaplasia.

Endoscopic Grading System for GERD

- **Grade 0:** Macroscopically normal esophagus, histologic evidence of GERD
- **Grade 1:** One or more non-confluent lesions with erythema or exudates above the GE junction
- **Grade 2:** Confluent, non-circumferential, erosive and exudative lesions
- **Grade 3:** Circumferential erosive and exudative lesions
- **Grade 4:** Chronic mucosal lesions (ulceration, stricture or Barrett's esophagus).

Savary-Miller Classification (Fig. 10.11C)

- **Grade 1:** Single erosion above gastroesophageal mucosal junction
- **Grade 2:** Multiple non-circumferential erosions above gastroesophageal mucosal junction
- **Grade 3:** Circumferential erosion above mucosal junction
- **Grade 4:** Chronic change with esophageal ulcerations and associated stricture
- **Grade 5:** Barrett's esophagus with histologically confirmed intestinal differentiation within columnar epithelium.

Los Angeles Classification of GERD (Fig. 10.11D)

- *Grade 1:* One or more mucosal breaks confined to the mucosal folds, each no longer than 5 mm.
- *Grade 2:* At least one mucosal break more than 5 mm long confined to the mucosal folds and not continuous between the tops of two folds.
- *Grade 3:* At least one mucosal break continuous between the tops of two or more mucosal folds but not circumferential.
- *Grade 4:* One or more circumferential mucosal breaks.

Complications

Although this esophagitis is superficial, it may result in:
- Stricture
- Metaplastic changes (Barrett's esophagus), which is a precursor of adenocarcinoma at that region.

Management

- *Medical*
  - *Position (head elevation)* in the postprandial period for gravitational effect on the gastric contents is effective

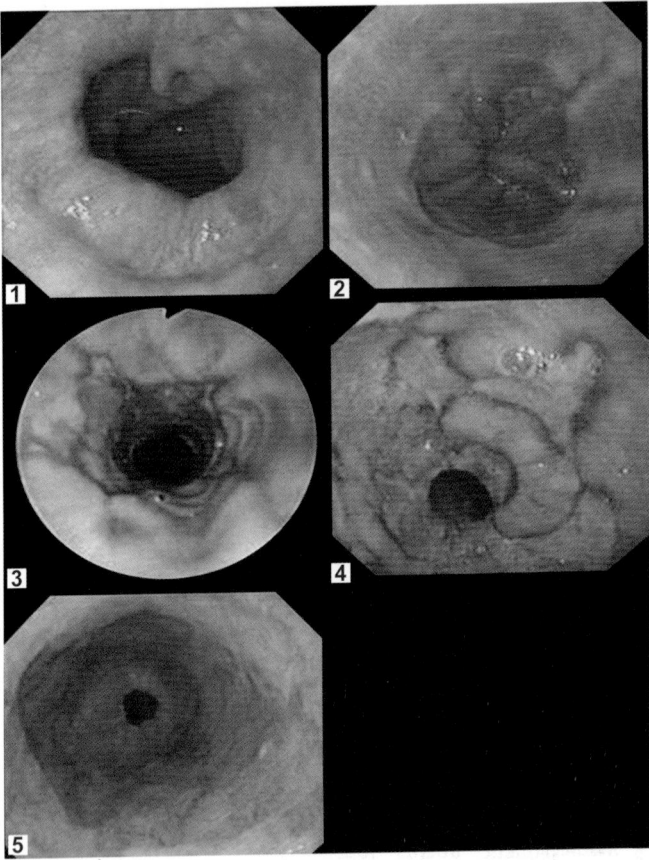

Fig. 10.11C: Savary–Miller classification

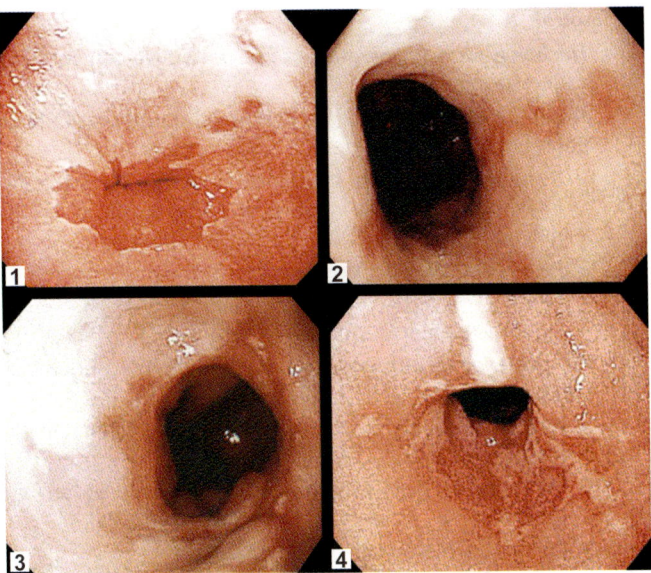

Fig. 10.11D: Los Angeles classification

- *Weight reduction in the obese*
- *Abstinence from smoking*
- *Small quantity meals and not to eat in the 2 hours preceding to going to bed*
- *H_2 blockers, proton-pump inhibitors* to reduce the acid contents and its effect on the esophagus
- *Liquid antacids after every meal and at bedtime*
- *Prokinetic agents (bethanechol, metoclopramide, levosulpiride)* before meals and at bedtime helps due to accelerated gastric emptying.

- *Surgical*
  - ***The Belsey Mark IV operation*** can be performed only through a thoracotomy.
  - ***Nissen fundoplication*** can be performed transthoracically or transabdominally
    - Restores or recovers the function of the mechanically incompetent LES and narrows or calibrates the distal GE junction
    - Increases resting LES pressure, decreasing the frequency of reflux
    - Optimizes sphincteric competence
  - ***Hill posterior gastropexy*** is done through the abdominal approach
    - Fixes the abdominal esophagus below the diaphragmatic hiatus
    - Maintains the distal esophagus subject to intra abdominal pressure
    - Prevents paraesophageal hiatus hernia.

Clinical Pearls

- Abrupt filling of the oral cavity with large gastric secretions due to GERD is called **'Water brash'**
- Though heartburn is the commonest presentation of GERD, not everyone with heartburn has GERD
- Esophageal function testing is not to be done in all patients of GERD but reserved only to those who fail to respond to medical management.

Surgical Therapy for GERD

Principles of Surgical Therapy

Though the surgical approaches have similar principles, for it to be successful, it should restore the normal or somewhat exaggerated length of intra-abdominal esophagus. This follows the Laplace's law of wall tension of tubes. The intra-abdominal narrow diameter esophagus entering the large diameter gastric pouch within a common pressure chamber, and this causes the smaller tube to remain closed and requires greater force to distend the lumen than is the case for the larger diameter stomach.

Advantages of Surgical Therapy over Medical Therapy

- Effectively corrects the defective valve mechanism
- Prevents transient loss of the sphincter and gastric distension
- Stops symptoms of heartburn and regurgitation
- Heals esophagitis, prevents progression of the disease.

Preoperative Assessment **(Table 10.2)**

Indications of Antireflux Surgery

- Patients requiring long-term medical therapy
- Recurrence of symptoms after discontinuation of therapy
- Requiring increasing doses of PPIs and not getting relieved over approximately 6 months of rigorous treatment
- Patients with high risk of complications of GERD (ulcerative esophagitis, stricture and bleeding)
- As an adjunct to upper abdominal surgical procedures
- Children with documented GERD causing esophagitis, recurrent pneumonia and failure to thrive
- Children with grade III esophagitis.

Table 10.2: Preoperative assessment for antireflux surgery

Parameter to be assessed	Relevant investigations
Establish that GERD is the cause of the symptoms	Ambulatory 24-hour esophageal pH testing
Determine the risk of progression of disease	• Ambulatory 24-hour esophageal pH testing for exposure to duodenal contents (Bilitec monitoring) • Esophageal motility studies
Determine the presence or absence of esophageal shortening and Barrett's esophagus	• Video contrast studies of esophagus • Endoscopy • Large hiatal hernia is usually associated with shortening
Evaluate esophageal body function and gastric emptying capacity	When peristalsis is absent or severely distorted or the amplitude of contraction in the lower half of the esophagus is globally less than 20 mm Hg, partial fundoplication is necessary

Contraindications

- Association of scleroderma (as results are poor due to progression of disease)
- Association of severe motility disorder (as they progress to stricture and aspiration pneumonia)
- Long or short segments of Barrett's esophagus (as they may progress to malignancy, and esophageal resection is acceptable).

Approaches

- Transthoracic
- Transabdominal (open or laparoscopic).

There are a variety of operations of gastric wrap (**Table 10.3**) are practised, and the choice of operation is often decided more by the experience and credentials of the surgeon rather than by the needs of the patient, but there are definite indications for choice of operation.

Table 10.3: Surgical procedures for correcting GERD

Procedure	Type of wrap
Total fundoplication	Nissen (360°)
	Rossetti-Hill modification (division of short gastric vessels)
Partial fundoplication	Belsey Mark IV (270° anterior— transthoracic)
	Dor (180°–200° anterior)
	Toupet (270° posterior)
	Thal (90° anterior)
	Watson (120° anterolateral)
Esophago-gastropexy	Hill repair (90° lesser curve plication)

- *Belsey Mark IV operation* can be performed only through a thoracotomy
- *Nissen fundoplication* can be performed transthoracically or transabdominally
- *Hill posterior gastropexy* is done through the abdominal approach.

Indications of Thoracic Approach

- Repeat operation
- Short esophagus
- Thoracotomy for another reason
- Obese patient.

Which Transthoracic Procedure

The procedure is decided on the presence of esophageal length.
- Nissen fundoplication—esophageal body function and length are normal
- Belsey Mark IV—esophageal body function is severely diminished
- Collis gastroplasty with partial fundoplication—esophageal length is shortened.

TRANSTHORACIC BELSEY MARK IV OPERATION

Procedure

Anesthesia

Double lumen endobronchial anesthesia.

Incision

Left posterolateral thoracotomy in sixth intercostal space (causes less pain due to less rib motion, and helps in mobilization of esophagus especially up to the aortic arch).

Surgical Procedure (**Fig. 10.12A**)

- Pulmonary ligament is divided
- Esophagus is mobilized from the diaphragm to aortic arch
- Vagi to be preserved
- Left superior and inferior bronchial arteries (branches of proximal descending aorta) are to be divided
- Cardia is separated from the diaphragmatic hiatus by blunt finger dissection (using thumb, index and middle fingers and using the other hand to retract the esophagus and protect the vagal trunks)
- The phrenoesophageal membrane is incised circumferentially, an ascending branch of inferior phrenic artery is encountered close to the left vagus, which is divided between ligatures
- Medially the hepatic branch of vagus is encountered, which is preserved
- Just posterior to the above, ascending communicating branch of left gastric artery (Belsey's artery) is encountered and it is divided between ligatures

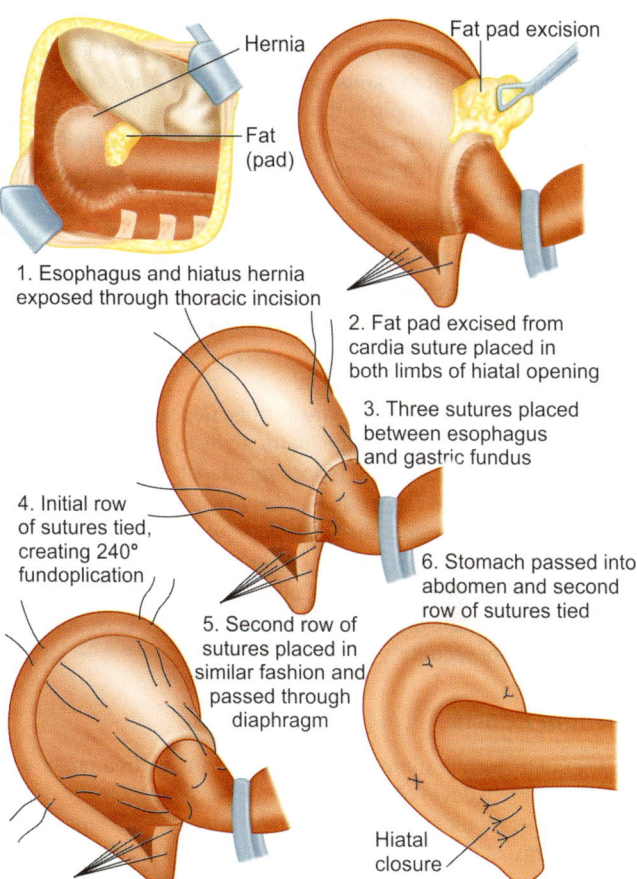

Fig. 10.12A: Belsey Mark IV operation

- Short gastric vessels are divided between ligatures
- The fundus and body of stomach are drawn up into the chest
- Vascular fat pad at the anterolateral surface of the cardia should be excised (this will help in the synechiae formation at this area)
- The right and the left crurae of the diaphragm are identified and approximated with figure of 8 sutures, and knots are not tied at this juncture
- **Plication**
    - Fundus is plicated around the anterior two-thirds of lower 4 cm of esophagus in two rows
    - First row—at 1.5 cm above the cardia to obtain good tissue opposition
    - Second row—at 2 cm above the first row
    - The second row sutures are further tied at the esophageal hiatus passing through the hiatus, to fix to the hiatus (sutures are placed at 4, 8 and 12 o'clock positions)
- The reconstructed fundus is massaged into the abdomen, and once in the abdomen it should lie without tension
- The integrity is tested by gently pulling into the chest (if it props into the chest, this will require Collis gastroplasty)
- Once satisfied, the untied crural sutures are tied by double knot technique for security.

Clinical Pearls

- Adequate mobilization is necessary for tension free repair and prevent breakdown of repair and return of symptoms
- The hiatus should be retracted well to protect the intraabdominal structures.

TRANSTHORACIC NISSEN FUNDOPLICATION

Principles

The 360° full fundoplication should be at least 60 F in diameter, only 1.5–2 cm long and held in permanent reinforced sutures **(Fig. 10.12B)**.

Surgical Procedures

- Steps are the same as in Belsy Mark IV procedure, up to adequate mobilization of esophagus
- When completely mobilized, the gastric fundus is kept in its left lateral relationship, and plicated around the distal esophagus
- The anterior and posterior fundic walls are pulled together using Babcock clamps
- A 60 F bougie is passed by the anesthesiologist into the esophagus

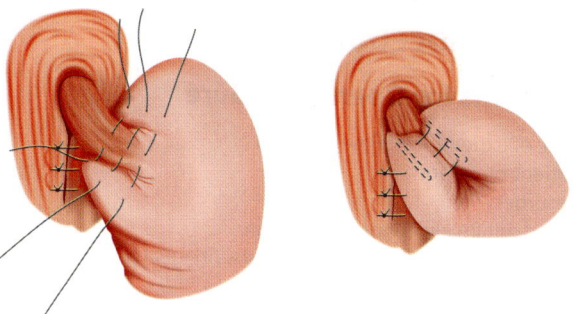

Fig. 10.12B: Nissen fundoplication

- The lips of the fundoplication are held with a U stitch using double arm polypropylene stitch over a PTFE pledget, so that the esophagus gets sandwiched between the lips
- The fundoplication should be placed 1 cm above the gastroesohageal junction, on the anterior-lateral wall of the esophagus
- The tightness is checked by inserting the index finger, which should enter snugly
- The completed, the fundoplication is massaged into the abdomen as in Belsy Mark IV procedure
- No sutures are required to hold the repair in the abdomen
- The fundus should not ride out of the hiatus, if it does so, Collis gastroplasty may be required (intrathoracic gastric pouch is subject to ulcerations, bleeding and perforation)
- The hiatus needs to be closed with sutures
- A nasogastric tube should comfortably pass through into the stomach.

NISSEN'S FUNDOPLICATION (OPEN PROCEDURE)

Indications for Open Procedure

- Lack of experience of the surgeon
- Patient preference
- Resurgery
- Failed minimally invasive procedure
- Association of giant mixed or paraesophageal hernia.

Position

- Supine, hips flexed (20°), extension of neck (20°).

Anesthesia

Endotracheal general.

Incision

Upper midline with sternal retraction with retractor or Rochard double blade retractors to retract the costal margins, Balfour retractor for the abdominal wound.

Surgical procedures

- Liver is retracted forward
- Stomach is retracted downwards
- Lesser omentum is opened above and below the hepatic branch of vagus to display the caudate lobe of liver and right hiatal pillar
- Both layers of phrenoesophageal ligament is divided to expose the left hiatal pillar
- Care is taken to preserve both vagus nerves
- Distal 4–6 cm esophagus is displayed well
- Posterior part of upper stomach is also separated well
- Esophagus is fully-mobilized by blunt dissection (take care of accessory left gastric artery, which runs along the hepatic branch of vagus, and left inferior phrenic artery a branch of left gastric artery)
- Upper short gastric vessels may be divided between ligatures if necessary
- The hiatal pillars are sutured behind the esophagus (around a esophagus with a 52 H bougie)
- Fundoplication is done by wrapping the anterior surface of the stomach without excessive tension on the stomach

- Nonabsorbable sutures are used for suturing, and the fundoplication should be 1–3 cm in length
- The stomach should be sutured to the margins of the hiatus to prevent intrathoracic herniation (intrathoracic gastric pouch is subject to ulcerations, bleeding and perforation).

Postoperative Care

- NG tube is not necessary
- Barium swallow is performed on the 2nd postoperative day, to establish free flow of barium
- Diet
- Vitaminized food for 3 weeks
- Normal diet 3–8 weeks
- For 3 months, food should be chewed well and fizzy drinks should be avoided.

Complications

- Injury to spleen (usually caused by retractors, which may be prevented by keeping a moist pad between the spleen and retractor blades)
- Injury to vagi (usually ignored as the side effects are few and take a long-time, but some prefer to do pyloroplasty)
- Esophageal perforation
- Difficult belching (gas bloat syndrome)
- Dysphagia (full fundus mobilization and division of short gastric vessels reduce the incidence of dysphagia)
- Wrap slippage—revision surgery (in spite of anatomic recurrence, only a small percentage of people develop symptoms).

MODIFIED HILL REPAIR

Principles

Lucisus Hill recommended the placement of anchoring sutures through the median arcuate ligament, which is formed by the condensation of the preaortic fascia and is located on the anterior surface of the aorta just superior to celiac axis. The modification describes the anchoring of GE junction to the strong crural musculature and underlying preaortic fascia (**Fig. 10.12C**). This fixation prevents the repair to be pulled into the chest, and advantageous when dealing with short esophagus and paraesophageal hernias.

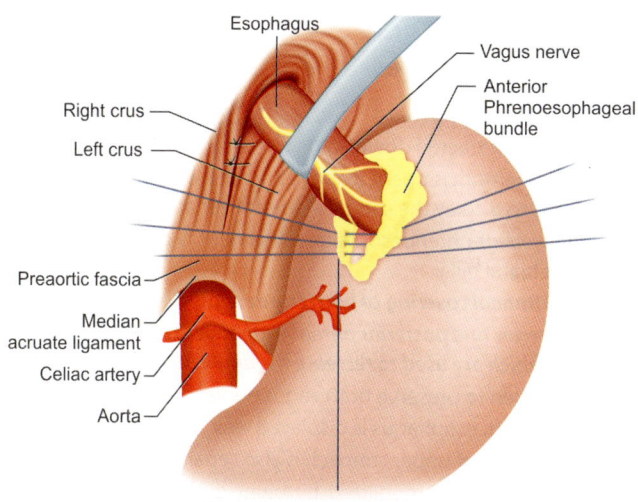

Fig. 10.12C: Modified Hill repair

Position

- Supine, hips flexed (20º), extension of neck (20º).

Anesthesia

- Endotracheal general.

Incision

- Upper midline with sternal retraction with retractor or Rochard double blade retractors to retract the costal margins, Balfour retractor for the abdominal wound.

Surgical Procedures

- Liver is retracted forward
- Stomach is retracted downwards
- Lesser omentum is opened above and below the hepatic branch of vagus to display the caudate lobe of liver and right hiatal pillar
- Both layers of phrenoesophageal ligament is divided to expose the left hiatal pillar
- *The peritoneal covering of both crurae should be preserved*
- *The anterior and posterior phrenoesophageal bundles should be intact, which are used to recreate the angle of His*
- Care is taken to preserve both vagus nerves
- Distal 4–6 cm esophagus is displayed well
- Posterior part of upper stomach is also separated well
- Esophagus is fully mobilized by blunt dissection (take care of accessory left gastric artery, which runs along the hepatic branch

of vagus, and left inferior phrenic artery a branch of left gastric artery)
- Upper short gastric vessels may be divided between ligatures if necessary
- The hiatal pillars are sutured behind the esophagus so as to close the hiatus snugly only to introduce the index finger
- *Plication*
  - Anterior phrenoesophageal bundle with gastric serosa is fixed anterior to the anterior vagus
  - Posterior phrenoesophageal bundle with gastric serosa is fixed posterior to posterior vagus
  - The first two sutures are fixed to the crural musculature, which deepens the angle of His and causes a good GE valve
  - Manometric measurements are done
  - The GE junction is now fixed posteriorly.

Postoperative Care

- NG suction is used to prevent gastric distension as this can disrupt the repair
- Barium swallow is performed on the 6th postoperative day, to establish free flow of barium
- Patient may experience transient dysphagia, which usually subsides.

What do These Procedures should Achieve?

- Appropriate length of esophagus intraabdominally
- Hold the intra-abdominal esophagus within the abdomen
- Restore the angle of His.

Postoperative Results

Though all procedures show near to equal success, a 4 cm segment of intraabdominal esophagus restoration and early postoperative standard acid reflux tests or 24-hour pH monitoring prove to be effective.

Recurrences may develop at any time following surgery, even after 10 years. However, when satisfactory antireflux repair is done, it can be expected that at least 85% of patients will have long-term relief from symptoms and complications of reflux.

COLLIS GASTROPLASTY

A gastric tube is created along the lesser curvature of stomach, in continuity with the distal esophagus (**Fig. 10.12D**) and for a length of 4–5 cm over a 48 F Maloney bougie. This tube can be constructed using a GIA stapler, and the suture line needs to be oversewn with sutures. The diameter of this tube should be the same as the diameter of the esophagus and should not flare out as it enters the stomach to avoid an inverted funnel effect, which causes reflux.

Clinical Pearls

Hill Repair
- Since it is attached posteriorly to the phrenoesophageal ligament, it might stay at the place it is required, but since the membrane itself is not a defined membrane and is present in only 50% of patients, this fixation is quite questionable
- Fixing to the phrenoesophageal ligaments and the median arcuate ligament is not really anatomical, and is as good as fixing it to the diaphragm like in the original Allison repair, which had a high recurrence rate of 80%. Moreover, this area is extremely close to the celiac axis and inadvertent injury will be a disaster.

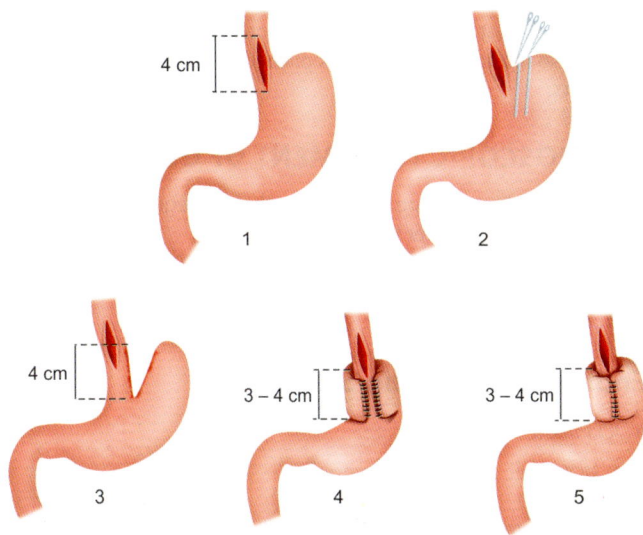

Fig. 10.12D: Collis gastroplasty

Nissen Repair

- It is held more by the bulk and the high incidence of gas bloat syndrome is disturbing. The wrap is around the serosa deficient esophagus and is held with pledgets, and holding this in place is quite questionable, and this wrap is fairly tight
- Though exact criteria are available to identify and quantify the appearance, ten valve criteria such as lip, body, anterior groove, posterior groove, lesser curvature, adherence to the scope, opening during respiration, flap, intraabdominal location, proper

repair position and the S-shaped lip, but correlating these with results are not available in the literature
- It is also felt that open Nissen's plication seems to have the best results.

ENDOSCOPIC TREATMENT OF GERD

Endoluminal therapies are divided into three categories treating the GE junction reflux barrier through:
1. Endoscopic suturing/stapling
2. Radiofrequency treatment
3. Injectable prostheses.

Endoscopic Suturing/Stapling

NDO Plicator

The NDO full thickness plicator restores the antireflux barrier with a single plication of the cardia. The plication consists of a pretied implant that secures a full thickness serosa-to-serosa apposition.

The procedure uses a specialized endoscope with a tissue retractor, which engages the gastric wall mucosa 1 cm distal to the Z line. The suture is placed over two bolsters and two titanium retention bridges keep it in place (**Fig. 10.13A**).

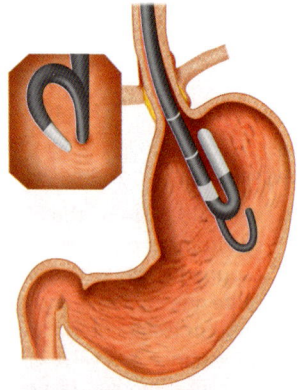

Fig. 10.13A: NDO plicator

Stretta Procedure

A method, which produces temperature, controlled radio-frequency energy to the muscle layer of the GE junction. This improved the objective and subjective parameters of GERD, by decreasing the transient lower esophageal sphincter relaxations by causing nerve ablation and collagen deposition, which thickens the GE junction.

The equipment consists of a Stretta catheter, which consists of a soft tip followed by a balloon with four needle electrodes to deliver radiofrequency energy. The treatment consists of four applications, each lasting 90 seconds, extending 1 cm above the Z-line to 0.5 cm below the Z-line. Two additional levels of application are done in the cardia, using a pull-back technique (**Fig. 10.13B**).

Contraindications for this procedure are:

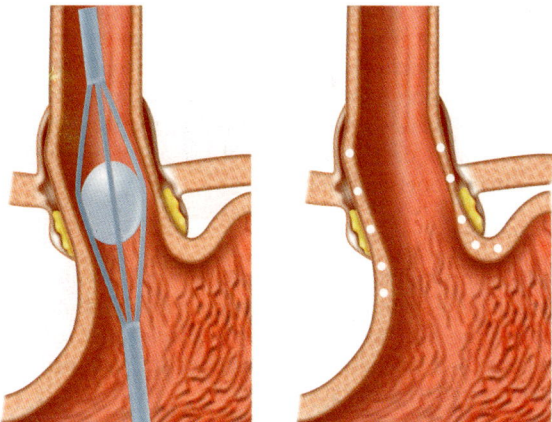

Fig. 10.13B: Stretta procedure

- Barrett's esophagus
- Subnormal lower esophageal sphincter pressures
- Significant hiatus hernia (>2 cm).

Many studies have found this procedure to be very effective at least in the first 3 years and has helped in not taking PPIs and also remaining symptom free. It appears that Stretta treatment seems to be an effective alternative to Nissen fundoplication. When cost effectiveness is considered, PPIs score over this procedure.

Gatekeeper Reflux Repair System

This uses a radiopaque hydrogel prosthesis that is delivered through an endoscope into the submucosa of the lower esophageal sphincter.

The procedure consists of passing a 16 mm tube over a wire into the esophagus. Suction is applied to catch the mucosa, and after injecting saline into the mucosa, the dry implant is placed into the submucosa **(Fig. 10.13C)**. Likewise, three hydrogels are placed. The position is checked by miniprobe endoscopic ultrasound.

Majority of patients have shown symptomatic improvement by this procedure. This was also corroborated by the study by Cicala who demonstrated decreased proximal spread of acid reflux in patients with hydrogel implantation.

EndoCinch Suturing System

Bard EndoCinch suturing system is in other words an endoscopic sewing machine, requiring two endoscopes for repeated intubations to complete the plications. A suturing capsule uses suction to capture tissue 1–2 cm below the Z-line, which is sutured and a plication is created **(Fig. 10.13D)**.

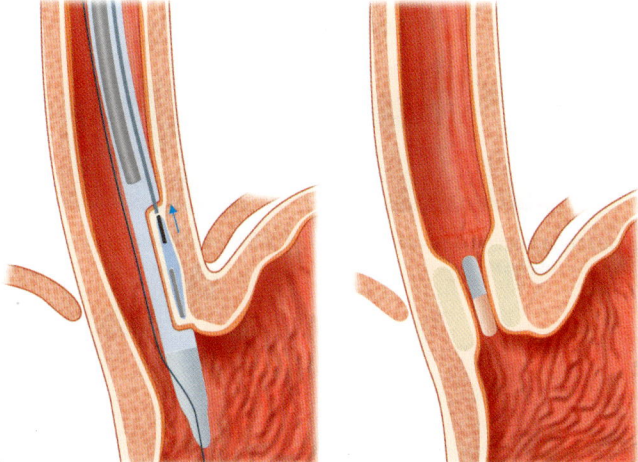

Fig. 10.13C: Gatekeeper reflux repair system

Summary

Of the many surgical procedures available for correcting the gastroesophageal reflux, only a few have gained popularity, and the procedure of choice is based on certain parameters. Endoscopic treatment for GERD is gaining popularity in recent times, but cost is a limiting factor. However, many patients seem to be on medical management for GERD in spite of the availability of surgical and endoscopic treatments.

The treatment algorithm is given in **Figure 10.13E**.

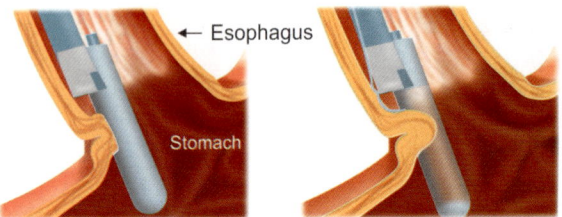

Endoscope suction a portion of the wall of the esophagus and sutures

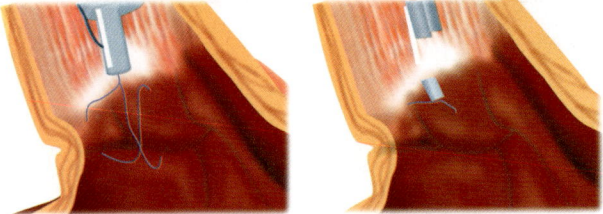

The sutures are pulled together and a fastener attached

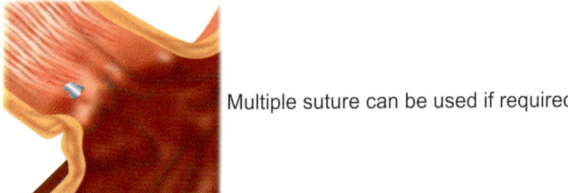

Multiple suture can be used if required

Fig. 10.13D: EndoCinch suturing system

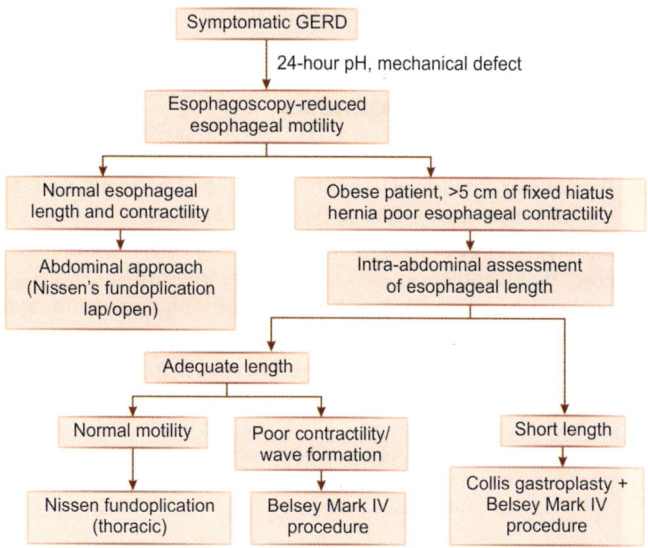

Fig. 10.13E: Treatment algorithm for GERD management

BARRETT'S ESOPHAGUS

Introduction

- It is an acquired condition in which the distal squamous epithelium of the esophagus is replaced by columnar mucosa containing intestinal metaplasia due to chronic gastro-esophageal reflux disease, and the intestinal metaplasia is recognized by the presence of goblet cells

- It is a premalignant condition with annual incidence of adenocarcinoma of 0.5–0.8%.

Etiology and Pathogenesis

There are two metaplastic events. They are:

1. *Phenotypic:* Phenotypic transformation of squamous cells to cardiac mucosa secondary to chronic acid reflux.
2. *Genotypic:* Appearance of intestinal goblet cells without the normal absorptive capacity (incomplete intestinal metaplasia), believed to be secondary to duodenoesophageal reflux and genetic predisposition.

Evolution of Barrett's esophagus to adenocarcinoma can be depicted as:

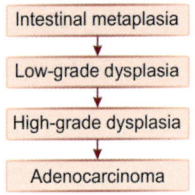

Types of Barrett's Esophagus

- **Short segment Barrett's esophagus:** Length of intestinal metaplasia <3 cm
- **Long segment Barrett's esophagus:** Length of intestinal metaplasia >3 cm.

Diagnosis

Symptoms and Signs
- Symptoms of gastroesophageal reflux.

Investigations
Endoscopy
- It is diagnosed only by endoscopy and multiple biopsies. Endoscopically, Barrett's mucosa appears salmon pink in color identical to gastric mucosa. The columnar lined mucosa extends proximally up the esophagus in irregular, finger like or tongue like projections (Refer Fig. 10.11B). Histologically, the presence of goblet cells in cardiac mucosa stained with Alcien blue pH 2.5 confirms the existence of Barrett's esophagus.

Principles of Therapy in Barrett's Esophagus
- Control acid reflux
- Heal erosive esophagitis
- Prevent adenocarcinoma.

Management

The main aim is to make the patient symptom free and to heal esophagitis.
- *Medical*: Proton pump inhibitors
- *Surgical*
  - *Cardia intestinal metaplasia:* Laparoscopic antireflux surgery
  - *Short segment BE:* Laparoscopic antireflux surgery
  - *Complicated long segment BE:* Laparoscopic surgery (*vagotomy + gastrectomy* to reduce acid production, *Roux-en-Y anastomosis* to prevent duodenal reflux and *fundoplication*

to diminish gastroesophageal reflux (**Fig. 10.14**)
  - ***High-grade dysplasia or adenocarcinoma:*** Esophagectomy.
- ***Ablative***
  - Thermal ablation using Nd:YAG laser
  - Photodynamic therapy.

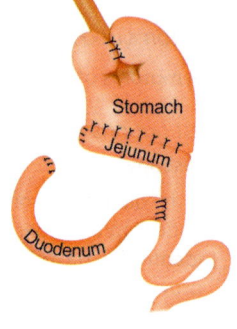

Fig. 10.14: Vagotomy + gastrectomy + R-en-Y + fundoplication

Clinical Pearls

- Adenocarcinoma is more likely to develop in long segment Barrett's esophagus
- Nissen fundoplication is an excellent operation for patients with short segment BE, with regression of intestinal metaplasia is about 50% patients, but not completely
- Medical or surgical therapy for Barrett's esophagus does not reverse the pathology completely
- **Surveillance:** Patients undergoing surveillance should have endoscopy at 2 cm intervals in four quadrants in the length of visible abnormal epithelium. The biopsy is reported as grades of dysplasia. Negative, indefinite, low grade, high grade and carcinoma.
  - ***Negative:*** 2 endoscopies at 6 monthly intervals: both negative: 3 yearly intervals endoscopy
  - ***Indefinite:*** 2 endoscopies at 6 monthly intervals: both negative: 2 yearly intervals endoscopy
  - ***Low grade:*** 2 endoscopies at 6 monthly intervals: both low grade: yearly endoscopy
  - ***High grade:*** confirm: endoscopic ablation, esophagectomy
  - ***Carcinoma:*** Radical esophagectomy.

STRICTURES OF ESOPHAGUS

Etiology

Strictures are caused by:
- Corrosives
- Surgery
- Radiotherapy
- Reflux esophagitis.

Diagnosis

Symptoms

Dysphagia, particularly to solids.

Investigations
- *Barium swallow* **(Figs 10.15A and B)** is the best investigation and is diagnostic
- *CT with oral contrast* **(Fig. 10.15C)** is useful in determining the esophageal wall thickness
- *Endoscopy* **(Figs 10.15D and 10.15E)** is confirmatory and useful in obtaining biopsy if needed.

Management
- *Endoscopic dilatation* where possible
- *Bypass procedures using stomach and colon* are reserved for impassable strictures.

Clinical Pearls

- Esophageal strictures and rings are distinguished by its thickness. Thickness >3 cm are called strictures and <3 cm are called rings.

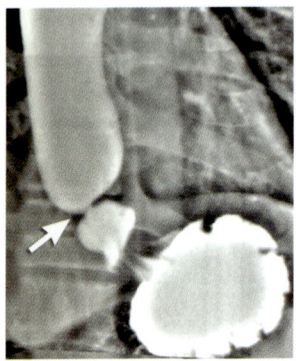

Fig. 10.15A: Barium swallow—Stricture esophagus

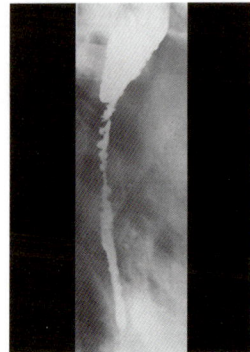

Fig. 10.15B: Barium swallow—**Corrosive strictures** esophagus

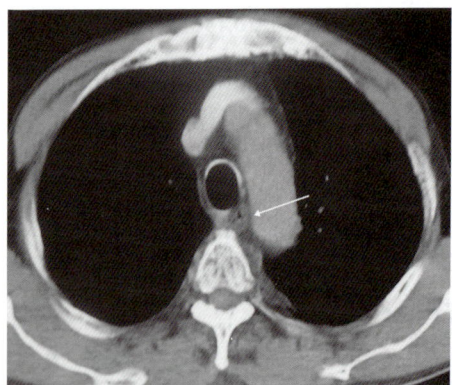

Fig. 10.15C: CT—Stricture esophagus after radiotherapy for **malignancy**

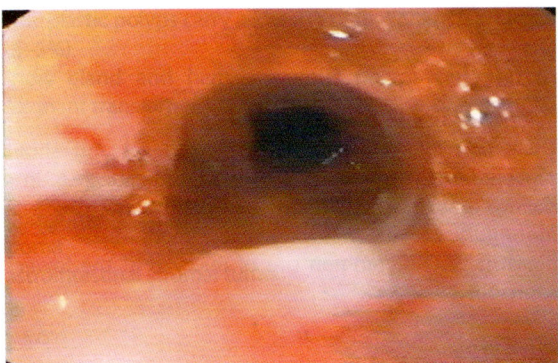

Fig. 10.15D: Esophagoscopy—Stricture of cervical esophagus

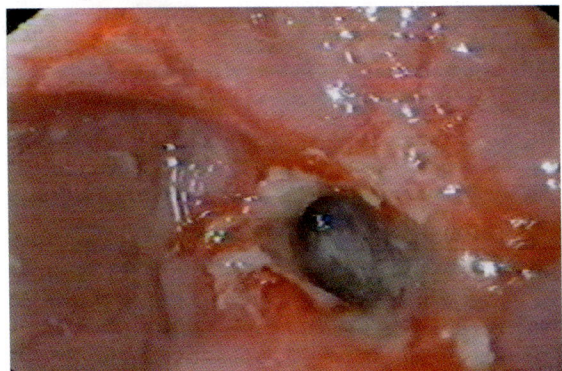

Fig. 10.15E: Esophagoscopy—Stricture of lower esophagus with ulcer

ESOPHAGEAL INJURY

Introduction

Esophageal injuries are caused by:
- ***Penetrating injury*** may occur at any level and should be suspected when the injury crosses the midline (e.g. in sword swallowers as circus act), during esophagoscopy
- ***Blunt injury:*** Usually following severe blow to the sternum or epigastrium. The common site of injury is at the lower 1/3rd esophagus.

Diagnosis

Symptoms and Signs

- Fever, dyspnea (due to mediastinitis or mediastinal emphysema) or tachypnea
- Features of surgical emphysema (spread of mediastinal emphysema to neck, face and chest wall) may supervene, with signs of hypoxia about 3–4 days later.

Investigations

- ***X-ray chest*** may reveal:
  - Pneumomediastinum
  - Air in the prevertebral space
  - Left pleural effusion
  - Hemo or pneumothorax in the absence of rib fracture
- ***Gastrograffin swallow*** may show the leak **(Fig. 10.16)**

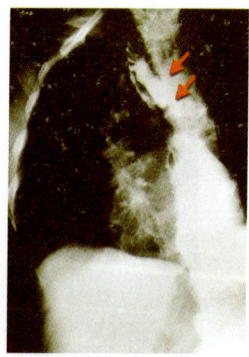

Fig. 10.16: Gastrograffin swallow—leaking dye in esophageal perforation

- ***Esophagoscopy*** may show the injury
- ***Intercostal drainage*** shows particulate food matter, and air leak during both phases of respiration.

Management

- ***Intercostal drainage*** is mandatory
- ***Early operative repair of the esophageal tear*** is necessary.

INFECTIONS OF ESOPHAGUS

Introduction

- The most common infections of esophagus are *Candida albicans*, herpes simplex virus (HSV) and cytomegalovirus (CMV)
- *Candida* and HSV infections can be seen in persons with normal immunity, but CMV infections are found in immunocompromised persons
- Infections cause severe edema of the esophageal mucosa
- It can be a presentation in AIDS
- Rarely, viruses like varicella zoster virus (VZV) and Epstein Barr virus (EBV) can infect the esophagus
- Fungi are known to cause inflammation of esophagus. *Candida albicans*, which is considered a normal flora in the oral cavity, infects the esophagus by a two-step process. The first is colonization, which involves adherence to the mucosal surface and proliferation. The second step is associated with impaired host defenses and results in invasion of mucosa. This is seen as white plaques or exudates. The above process is initiated and augmented by antibiotics and steroids, which alter the normal gut flora.

Diagnosis

Symptoms and Signs
- Dysphagia associated with pain (odynophagia)
- Heartburn, chest pain, nausea, dysgeusia and bleeding can also occur
- The fungal infection concomitantly occurs in the oral cavity, and presents with glossitis and pharyngitis with ulcers in the oral cavity.

Investigations
Fungal cultures and swabs taken through esophagoscopy (Fig. 10.17) are useful in making the diagnosis (affected areas appear as white patches).

Management

- ***Fungal infections*** require antifungal agents (fluconazole 100 mg/day/Itraconazole 200 mg/day for 15 days)

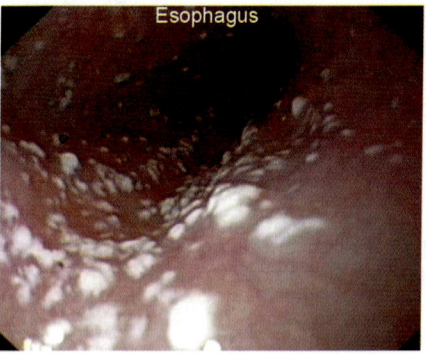

Fig. 10.17: Esophagoscopy—Candidiasis of esophagus

- **HSV esophagitis** is self-limiting and may not require any therapy. Antivirals like acyclovir (250 mg/m^2) every 8 hours till the patient is able to swallow, followed by Valacyclovir 100 mg thrice daily for a total of 10 days, are useful in severe cases
- **CMV esophagitis** is treated with ganciclovir and forcarnet.

DIFFUSE ESOPHAGEAL SPASM

Introduction

Exact etiology is not known.

Diagnosis

Symptoms and Signs

Chest pain (mimicking a cardiac pain) and dysphagia.

Investigations

- **Contrast studies** may show exaggerated esophageal contractions giving a *'corkscrew'* appearance (**Fig. 10.18**)
- **Esophageal manometry** is diagnostic.

Management

- **Drugs like nitrates and calcium channel blockers,** which reduce smooth muscle contractions are used
- **Long esophageal myotomy** in which all layers (excepting mucosa) are divided may be helpful.

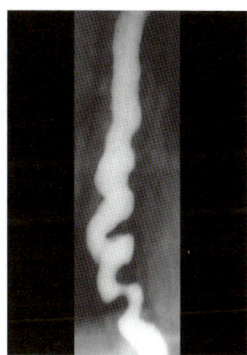

Fig. 10.18: Barium swallow—Corkscrew esophagus

FOREIGN BODIES OF ESOPHAGUS

Introduction

- Swallowing of foreign bodies like coins is common in small children, the dentures in the very elderly
- Accidental swallowing occurs in children and intentional swallowing is seen in patients with psychiatric illness and mental retardation
- Foreign bodies in the esophagus, especially large ones, get impacted at normal anatomic levels of narrowing (cricopharyngeus, arch of aorta, left mainstem bronchus, pylorus, esophagogastric junction) and pathologically narrowed areas (strictures, rings)
- Most blunt objects pass without difficulty, whereas sharp objects have a tendency to get impacted.

Diagnosis

Symptoms and Signs

- Most patients describe the sensation of obstruction in the throat, which does not correspond to its exact location
- Some patients present with dysphagia of acute form.

Investigations

Radiology

- *Plain radiographs* (Fig. 10.19) are useful in identifying radiopaque objects.

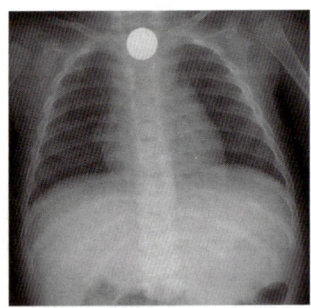

Fig. 10.19: X-ray—Foreign body esophagus

Endoscopy

- ***Esophagoscopy* (Figs 10.20A to C)** is useful in identifying the obstructing agent and removal of the same.

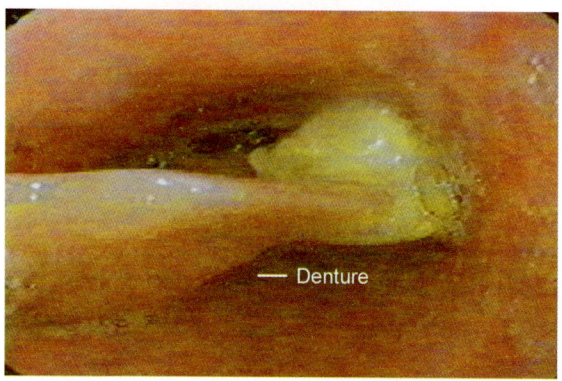

Fig. 10.20A: Esophagoscopy—Denture in thoracic esophagus

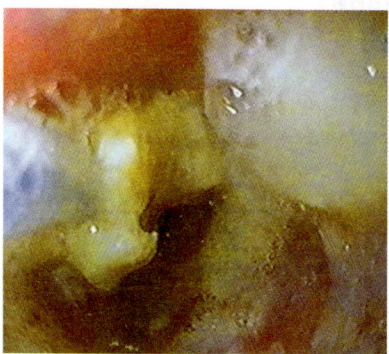

Fig. 10.20B: Esophagoscopy—Foreign body (corn)

Snapshots in Gastroenterology

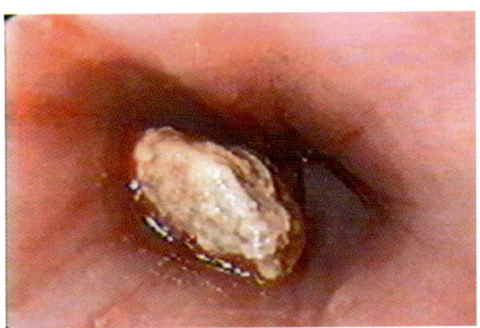

Fig. 10.20C: Esophagoscopy—Foreign body

Complications

- Obstruction
- Perforation of esophagus.

Management

- *Small objects pass without any difficulty*
- *Obstructed large foreign bodies like coins should be removed using an endoscope*
- *Sharp and pointed objects should be removed, as they may not be able to negotiate the entire GIT*
- *Long objects like pen, toothbrush etc., should be removed as they may not be able to negotiate the duodenal sweep*
- *Rarely, surgery is required to remove the foreign bodies.*

Clinical Pearls

- Oral contrast studies should be avoided for the fear of aspiration.

ESOPHAGEAL VARICES

Introduction

- Occurs usually due to portal hypertension secondary to cirrhosis of liver
- Any disease causing portal hypertension (e.g. portal vein thrombosis, idiopathic portal hypertension, non-cirrhotic portal fibrosis) can cause esophageal varices.

Diagnosis

Symptoms and Signs
- Sudden and massive upper GI bleed
- Chronic blood loss due to bleeding varices is rare
- Recurrent bleeds are common.

Investigations
- ***Barium swallow*** **(Fig. 10.21A)** is informative
- ***Esophagoscopy*** **(Fig. 10.21B)** is diagnostic
- ***Other investigations*** related to liver pathology should be performed to identify the cause of varices.

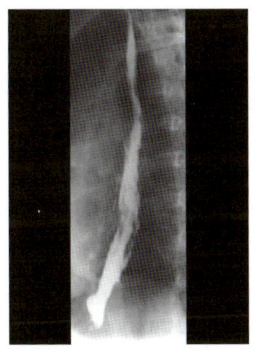

Fig. 10.21A: Barium swallow — Esophageal varices

Management

Medical

Acute bleeds require medical management with measures to stop

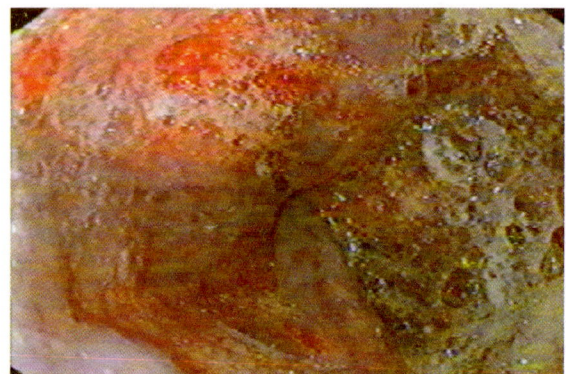

Fig. 10.21B: Esophagoscopy—Bleeding esophageal varices

the bleeding (compression with Sengstaken–Blakemore tube) and blood transfusions, in ICU.

Interventional Nonsurgical

Once the acute crisis is managed, ***esophagoscopy and sclerotherapy*** to control the bleeding.

Surgical

Surgical procedures are required to prevent recurrences.

Minimally invasive

Transjugular intrahepatic portosystemic shunt (TIPSS)— a percutaneous technique that creates a shunt within the liver between the portal and hepatic veins.

MALLORY–WEISS TEAR OF ESOPHAGUS

Introduction

- Refers to a longitudinal tear in the region of gastroesophageal junction, majority just below the junction
- The tear follows retching and related to alcohol intake.

Diagnosis

Symptoms and Signs

Retching and vomiting of normal gastric contents followed by hematemesis and or melena.

Investigations

Endoscopy

- *Esophagoscopy* (Fig. 10.22) is diagnostic.

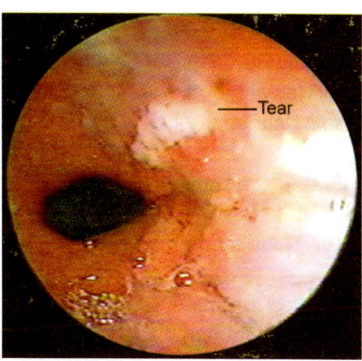

Fig. 10.22: Esophagoscopy—Bleeding from Mallory–Weiss tear

Management

- *Initial treatment is supportive and expectant*
- *Minor tears can be treated endoscopically*
- In a small minority of cases, persistent bleeding requires ***suturing of laceration through gastrotomy***

BENIGN TUMORS

Introduction

Benign tumors of esophagus are classified based on the layer of origin.

- *Mucosa*
  - ***Epithelium:*** Papilloma, adenoma
  - ***Lamina propria:*** Mucus retention cyst, fibrovascular polyp
  - ***Smooth muscle:*** Leiomyoma
- *Submucosa*
  - ***Mucous gland:*** Mucous retention cyst, adenoma
  - ***Connective tissue:*** Fibrovascular polyp
  - ***Blood vessels:*** Hemangioma
  - ***Nervous tissue:*** Neurilemmoma, granular cell tumor
- *Muscularis*
  - ***Striated muscle:*** Rhabdomyoma
  - ***Smooth muscle:*** Leiomyoma
  - ***Nervous tissue:*** Neurilemmoma, granular cell tumor
- *Adventitia*
  - ***Connective tissue:*** Fibroma
  - ***Neural tissue:*** Neurilemmoma.

Among these leiomyomas are the most common.

Diagnosis

Symptoms and Signs

- Generally asymptomatic
- Large lesions cause dysphagia.

Investigations

- **CT and EUS** are useful in differentiating from malignancy
- **Barium swallow (Fig. 10.23A) and esophagoscopy (Fig. 10.23B)** are diagnostic.

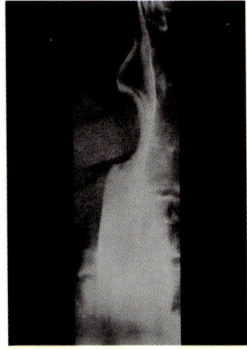

Fig. 10.23A: Barium swallow —Leiomyoma of esophagus

Management

Simple enucleation is the treatment of choice.

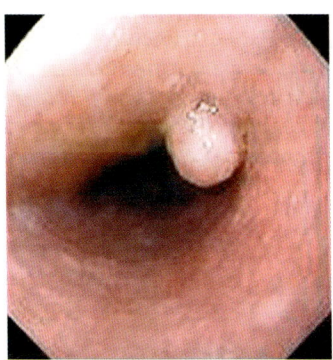

Fig. 10.23B: Esophagoscopy—Lipoma of esophagus

ESOPHAGEAL MALIGNANCY

Introduction

- Affects males more than the females
- Frequency increases with age, peaking in the sixth decade
- Common in the middle (40–50%) and lower (40–50%) third of esophagus.

Etiology

Risk Factors for Squamous Cell Carcinoma

- Smoking
- Alcohol consumption
- Dietary deficiency (low fruits and vegetables)
- Fungal infections
- Paterson Kelly (Plummer–Vinson) syndrome
- Achalasia cardia
- Esophageal diverticula
- Chronic esophagitis
- Human papilloma virus types 16 and 18.

Risk Factors for Adenocarcinoma

- Barrett's esophagus
- GERD
- Obesity.

Pathological Features

- Macroscopically, the tumor appears:
  - Nodular

- Ulcerative
- Diffusely infiltrative (results in stricture with proximal dilatation).
- Microscopically, it may be:
  - Squamous cell carcinoma (common)
  - Adenocarcinomas (in the lower end in uncorrected reflux disease, against a background of glandular metaplasia of Barrett's esophagus)
  - Stromal tumors and lymphomas (rare).

Spread of Esophageal Malignancy

- Esophageal cancer spreads by various routes:
  - ***Longitudinally and circumferentially*** within the esophagus
  - ***Submucosal spread*** leads to diffuse infiltration and also skip lesions
  - ***Direct spread*** to mediastinal structures like trachea, main bronchi, lungs, pleura, vertebrae and great vessels
  - ***Lymphatic spread***
    - Upper third tumors to deep cervical and supraclavicular nodes *(Virchow's nodes)*
    - Middle third tumors to mediastinal, paratracheal and subcarinal nodes
    - Lower third tumors to celiac nodes below the diaphragm
  - ***Hematogenous spread*** to liver, lungs, and bones, liver being the most common.

TNM Classification

It is given in Table 10.4.

Table 10.4: TNM classification of esophageal malignancy

Tumor status	
T_X	Primary tumor cannot be assessed
T_0	No evidence of primary tumor
T_{is}	Carcinoma in situ
T_1	Tumor invading lamina propria or submucosa
T_2	Tumor invading muscularis propria
T_3	Tumor invading adventitia
T_4	Tumor with invasion of adjacent structures
Lymph node status*	
N_X	Regional lymph nodes cannot be assessed
N_0	No regional node metastasis
N_1	1–2 Regional lymph node metastases
N_2	3–6 Regional lymph node metastases
N_3	7 or more regional lymph node metastases
Metastatic status	
M_0	No distant metastasis
M_1	Distant metastasis (includes ipsilateral supraclavicular lymph nodes)

Stage grouping			
Stage 0	T_{is}	N_0	M_0
Stage 1 A	T_1	N_0	M_0
Stage 1 B	T_2	N_0	M_0
Stage II A	T_3	N_0	M_0
Stage II B	T_1, T_2	N_1	M_0
Stage III A	T_{4a}	N_0	M_0
	T_3	N_1	M_0
	T_1, T_2	N_2	M_0
Stage III B	T_3	N_2	M_0
Stage III C	T_{4a}	N_1, N_2	M_0
	T_{4b}	Any N	M_0
	Any T	N_3	M_0
Stage IV	Any T	Any N	M_1

*For the cervical esophagus, cervical and supraclavicular lymph nodes are considered regional; for the thoracic esophagus, mediastinal and perigastric lymph nodes (including celiac nodes) are considered regional

Diagnosis

Symptoms

- Progressive dysphagia (for solids to start with and to liquids later)
- Retrosternal discomfort
- Weight loss
- Anemia
- Loss of appetite is a very common symptom.

Signs

- Signs of undernutrition
- Stigmata of chronic liver disease in alcoholics
- Hepatomegaly may suggest hepatic metastases
- Enlarged supraclavicular lymph nodes if there is spread *(Troisier's sign).*

Investigations

Blood Tests

- *Hematocrit to evaluate anemia*
- *Proteins to assess undernutrition.*

Radiology

- *Barium swallow (Figs 10.24A and B), CT (Fig. 10.24C) and MRI* of thorax are diagnostic. They may show it as an exophytic mass, nodularity or stricture
- *X-ray chest* to assess aspiration pneumonitis, and intrathoracic metastases
- *CT and MRI scans of upper abdomen and PET scan* for assessment of hepatic and distant metastases.

Snapshots in Gastroenterology

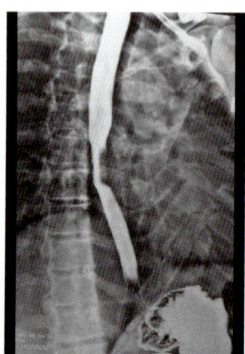

Fig. 10.24A: Barium swallow—Esophageal malignancy mid-third

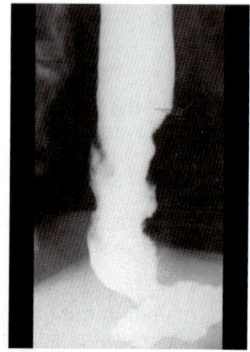

Fig. 10.24B: Barium swallow—Esophageal malignancy lower third

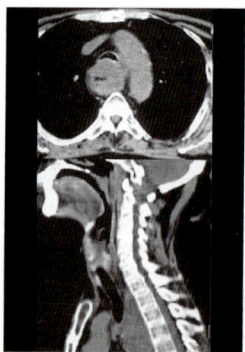

Fig. 10.24C: CT—Esophageal malignancy upper-third

Endoscopy

- ***Esophagoscopy (Figs 10.25A and B) with biopsy*** is confirmatory
- ***Bronchoscopy*** to exclude invasion of posterior tracheal wall and left main bronchus.

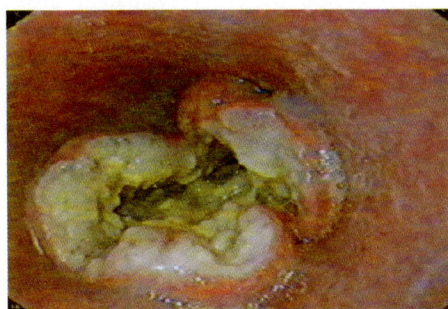

Fig. 10.25A: Esophagoscopy—Malignant growth (Thoracic esophagus)

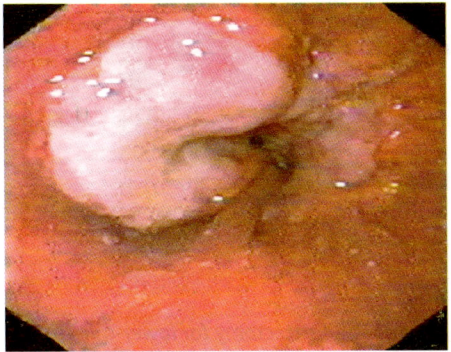

Fig. 10.25B: Esophagoscopy—Malignant growth (OG junction)

Ultrasonography

- *Endoscopic ultrasound* is useful in regional staging, which shows esophageal cancer as a hypoechoic interruption of layers of the esophagus, and delineates the depth of tumor involvement better than CT. Also useful in evaluating the mediastinal lymph nodes (Large nodes that are uniformly hypoechoic are suspicious). This procedure can be used for obtaining biopsy of lymph nodes also.

Laparoscopy

- *Diagnostic laparoscopy* is the standard in advanced adenocarcinoma of distal esophagus before embarking on therapy.

Complications

- Esophageal obstruction
- Tracheoesophageal fistula
- Malnutrition

Management

- *Limited disease*
- T_{is}, $T_1/N_0/M_0$: Endoscopic mucosal resection (ablative therapies like radiofrequency ablation are used by some
- T_1, $T_2/N_0/M_0$: Surgery (esophagectomy) alone
- *Extensive disease:* Surgery and chemoradiation (neoadjuvant therapy is used in some cases).

Curative Surgery

- *Surgery (esophagogastrectomy for lower-third tumors) and Ivor Lewis two stage esophagectomy for middle-third tumors)/or radiotherapy* is the treatment of choice

Palliative Procedures

- **Combined chemoradiation (CRT)** is used for inoperable tumors
- **Chemotherapy as a curative treatment is not advised excepting for synchronous CRT**
- **Dilatation and stenting** are for inoperable malignancies
- **Laser application** is useful for restoration of passage, in very advanced cases *(Laser rebore)*
- **Feeding gastrostomy** is done as palliation for impassable strictures or for nutritional supplementation during radiotherapy.

ESOPHAGEAL RESECTIONS

Resections of Esophagus (Fig. 10.26)

- Transhiatal esophagectomy
- Three hole esophagectomy
- Right posterolateral esophagectomy
- Left thoracotomy approach.

Reconstructions after Resections (Fig. 10.27)

- Cervical gastroesophagostomy (Stapled or handsewn)
- Ivor Lewis approach (esophagogastrostomy in the apex of right chest)
- Colonic interposition.

Indications

- Benign strictures of esophagus
- Malignancy of esophagus.

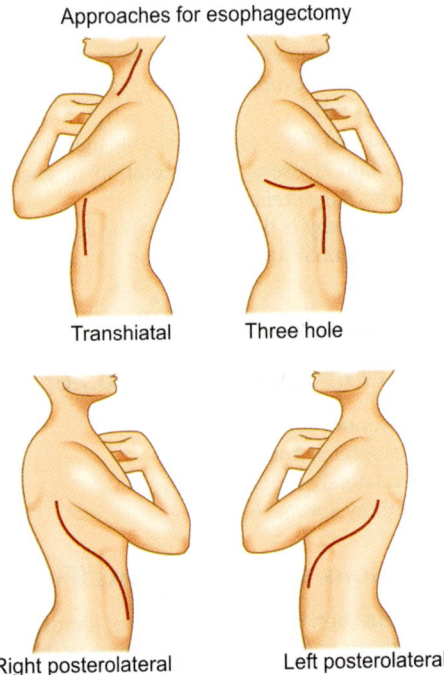

Fig. 10.26: Esophageal resections

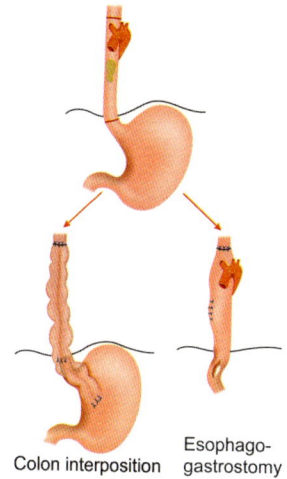

Fig. 10.27: Reconstructions

Colon interposition   Esophago-gastrostomy

TRANSHIATAL ESOPHAGECTOMY

Surgical Technique (Fig. 10.28)

This consists of three phases:
- *Abdominal dissection*
  - Upper midline abdominal incision
  - Mobilization of stomach based on the right gastroepiploic and right gastric arteries
  - Enlargement of esophageal hiatus
  - With downward traction on the esophagus, it is mobilized by finger dissection
  - Kocher's maneuver and pyloroplasty are necessary.

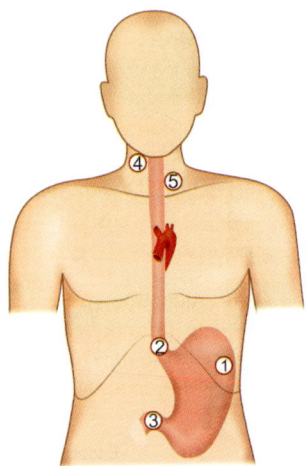

Fig. 10.28: Surgical technique

- *Cervical dissection*
    - Left cervical incision along the anteromedial border of sternomastoid
    - Reflection of thyroid medially, sternomastoid and carotid sheath laterally
    - Blunt dissection using finger to separate the esophagus from the prevertebral fascia, with upward traction.

The fingers from top and bottom should meet and completeness of mobilization assessed

Transection of Esophagus

- Transection of cervical esophagus with staples
- Gastroesophageal transection done with gastric tube formation with staples

- *Reconstruction*
  - Stomach is passed through esophageal bed
  - Esophagogastric anastomosis done in the neck.

POSTESOPHAGECTOMY COMPLICATIONS

- *Anastomotic leak*—occurs around the 2nd postoperative day, manifests with fever, chest pain and dyspnea, X-ray may show pleural effusion. Contrast study may show the leak (Refer Fig. 10.16). Minor leaks may require chest drainage with delayed oral intake, while major leaks require resurgery with feeding jejunostomy
- *Dysphagia*—in the early postoperative period may be due to edema (**Fig. 10.29**), which usually subsides spontaneously. Persistent dysphagia may be due to anastomotic stricture or a recurrent malignancy. Both require operative management or dilatations. Stents can be applied for impassable strictures

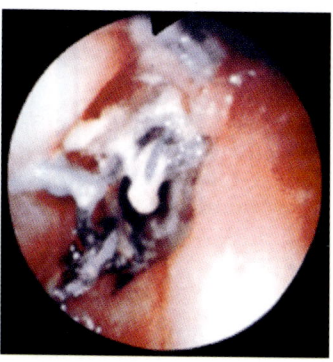

Fig. 10.29: Edema and inflammation of esophagojejunal anastomosis

- *Hoarseness of voice*—may be transient due to traction on the recurrent laryngeal nerves, which recovers in due course of time.

Clinical Pearls

- Operation with cervical anastomosis is preferred to thoracic anastomosis, as it carries much less mortality comparatively.

Chapter 11

Stomach and Duodenum

SURGICAL ANATOMY

Stomach is the most proximal abdominal portion of the gastrointestinal tract. This is a very distensible organ and continues from the esophagus. The junction has a lower esophageal sphincter, which does not allow the gastric contents to regurgitate into the esophagus. The angle at which the left border of the stomach meets the esophagus is called the angle of His.

Stomach is divided into fundus (part of the stomach above the GE junction), body (part of the stomach below the GE junction extending up to the incisura angularis), antrum (part below the incisura angularis) up to the first part of the duodenum.

The organs, which are closely related to the stomach are:
- Liver
- Transverse colon
- Spleen
- Pancreas

The lesser curvature is attached to the liver by hepatogastric ligament (lesser omentum).

The greater curvature is attached to the transverse colon by gastrocolic omentum.

Arterial supply to the stomach comes from the celiac axis via its four major arteries:
- Left gastric artery (arises directly from the celiac axis) and right gastric artery (branch of hepatic artery) form an arcade along the lesser curvature

- Left gastroepiploic artery (branch of splenic artery) and right gastroepiploic artery (branch of gastroduodenal artery) form an arcade along the greater curvature
- From the above two arcades, branches arise to supply the stomach along the curvatures
- Short gastric arteries (branches of splenic artery) supply the fundus of the stomach.

Venous drainage follows the arterial supply.

Lymphatic drainage of the stomach is parallel to the blood vessels, and they are grouped and named by various classifications.

Classification of lymph nodes relevant to gastric malignancy based on Japanese Research Society for Gastric Cancer (JRSGC).

It is shown in **Box 11.1**.

Box 11.1: Regional lymph nodes of stomach	
No. 1	Right paracardial LN
No. 2	Left paracardial LN
No. 3a	LN along the left gastric vessels
No. 3b	LN along the right gastric vessels
No. 4sa	LN along the short gastric vessels
No. 4sb	LN along the left gastroepiploic vessels
No. 4d	LN along the right gastroepiploic vessels
No. 5	Supra pyloric LN
No. 6	Infra pyloric LN
No. 7	LN along the left gastric artery
No. 8a	LN along the common hepatic artery (anterosuperior group)
No. 8b	LN along the common hepatic artery (posterior group)
No. 9	LN along the celiac artery

Contd....

Contd....

No. 10	LN at the splenic hilum
No. 11p	LN along the proximal splenic artery
No. 11d	LN along the distal splenic artery
No. 12a	LN in the hepatoduodenal ligament (along the hepatic artery)
No. 12b	LN in the hepatoduodenal ligament (along the bile duct)
No. 12p	LN in the hepatoduodenal ligament (behind the portal vein)
No. 13	LN on the posterior surface of the pancreatic head
No. 14v	LN along the superior mesenteric vein
No. 14a	LN along the superior mesenteric artery
No. 15	LN along the middle colic vessels
No.16a1	LN in the aortic hiatus
No.16a2	LN around the abdominal aorta (from the upper margin of the celiac trunk to the lower margin of the left renal vein)
No.16b1	LN around the abdominal aorta (from the lower margin of the left renal vein to the upper margin of the inferior mesenteric artery)
No.16b2	LN around the abdominal aorta (from the upper margin of the inferior mesenteric artery to the aortic bifurcation)
No. 17	LN on the anterior surface of the pancreas head
No. 18	LN along the inferior margin of the pancreas
No. 19	Infradiaphragmatic LN
No. 20	LN in the esophageal hiatus of the diaphragm

According to this classification, lymph nodes surrounding stomach are divided into 20 stations and these are classified into three groups depending upon the location of the primary tumor. This grouping system is based on the results of studies of lymphatic flow at various tumor sites, together with the observed survival associated with metastasis to each nodal station.

This has three groups of lymph nodes called stations.
- Group 1—station 1 to 6 **(Fig. 11.1A)**
- Group 2—station 7 to 12 **(Fig. 11.1B)**
- Group 3—station 13 to 20 **(Fig. 11.1B)**.

Nerve supply comes from the extrinsic and intrinsic nerve plexuses. The extrinsic innervation comes from the parasympathetic system through vagus nerves, and acetylcholine is the most important neurotransmitter. In the abdomen, the vagus nerves (anterior and posterior) give off the hepatic branch and continue as the nerves of Latarjet along the lesser curve. Posterior vagus gives off the nerve to the fundus called the criminal nerve of Grassi. Nerves of Latarjet give of the anterior and posterior branches to the stomach and ends near the incisura angularis as the "crow's foot". The extrinsic sympathetic nerve supply comes from spinal levels T5 through T10 and travels in the splanchnic nerves to the celiac ganglion. Post-ganglionic nerves travel along the blood vessels to the stomach. The sympathetic neurotransmitter is epinephrine.

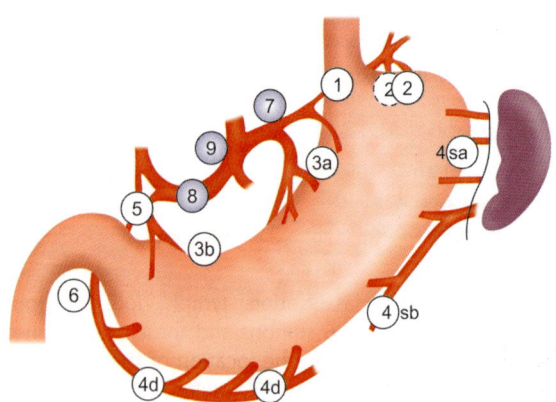

Fig. 11.1A: Lymph nodes of stomach

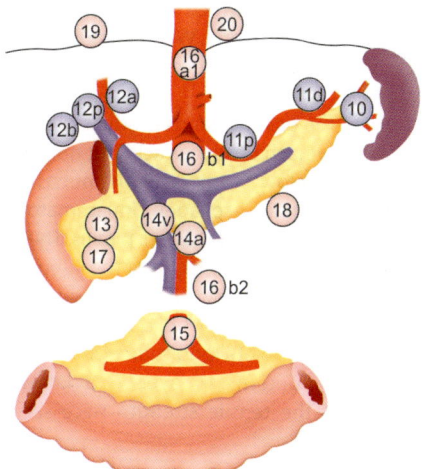

Fig. 11.1B: Lymph nodes of stomach

Histologically, the gastric wall has four distinct layers: mucosa, submucosa, muscularis propria and serosa.

- ***The mucosa*** (consist of epithelium, lamina propria and muscularis mucosa) is lined by columnar glandular epithelium and gastric glands open into it. The gastric glands are lined with different types of epithelial cells, depending upon the location and have different functions.
    - ***In the cardia,*** the gastric glands secrete mucus and bicarbonate with very little acid
    - ***In the fundus and body,*** gastric glands consist of the ***parietal cells*** (occupying the mid portion of the gastric glands) secrete acid and intrinsic factor into the gastric lumen and bicarbonate in the intercellular space. The other cells called ***chief cells*** (also

called zymogenic cells), which occupy the base of the gastric glands secrete pepsinogen I. When stimulated, the chief cells produce the pepsinogen proenzymes, pepsinogen I and some pepsinogen II

– *In the antrum,* the gastric glands produce gastrin and no acid.

Note: The proximal stomach produces acid but no gastrin.

- *The submucosa* is below the muscularis mucosa and is rich in blood vessels, lymphatics, collagen, inflammatory cells, nerve fibers and ganglion cells of Meissner's plexus. The strength to an anastomosis is given by the collagen of the submucosa.
- *The muscular propria* is below the submucosa and consist of three layers—incomplete inner oblique layer, complete middle circular layer and a complete longitudinal layer.
- *The serosa* is the outermost layer also known as visceral peritoneum, gives the tensile strength necessary for a strong gastric anastomosis.

Physiology

The stomach stores food and aids in the digestion through secretory and motor functions. It secretes acid, pepsin, intrinsic factor, mucus and a variety of GI hormones. Motor functions include food storage, grinding and mixing and controlled emptying of ingested food. Proximal stomach stores food for a short time and helps in regulation of basal intragastric tone, and distal stomach mixes and grinds the food. Distal stomach further breaks up solid food and helps in gastric emptying of solids.

Acid Secretion

The parietal cell is stimulated to secrete acid when one or more of three membrane receptors are stimulated by acetylcholine by vagal stimulation, gastrin from D cells and histamine from enterochromaffin like (ECL) cells. *The enzyme H^+/K^+ ATPase is the proton pump.* PPIs interfere with the function of the proton pump. Hydrochloric acid aids in the physical and biochemical breakdown of ingested food. Pepsin and acid together aid in the proteolysis. Gastrin, acetylcholine and histamine stimulate the parietal cell to secrete hydrochloric acid.

The acid secretory response occurs after a meal and is divided into three phases:
1. Cephalic or vagal phase (stimulated by thought, smell, sight or taste).
2. Gastric phase (stimulated by the food in the stomach).
3. Intestinal phase (stimulated by food in the proximal small intestine mediated by some hormone).

Pepsinogen Secretion

The most potent stimulus for pepsinogen secretion by chief cells is food in the stomach, and acetylcholine is the chief mediator.

Intrinsic Factor

In addition to hydrochloric acid, the parietal cells secrete intrinsic factor by the stimulus same as for acid secretion. Intrinsic factor binds to luminal vitamin B_{12} and this complex is absorbed in the terminal ileum. Vitamin B_{12} deficiency and pernicious anemia are common after total gastrectomy, for this reason.

Gastric Mucosal Barrier

There are various components and mediators which protect the gastric mucosa from autodigestion. They are given in **Table 11.1**.

Gastric Hormones

- ***Gastrin:*** A major hormonal stimulus for acid secretion, which has three components (big gastrin—G34, little gastrin—G17, and

Table 11.1: Various components and mediators protecting the gastric mucosa

Components	Mediators
Mucous barrier	Prostaglandins
Epithelial barrier	Epidermal growth factor
Bicarbonate secretion	Hepatocyte growth factor
Microcirculation	Nitric oxide
	Gastrin releasing peptide

minigastrin—G14). Majority of gastrin is G17 and is blocked by H_2 antagonists. Luminal peptides and amino acids stimulate gastrin release and luminal acids inhibit gastrin release.
- *Somatostatin:* Produced by D cells present throughout gastric mucosa. The predominant form is somatostatin 14, its release is stimulated by antral acidification, and acetylcholine from vagal stimulation inhibits its release.
- *Gastrin releasing peptide (GRP):* Stimulates both gastrin and somatostatin release by binding to G and D cell receptors.
- *Leptin:* A protein primarily synthesized by adipocytes, and takes part in reducing the food intake via vagally mediated pathways
- *Ghrelin:* A regulator of appetite.

APPROACH TO A PATIENT WITH UPPER GASTROINTESTINAL PATHOLOGY

Signs and Symptoms

The most common symptoms of gastric diseases are:
- Abdominal pain
- Weight loss

- Early satiety
- Anorexia
- Nausea/vomiting
- Upper abdominal fullness
- Anemia.

Signs of gastric disease are:
- Tenderness
- Lump.

Investigations

- Esophagogastroduodenoscopy
- Radiologic tests
  - Plain X-rays
  - Contrast studies
- CT scan and MRI
- Ultrasound
  - Transabdominal ultrasound
  - Endoscopic ultrasound
- Gastric secretory analysis
- Antroduodenal motility tests and electrogastrography.

GASTRIC VOLVULUS

Introduction

- **Gastric volvulus** or **volvulus of stomach** is twisting of all or part of the stomach by more than 180° with obstruction of the flow of material through the stomach, with variable loss of blood supply and possible tissue death.

- They are more common in the 5th decade, with equal sex incidence. In about 25%, children less than 1 year are affected.

Etiology

- Elevated left hemidiaphragm (diaphragmatic hernia)
- Adhesion
- Gastric tumors
- Mass in adjacent organs
- Hiatus hernia.

Pathogenesis

Normally the stomach is fixed to the posterior by ligamentous attachment to spleen, liver and diaphragm. The duodenum is fixed to the retroperitoneum.

The twisting can occur around two axes,
1. The long axis of the stomach, called *organoaxial.*
2. Around the axis perpendicular to this, called *mesenteroaxial.*

In organoaxial variety, the twist occurs along the long axis of the stomach (line extending from esophagogastric junction or fundus of stomach to gastropyloric junction).

- ***When the axis passes through the EG junction***, the antrum rotates anteriorly and superiorly and the fundus posteriorly and inferiorly.
- ***When the long axis passes through the body of the stomach***, greater curvature of both antrum and fundus rotates anteriorly and superiorly.

In mesenteroaxial variety, the stomach folds on its straight axis running across the lesser curvature to the greater curvature, with antrum twisting anteriorly and superiorly. This is more likely to be incomplete, intermittent and transient with chronic symptoms. Mixed varieties also occur (**Fig. 11.2**).

- Organoaxial variety is more common (60%) than the mesenteroaxial.

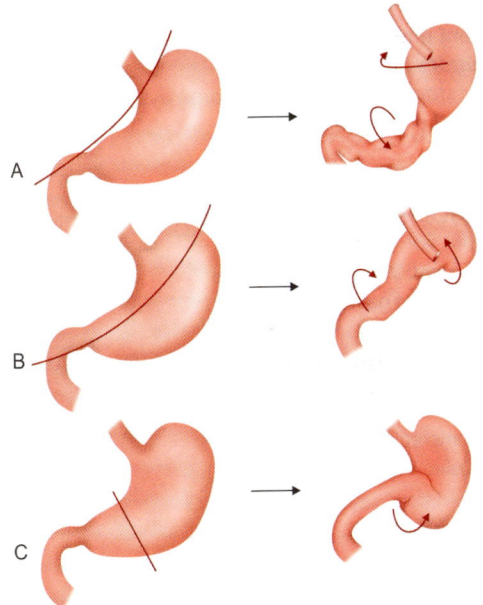

Fig. 11.2: Gastric volvulus. (A and B) Organoaxial; (C) Mesenteroaxial

- Obstruction is more likely in organoaxial twisting than with mesenteroaxial while the latter is more associated with ischemia.

Diagnosis

Symptoms and Signs

- **Acute stage:** Severe upper abdominal pain or lower chest, persistent unproductive retching, impossible to pass Ryle's tube **(Borchardt's triad)**
- **Chronic stage:** No specific symptoms, dyspepsia, epigastric pain, bleeding, hematemesis, PP pain.

Investigations

- **X-ray:** Gas filled stomach in the chest, large diaphragmatic hernia in chronic volvulus
- **Barium meal:** Stomach in the chest
- **Scopy:** Twisted gastric folds.

Differential Diagnosis

- Acute myocardial infarction
- Acute pancreatitis
- Biliary colic.

Management

- Emergency
- NG decompression if possible
- Acute endoscopic detorsion under fluoroscopy
- Surgery—open or laparoscopic

GASTRITIS

Introduction

It is defined as inflammation of gastric mucosa. This is best appreciated by histology. However, endoscopy also can identify this with characteristic findings.

Classification

It is classified as acute and chronic and the causes vary (**Table 11.2**).

Helicobacter pylori Gastritis

Introduction

The most common etiology of gastritis is *Helicobacter pylori* infection. This is acquired usually in infancy or early childhood and is

Table 11.2: Classification and causes of gastritis

Acute gastritis	Chronic gastritis
Toxic agents	*Helicobacter pylori*
• NSAIDs	
• Alcohol	
Stress	Autoimmune
Viruses	Nonspecific
Bacteria	Bile reflux
	Lymphocytic
	Granulomatous
	Eosinophilic
	Menetrier's disease

more common in underdeveloped countries. It is believed to spread by fecal–oral or oral–oral routes and it can be cultured in the stools of patients with acute diarrheal disease. Since this remains alive in water for many days, contaminated water may be the prime source.

H. pylori have an inhibitory effect on antral D cells that secrete somatostatin, a potent inhibitor of antral G-cell gastrin production. This leads to local alkalization of antrum (antral acidification is the most potent antagonist to antral gastric secretion) and increases local mediators and cytokines. This hypergastrinemia probably leads to parietal cell hyperplasia, ultimately leading to duodenal metaplasia. This allows colonization of *H. pylori* in the duodenal mucosa and duodenal ulcer forms. Additionally, *H. pylori* can induce gastroduodenal injury by producing toxins (vacA and cagA), local elaboration of cytokines particularly interleukin-8, recruitment of inflammatory cells and activation of local immune factors, which ultimately weaken the mucosal defense.

Diagnosis

Symptoms and Signs

Symptoms occur in later life. Non-ulcer dyspepsia is predominant.

Investigations

The diagnosis can be made by:
- Noninvasive (nonendoscopic) tests
  - Serology
  - Urea breath test
  - Stool antigen test
- Invasive (endoscopic) tests
  - Rapid urease assay
  - Histology
  - Culture.

Serology: When chronically infected, patient will have IgG antibodies and IgA antibodies when IgG is negative. IgM antibodies are found only in the early phase of infection. Since antibody titers remain elevated for long periods, this is a reliable test for those who have not been treated for *H. pylori* infection.

Urea breath test: Since this is positive in acute infective stage, it can be used for diagnosing primary infection, reinfection and treatment response. The patient ingests carbon labeled urea (^{13}C or ^{14}C), and the urease of *H. pylori* hydrolyzes the urea to produce labeled carbon dioxide, which can be collected and quantified in breath samples. This test has a sensitivity of 95%. Care should be taken to stop all medications (antibiotics, PPIs, bismuth containing compounds) about 2 weeks before testing to get reliable results.

Stool antigen test: This test is based on ELISA of specific *H. pylori* antigens excreted in stool samples, and has a sensitivity of 95–98%. Like in urea breath test, care should be taken to stop all medications (antibiotics, PPIs, bismuth containing compounds) about 2 weeks before testing to get reliable results.

Management

The treatment of chronic *H. pylori* infection is by antibiotics combined with acid suppression.
- ***Triple drug therapy***: Amoxicillin, clarithromycin, PPI (14 days)
- ***Quadruple therapy:*** Bismuth subsalicylate, tetracycline, metronidazole and PPI (14 days)
- ***Sequential therapy:*** PPI and amoxicillin for 5 days, followed by PPI, clarithromycin and tinidazole for 5 days.

Clinical Pearls

- Flagellated *H. pylori* alone can be pathogenic and the mutant strains of *H. pylori* which are unflagellated and which do not produce urease are nonpathogenic
- *H. pylori* infection if found should be treated
- Failure of eradication is usually due to non-compliance and reinfection is seen in only less than 5%
- There is no evidence that *H. pylori* infection causes GERD
- Those who fail to initial triple therapy should not be treated again with clarithromycin because of macrolide resistance and quadruple therapy is preferred
- Persistent infections may require more courses of therapies
- Refractory cases can be treated with quinolone, rifabutin or furazolidone based therapies
- Patients with increased risk of gastric cancer if found to be infected by *H. pylori* require vigorous treatment
- Patients with *H. pylori* infection develop gastric or more commonly duodenal ulcer disease. Less commonly, B cell lymphoma and adenocarcinoma are associated with this infection.

Stress Gastritis

Gastritis occurring during periods of stress, more commonly in the ICU patients, especially those requiring mechanical ventilation and those with coagulopathy, renal failure, severe burns, sepsis and CNS injury is called stress gastritis They may develop into frank ulcers with hemorrhage and perforation. Administration of H_2 blockers and PPIs prophylactically significantly reduces the incidence of stress ulcers, by inactivating the proteolytic enzyme pepsin.

Bile Reflux Gastritis

This occurs due to reflux of bile most commonly seen after gastrectomy, pyloroplasty or cholecystectomy. During endoscopy, large amounts of bile are found in the stomach. The gastric mucosa looks granular and intensely erythematous with a brick red color or greenish yellow discoloration. Diversion surgery is the choice when medical management fails.

Lymphocytic Gastritis

This is characterized by accumulation of intraepithelial lymphocytes containing cytotoxic granules in the surface and foveolar epithelium. When the number of such lymphocytes exceeds 30, it is diagnostic. This gastritis is asymptomatic. There is no specific therapy to this gastritis.

Autoimmune Gastritis

An uncommon variety of gastritis usually found in patients with megaloblastic anemia. They produce antibodies against parietal cells, which affect the gastric acid secretion and intrinsic factor. Gastric acid in turn reduces the gastrin levels. Parietal cell destruction results in achlorhydria and decreased levels of intrinsic factor leading to high serum gastrin levels and vitamin B_{12} malabsorption. They are usually asymptomatic. Endoscopic appearance is that of severe atrophy with marked flattening of gastric rugae and visible submucosal vasculature, which is typically found in the fundus and body of the stomach. In the early stages, inflammatory changes are seen, which get replaced by intestinal metaplasia. Patients with gastric atrophy and intrinsic factor antibodies should be followed for the development of pernicious anemia and gastroscopy for gastric polyps or carcinoma. Gastroscopy should be performed at 3–5 years intervals.

Granulomatous Gastritis

Usually occurs in patients with granulomatous diseases like sarcoidosis, Wegener's granulomatosis, and severe systemic granulomatosis, more commonly with Crohn's disease. They present with gastric outlet obstruction. Endoscopy reveals aphthous ulcers and histologic confirmation is difficult.

Eosinophilic Gastritis

Usually occurs as a part of eosinophilic gastroenteritis. Symptoms are usually of acid peptic disease or irritable bowel syndrome. Depth of eosinophilic infiltration of stomach wall determines the severity of symptoms. Corticosteroids are useful in certain cases.

ACID PEPTIC DISEASE

Introduction

Acid peptic disease (APD) is a very general term representing a variety of overlapping symptoms of the upper abdomen caused by an imbalance between mucosal defenses and acid peptic injury.

Risk Factors

- Excessive usage of NSAIDs
- Stress factors (e.g. trauma, burns)
- *H. pylori* infections
- Acid hypersecretion

Stomach and Duodenum

- Genetic factors
- Use of tobacco, alcohol, and caffeine
- Blood group O
- Unchecked gastric secretion (Zollinger–Ellison syndrome).

Results of High Acidity in the Stomach

- Reflux esophagitis
- Gastritis
- Duodenitis
- Gastric and duodenal erosions
- Gastric ulcer
- Duodenal ulcer.

Classification of Gastric Ulcers

Modified Johnson's classification of gastric ulcer is based on its anatomic location (**Fig. 11.3A**) (**Table 11.3**). The incidence varies between different types of gastric ulcers (**Fig. 11.3B**).

A giant gastric ulcer is defined as an ulcer of size more than 3 cm in size, along the lesser curvature and carries the malignant potential of about 30%, and they require surgical resection.

Diagnosis

Symptoms and Signs

Patients with APD present with the following symptoms (**Table 11.4**).
- *Pain:* Burning in nature, more in the epigastrium, intermittent and always related to food.
- *Periodicity:* Pain-free intervals is a characteristic feature.
- *Vomiting:* Sometimes a feature and has influence on pain, blood stained vomiting (hematemesis) may occur.

- ***Weight:*** Duodenal ulcer patients gain weight, and gastric ulcer patients lose weight.
- ***Dyspepsia:*** A feature of gastric ulcer and not that of duodenal ulcer.
- ***Anemia:*** May be a feature of gastric ulcer (malignant), duodenal ulcer (bleeding).

Investigations

- ***Barium meal* (Fig. 11.4)** may be diagnostic

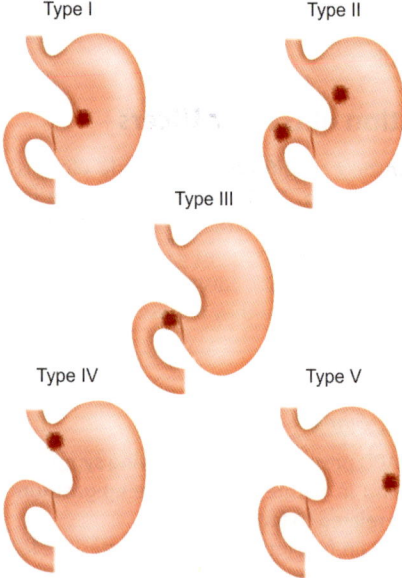

Fig. 11.3A: Types of gastric ulcers

Stomach and Duodenum

Table 11.3: Modified Johnson's classification of gastric ulcers

Type	Incidence	Location of ulcer	Acid secretion
Type I	50%	Ulcer in the body of stomach along the lesser curvature at the incisura	Low
Type II	25%	Ulcer in the body of the stomach along the lesser curvature + duodenal ulcer	High
Type III	20%	Ulcer in the prepyloric region	High
Type IV	<10%	Ulcer high along the lesser curvature near OG junction	Low
Type V		Ulcer anywhere in the stomach (NSAID induced)	High

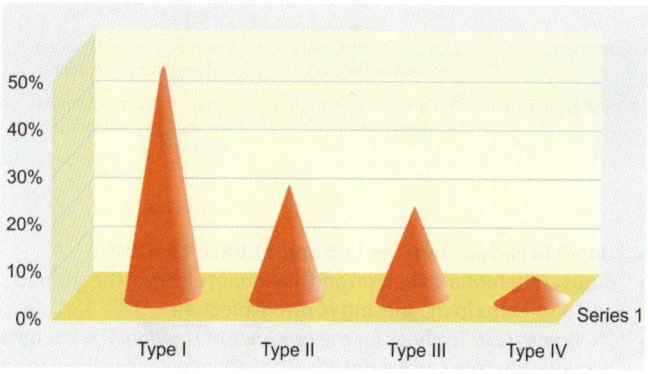

Fig. 11.3B: Incidence of gastric ulcers

Table 11.4: Clinical features of acid peptic disease

Clinical feature	Pathology	
	Gastric ulcer	**Duodenal ulcer**
Pain	Upper abdominal pain (epigastric), when penetrates the pancreas—develops back pain	Upper abdominal pain (epigastric or right hypochondrial) on empty stomach (hunger pain), common at night (12 to 2 AM)—'Nocturnal cries'
Relationship to food	Food intake increases pain	Food intake relieves pain
Appetite	Normal or reduced	Increased
Body weight	Loss due to reduced intake of food	Gain due to increased intake of food
Vomiting	Spontaneous, relieves pain	Occurs when gastric outlet obstruction occurs
Hematemesis or melena	Not uncommon, bleeds are small and lead to anemia	Common in posterior ulcers, and bleeds are large, presents as emergency
Perforation	Not uncommon, and presents as peritonitis	Common in anterior ulcers, and presents as peritonitis
Clinical examination	Tenderness in epigastrium on deep palpation	Tenderness in epigastrium and right hypochondrium on palpation

- *Upper GI endoscopy* **(Figs 11.5 and 11.6A)** is conclusive
- *Biopsy* differentiates benign and malignant ulcers of the stomach, and also helps in diagnosing *H. pylori* infection
- *^{14}C breath test:* To check for the presence of *H. pylori*. The bacteria convert urea into carbon dioxide. The test involves swallowing an

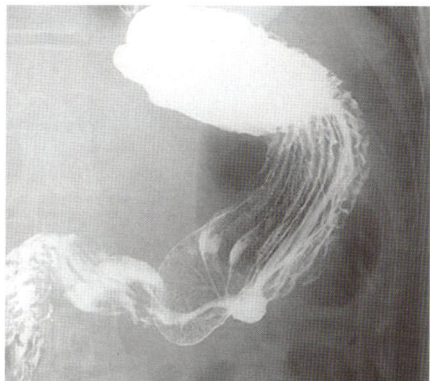

Fig. 11.4: Barium meal—Gastric ulcer

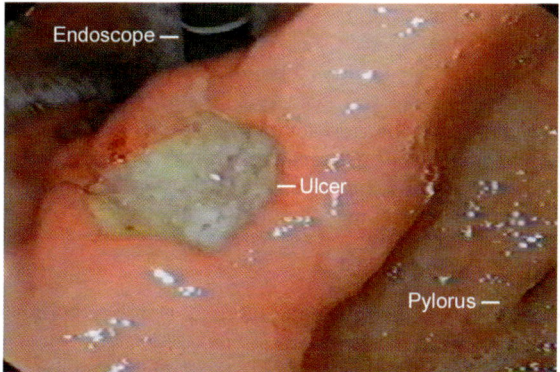

Fig. 11.5: Endoscopy—Chronic gastric ulcer

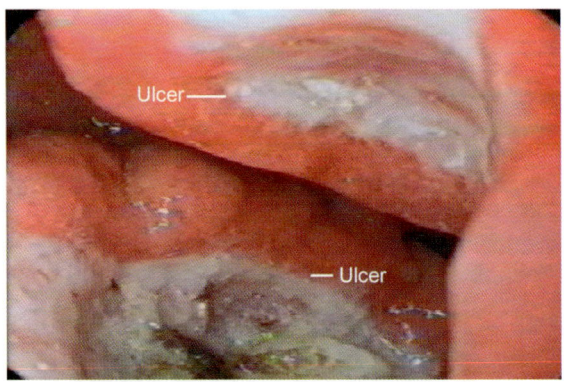

Fig. 11.6A: Endoscopy—Chronic duodenal ulcer

amount of radioactive carbon (^{14}C) and testing the air exhaled from the lungs. A non-radioactive test can be used for children and pregnant women
- ***Serology:*** ELISA can detect both immunoglobulins, IgG and IgA antibodies directed against *H. pylori*. The sensitivity of most serologic tests is approximately 95%
- ***Fecal antigen test:*** The detection of *H. pylori* in feces is emerging as a noninvasive method of detection. This test has mainly been used in pediatric settings.

Complications

The three most common complications of acid peptic disease in decreasing order of frequency are:
1. Hemorrhage (most common) due to *H. pylori* infection and NSAIDs.
2. Perforation.
3. Obstruction due to cicatrization of ulcer.

Hemorrhage: Patients with bleeding ulcers typically present with melena and/or hematemesis. Usually the bleeding is not massive, unless on anticoagulants, and they respond to acid suppression and nothing by mouth. A quarter of patients will continue to bleed or will rebleed after a quiescent period. High-risk patients are identified by the factors like large hemorrhage, shock, transfusion requirement of 4 units in 24 hours and endoscopic appearance of the ulcer size (>1 cm) and ulcer bed. They are benefited from endoscopic procedures like epinephrine injection and electrocautery. Surgery may be indicated for persistent bleeders or those who rebleed. The bleeding ulcers can be graded by Forrest classification (**Refer Table 9.3**).

Perforation: Perforation (**Fig. 11.6B**) is commonly associated with NSAID use and presents clinically as acute abdomen, and chemical peritonitis results, which may progress to bacterial peritonitis making this a surgical emergency. Presence of gas under the domes

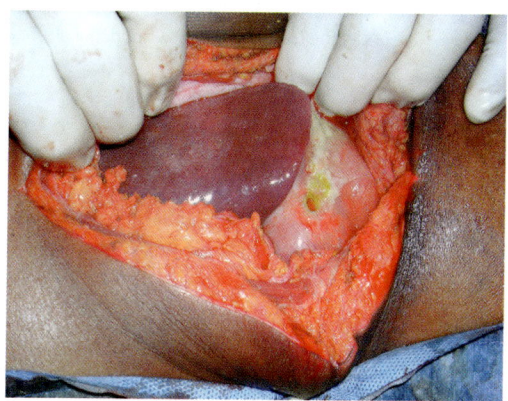

Fig. 11.6B: Duodenal ulcer perforation

of the diaphragm in the erect X-ray chest (**Fig. 11.6C**) confirms the diagnosis. Surgery is to close the perforation with an omental patch (**Fig. 11.6D**)—***Graham closure***, with thorough peritoneal toileting.

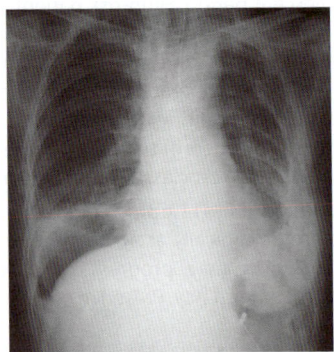

Fig. 11.6C: X-ray—Gas under the diaphragm due to duodenal ulcer perforation

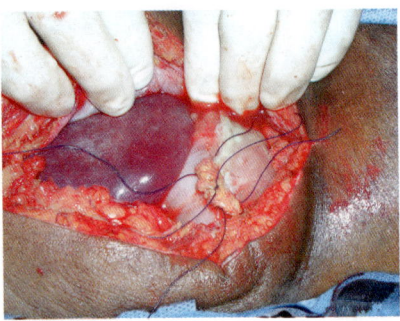

Fig. 11.6D: Closure of duodenal perforation with omental patch

Obstruction: Gastric outlet obstruction occurs in small percentage of patients with duodenal ulcer, and they present with nonbilious vomiting and electrolyte disturbances, like hypokalemic hypochloremic metabolic alkalosis. Succussion splash is a constant finding and visible gastric peristalsis may be seen. After initial resuscitation, vagotomy and a bypass procedure (gastrojejunostomy) is performed.

Management

Medical

- ***Diet*** at regular intervals
- ***Avoidance of aspirin and NSAIDs***
- ***Antacids*** to neutralize gastric pH, which can alleviate symptoms
- ***H_2 receptors***—inhibit gastric hypersecretion
- ***Proton pump inhibitors (PPIs)***—block the hydrogen-potassium adenosine triphosphatase pump in the gastric parietal cells and inhibit hydrogen ion activity
- ***Sucralfate***—coats the ulcer (antacids/proton-pump inhibitors/ H_2 receptor antagonist is mandatory)
- ***Anti-H. pylori treatment*** for *H. pylori* positive cases
- ***Supportive treatment with blood transfusions*** may be required to treat large bleeds.

Endoscopic

- Endoscopic balloon dilatation for obstructing peptic ulcer
- Endoscopic treatment for bleeding peptic ulcers
    - ***Injection therapy*** (epinephrine as vasoconstrictor, ethanol, ethanolamine and polidocanol as sclerosants, thrombin and fibrin as hemostatics)
    - ***Thermocoagulation*** (heat or electrocoagulation using a probe)
    - ***Mechanical therapy*** (endoclip application or band ligation)

Surgical

- **Surgery** is indicated when
  - Ulcers are intractable or non-healing—Truncal vagotomy + drainage (gastrojejunostomy/pyloroplasty) or truncal vagotomy and antrectomy or highly selective vagotomy (HSV)
  - Medical management fails/for ulcer bleed—***Oversewing the bleeding vessel/ulcer excision/gastric resection. After oversewing the vessel, the pylorus is closed using a technique of pyloroplasty (Heinecke–Mikulicz/Finney/Jaboulay type) (Figs 11.7 to 11.9)***

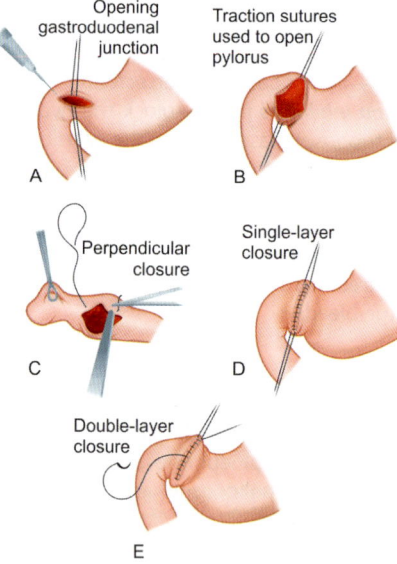

Fig. 11.7: Heinecke–Mikulicz pyloroplasty

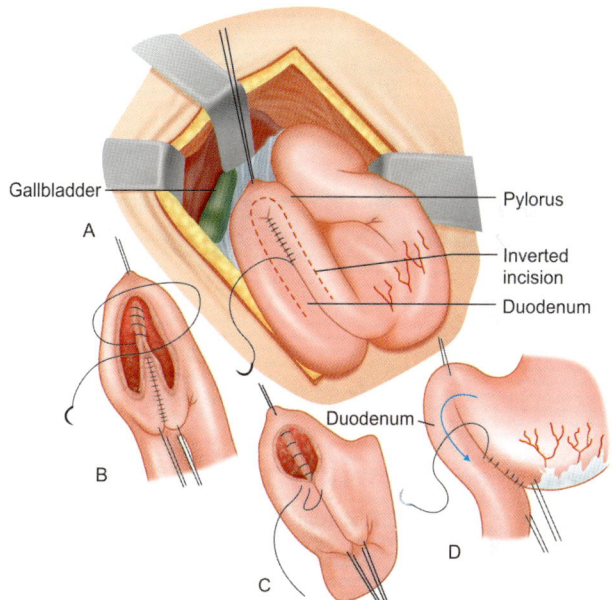

Fig. 11.8: Finney's pyloroplasty

- Perforation—simple closure with or without omental patch *(Graham closure)*
- Obstruction is caused by cicatrized ulcer—Vagotomy + ***Gastrojejunostomy/antrectomy***
- ***Vagotomy was considered essential and today it is not done as a routine by many surgeons, probably due to the decreasing experience of the surgeon and reliance on PPIs to decrease acid secretion.***

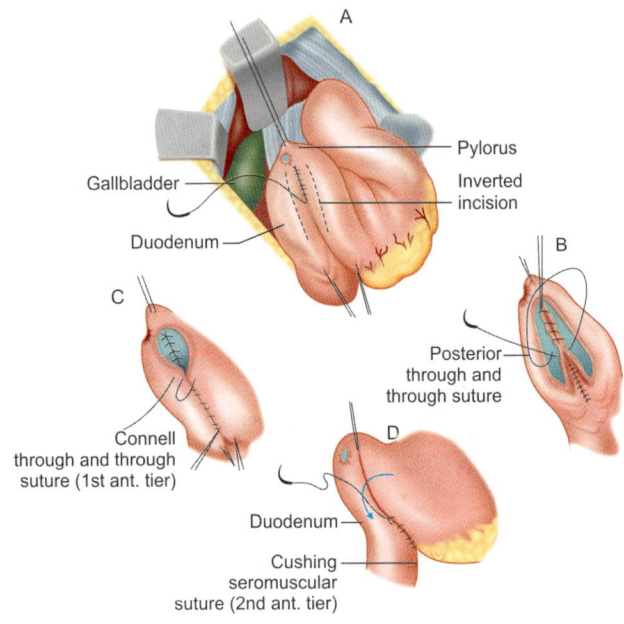

Fig. 11.9: Jaboulay pyloroplasty

Clinical Pearls

- In young patients with dyspepsia or epigastric pain, it may be appropriate to start with empiric PPI therapy without an endoscopy
- Patients of over 45 years with upper abdominal symptoms should be subjected to endoscopy to rule out malignancy

- Once ulcer is diagnosed either radiologically or endoscopically, the possible causes should be considered and appropriate measures like biopsy becomes mandatory, including for *H. pylori*
- In acute peptic ulcer disease, the obstruction caused by edema resolves by gastric decompression and intense medical management
- Chronic peptic ulcer disease causing obstruction, is unlikely to resolve with medical management
- Endoscopic dilatation offers excellent symptomatic relief in patients with obstructing peptic ulcer, but it is often transient
- Truncal vagotomy denervates the antropyloric mechanism and a drainage procedure becomes necessary.
- Following antrectomy, Billroth I or II anastomosis is preferred. Roux-en-Y reconstruction [Csendes' procedure (Fig. 11.10)] is avoided as marginal ulcers are common due to the large gastric remnant, but is the procedure of choice in type IV gastric ulcers, as the ulcer is highly placed and the residual gastric remnant is small
- HSV—highly selective vagotomy (parietal cell vagotomy/proximal gastric vagotomy), which denervates the proximal two-thirds of the stomach where majority of parietal cells are located and preserves the innervation of

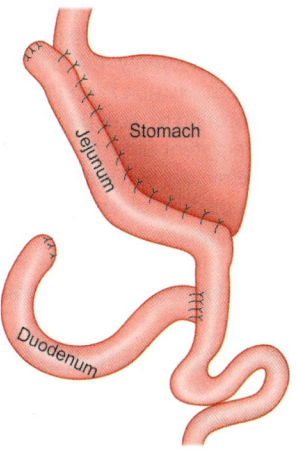

Fig. 11.10: Csendes' procedure

the rest of the GIT is a safe procedure, but recurrence rates are high.
- In today's scenario of peptic ulcer disease, the use of PPIs, H_2 blockers and effective anti-*H. pylori* treatment, peptic ulcer disease is no longer the primary cause of gastric outlet obstruction, but it is malignancy
- Pyloroplasty is not preferred as a drainage procedure in obstructing peptic ulcer disease
- Once free air is found in the abdominal X-ray, no further investigation is necessary and surgery should be undertaken immediately
- Vagotomy and antrectomy should be avoided in hemodynamically unstable patients and patients with peritonitis
- Types I and IV gastric ulcers require gastrectomy without vagotomy due to low acidity, types II and III require gastrectomy and vagotomy due to high acidity
- Ulcer excision is preferred for bleeding gastric ulcers and direct suturing of ulcer bed is preferred for bleeding duodenal ulcer
- Persistent ulcer of >12 weeks of medical therapy is considered refractory and requires surgical treatment
- Refractory ulcers especially in the elderly are suspected to be malignant
- All surgical procedures required for acid peptic disease can be performed by laparoscopic method.

ZOLLINGER–ELLISON SYNDROME (ZES)

Introduction

- This syndrome is caused by uncontrolled excessive secretion of abnormal amounts of gastrin by duodenal or pancreatic neuroendocrine tumor (gastrinoma)

Stomach and Duodenum

- Majority are sporadic and about a quarter are inherited
- Inherited tumors form a part of MEN I (parathyroid, pituitary and pancreatic tumors)
- Gastrinomas of MEN I are multiple in number
- Sporadic gastrinomas are usually solitary
- Half the gastrinomas are found to be malignant, metastasizing to lymph nodes, liver and other distant organs
- Larger the size of the gastrinoma, higher the chances of metastases
- 80% of the tumors are found in the gastrinoma triangle.

Diagnosis

Symptoms and Signs

- Epigastric pain, GERD and diarrhea.

Investigations

Blood Test

- ***Serum gastrin levels are elevated—>500 pg/mL (Normal <200 pg/mL).*** In borderline cases (gastrin levels 200–500 pg/mL), administration of IV bolus of secretin (2U/kg) will increase gastrin level by 150 pg/mL within 15 minutes of administration, which will confirm ZES.

Endoscopy

- *Endoscopy* reveals multiple ulcers commonly in the duodenum, rarely in the jejunum.

Radiology

- *CT and MRI* will localize tumors of size more than 2 cm
- *EUS* is more sensitive than the other investigations, but can be mistaken with the lymph node enlargements.

Management

- A gastrinoma when located, surgery is the best option
- If multiple tumors are located, the largest tumor is excised
- Inoperable tumors in the liver, can be treated by
  - Debulking surgery
  - Radiofrequency ablation
  - Chemoembolization
  - Liver transplantation.

Clinical Pearls

- Thorough intra-abdominal exploration is essential to locate the tumor
- Intraoperative ultrasound may be used to locate the tumor
- When tumor is not located, a generous duodenotomy should be done to locate the mucosal tumors
- All lymph nodes should be sampled
- Excision of gastrinomas of MEN I is difficult and never complete as they are multiple and small
- Acid secretion due to gastrinomas can always be managed by high dose PPIs
- Gastrectomy for ZES is no longer indicated.

GASTROPARESIS

Introduction

- This is defined as delay in gastric emptying.
- This is a derangement of the gastric function, which is to act as a food reservoir and to deliver it in a controlled manner into the intestine.

Etiology

The basic pathology is impaired motility, without any mechanical obstruction. The causes are many:
- Autonomic neuropathy (diabetes)
- Infiltrative (amyloidosis)
- Collagen vascular disease (scleroderma)
- Postsurgical (vagotomy)
- Drugs (anticholinergics, opiates, antidepressants)
- Others (pregnancy, Parkinson's disease, viral infections).

Diagnosis

Symptoms and Signs

- Postprandial fullness
- Bloating
- Nausea
- Vomiting.

Investigations

- ***Endoscopy or contrast studies*** to eliminate mechanical obstruction
- ***Scintigraphy*** is highly useful
- ***Electrogastrography***

Management

- ***Prokinetic drugs*** (metoclopramide, domperidone)
- ***Macrolides*** (erythromycin)
- ***Mosapride and itopride***

GASTRIC POLYPS

Introduction

- Gastric polyps are small, benign hyperplastic growths of epithelial tissue
- They may be single or multiple and occur anywhere in the stomach
- They may be sessile or pedunculated
- They are potentially malignant

Classification of Gastric Polyps and their Incidence

1. Fundic gland polyps (80%)
2. Hyperplastic polyps (17%)
3. Adenomatous polyps (1%)
4. Hamartomatous polyps
5. Others
   - Polypoid adenocarcinoma
   - Inflammatory polyps
   - Carcinoids
   - Pancreatic rests

Diagnosis

Symptoms and Signs

Generally asymptomatic, but rarely presents with minor bleeds.

Investigations

Found incidentally on barium studies or endoscopy (**Figs 11.11A and B**).

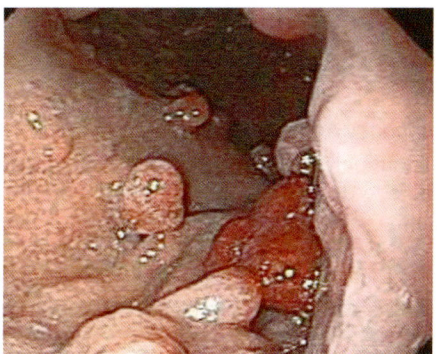

Fig. 11.11A: Gastroscopy—Gastric polyps

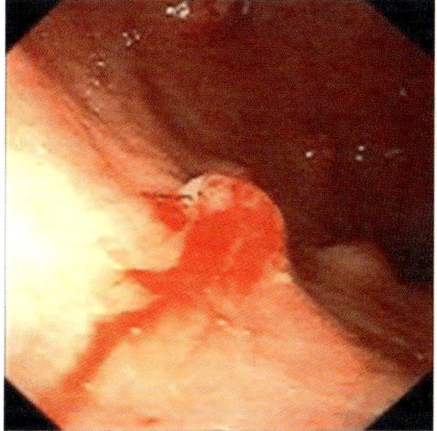

Fig. 11.11B: Gastroscopy—Bleeding from polyp of stomach

Endoscopic and Histologic Features of Gastric Polyps

The endoscopic and histologic features of gastric polyps are given in **Table 11.5**.

Risk of Malignancy Associated with Gastric Polyps
- Adenomatous polyps have high risk of malignant transformation (75%) and size dependent; polyps of size more than 2 cm are significant

Table 11.5: The endoscopic and histologic features of gastric polyps

Type of polyps	Endoscopic appearance	Histologic appearance
Fundic gland polyps	Large in number (usually more than 5), small (3–5 mm), pale and hemispheric in appearance, arise in the gastric fundus	Contain hypertrophied gastric gland mucosa
Hyperplastic polyps	Typically pedunculated and erythematous, vary in number (1–many) and size (5–20 mm), occur anywhere in the stomach	Hyperplastic, elongated gastric glands with edematous stroma. Glandular portions show cystic dilatation with no alteraton in the cellular configuration
Adenomatous polyps	Solitary and 5–20 mm in size. Sessile or pedunculated and resemble hyperplastic polyps	True neoplastic growths showing dysplastic epithelium. Cells have hyperchromatic, elongated nuclei arranged in picket fence pattern with increased mitotic figures
Hamartomatous polyps	Resemble hyperplastic and adenomatous polyps	Show branching bands of smooth muscle surrounded by glandular epithelium, with normal lamina propria

- Hyperplastic polyps carry a low risk of malignant transformation (0.5–5%)
- Fundic gland and hamartomatous polyps carry no risk of malignant transformation.

Differential Diagnosis

- Leiomyoma
- Lipoma
- Gastrointestinal stromal tumor (GIST)

Management

- ***Endoscopic excision*** is the treatment of choice. When found, a gastric polyp should be excised as the histology cannot be determined by the endoscopic appearance and also sampling errors are common. When the polyps are large in number, larger lesions should be excised and biopsied. Endoscopic surveillance should be done every 2–3 years in the absence of dysplasia.
- Since *H. pylori* infection is commonly associated, its eradication should be done as this is known to reduce the polyps or its recurrence.

Clinical Pearls

- Since adenomatous and hyperplastic polyps occur in the background of chronic gastritis, the risk for malignant transformation is raised
- Hyperplastic, adenomatous and fundic gland polyps have an increased potential to be a part of familial adenomatous polyposis and attenuated FAP syndromes, and hence general screening for associated conditions should be undertaken

- Patients with Gardner's syndrome have a preponderance for hyperplastic polyps
- Patients with Peutz-Jegher's syndrome and Juvenile polyposis syndromes have hamartomatous polyps in the stomach.

GASTRIC MALIGNANCY

- Commonly they are adenocarcinomas
- Less commonly they can be lymphomas, stromal tumors, carcinoids and metastatic tumors.

Adenocarcinoma

Introduction

- More common in men
- Common above the age of 50
- More common in the antrum or on the lesser curve, and less frequent on the corpus.

Risk Factors

- Achlorhydria and atrophic gastritis
- Use of preserved and packed food *(especially starchy food preserved in salt)*
- *H. pylori* infection of stomach
- Tobacco smoking
- Previous gastroenterostomy
- Blood group A
- Epstein Barr virus
- Gastric polyps
- Benign gastric ulcer
- Familial [familial adenomatous polyposis, E-cadherin gene (CDH1) mutation)].

H. pylori and Gastric Malignancy

H. pylori cause inflammation of stomach, which eventually may lead to atrophic gastritis and achlorhydria, caused by immune destruction of parietal cells. Antiparietal cell antibodies and elevated gastrin levels favor the development of malignancy probably due to 'proinflammatory host genotype'.

Macroscopic Appearances of Gastric Malignancy

Macroscopically the gastric cancer is of four types:
1. Polypoid fungating growth
2. Sessile lesion
3. Ulcerative
4. Diffuse infiltrative type (scirrhous)—Linitis plastica (**leather bottle stomach).**

Microscopic Variety of Gastric Malignancy

- Microscopically, they are adenocarcinomas of columnar or cuboidal type.

Early gastric cancer is defined as the adenocarcinoma confined to the mucosa or submucosa, independent of nodal status. They are classified by ***Japanese classification*** (**Fig. 11.12**).

- **Type I**—exophytic lesion extending into the gastric lumen
- **Type II** superficial variant
    - **IIA**—elevated lesion with a height no more than the thickness of the adjacent mucosa
    - **II B**—Flat lesion
    - **IIC**—depressed lesion with an eroded but not deeply ulcerated appearance
- **Type III**—excavated lesion that may extend into the muscularis propria without invasion of this layer by cancer cells.

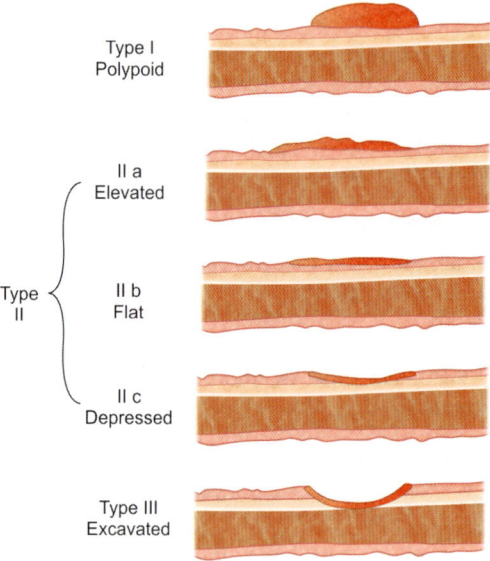

Fig. 11.12: Japanese classification of gastric cancer

Classification of advanced gastric cancer according to *Borrmann* **(Fig 11.13)** is as follows:
- **Type I:** Polypoid, fungating
- **Type II:** Ulcerative with elevated distinct borders
- **Type III:** Ulcerative with indistinct borders
- **Type IV:** Diffuse, indistinct borders

Note: Type I and II: localized types, types III and IV: infiltrative types.

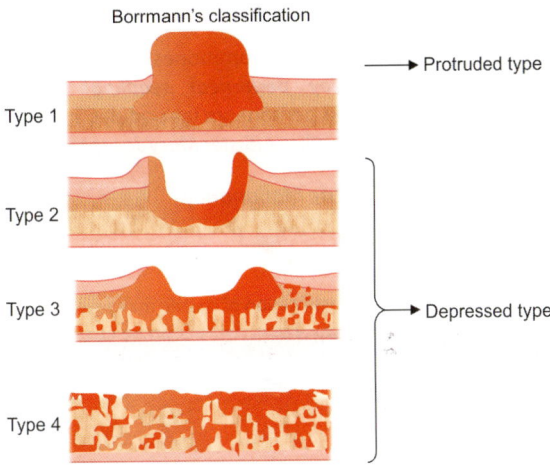

Fig. 11.13: Borrmann's classification of advanced gastric cancer

Spread of Gastric Cancer

Gastric cancer spreads by various routes:
- ***Longitudinally and circumferentially*** within the walls of the stomach
- ***Submucosal spread*** leads to diffuse infiltration of the whole stomach leading to luminal narrowing and rigidity of stomach (linitis plastica)
- ***Direct spread*** to contiguous structures like pancreas, transverse colon, left lobe of liver occurs when the muscle layer and serosa are invaded

- **Lymphatic spread** to celiac nodes and to left supraclavicular nodes *(Virchow's nodes)*
- **Hematogenous spread** to liver (commonest), lungs, and brain
- **Transcelomic spread *(by peritoneal seedling)*** to ovaries *(Krukenburg's tumor)* and peritoneum (as nodules and ascites)
- **Retrograde spread** to umbilicus *(Sister Mary Joseph's nodules).*

TNM Classification of Gastric Malignancy

It is given in **Table 11.6**.

Table 11.6: TNM classification of gastric malignancy

Tumor status	
T_X	Primary tumor cannot be assessed
T_0	No evidence of primary tumor
T_{is}	Carcinoma *in situ*
T_1	Tumor invading lamina propria muscularis mucosae or submucosa
T_{1a}	Tumor invading lamina propria or muscularis mucosae
T_{1b}	Tumor invading submucosa
T_2	Tumor invading muscularis propria
T_3	Tumor penetrates subserosa (visceral peritoneum) without invasion of adjacent structures
T_4	Tumor with invasion of adjacent structures
T_{4a}	Tumor invading serosa
T_{4b}	Tumor invading adjacent structures
Lymph node status	
N_X	Regional lymph nodes cannot be assessed
N_0	No regional node metastasis

Contd....

Contd....

N_1	Metastasis in 1–2 regional nodes
N_2	Metastasis in 3–6 regional nodes
N_{3a}	Metastasis in 7–15 regional nodes
N_{3b}	Metastasis in 16 or more nodes

Metastatic status

M_0	No distant metastasis
M_1	Distant metastasis (includes ipsilateral supraclavicular lymph nodes)

Stage grouping

Stage	T	N	M
0	T_{is}	N_0	M_0
IA	T_1	N_0	M_0
IB	T_1	N_1	M_0
	T_2	N_0	M_0
II A	T_1	N_2	M_0
	T_2	N_1	M_0
	T_3	N_0	M_0
II B	T_1	N_3	M_0
	T_2	N_2	M_0
	T_3	N_1	M_0
III A	T_2	N_3	M_0
III B	T_{4b}	N_0, N_1	M_0
	T_{4a}	N_2	M_0
	T_3	N_3	M_0
III C	T_{4b}	N_2, N_3	M_0
	T_{4a}	N_3	M_0
IV	T_4	N_{1-3}	M_0
	T_{1-3}	N_3	M_0
	Any T	Any N	M_1

Diagnosis

Symptoms and Signs

- Early lesions are without symptoms, however, loss of appetite and early satiety are early symptoms of gastric cancer
- Symptoms and signs of cancer stomach are given in **Table 11.7** in the order of occurrence.

Table 11.7: Symptoms and signs of gastric malignancy

Symptom	Sign
Appetite loss	Weight loss
Weight loss	Abdominal lump in the epigastrium or right hypochondrium (local fixity indicates local invasion)
Nausea	Abdominal tenderness
Vomiting (in cancers of the pyloric region producing gastric outlet obstruction)	Irregular hepatomegaly (due to liver metastases)*
Upper abdominal discomfort, early satiety, postprandial fullness after small feeds	Rectal shelf mass–Blumer's shelf (due to pelvic deposits in the rectovesical or rectovaginal pouch–Pouch of Douglas)*
Upper gastrointestinal hemorrhage (ulcerative lesions)	Troisier's sign—cervical lymphadenopathy (Virchow's nodes)*
Upper abdominal pain (usually indicates local infiltration)	Ascites (due to peritoneal spread)*
Melena (ulcerative lesions)	Umbilical nodules (Sister Mary Joseph's nodules) due to retrograde spread*
Dysphagia (tumors near OG junction)	Lung secondaries*
Jaundice (liver metastases)*	Pathological fractures*
	Migrating thrombophlebitis (Trousseau's sign)*

* Indicates advanced disease

Stomach and Duodenum

Investigations

Endoscopy
- *Upper GI endoscopy* (**Fig. 11.14**) is diagnostic for primary lesion

Radiology
- *US and CT abdomen* (**Figs 11.15A and B**) are useful is diagnosing liver, lymph nodal and peritoneal metastases
- *EUS* is useful in detecting the T and N staging more accurately, and has the advantage of obtaining biopsy. It is useful in detecting small amounts of ascites, which suggests unresectability
- *X-rays and CT of chest* are useful in diagnosing lung metastases.

Management

Management is multimodal, surgery being the primary mode of management.

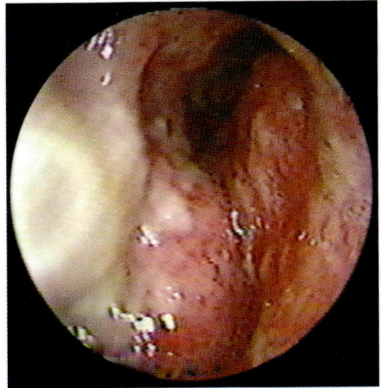

Fig. 11.14: Endoscopy—Malignant growth stomach

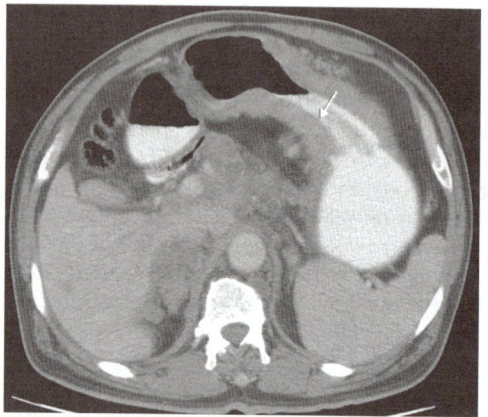

Fig. 11.15A: CT—Carcinoma stomach

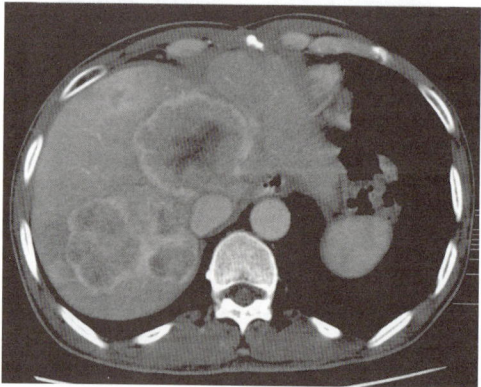

Fig. 11.15B: CT—Carcinoma stomach with liver metastases

Curative Treatment

- **Radical (clearance) surgery** depending on the location of the tumor is the treatment of choice, **followed by chemotherapy and sometimes radiotherapy**
  - Tumors located in the proximal or middle third of the stomach, **total gastrectomy** is the procedure of choice
  - For distal tumors, **subtotal gastrectomy** is preferred.

Note

- D1 gastrectomy is defined as dissection of all the group 1 nodes, and D2 is defined as dissection of all the nodes of groups 1 and 2. D3 gastrectomy is defined as dissection of nodes belonging to all the three groups
- Spleen preservation versus splenectomy; preservation of the pancreas versus left-sided pancreatectomy; and limited D1 resection versus extended D2/D3 lymphadenectomy are controversial. However, D2 gastrectomy is becoming accepted as a safe treatment for gastric cancer at experienced centers, in western countries.

Palliative Treatment

- **Surgery**—gastrojejunostomy to relieve gastric outflow obstruction
- **Radiotherapy**—to relieve local symptoms like obstruction, hemorrhage and pain and has no curative role
- **Chemotherapy**—confers marginal survival advantage
- **Endoscopic procedures**—laser therapy (for bleeding tumors) and endoprosthesis (for obstructive tumors) of esophagogastric junction
- **Preoperative chemoradiation** (CRT) is useful in advanced lesions.

Note: Endoscopic mucosal or submucosal resection may be appropriate for selected patients with early gastric adenocarcinoma.

Clinical Pearls

- To diagnose cancer stomach in its early stage, high degree of suspicion is needed
- Signet ring carcinomas are adenocarcinomas in which more than 50% of malignant cells have intracytoplasmic mucin. They tend to infiltrate and produce a desmoplastic reaction, and is very aggressive in behavior
- The goal of surgical cure is resection of all tumors (R0 resection). A clear margin of 5 cm is to be provided and all margins should be tumor free
- Though the lymphatics have very rich anastomotic network, they drain in a very unpredictable fashion, and skipping node stations are also possible.

Gastric Lymphoma

Introduction

- Represent 5% of all GI malignancies
- Peak incidence is between 50 and 70 years
- Male predominance 2:1
- Malignant transformation of mucosa associated lymphatic tissue (MALT) is important
- Lymphomas constitute about 10% of gastric malignancies, and *H. pylori* infection is closely associated with the lymphoid hyperplasia, which may progress to lymphoma
- They infiltrate the stomach wall diffusely.

Risk Factors for GI Lymphomas

- Atrophic gastritis
- *H. pylori* infections

- α-chain disease
- Celiac disease
- Dermatitis herpetiformis
- Autoimmune disorders
- Crohn's disease
- Immunodeficiency syndromes including AIDS.

MALT Lymphoma

It can occur in any mucosal location, both inside and outside the GIT. In the stomach, this is associated with *H. pylori* infection. The organism is believed to cause chronic inflammation (T cell response to bacterial antigens), which in turn leads to monoclonal (B cell) neoplasm of inflammatory cells. These tumor cells express surface membrane immunoglobulins and B-cell associated antigens like CD20. They are low grade B-cell lymphomas and are rarely aggressive. Histologically, lymphoid follicles will be enlarged and plenty, with a dense B–cell lymphocytic infiltrate, plasma cell infiltrate and lymphoepitheloid lesions. Clinically, they may present with bleeding due to ulceration or simply as thickened folds in endoscopy and CT. Majority of MALTomas are low-grade lesions, but some may progress to invasive lymphoma. EUS assesses the depth of involvement and wall layer disruption. Anti-*H. pylori* treatment with antibiotics seems to be curative for low-grade MALT lymphoma. EUS is useful in assessing the regression.

Pathological Types of GI Lymphomas

Pathologically, the three main types are:
1. Non-Hodgkin's lymphoma
2. Primary lymphoma associated with celiac disease (T-cell lymphoma)
3. Mediterranean lymphoma associated with α-chain disease.

Musshoff Classification of Ann Arbor Staging of Gastric Lymphomas

- **Stage IE**—stomach only
  - **Stage IE i**—involvement of mucosa and submucosa
  - **Stage IE ii**—involvement of stomach surpassing stage IEi
- **Stage IIE i**—perigastric nodes
- **Stage IIE ii**—para-aortic nodes
- **Stage III**—spleen
- **Stage IV**—distant sites (usually bone marrow)

'E' denotes extralymphatic involvement.

Diagnosis

Symptoms

- Epigastric pain
- Dyspepsia
- Upper GI bleed
- Constitutional symptoms
  - Weight loss
  - Fatigue
  - Fever
  - Night sweats
- Abdominal mass (rare)
- Anemia.

Investigations

- ***Endoscopy*** (upper GI) (**Fig. 11.16**) and ***biopsy*** (for histologic type of lymphoma and the presence of *H. pylori*) is most specific
- ***CT abdomen*** is useful for staging the disease
- ***Chest X-ray and bone marrow biopsy*** are useful in staging the disease.

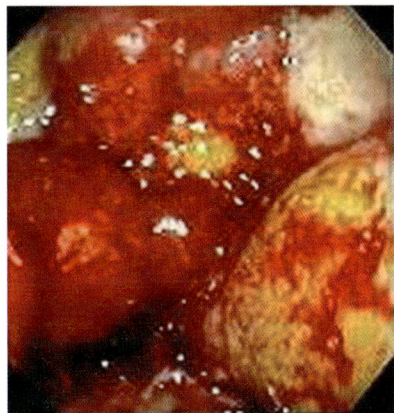

Fig. 11.16: Gastroscopy—Bleeding gastric lymphoma

Management

Since most gastric lymphomas are infected by *H. pylori*, a 2-week anti-*H. pylori* treatment is necessary, but high-grade lymphomas may not respond to therapy.

Low-grade Lymphomas
- Low-grade lymphomas resolve by *H. pylori* eradication
- Gastric MALT lymphomas which are negative for *H. pylori* or those infected with *H. pylori* not responding to bacterial eradication therapy require other methods of treatment
    - Radiotherapy (30 Gy in 150 cGy fractions over 4 weeks)
    - Oral cyclophosphamide—100 mg/day (6–12 months)
    - Monoclonal antibodies (rituximab (375 mg/m^2 weekly for 4 weeks).

High-grade Lymphomas

- *Stage IE*–*H. pylori* eradication (persistent disease needs R-CHOP therapy)
- *Stage II–IV*–R-CHOP therapy and bulky or residual tumor requires radiotherapy.

Clinical Pearls

- When Maltoma is superficial and of low histologic grade, *H. pylori* eradication cures in 90% of cases
- Some cases of conjunctival MALTomas have been reported to be associated with *H. pylori* infection
- The majority of gastric lymphomas are non-Hodgkin's lymphoma of B-cell origin. These tumors may range from well-differentiated, superficial involvement (MALT) to high-grade, large-cell lymphomas
- Sometimes, it is difficult to differentiate poorly differentiated high grade B-cell gastric lymphoma from gastric adenocarcinoma clinically or radiologically, yet histopathology with immunohistochemistry is recommended to stain specific markers on the malignant cell that favor the diagnosis of lymphoma. Immunohistochemistry stains specific clusters of differentiation that are present on B-cells like CD20. Cytokeratin is also a surface marker that is presented on epithelial cells, is stained histochemically and favors the diagnosis of epithelial tumors like adenocarcinoma
- Differentiating poorly differentiated gastric adenocarcinoma from lymphoma is a must because the prognosis and modalities of treatment differ significantly
- Other lymphomas involving the stomach include mantle cell lymphoma and T-cell lymphomas, which may be associated with

enteropathy; the latter usually occur commonly in the small bowel but have been reported in the stomach
- The clinical diagnosis of gastric lymphomas is almost impossible without a tissue biopsy
- *H. pylori* infection resistant to therapy needs a change in antibiotic
- Histologically, the resolution of MALT lymphoma require about 3–6 months or even longer. Repeat endoscopies are required every 3 months till complete resolution and this surveillance should be continued every 6–12 months as microscopic relapses are seen in about 20% of cases
- Histologic recurrent disease does not require active treatment at the first instance, and wait and watch approach may be sufficient, as they may resolve spontaneously
- Macroscopic recurrence after successful resolution is rare, unless there is recurrent *H. pylori* infection.

CONGENITAL PYLORIC STENOSIS

Introduction

- Congenital anomaly of babies of 2 to 4 weeks of age
- Stenosis of the pylorus due to muscle hypertrophy, which spasms when the stomach empties. **(Fig. 11.17)**
- First described by Hirschprung in 1888
- Ramstedt **(Fig. 11.18)** described the operative procedure in 1907
- 3/1000 live births
- More common in males in firstborn
- Associated with other congenital defects—TEF
- Elevated serum prostaglandins, reduced levels of pyloric nitric oxide synthetase and infant hypergastrinemia have been found.

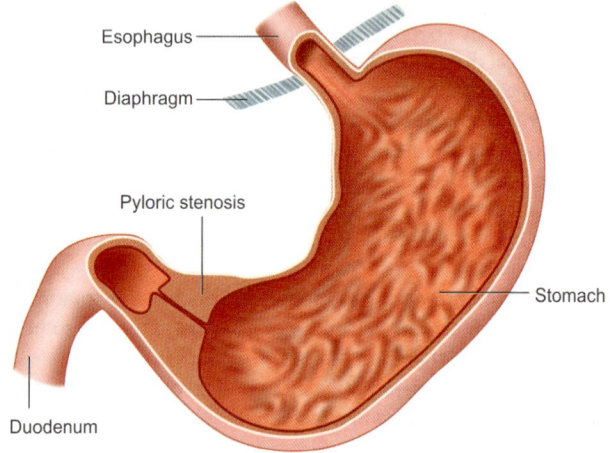

Fig. 11.17: Congenital pyloric stenosis

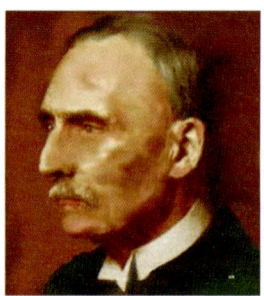

Fig. 11.18: Conrad Ramstedt

Etiology and Pathogenesis

- Cause not known
- Abnormal muscle innervation and maternal stress in third trimester are suggested.

Diagnosis

Symptoms

- Projectile *non-bilious vomiting* is a constant symptom
- After vomiting the infant is hungry and wants a feed.

Signs

- Dehydration and shrunken appearance
- A firm movable palpable lump of about 2 cm long (olive shaped) in the epigastrium
- Visible gastric peristalsis is prominent.

Investigations

- ***Ultrasonography*** is 90% specific—pyloric muscle thickness more than 4 mm and overall pyloric muscle length of 14 mm is diagnostic
- ***Barium meal*** (**Fig. 11.19**) shows the abrupt termination of contrast at the pylorus.

Management

Pyloromyotomy or Ramstedt's operation—pyloric muscle mass is cut without incising the mucosa (**Fig. 11.20**).

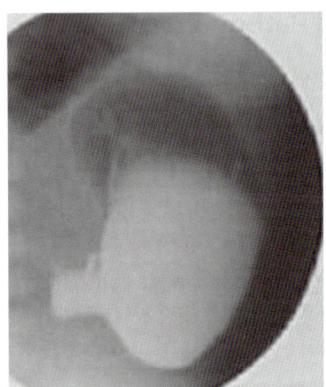

Fig. 11.19: Barium meal—Congenital pyloric stenosis

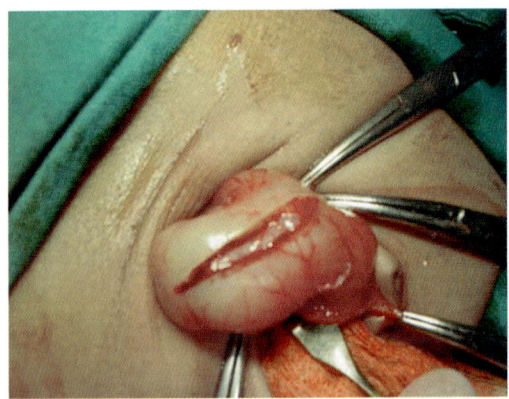

Fig. 11.20: Pyloromyotomy

INJURIES OF DUODENUM

Introduction

- Duodenum can be injured both by penetrating and non-penetrating abdominal trauma
- The duodenum can rupture:
  - ***Intraperitoneally*** and cause immediate chemical irritation of the peritoneum due to the highly alkaline duodenal content
  - ***Retroperitoneally*** (more common with blunt trauma such as steering wheel injuries).

Diagnosis

Symptoms and Signs

- ***Intraperitoneal rupture***
  - Abdominal pain, fever and distension with vomiting
  - Examination shows marked tenderness in the upper abdomen and later signs of generalized peritonitis.
- ***Retroperitoneal rupture***
  - Pain in the epigastrium and back, with pronounced vomiting
  - Testicular pain is a common feature of retroperitoneal rupture of duodenum.

Investigations

- ***X-ray abdomen*** may show air under the domes of diaphragm (intraperitoneal rupture) or large accumulation of air above the right kidney (retroperitoneal rupture). Diagnostic accuracy can be increased by injecting air in the Levine's tube to increase the air collections. Water soluble dye injections in the tube can make the diagnosis more precise
- ***CT with contrast*** is conclusive

- **Paracentesis** may show bile-stained fluid, if the rupture is intraperitoneal.

Management

- *Simple suturing* may be adequate in many cases
- *Supplementary gastroenterostomy* is required for large tears
- *Rarely, even a pancreatoduodenectomy* may be necessary for extensive trauma involving the periampullary region.

BEZOARS

Introduction

- Bezoars are collected or collection of undigested foreign material that accumulates and coalesce in the GIT, usually in the stomach.
    - *Phytobezoar*—vegetable matter
    - *Trichobezoar*—hair
    - *Pharmacobezoars*—medicines
    - *Lactobezoars*—milk and curd
    - *Trichophytobezoar*—hair and vegetable matter.

Diagnosis

Symptoms and Signs

- Chronic abdominal pain and vomiting may be present
- Acute pain may be predominant when obstruction occurs.

Investigations

- *Plain radiographs, US, barium meal* (Fig. 11.21), *and endoscopy* (Fig. 11.22) are diagnostic
- *CT* may be useful.

Stomach and Duodenum

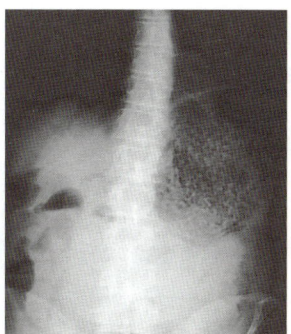

Fig. 11.21: Barium meal—Trichobezoar

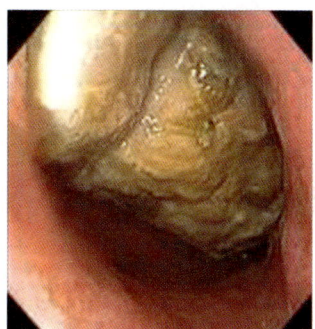

Fig. 11.22: Gastroscopy—Phytobezoar

Management

Medical

- Antacids
- Surfactants

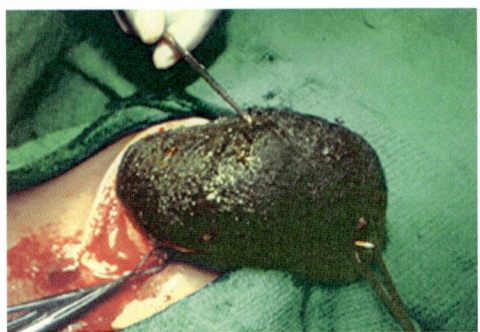

Fig. 11.23: Removal of trichobezoar by laparotomy
(*Courtesy:* Dr R Surendran)

- Cholestyramine
- ***Digestive agents*** (e.g. papain, cellulose) may be tried in dissolving vegetable matter.

Surgical

- ***Endoscopic or surgical removal* (Fig. 11.23)** may be necessary for hairballs.

DIEULAFOY'S ULCER

Introduction

It is a tiny mucosal ulcer forming over a very large submucosal blood vessel. The ulcer forms when the mucosa is compromised by the mechanical effects of the large vessel close to it. The usual sites of Dieulafoy's ulcer are:
- Proximal stomach (75%)

- Distal stomach (13%)
- Proximal duodenum (12%).

Diagnosis

Symptom

- Upper GI bleeding.

Investigation

- ***Endoscopy*** is the only method to diagnose the ulcer (**Fig 11.24**).

Management

- ***Endoscopic coagulation*** of bleeding vessel is the treatment of choice
- ***Heater probe, sclerotherapy, hemoclipping, band ligation and laser*** are effective modes of therapy

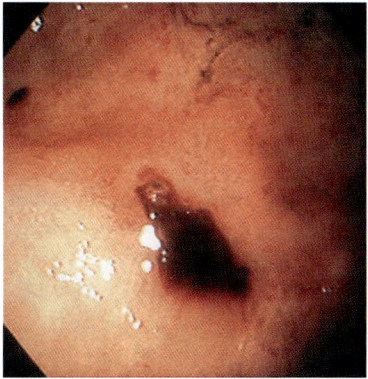

Fig. 11.24: Gastroscopy—Dieulafoy lesion

- When endoscopic treatment fails, ***surgery with limited wedge resection*** using intraoperative endoscopic guidance is appropriate.

MENETRIER'S DISEASE

Introduction

This disease is characterized by giant hypertrophic gastric folds, involving mainly the gastric fundus. It may be associated with hypochlorhydria, hypergastrinemia, hypoalbuminemia and excess mucus production.

Diagnosis

Symptoms and Signs

- Epigastric pain
- Nausea
- Anorexia
- Weight loss
- Peripheral edema

Investigations

- ***Gastroscopy and full thickness biopsy***—marked foveolar hyperplasia, glandular atrophy and increased mucosal thickness.

Management

Medical

- Proton pump inhibitors, corticosteroids, octreotide
- Monoclonal antibodies against EGF receptor.

Surgical
- Partial gastrectomy for refractory cases or severe hypoproteinemia or cancer.

BARIATRIC SURGERY

Introduction

Obesity is defined as the accumulation of excess body fat which is quantified as body mass index (BMI), weight in kilograms divided by height in meters square (kg/m^2).

Classification of Obesity

It is tabulated in **Table 11.8**.

Types of Bariatric Surgery Procedures (Fig. 11.25)

- *Restrictive procedures*
  - Laparoscopic adjustable gastric banding (LAGB)
  - Laparoscopic sleeve gastrectomy (LSG)
  - Vertical banded gastroplasty (VBG).

Table 11.8: Classification of obesity

Severity	Body mass index (BMI)
Overweight	25–29.9
Obesity (Class I)	30–34.9
Moderate obesity (Class II)	35–39.9
Severe obesity (Class III)	40–49.9
Super morbid obesity	>50

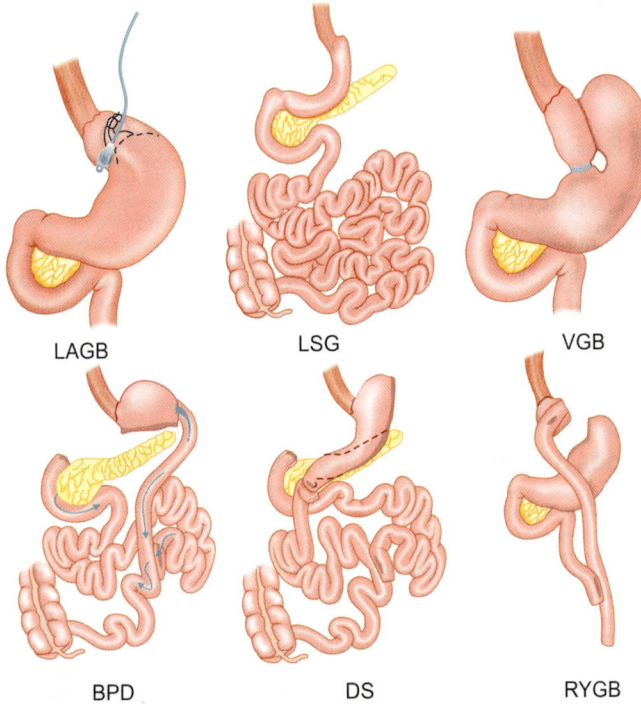

Fig. 11.25: Bariatric surgery procedures

- *Malabsorptive procedures*
  - Biliopancreatic diversion (BPD)
  - Duodenal switch (DS).
- *Combined procedures*
  - Roux-en-Y gastric bypass (RYGB).

Stomach and Duodenum

Indications for Bariatric Surgery

- BMI ≥ 40 kg/m^2
- BMI ≥ 35 kg/m^2 with significant obesity related comorbid conditions
- People in whom dietary attempts at weight control have been ineffective.

Advantages and Complications of LAGB

Advantages

- Gastric pouch can be adjusted to weight loss and symptoms (reflux, dysphagia, vomiting, maladaptive eating habits)
- Safest with least morbidity and mortality rates.

Complications

- Device related problems (band slippage, band erosion).

Advantages and Complications of LSG

Advantages

- Safe and simple procedure for high-risk patients
- No devices or ports used
- Patients are able to eat most types of food but in small quantities
- Incidence of dumping or malabsorption are less, as the stomach openings are intact
- Low complication rate.

Complications

- Strictures
- Bleeding
- Staple line leaks.

Complications of VBG

- Inferior weight loss
- Severe gastroesophageal reflux
- Nausea and vomiting.

Advantages and Complications of BPD

Advantages

- Excellent long-term weight loss
- Patients can consume relatively normal quantity of food
- Good resolution of comorbid conditions.

Complications

- Anastomotic leaks
- Bleeding
- Stenosis
- Marginal ulcers
- Bowel obstruction
- Protein calorie malnutrition
- Anemia
- Micronutrient deficiency
- Diarrhea
- Stomal ulceration
- Metabolic bone disease

Advantages and Complications of RYGB

Advantages

- Excellent long-term weight loss
- Patients can consume relatively normal quantity of food
- Good resolution of comorbid conditions.

Complications

- Anastomotic leaks
- Bleeding
- Stenosis
- Marginal ulcers
- Bowel obstruction
- Protein calorie malnutrition
- Anemia
- Micronutrient deficiency
- Diarrhea
- Stomal ulceration
- Metabolic bone disease

SURGERIES OF STOMACH AND DUODENUM (TABLE 11.9)

- Gastrostomy (connect stomach to the exterior) **(Fig. 11.26)**
- Gastrectomy (excision of stomach) **(Fig. 11.27)**
    - Upper partial (excision of upper half of stomach)
    - Lower partial (excision of lower half of stomach)
    - Subtotal (excision of lower 2/3 or 3/4 of stomach)
    - Total (excision of whole of stomach)
- Gastrotomy (opening and closing the stomach)
- Gastrojejunostomy (joining stomach and jejunum side to side) **(Fig. 11.28A)**

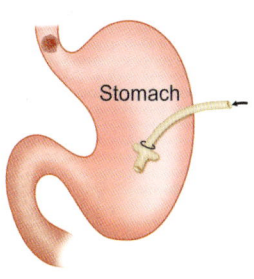

Fig. 11.26: Gastrostomy

Table 11.9: Varieties of gastric surgery

Procedure	Variety	Reconstruction	Indication
Gastrectomy (Removal of stomach)	Total gastrectomy (100%)	Esophagojejunostomy (Roux-en-Y)—End to end or end to side	Carcinoma of stomach (Fundus and body) (Linitis plastica) or multiple ulcers of stomach
	Upper partial gastrectomy (Upper 50%)	End to end esophago-gastrostomy	Carcinoma of stomach (Fundus)
	Subtotal gastrectomy (Lower 85%)	End to side gastrojejunostomy and duodenal stump closure (Billroth II)	Carcinoma of stomach (any part of the stomach excepting the fundus)
	Lower partial gastrectomy (Lower 50%)	End to side gastrojejunostomy and duodenal stump closure (Billroth II)	Benign ulcers of antrum, pylorus and I part of duodenum
		End to end gastroduodenostomy (Billroth I)	Benign ulcer disease of gastroduodenum
Excision of ulcer		Primary closure	Benign gastric ulcer
Gastrojejunostomy	Retrocolic	Side to side	Duodenal ulcer
	Antecolic	Side to side	Non-resectable malignancy of antrum and duodenum
Gastrostomy	Connect the stomach to the exterior		Feeding in oropharyngeal or esophageal obstructive lesions
Gastrotomy	Opening and closing the stomach		To remove foreign bodies or bezoars
Pyloroplasty	Pylorus relaxing operations	Gastroduodenostomy	To overcome the pyloric obstruction or as a drainage procedure

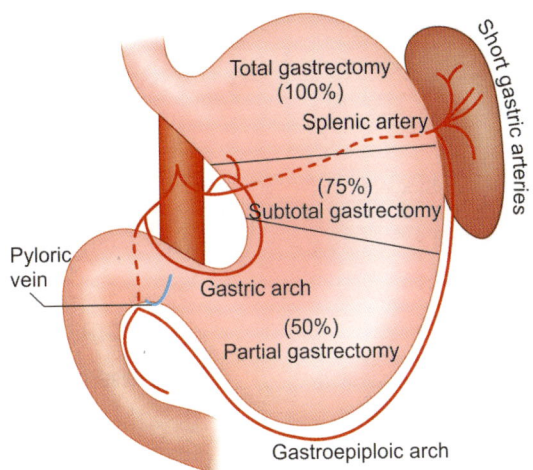

Fig. 11.27: Varieties of gastrectomies

- Pyloroplasty (relaxing procedure of pyloric sphincter) **(Fig. 11.28B)**
    - *Heinicke Mikulicz method*—pyloroduodenal incision is done in longitudinal axis and closed transversely **(Refer Fig. 11.7)**
    - *Finney's method*—gastroduodenostomy by separate incisions one in the stomach and the other in the duodenum **(Refer Fig. 11.8)**
    - *Jaboulay's method*—gastroduodenostomy by a curved single incision in the stomach and duodenum **(Refer Fig. 11.9)**.

Preoperative Management

The preoperative management of patients for surgery of the stomach is for any gastrointestinal surgery in general. The points to remember are:

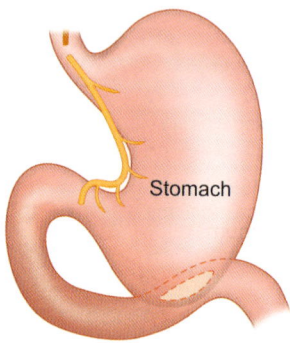

Fig. 11.28A: Gastrojejunostomy

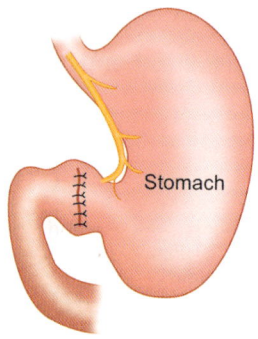

Fig. 11.28B: Pyloroplasty

- Nasogastric aspiration is required in patients with outlet obstructive lesions of the stomach, to keep the stomach decompressed so that the restoration of the gastric motility is not delayed in the postoperative period
- Since nasogastric aspiration is done on continuous basis for prolonged periods of time, replacement of water and electrolytes is important so that the imbalance is avoided, which may hamper the restoration of intestinal motility.

PARTIAL/SUBTOTAL GASTRECTOMY

Surgery Steps (Figs 11.29A and B)

Incision: Upper midline (most popular)
- Good exposure of abdominal cavity

- Step 1—Division of greater omentum and entry into the lesser sac and assess resectability
- Step 2—Mobilization of greater curvature and marking the line of resection on the stomach
- Step 3—Division of left gastroepiploic vessels at the marked place
- Step 4—Division of right gastroepiploic vessels at its origin from gastroduodenal artery
- Step 5—Division of right gastric vessels
- Step 6—Division and closure of duodenum
- Step 7—Division of gastrohepatic omentum
- Step 8—Division of left gastric artery

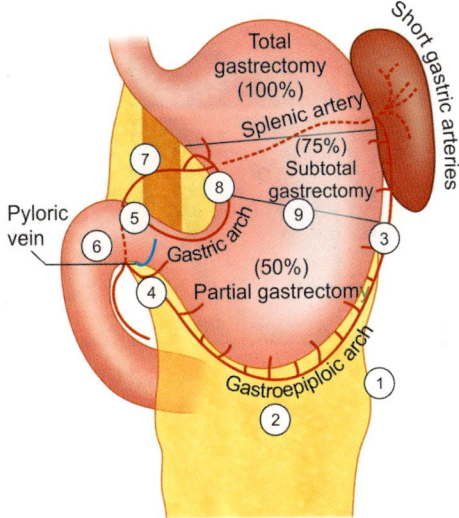

Fig. 11.29A: Surgical procedure

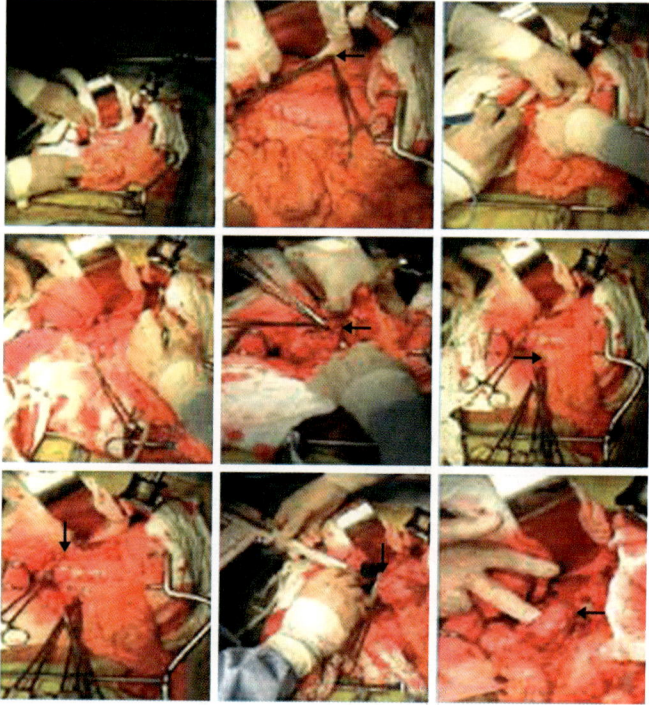

Fig. 11.29B: Steps of gastrectomy

- Step 9—Transection of stomach and removal of resected stomach
- Establishment of pathway by reconstruction.

The stomach can also be removed after the gastrojejunal anastomosis.

Reconstructions after Gastrectomy

After removal of stomach, the continuity is established in many ways. They are:
- After partial gastrectomy, end to end gastroduodenostomy (Billroth I) or end to side gastrojejunostomy (Billroth II) **(Fig. 11.30A)**

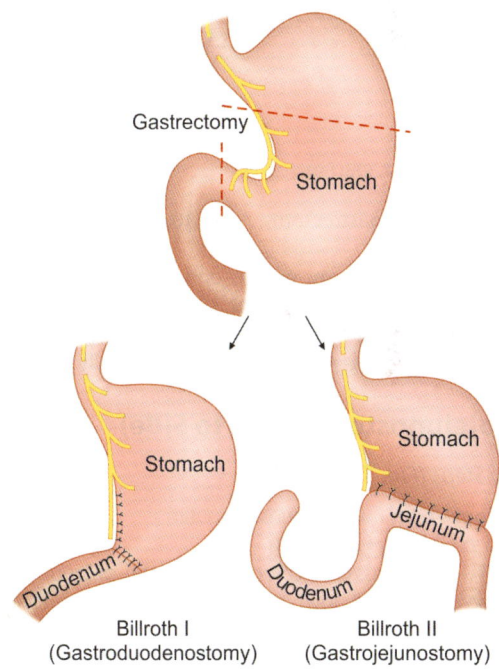

Fig. 11.30A: Methods of reconstructions after gastrectomy

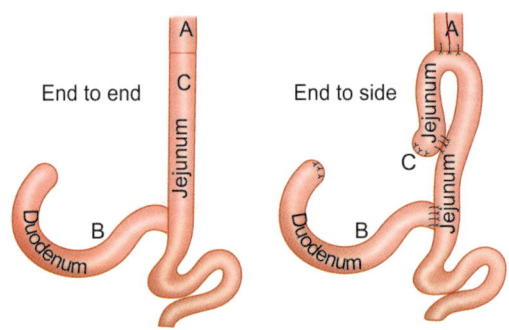

Fig. 11.30B: Esophagojejunostomy (Roux-en-Y)

- After subtotal gastrectomy, end to side gastrojejunostomy (Billroth II)
- After total gastrectomy, end to end or end to side esophagojejunostomy (Roux-en-Y) **(Fig.11.30B)**

The steps for open procedure are shown in **Fig. 11.31A** and the same procedure can be performed laparoscopically **(Fig. 11.31B)**.

Gastrojejunostomy (Side to Side)

Surgery Steps (Fig. 11.31A)

- **Incision:** Upper midline (most popular)
- Good exposure of abdomen
- Step 1—the transverse colon is lifted, the posterior surface of stomach is brought down through a rent in the transverse colon created to the right of middle colic artery
- Step 2—the jejunum is picked at the antimesenteric border and kept along with the posterior surface of stomach **(Fig. 11.31A1)**

Stomach and Duodenum

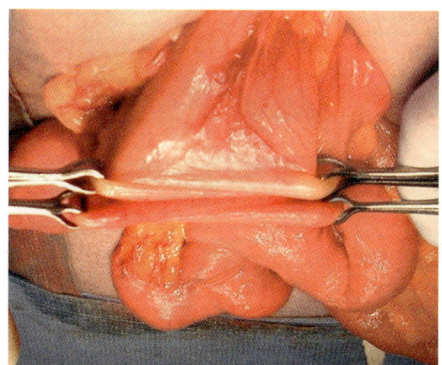

Fig. 11.31A1: Approximation of stomach and jejunum

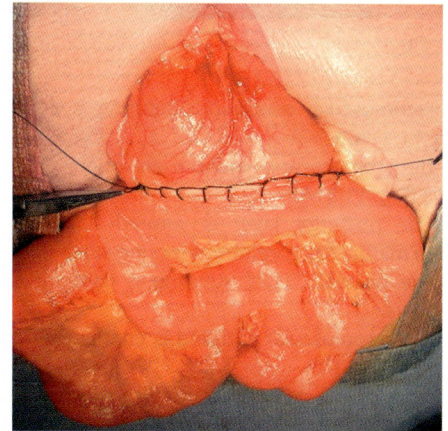

Fig. 11.31A2: Seromuscular suturing

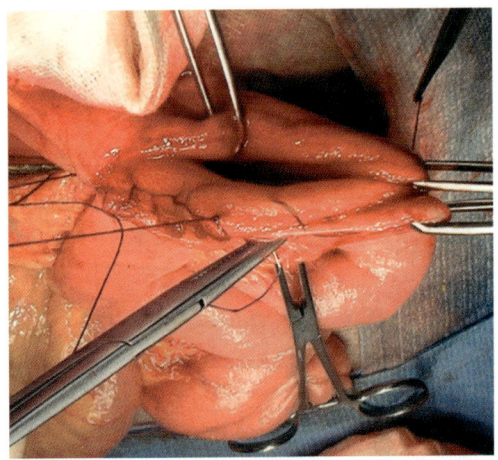

Fig. 11.31A3: Opening of stomach and jejunum

- Step 3—seromuscular continuous suturing is done for about 7 cm (**Fig. 11.31A2**)
- Step 4—the stomach and jejunum are opened lateral to the suture line (**Fig. 11.31A3**)
- Step 5—the posterior layer is sutured full thickness with absorbable material as continuous locking stitch (**Fig. 11.31A4**)
- Step 6—the posterior layer suturing is continued along the anterior layers
- Step 7—the seromuscular suturing is continued from the first layer (**Fig. 11.31A5**)
- Step 8—stomach is fixed to the transverse mesocolon to prevent internal herniation (**Fig 11.31A6**).

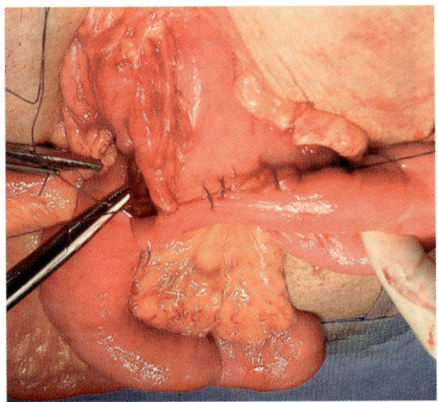

Fig. 11.31A4: Full thickness suturing of both layers

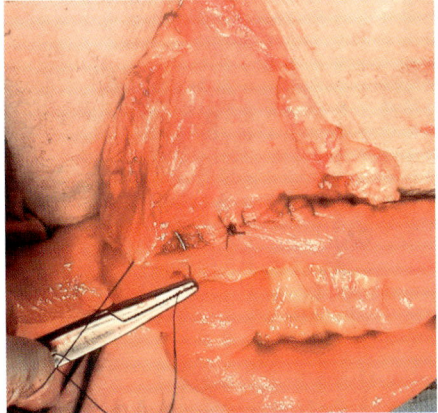

Fig. 11.31A5: Completion of anastomosis

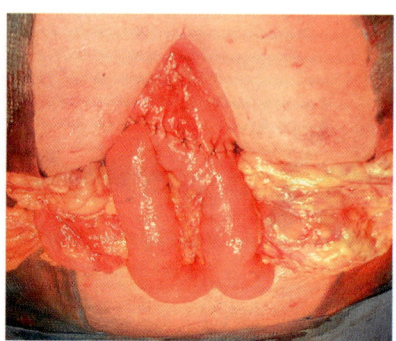

Fig. 11.31A6: Completed anastomosis and fixed to transverse mesocolon

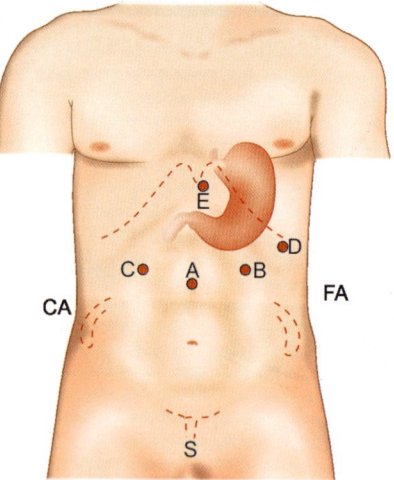

Fig. 11.31B1: Ports for gastrectomy

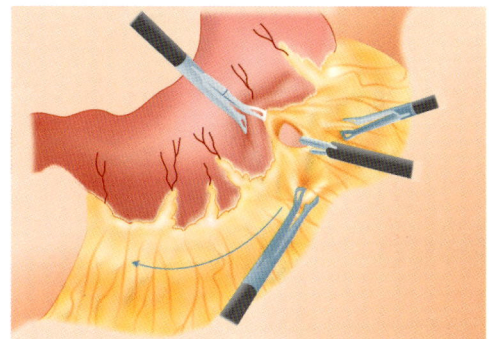

Fig. 11.31B2: Division of left gastroepiploic vessel

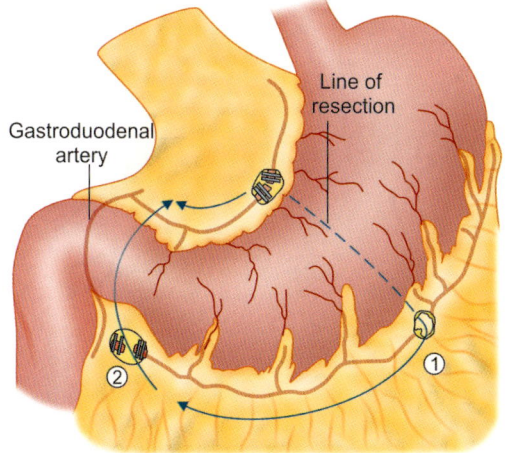

Fig. 11.31B3: Progression of steps

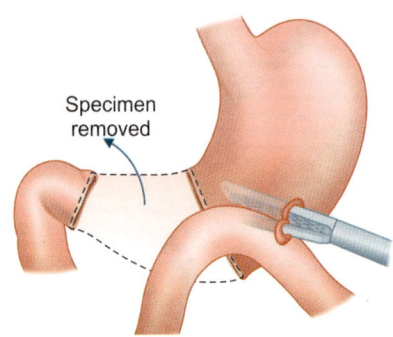

Fig. 11.31B4: Gastrojejunostomy after removal of distal stomach

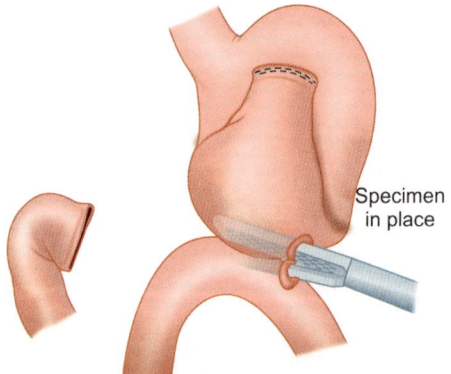

Fig. 11.31B5: Gastrojejunostomy before removal of distal stomach

The Billroth II reconstruction (end to side gastrojejunostomy) follows the same principles of side to side gastrojejunostomy, and the gastrectomy with Billroth II reconstruction can be done

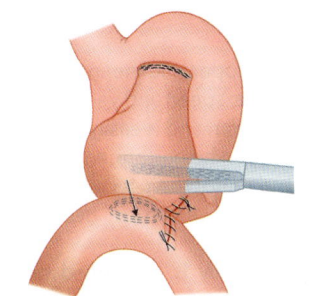

Fig. 11.31B6: Removal of distal stomach after GJ

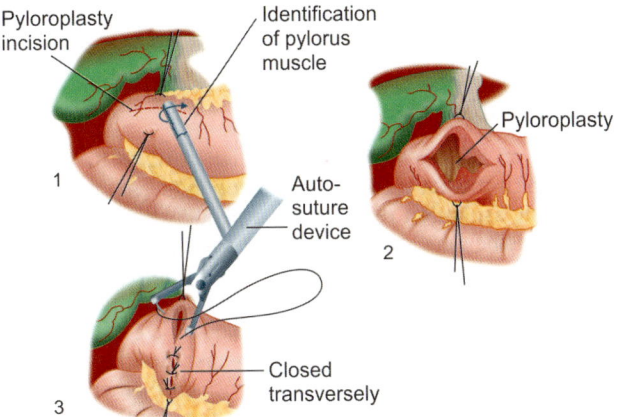

Fig. 11.31C: Laparoscopic pyloroplasty

laparoscopically (**Fig 11.31B**). So also, the pyloroplasty can be done laparoscopically (**Fig 11.31C**).

Clinical Pearls

- During laparotomy, upper midline incision is preferred as it has the advantage of ease, speed and versatility and allows access to stomach and duodenum and is easily extendable when needed
- All the anastomosis can be performed by hand sewn and stapled techniques and by laparoscopic technique
- No ligation of blood vessels is needed in simple gastrojejunostomy
- When gastrojejunostomy is performed behind the transverse colon, it is called retrocolic posterior gastrojejunostomy (anastomosis of posterior surface of stomach to jejunum), and when it is done anterior to the transverse colon, it is called antecolic anterior gastrojejunostomy (anastomosis of anterior surface of stomach to jejunum).

Postoperative Management

A period of ileus is anticipated in the postoperative period, during which the patient is maintained on intravenous fluids, and **nasogastric aspiration** regularly for a period of about 48 hours. The nasogastric tube can be removed when bowel sounds return, the volume of aspirate drops below 500 mL and there is passage of flatus. *Peristalsis returns to the small bowel before the stomach and colon regain their motility*. Clear liquids are begun and if tolerated, the diet is advanced to normal intake over the next 2 days. If restoration of oral feeding is delayed, consider whether a period of parenteral nutrition would be appropriate. Remove the drain when fluid loss diminishes, generally at 2–3 days.

- **Intravenous fluids** are maintained until the patient is taking sufficient fluids orally.

- **Urinary catheter** is normally discontinued between the second and fourth day of surgery.
- **Antibiotic prophylaxis** is continued for 24 hours in clean cases and continued for a reasonable time of about 5–7 days in contaminated cases till the evidence of sepsis disappears.
- **Intra-abdominal drains** kept near the anastomosis are removed when the motility of the bowel returns to normal with the passage of flatus and or feces. If there is evidence of infection or sepsis without an obvious etiology, the surgeon must **suspect a leaked anastomosis**.
- Patients who have generally recovered sufficiently, are discharged 6–8 days after surgery.

COMPLICATIONS OF GASTRIC SURGERY AND MANAGEMENT

All gastric surgeries derange gastric function, and during the first few weeks or months after surgery, almost all patients experience some adverse effects, which may be mild or severe, depending on the type of operation. In most patients, symptoms decrease with time due to physiological and psychological adaptation. For this reason, the outcome and sequelae of gastric surgery should be assessed at least 6 months after surgery, or even later.

Post-gastrectomy syndromes appear as combinations of signs and symptoms brought about primarily by the changes in the motor function of the stomach and upper small bowel secondary to the operations.

---

*Proximal gastric vagotomy impairs the compliance of proximal stomach and decreases its reservoir function

The motor functions of the stomach include:
- Accept and store bolus of ingested food—contributed by vagal function*
- Reduce large particles to smaller size—Peristalsis of stomach and pylorus**
- Transport the food into small bowel for further digestion and absorption—intact pylorus and activation of neural and hormonal mechanisms provided by the upper small bowel.***

There are unfortunately few specific tests, and those that are specific are of little help in clinical practice. Thus, a careful history is still the most reliable way of making a diagnosis on which to base treatment.

Post-gastrectomy complications can be classified as early and late. Early complications occur in the early postoperative period that is, within a week after surgery. They are given in **Box 11.2**.

> **Box 11.2:** Early complications of gastric surgery (Fig. 11.31D)
> - Early intragastric hemorrhage
> - Late intragastric hemorrhage
> - Extragastric hemorrhage
> - Duodenal stump leakage
> - Anastomotic leak
> - Gastric remnant necrosis
> - Stomal obstruction
> - Acute afferent loop obstruction
> - Jejunal loop herniation
> - Intra-abdominal abscess
> - Postoperative pancreatitis

**Removal of gastric segments impairs this function.
***Distal gastric vagotomy and distal gastric resection including pyloric resection decrease the mechanical-digestive function, removal of pylorus may allow reflux of intestinal contents into the stomach and varieties of gastroenterostomy may mechanically or functionally affect transporting function of the stomach.

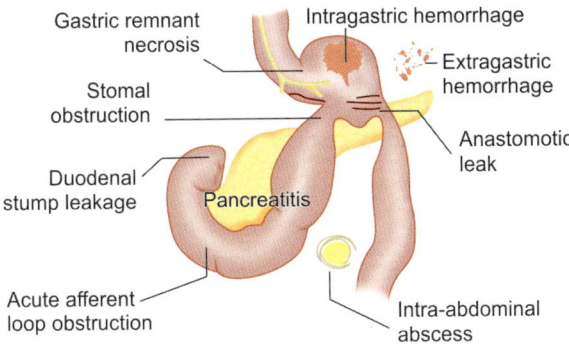

Fig. 11.31D: Early complications of gastrectomy

Early Intragastric Hemorrhage

Introduction

This complication is a sequel to the bleeding from a site in the anastomotic area (more common) or a small bleeding ulcer in the proximal gastric pouch.

Diagnosis

Symptoms and Signs

Immediately after gastric resection, it is usual to aspirate bloody or blood-stained fluid from the nasogastric tube. The color should clear in about 48 hours and the aspirate should become bilious in nature. The persistence of bloody aspirate beyond 48 hours is a major concern and needs to be attended to.

Investigation

It is difficult to assess the amount of blood loss by measuring the bloody nasogastric aspirate, as there may be retained blood clots in the stomach, which cannot be aspirated, and also some blood is bound to travel down the intestine.

Management

Medical

a. Ice cold saline lavage
b. Blood transfusions.

Surgical

Reoperation should not be postponed when faced with continuous bleeding. The gastric pouch should be opened much above the gastroenterostomy or gastroduodenostomy using a transverse incision and blood clots should be evacuated. Saline irrigations are done and enough suction should be applied to clear the stomach pouch well. Manual pressure on the distended gastric pouch is quite effective in evacuating the clots. Saline irrigations and moist saline packs are applied to the gastric mucosa to remove small clots and debris. *Care should be taken not to damage the mucosa while suction, especially the use of metal tips, as it may result in diffuse gastric mucosal bleeding.* The bleeding site is usually a single vessel at the lesser curvature or at the anastomosis. A single *'figure of 8'* suture will usually control the bleeding. The nasogastric aspiration should be done to clear the blood remnants and the tube flushed well to be sure that the aspirate is clear or only mildly tinged.

Delayed Intragastric Hemorrhage

Introduction

Such bleeding may result from a duodenal ulcer deliberately not removed or from inadequate undersewing of a bleeding ulcer at the time of original operation.

Diagnosis

Clinical Presentation

Intraluminal bleeding may occur in the recovery room or several days postoperatively, after removal of the nasogastric tube, presenting in the form of hematemesis and melena.

Investigations

It is difficult to assess the amount of blood loss by nasogastric aspirate, as there may be retained blood clots in the stomach, which cannot be aspirated, and also some blood is bound to travel down the intestine. Gastroduodenoscopy may be done, if it is more than 15 days after surgery.

Management

Medical

a. Ice cold saline lavage
b. Blood transfusions

Endoscopic

Coagulation of the bleeding vessel is possible through endoscope.

Surgical

Reoperation should not be postponed when faced with continuous bleeding, in spite of medical management. The patient's general condition should be assessed very closely and if hemorrhage does not abate even after three units of blood transfusion, reoperation should be done. The decision demands sound surgical judgment and has various alternatives. They are:

a. For the bleeding ulcers distal to the point of resection in the retrobulbar duodenum, a *Horsley's slit* (**Fig. 11.32**) on the

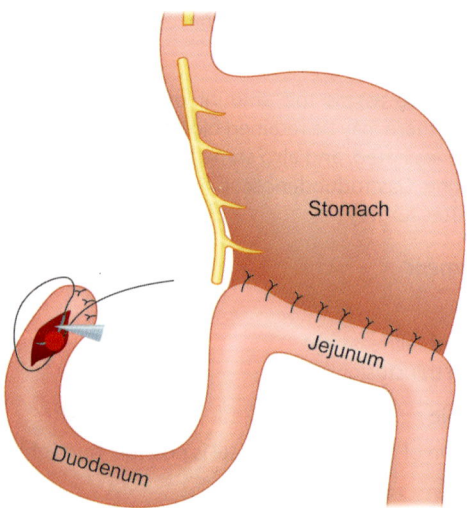

Fig. 11.32: Horsley's slit and oversewing of ulcer

Stomach and Duodenum

anterior duodenal wall is done to gain access to the ulcer crater and obliterate the ulcer with several "figure of 8" sutures with 2–0 silk.

b. Billroth II reconstruction or Roux-en-Y diversion if the gastric chyme is to be prevented to traverse the duodenal outflow.
c. If the original operation is Billroth I reconstruction, the revision surgery should be Billroth II reconstruction or Roux-en-Y diversion.
d. If the original operation is Billroth II reconstruction or primary Roux-en-Y reconstruction, the duodenal stump is reopened, the bleeding ulcer transfixed, and either **catheter duodenostomy (Fig. 11.33)**

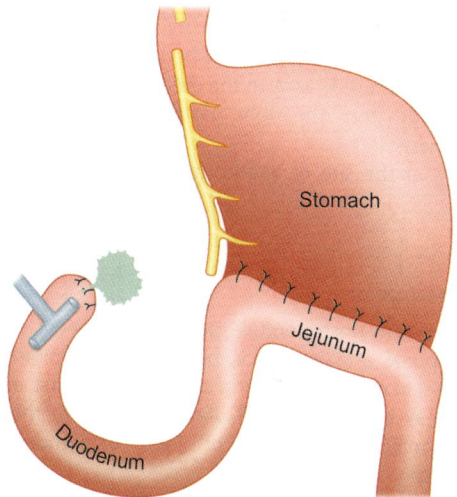

Fig. 11.33: Catheter duodenostomy for duodenal stump leakage

or reclosure of the duodenal stump is performed depending upon the duodenal tissue's appearance and integrity.
e. If the original operation is pyloroplasty, antral resection with removal or suture control of the ulcer, followed by either a Billroth I, Billroth II or Roux-en-Y reconstruction.

Extragastric Hemorrhage

Introduction

Hemorrhage from outside the stomach or intraperitoneal hemorrhage can occur in the first 48–72 hours due to:
1. Laceration of spleen
2. Injury to the liver by the use of retractors
3. Injury to the vasa brevia
4. Hemorrhage from the pancreatic bed
5. Improperly secured vessel in the greater or lesser omentum.
6. Hemorrhage from the right gastric artery and right gastro-epiploic vessels.
7. Bleeding at the site of vagotomy from the subdiaphragmatic vessels.

Diagnosis

Clinical Presentation

In the immediate postoperative period, the patient may present with rapid pulse, a falling blood pressure and diminished urinary output. The skin may be moist and clammy and at first, a myocardial infarction may be suspected. If drains are kept in the peritoneal cavity, they may show drainage of bloody or blood-stained fluid, and *clear nasogastric aspirate.*

Stomach and Duodenum

Investigations

CT scan of the abdomen is useful in such circumstances.

Management

If vital signs are not promptly restored after four units of blood, exploratory laparotomy is indicated. The splenic laceration is sutured and all attempts should be made to preserve the spleen unless a major splenic fracture or multiple fractures are present. The bleeding vessel if any, is identified and ligated.

Duodenal Stump Leakage

Introduction

One of the serious complications that may follow Billroth II gastrectomy. Several factors are responsible for the duodenal stump leakage. They are:
- Severely diseased and scarred duodenal bulb precluding adequate closure
- Excessive suture closure leading to tissue necrosis
- Postoperative pancreatitis with acute inflammatory exudate in the area of the closed stump, which may retard stump healing
- Poor nutritional state
- Improper surgical technique
- Localized infection and sepsis.

Diagnosis

Clinical Presentation

These patients present with a bile leak through the drain left near the closed duodenal stump. This occurs usually from the 2nd to 5th postoperative day. The patient experiences severe abdominal pain and fever, and a shock-like picture. Sometimes, symptoms may be relatively subtle, with only a moderate degree of pain, fever and leukocytosis, rarely with jaundice.

Investigations

The leak may be demonstrated by CT scan, which may reveal intraluminal fluid or gas in the right upper abdomen.

Management

It consists of the establishment of prompt and adequate sump drainage of the right upper quadrant, along with internal drainage of the afferent jejunal loop via either a tube gastrostomy, jejunostomy or nasogastric intubation. A catheter duodenostomy (**Fig. 11.33**) may be performed. *The aim is to create a controlled external fistula.* Exploration and corrective surgery may be needed if obstruction is identified.

Clinical Pearl

Although the morbidity is high following a duodenal stump fistula, with prompt diagnosis and surgical drainage, most cases recover and the prognosis is favorable.

Suture Line Leak

This occurs when the gastroduodenal or gastrojejunal anastomosis is performed in the presence of a severely diseased and scarred duodenum or jejunum, due to jeopardized blood supply.

Diagnosis

Clinical Presentation

These patients present with a bile stained fluid leak through the drain left near the anastomosis. This occurs usually from the 2nd to 5th postoperative day. The symptoms may be relatively subtle, with only a moderate degree of pain, fever and leukocytosis.

Investigations

Gastrograffin study may be done. The leak may be demonstrated by CT scan, which may reveal intraluminal fluid or gas in the right upper abdomen.

Management

Medical

Small leaks cease by 24–48 hours and need only nasogastric suction and supportive therapy.

Surgical

Failure of medical management warrants surgical intervention.
- If the leak is minimal or moderate with minimal signs of peritoneal irritation, and not responding to medical management, the rent may be closed with an omental patch.
- If the rent or the disruption and the leak are large, with closure of the rent, Billroth I reconstruction should be converted into Billroth II or a Roux-en-Y, supplemented by a feeding jejunostomy.
- If the original operation is pyloroplasty, distal gastric resection with closure of the duodenal stump with either a Billroth II or Roux-en-Y reconstruction, as Billroth I reconstruction would not

be feasible due to edema and reaction at the pyloroplasty site. Suture obliteration of the pyloroplasty with gastrojejunostomy is an option.

Clinical Pearls

- The leakage from a gastroduodenal anastomosis is associated with less morbidity than the duodenal stump leakage
- Leaks from gastrojejunostomy and pyloroplasty are very unusual.

Gastric Remnant Necrosis

Introduction

This occurs due to the ischemic necrosis of the gastric remnant due to ligation of the left gastric artery at its base and a concomitant splenectomy. With only phrenic arterial branches intact, the remnant is severely devascularized. When the left inferior phrenic artery itself arises from the left gastric artery, necrosis becomes inevitable.

Diagnosis

Clinical Presentation

These patients present with a drainage of dark brown fluid through the drain kept near the anastomosis. This occurs usually from the 2nd to 3rd postoperative day. The patient experiences severe abdominal pain and fever, and presents a shock-like picture.

Investigations

- *Endoscopy and gastrograffin* examination would be useful
- *CT* may be useful.

Management

Treatment is always surgical and the available options are:
a. When there is a small viable proximal gastric remnant, excision of gangrenous segment with Roux–en-Y (side to side gastrojejunostomy) reconstruction is made (**Fig. 11.34A**).
b. When the entire gastric remnant has questionable viability, total gastrectomy with esophagojejunostomy (Roux-en-Y) should be performed (**Fig. 11.34B**).
c. If the necrosis extends to the esophagus, cervical esophagostomy + feeding jejunostomy is performed followed by colonic interposition through the substernal route, at a later date (**Fig. 11.34C**).

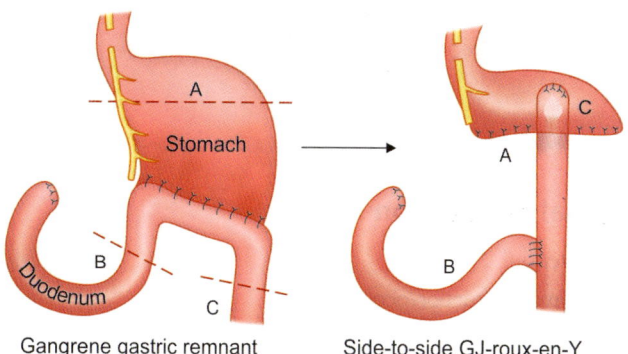

Fig. 11.34A: Side-to-side Roux-en-Y gastrojejunostomy

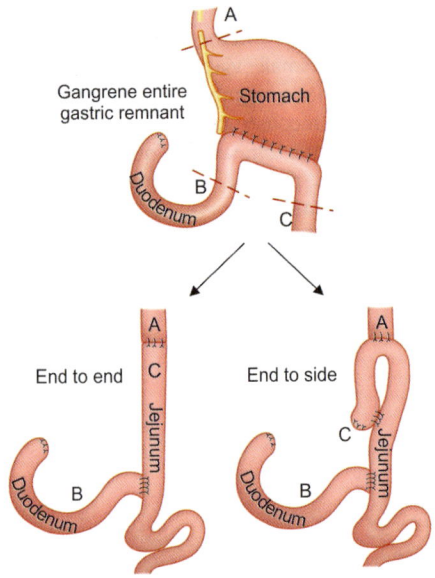

Fig. 11.34B: Esophagojejunostomy (Roux-en-Y)

Stomal obstruction

Introduction

The stomal obstruction occurs due to:
- Stomal edema
- Improper surgical technique
- Extensive duodenal pathology

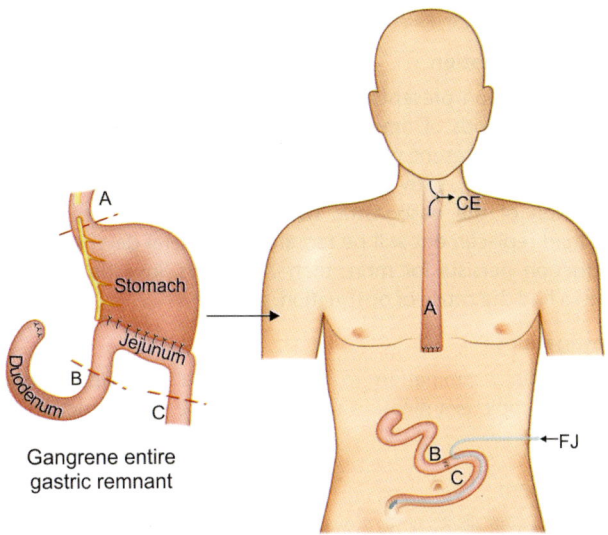

Fig. 11.34C: Cervical esophagostomy, jejunojejunostomy with feeding jejunostomy

- Postoperative suture line bleeding
- Anastomotic leakage
- Acute pancreatitis
- Inflammatory adhesions (after Billroth II reconstruction)
- Mesocolic herniation involving the afferent and efferent loops
- Extensive fat necrosis
- Inflamed omentum.

Diagnosis

Clinical Presentation

This complication presents with excessive nasogastric aspirate for prolonged periods of time. When the nasogastric tube has been removed, they present with upper abdominal discomfort, nausea and or vomiting, with inadequate gastric emptying, requiring reinsertion of the nasogastric tube. Continuous decompression with fluid replacement will be required for several days. When the obstruction persists for more than 7–10 days, investigations are done to find the cause of obstruction.

Investigations

Gastrograffin examination to determine the emptying pattern and endoscopic examination to find the cause of obstruction are required.

Management

Most cases will recover by conservative management, continuous nasogastric suction and intravenous fluids for several days, unless there is mechanical obstruction.

When the recovery takes more than 2 weeks, it is wise to operate. The options are:

a. To relieve the obstruction after a Billroth I reconstruction, dismantle the gastroduodenostomy and redo the same, or convert to Bilroth II or Roux-en-Y reconstruction.
b. To relieve the obstruction after a Billroth II reconstruction,
   – If kinking and adhesions are found, they are released and a feeding jejunostomy is performed
   – If both afferent and efferent loops are found herniated into the lesser sac, they are reduced and preventive measures taken

- If either loop be found non-viable, resection with Roux-en-Y reconstruction is done.

Acute Afferent Loop Obstruction

The commonest cause of leakage of a closed duodenal stump is afferent loop obstruction. The obstruction causes the intraduodenal pressure to raise as it becomes a closed loop, and when the pressure goes beyond the pancreatic ductal pressure, the serum amylase levels raise.

The reasons for mechanical obstruction of the afferent loop are:
a. Twist of the afferent loop
b. Volvulus of the afferent loop
c. Internal herniation
d. Jejunogastric intussusception
e. Kink at the gastrojejunostomy site.

Diagnosis

Clinical Presentation

The patient presents with severe upper abdominal pain, tenderness of the upper abdomen, leukocytosis, tachycardia and also shock like picture in the early postoperative period.

Investigations

Radiology

- *Gastrograffin meal* will show the non-entry of the contrast into the afferent loop
- *CT scan* may aid the diagnosis
- *A plain film* may reveal the presence of an enormously dilated afferent loop.

Endoscopy
- ***Endoscopy*** is rarely of help in diagnosis.

Management

Exploration will be needed and the treatment will depend upon the operative findings.
- If the patient is seriously ill, ***simple enteroenterostomy*** between the afferent and the efferent loops should be enough to decompress the afferent loop—***duodenojejunostomy*** **(Fig. 11.35)**
- If the patient is not seriously ill, and there is enough time for definitive surgery, and if a volvulus or a kink in the long afferent loop is found, the loop may be shortened and reanastomosed **(Fig. 11.36)**, or simply the afferent loop be divided near the gastroenterostomy stoma and a Roux-en-Y reconstruction **(Fig. 11.37)** is done

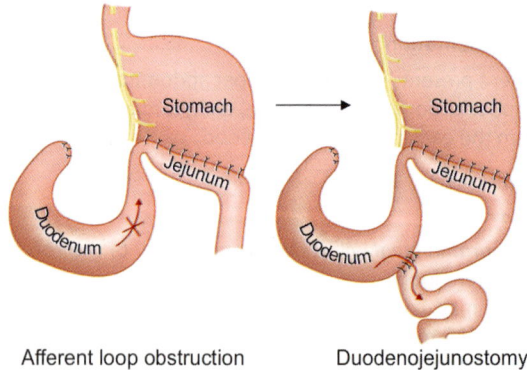

Afferent loop obstruction   Duodenojejunostomy

Fig. 11.35: Simple enteroenterostomy (duodenojejunostomy)

Stomach and Duodenum

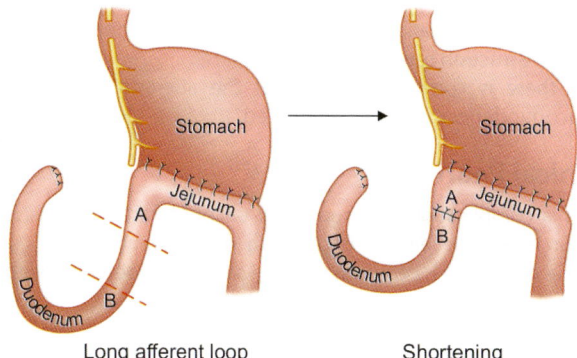

Fig. 11.36: Shortening of afferent loop and end-to-end anastomosis

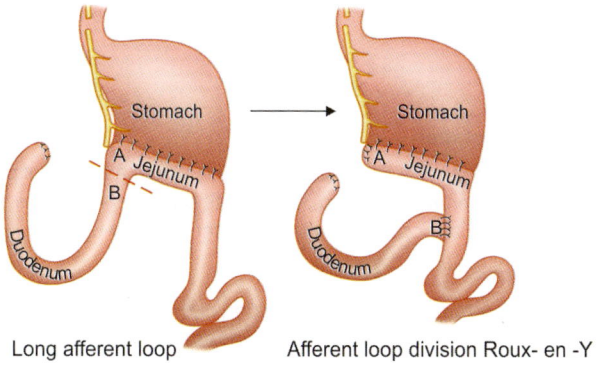

Fig. 11.37: Division of afferent loop and Roux-en-Y reconstruction

- If there is a delay in diagnosis and if the distal part of the afferent loop is found gangrenous, it may be resected and a Roux-en-Y reconstruction is done
- If there is complete necrosis of the afferent loop, pancreaticoduodenectomy will be required.

Clinical Pearls

- This complication is infrequently encountered today, as many surgeons have learnt not to leave a long afferent loop
- The raised levels of serum amylase should not deter the surgeon from operating on these patients.

Jejunal Loop (Efferent Loop) Herniation

Either the afferent or efferent jejunal loop may herniate behind the gastrojejunal anastomosis. When the afferent loop is fashioned short, the efferent loop may herniate to cause obstruction. If the afferent loop is long, it itself may herniate posterior to the efferent loop.

Diagnosis

Clinical Presentation

The patient presents with epigastric fullness, upper abdominal pain, nausea and vomiting, between 3rd and 7th postoperative days, but it is more prone to occur during the long-term follow-up.

Investigations

Gastrograffin study will show obstruction of the efferent loop, when supplemented by the CT scan, the diagnosis should be easy.

Management

Re-exploration is needed and during the surgery, the options available are:
- If the afferent loop is long, it should be divided at the gastroenterostomy and Roux-en-Y reconstruction is done (**Fig. 11.37**)
- If the efferent loop is gangrenous, it will require division and anastomosis (**Fig. 11.38**), or a Roux-en-Y reconstruction (**Fig. 11.39**).

Clinical Pearl

This complication can be prevented by fixing both the afferent and efferent loops to the parietal peritoneum during the first surgery.

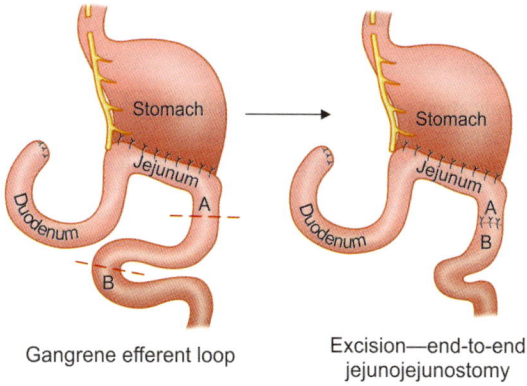

Fig. 11.38: Excision of gangrenous efferent loop and end to end anastomosis

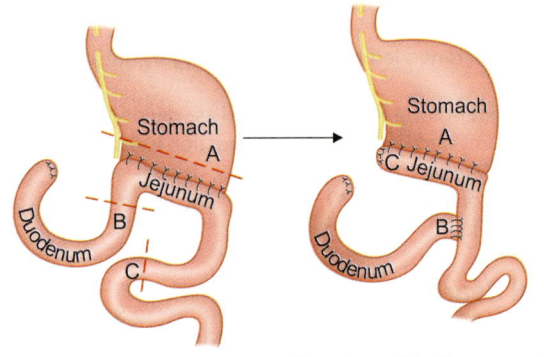

Gangrene efferent loop   Excision – GJ - Roux - en - Y

Fig. 11.39: Excision of efferent loop with Roux-en-Y reconstruction

Intra-Abdominal Abscess

Introduction

This complication occurs due to the spillage of duodenal, gastric or jejunal contents, into the peritoneal cavity. Anastomotic leaks are also a frequent cause of intra-bdominal abscess formation.

Diagnosis

Clinical Presentation

The patient presents with general malaise and the recovery and convalescence is not in a normal manner. The patient may be febrile. The acute picture may be subdued by the administration of antibiotics. Physical examination may not be of any value in most cases.

Investigations
- ***Leukocytosis*** may be present
- ***US and CT scan*** help in diagnosis and localizing the abscesses.

Management

The abscess should be drained early before the patient's condition deteriorates, and also prevent a general peritonitis which in turn deteriorate the condition. The drainage may be done either (1) transabdominally or posteriorly depending upon its location or (2) by percutaneous aspiration or catheter drainage under US or CT guidance, and by administration of appropriate antibiotics.

Clinical Pearl

Small spillages of the stomach, duodenal or jejunal contents into the peritoneum during the surgical procedures rarely lead to intraperitoneal sepsis and resolve in due course of time.

Postoperative Pancreatitis

Introduction

The inflammation of the pancreas can result due to
- Operative trauma to the head and proximal part of the pancreas
- Extensive dissections of the supracolic compartment.

Both create trauma to the pancreatic ductile system, which results in the escape of pancreatic juice into the peritoneal cavity, which causes local peritonitis. Only rarely, it is of the hemorrhagic variety.

Diagnosis

Clinical Presentation

- The patient presents with restlessness, diffuse abdominal pain, fever, abdominal tenderness and leukocytosis, within the first few postoperative days
- The patient may be seriously ill and may even die.

Investigations

Markedly elevated serum amylase level is diagnostic. CT scan is useful in determining the pancreatic inflammation and localization of abscesses.

Management

Medical

- Continuous nasogastric suction, fluid and electrolyte management, antibiotics, somatostatin or its analogue (octreotide).

Surgical

- The abscesses should be drained without hesitation.
- Extensive intraperitoneal drainage, debridement may also be needed.

Clinical Pearls

- Though unusual, external pancreatic fistulae can occur and need to be managed. If pseudocyst results, it may have to be drained internally, into the stomach (cystogastrostomy), duodenum (cystoduodenostomy) or a Roux-en-Y limb depending on its anatomic location.

Postoperative Jaundice

Introduction

Jaundice in the postoperative period occurs due to:
- Postoperative edema in the duodenal area, which may produce a transient and partial obstruction of the intrapancreatic part of the common bile duct
- Anastomotic leaks and the absorption of bile from the peritoneal cavity
- Overlooked common bile duct stones
- Accidental occlusion or division of the common bile duct
- Intravascular lysis
- Ascending cholangitis
- Sepsis.

Diagnosis

Clinical Presentation

The patient presents with mild icterus in the early postoperative period, which usually resolves in a few days, if there is no mechanical obstruction.

Investigations

Elevated levels of conjugated bilirubin will establish jaundice. The nature and level of obstruction may be determined by the US or CT scans.

Management

Medical

When no obstruction is demonstrated, medical management is advocated. Adequate antibiotic cover has to be established to prevent ascending cholangitis and hepatic failure.

Surgical

When obstructions like gallstones are found in the common bile duct, they have to be removed either by open surgery (choledochotomy) or by ERCP sphincterotomy and basketing.

LONG-TERM COMPLICATIONS OF GASTRIC SURGERY

Except a small percentage, majority of the patients who undergo gastric surgery especially gastrectomy, have a satisfactory and symptom-free postoperative period. The undesirable side effects in this 20 – 25% may take place for various reasons such as:

- Loss of gastric tissue
- Bypass, removal or alteration of pyloric sphincter mechanism

Vagotomy performed in addition to gastric surgery also contributes to the development of the complications for prolonged periods of time. It is to be noted that these symptoms form a symptom-complex and are patient-specific and the same symptom does not occur in similar patients and also one patient can experience combination of symptoms. The long-term complications are given in **Box. 11.3 (Fig. 11.40)**.

It should be noted clearly as the remedial operation, if need to be performed, should take care of all the symptoms. The severity of

Stomach and Duodenum

> **Box 11.3:** Long-term complications of gastric surgery
>
> - Alkaline reflux gastritis
> - Early dumping syndrome
> - Late dumping syndrome
> - Post-vagotomy diarrhea
> - Malabsorption
> - Weight loss
> - Anemia
>   - Microcytic anemia, iron deficiency anemia
>   - Megaloblastic anemia
> - Chronic gastric atony
> - Gastric stasis and bezoar formation (trichobezoar, phytobezoar, or both)
> - Small gastric remnant syndrome
> - Roux stasis syndrome
> - Gastric remnant carcinoma
> - Anastomotic ulcer
> - Recurrent ulcer
> - Gastrojejunocolic fistula
> - Chronic afferent loop obstruction
> - Chronic efferent loop obstruction
> - Internal hernia
> - Jejunogastric intussusception

symptoms after gastric operations and the success of treatment can be determined by Visick's classification **(Table 11.10)**.

Alkaline reflux gastritis

Introduction

The complication is due to the reflux of the duodenal contents (bile, pancreatic juice and duodenal content) irritating the gastric mucosa. The enterogastric reflux is said to occur due to the absence of pylorus in pylorus ablative (distal gastrectomy) or relaxing procedures (pyloroplasty).

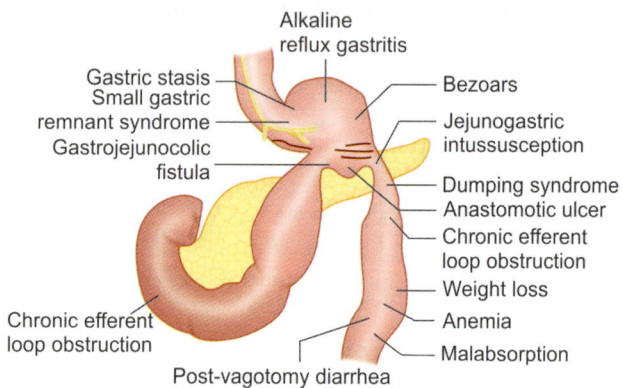

Fig. 11.40: Late complications of gastrectomy

Table 11.10: Visick's classification of gastric surgery symptoms

Grade	Characteristics
I	No symptoms
II	Mild-to-moderate symptoms
III	Moderate-to-severe symptoms
IV	Very severe or persistent symptoms affecting the quality of life requiring intense medical therapy/surgery

Diagnosis

Clinical Presentation

The patient presents with burning epigastric pain different from the original ulcer pain before surgery. The pain is worsened by food intake and bilious vomiting is constantly present, which does not relieve the pain. The vomitus often contains food mixed with bile. The symptoms may result in diminished caloric intake, weight loss and anemia.

Investigations

- The diagnosis is made by careful history taking.
- **Gastroscopy:** The gastroscopist sees bile refluxing into the stomach, which is lined by an acutely inflamed, even ulcerated mucosa. Gastroscopic biopsy of the gastric mucosa will show intestinalization of the gastric glands, inflammation, ulceration and hemorrhage.
- **Scintigraphy:** This is used to assess the magnitude of reflux by tagging bile with a radioactive marker and determining the percentage of the secreted isotope reflux into the stomach.

Management

Medical

Antispasmodics, H_2-blockers/proton-pump inhibitors, gastrokinetics like metoclopramide, mozapride are useful.

Surgical

- Roux-en-Y diversion is the operation of choice for the small percentage of patients who require operation, with completion of vagotomy if it is incomplete, and also excision of antrum to reduce the cephalic and humoral phases of gastric secretion, as Roux-en-Y procedure itself is ulcerogenic. To prevent this, the alkaline stream should be diverted from the gastroenterostomy at least 45–60 cm
- **Braun enteroenterostomy (Refer Fig. 11.35)** is useful in patients who have undergone Billroth II reconstruction

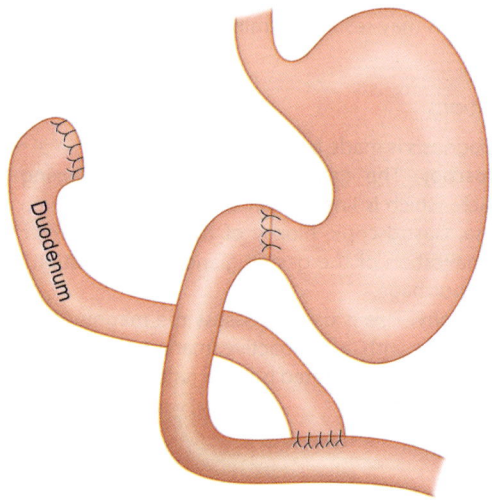

Fig. 11.41: Duodenal switch

- When the pylorus is intact, ***"duodenal switch"*** procedure **(Fig 11.41)** (it leaves the suprapapillary duodenum intact in continuity with the intact stomach preserving the normal gastric reservoir function, antropyloric function, the duodenal inhibition of gastric secretion and stimulation of the duodenal mucosa by gastric chyme) can be done.

Clinical Pearl

- This occurs more commonly after Billroth II type of construction, but may also occur after Billroth I reconstruction, gastrojejunostomy or pyloroplasty.

Early Dumping Syndrome

Introduction

Dumping syndrome is a bunch of postprandial symptoms varying in severity from annoying and irritating to disabling.

Etiology and Pathogenesis

- The symptoms are thought to occur due to the sudden rush of hyperosmolar gastric contents into the small bowel
- This rush is attributed to the loss or bypass of pyloric sphincter. Pyloromyotomy, pyloroplasty and distal gastrectomy are known to be associated with dumping syndrome
- Gastrointestinal and vasomotor symptoms occur within 10 to 40 minutes of food intake. This complex of symptoms occurs due to two postulated theories. They are:
    - ***Theory 1:*** Sudden entry of large amounts of carbohydrate rich liquid in the small bowel leads to fluid shifts from the intravascular space into the bowel lumen producing the vasomotor and gastrointestinal symptoms
    - ***Theory 2:*** The vasoactive intestinal hormones responsible for the vasomotor symptoms are serotonin, gastric inhibitory polypeptide (GIP), vasoactive inhibitory peptide (VIP) and neurotensin.

Diagnosis

Clinical Presentation

- The clinical presentation consists of gastrointestinal and vasomotor symptoms

- The symptoms begin within 10–30 minutes of food intake in response to the ingestion of hyperosmolar, carbohydrate rich food. They are:
  - ***Gastrointestinal symptoms***: Abdominal fullness, crampy abdominal pain, nausea, vomiting and explosive diarrhea
  - ***Vasomotor symptoms***: Diaphoresis, weakness, dizziness, flushing and palpitations.

Investigations

- Careful history taking is more useful than laboratory investigations
- There is no specific investigation to document early dumping excepting for motility studies by scintigraphy using both solid and liquid-phase markers to document rapid gastric emptying, but they are not very important. Levels of various hormones like neurotensin, vasoactive intestinal peptide, pancreatic polypeptide, insulin and glucagon are raised but they are not diagnostic.

Management

Medical Management

- Changes in dietary habits like the consumption of frequent small meals with reduction of carbohydrates, restriction of fluid intake with meals, and restriction of extra salt are useful in the management
- When dietary management is not beneficial, patient is started on octreotide 100 µg subcutaneously twice daily, which can be increased to 500 µg twice daily if necssary.

Surgical Management

There are various operations suggested by various authors who have shown good results, but only a small percentage of patients will require surgery. They are:

If the Original Reconstruction is Billroth I

- **Roux-en-Y reconstruction: Conversion to Billroth II or** Roux-en-Y reconstruction
- **Henley's operation:** Interposition of isoperistaltic segment of jejunum (20–25 cm) between the gastric remnant and the duodenum (**Fig. 11.42A**)
- **Poth's operation:** Interposition of two separate isolated jejunal segments (one isoperistaltic and the other antiperistaltic direction to the duodenum), each approximately 10–12 cm between the gastric remnant and the duodenum (**Fig. 11.42B**)

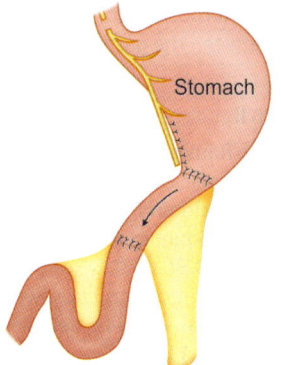

Fig. 11.42A: Henley's operation

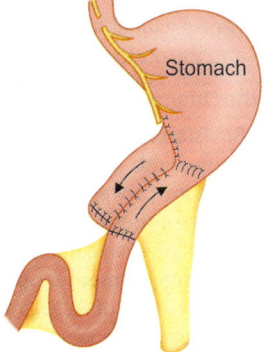

Fig. 11.42B: Poth's operation

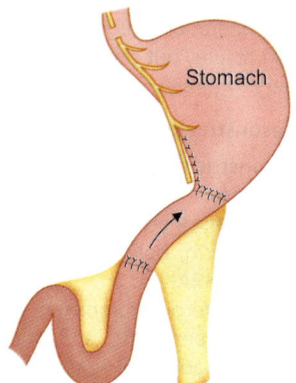

Fig. 11.42C: Reversed interposition

- **Reversed interposition of jejunum:** Interposition of single reversed jejunal segment interposed between the gastric remnant and the duodenum **(Fig. 11.42C)**.

If the Original Reconstruction is Billroth II

- **Revision of reconstruction:** Billroth II to Roux en Y reconstruction
- **Triple limb pouch operations:** Three plicated segments of jejunum converted into a single receptacle and placed either between the gastric remnant and the duodenum **(Fig. 11.43A)** or fashioned in a Roux-en-Y limb **(Fig. 11.43.B)**
- **Terrence Kennedy's operation:** Roux-en-Y reconstruction with interposition of 8–10 cm of reversed jejunal segment between the gastric remnant and the Roux-en-Y **(Fig. 11.43C)**.

Stomach and Duodenum

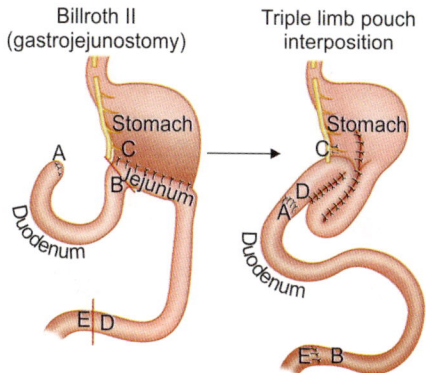

Fig. 11.43A: Triple limb pouch

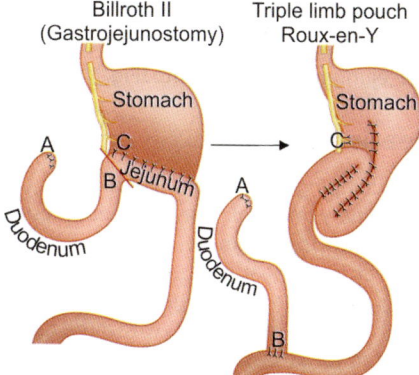

Fig. 11.43B: Triple limb Roux-en-Y

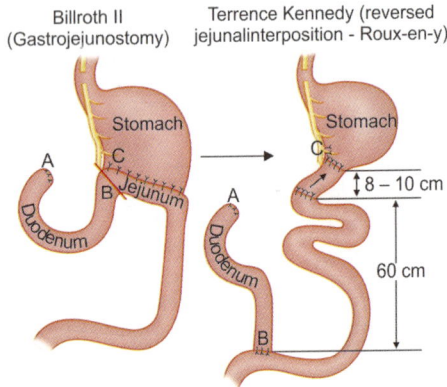

Fig. 11.43C: Terrence Kennedy operation

If the Original Reconstruction is Roux-en-Y

- **Christeas operation:** Interposition of 10 cm of antiperistaltic segment of jejunum in the Roux limb **(Fig. 11.44)**.

Clinical Pearls

- Diagnosis of dumping syndrome is clinical
- A multidisciplinary medical management is essential before jumping to surgical management
- A long follow-up is essential in assessing any operative procedure for dumping syndrome and surgery for dumping should be restricted only to those rare patients with more severe symptoms that have lasted for at least 1 year and are unresponsive to all

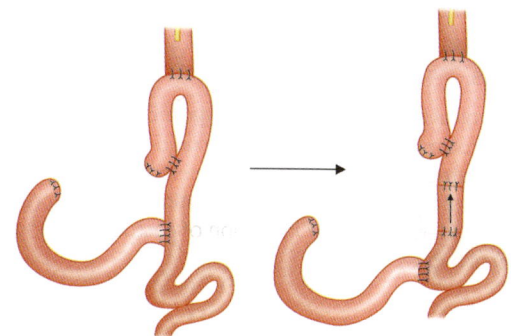

Fig. 11.44: Christeas operation

other forms of treatment. The interposition of an antiperistaltic jejunal segment often created gastric retention and is not advocated by many. It is mandatory to complete the vagotomy and antral resection in all cases
- These may be mild to moderate and may disappear with time
- The symptoms may be severe and refractory to medical treatment.

Late Dumping Syndrome

Introduction

The postprandial vasomotor symptoms occurring about 2–3 hours after a meal is called late dumping syndrome.

Etiology and Pathogenesis

The factors which cause late dumping syndrome are shown in **Figure 11.45**.

The four surgical factors which increase gastric emptying are:
1. Loss of proximal gastric receptive relaxation due to vagotomy.
2. Loss of gastric capacity due to gastric resection.
3. Loss of control of emptying due to ablation of the pylorus.
4. Loss of duodenal feedback inhibition of gastric emptying due to duodenal bypass.

Diagnosis

Clinical Presentation

The clinical presentation consists of vasomotor symptoms namely, sweating, weakness, palpitations, dizziness, flushing during the late

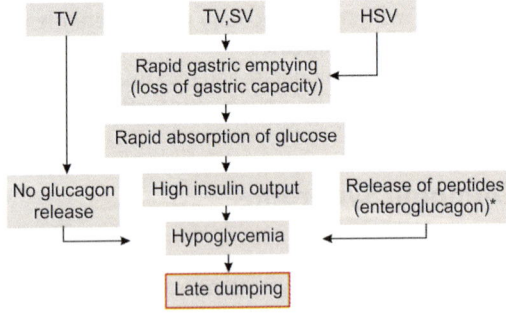

Fig. 11.45: Late dumping pathogenesis

*Release of enteroglucagon in response to carbohydrate diet, sensitizes β cell to stimuli and causes increased secretion of insulin producing hypoglycemia.

Stomach and Duodenum

postprandial period (2–4 hours following meals). *The gastrointestinal symptoms are absent.* The patients may decrease their food intake with resultant weight loss and malnourishment. These may be mild to moderate and may disappear with time.

Investigations

Careful history taking will give the diagnosis.

Management

Medical

- Frequent small quantities of food with reduced carbohydrate content with increased protein component. The attacks may be controlled by the intake of small quantities of glucose containing foods between meals
- In patients with striking symptoms, insulin may be administered before meals to correct the hyperglycemia and facilitate glucose absorption by the small intestine.

Surgical

The procedures described for the treatment of early dumping syndrome may be chosen in select cases, but the requirement is extremely rare.

Clinical Pearls

- As a rule, borborygmi and diarrhea do not accompany late dumping syndrome
- Few patients have both early and late dumping syndromes.

Post-Vagotomy Diarrhea

Introduction

Majority of gastric surgery patients complain of diarrhea, but the incidence is higher in patients who have undergone vagotomy, truncal vagotomy causing the maximum discomfort. Only a small percentage of patients are truly disturbed by this.

Etiology

Of the many hypotheses on etiology, it is felt that
- Gastric stasis produces bacterial overgrowth, enteritis with malabsorption, changes in the small intestinal epithelial content, decrease mesenteric blood flow
- Denervation of extrahepatic biliary tree and small intestine leading to rapid transit of unconjugated bile salts into the colon, and inhibition of water absorption.

Diagnosis

Clinical Presentation
- Watery stools (explosive diarrhea)
- Nocturnal stools
- Always associated with food intake.

Investigations
- Fecal white cell count and stool culture to eliminate infective pathology
- Fecal fat studies (to rule out malabsorption)
- Upper and lower GI endoscopy
- Barium followthrough studies.

Stomach and Duodenum

Management

Medical
- Diet (liquid and lactose restricted diet)
- Antidiarrheal (loperamide)
- Octreotide has some benefit.

Surgical
- Operations to delay intestinal transit (antiperistaltic segment of jejunum/ileum) rarely advocated.

Clinical Pearls

- In spite of the etiologies suggested, the diarrhea is more related to rapid transit without true malabsorption
- More than 90% of patients improve with medical management
- Surgery is avoided due to inconsistent results.

Malabsorption and Weight Loss

Introduction

- Weight loss is commonly seen in patients who have undergone gastric surgery and is almost proportional to the magnitude of resection
- After bariatric surgery, this is permanent and was intended to happen
- After antireflux surgery it is transient usually due to decreased intake of food and mild transient dysphagia
- After truncal vagotomy and gastrectomy, the weight loss is common and progressive loss should warrant thorough evaluation.

Etiology

The reasons for post-gastrectomy weight loss are varied (**Fig 11.46**).

Diagnosis

Clinical Presentation

The patients present with excessive weight loss, fatigue and anemia with or without diarrhea and usually in the absence of dumping symptoms.

Investigations

Investigations related to malabsorption and anemia may be needed to make the diagnosis.

Management

Medical

- Modification of diet and eating habits will be useful.
- Consumption of a balanced diet with adequate caloric content with addition of pancreatic enzymes will be useful

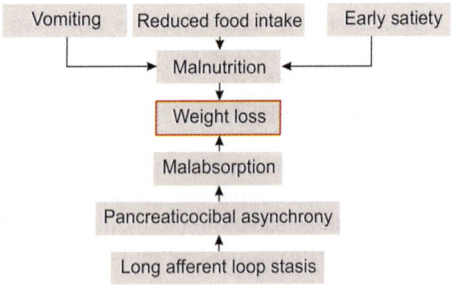

Fig. 11.46: Weight loss pathogenesis

Surgical

- Surgical correction consists of conversion of Billroth II to Billroth I or a Roux-en-Y diversion, but the surgery is extremely rarely required.

Clinical Pearls

- Of the many causes for weight loss after gastric surgery, decreased caloric consumption is the most common cause for weight loss due to small stomach, gastroparesis or self-imposed restrictions due to dumping or diarrhea
- Malabsorption is more prone to occur with Billroth II anastomosis if a long afferent loop is constructed, the stasis in the afferent loop may impair fat absorption and overgrowth of bacteria
- Ineffective mixing of pancreatic enzyme with food may occur due to the delay in emptying of the afferent loop.

Anemia

Introduction

- The anemia could be microcytic anemia or megaloblastic anemia, due to deficiency of iron and vitamin B_{12}, respectively
- Anemia is the most common metabolic side effect of gastric bypass or surgery for morbid obesity.

Etiology

- Iron absorption takes place in the proximal stomach in the presence of acidic environment. Intrinsic factor, which is essential for enteric B_{12} absorption, is made by the parietal cells of the stomach again in the acidic environment. When the acidic

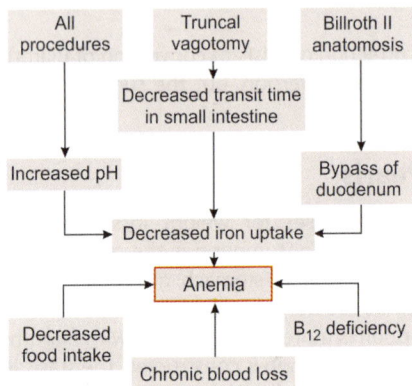

Fig. 11.47: Anemia pathogenesis

environment is changed in gastric operations, the bioavailability of iron and vitamin B_{12}
- Many other factors contribute to the absorption of these factors and precipitate anemia (**Fig. 11.47**).

Diagnosis

Clinical Presentation

These patients present with pale conjunctivae and skin.

Investigations

Determination of hemoglobin, packed cell volume, serum iron, transferrin, folate and B_{12} levels will help in the diagnosis.

Management

- Oral iron supplements in the form of Ferrous sulfate or Ferrous fumarate 100–200 mg daily is required in the treatment of microcytic anemia
- If the anemia is due to deficiency of vitamin B_{12} and folate, injections of cyanocobalamin 1 mg in the form of intramuscular injections and Folate as tablets 10–15 mg daily are required for treatment of megaloblastic anemia.

Clinical Pearls

- If the nutritional status is found to be marginal in a post-gastric surgery patient, correction using oral or parenteral supplementation is mandatory.

Chronic Gastric Atony

Introduction

Gastric atony leads to delayed gastric emptying.

Etiology

- This can be caused by gastric vagal denervation or it may have been preexisting and unrecognized before surgery
- Alternatively, it may be due to an obstruction like anastomotic stricture, efferent loop kink or proximal small bowel obstruction.

Diagnosis

Clinical Presentation

The patients complain of fullness and pain in the epigastrium and postprandial fullness, nausea and vomiting of partially digested food eaten hours or days before **(Fig. 11.48)**.

Investigations

The diagnosis is based on elimination of mechanical or functional causes of obstruction.
- **Contrast radiography** demonstrates a distended, flaccid gastric remnant without evidence of mechanical obstruction
- **Endoscopy** is performed to rule out any mechanical obstruction
- The diagnosis is confirmed by **scintigraphy,** which shows delayed gastric emptying especially of solids.

Management

Medical
- Prokinetic drugs like metoclopramide and erythromycin.

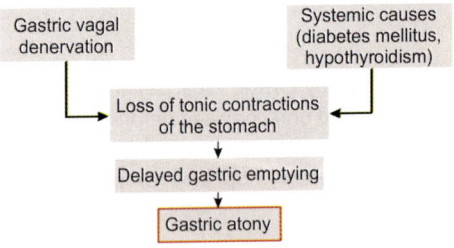

Fig. 11.48: Gastric atony pathogenesis

Surgical

- When medical treatment fail surgery is contemplated
- When the original surgery is vagotomy + pyloroplasty, antrectomy may be performed
- When the gastric remnant is distended massively, near total gastrectomy and Roux-en-Y reconstruction (to prevent bile reflux) may be needed
- Anastomotic stricture warrants revision of anastomosis.

Clinical Pearl

Less selective vagotomies have a high incidence of delayed gastric emptying.

Small Gastric Remnant Syndrome

Introduction

A complex of symptoms due to a residual small gastric remnant.

Diagnosis

Clinical Presentation

The patient may present with dumping, fullness, epigastric distress, weight loss and nutritional defects.

Investigations

Careful history taking is useful in diagnosis. Gastrograffin studies exhibit early emptying of stomach with no reservoir function.

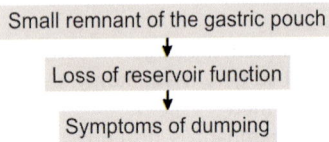

Management

Medical
Medical management is usually successful. Small feeds with enzyme supplements, iron, vitamins and antispasmodics are useful.

Surgical
- Patients with more severe symptoms not controlled by medical treatment may receive some benefit with a remedial surgery. This surgery is designed to restore the reservoir function of the gastric remnant and also to promote intestinal absorption. Various pouch operations are practiced. They are:
  - **Hunt–Lawrence pouch operation**: The afferent jejunal loop of the Billroth II reconstruction is divided 10–12 cm from the inteact gastrojejunostomy. The end of the 10–12 cm segment is closed and then anastomosed side-to-side to the efferent jejunal limb, creating a double-limb pouch just distal to the gastrojejunostomy. The proximal divided afferent jejunal limb is anastomosed to the efferent jejunal limb (Roux-en-Y) 60 cm distal to the gastrojejunostomy (**Figs 11.49A and B**)
  - If the original surgery was Billroth I reconstruction, the gastroduodenostomy is taken down and the duodenal stump closed. The jejunum is divided approximately 15 inches distal to the ligament of Treitz and the distal end is closed. The long efferent loop is folded back upon itself and the two adjacent

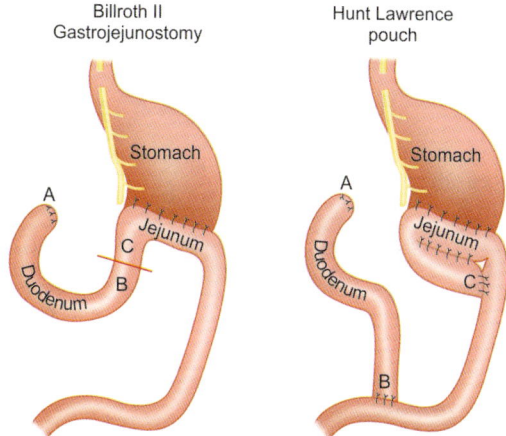

Fig. 11.49A: Hunt–Lawrence pouch—Schematic

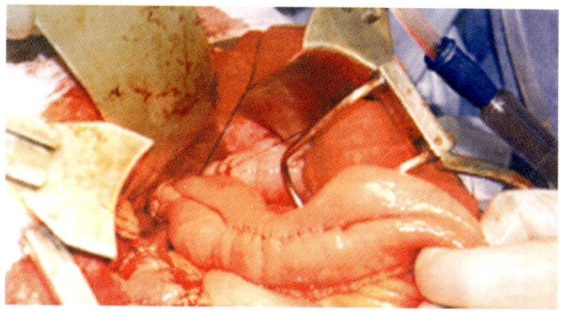

Fig. 11.49B: Hunt–Lawrence pouch

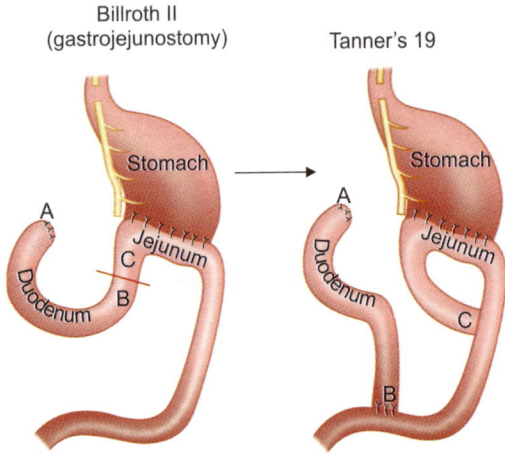

Fig. 11.50: Tanner's 19 reservoir operation

limbs are converted into a single pouch approximately 10–12 cm in length. The pouch is anastomosed to the small gastric remnant. The afferent jejunal limb is anastomosed end-to-side to the efferent loop approximately 60 cm below the pouch
- *The Tanner's 19 reservoir pouch* is a circular pouch connected to the remnant of the stomach, in Roux principle (**Fig. 11.50**).

Roux Syndrome

Introduction

A small group of patients who have had reconstruction as Roux-en-Y gastrojejunostomy after distal gastrectomy may face with the difficulty in gastric emptying, in the absence of mechanical obstruction. Patients develop a complex of symptoms called Roux syndrome.

Etiology and Pathogenesis

- The exact pathology is not clear, but both the vagotomized gastric remnant and the Roux-en-Y reconstruction seem to have a role in the development of this syndrome
- The length of the Roux limb is found to have definite correlation with delayed transit time through the intestinal segment.
- Transection of the jejunum in the construction of the limb prevents the propagation of pacesetter potentials resulting in slower transit. Ectopic pacemaker potentials, which act retrogradely contribute to this delayed transit.
- Phase III of the interdigestive motor complex are irregular and their propagation isoperistaltically is improper resulting in the delayed transit. Phase III is a cyclically recurring pattern of organized intense motor activity in the fasting state, which is thought to sweep the bowel clear of all residue after the digestion is complete.
- Truncal vagotomy results in the loss of vagal innervation of the jejunum, which results in diminished strength in jejunal contractions.

Diagnosis

Clinical Presentation

The patients present with epigastric fullness, abdominal pain, nausea and vomiting of food, and in severe cases with malnutrition and weight loss.

Investigations

- Investigations to rule out mechanical causes like contrast radiography and endoscopy are essential
- Scintigraphic imaging is the best way to quantitate the delayed emptying of solids and liquids through the gastric remnant and the Roux limb
- GI motility testing will show abnormal motility in the Roux limb, with propulsive activity toward the stomach. Gastric motility will also be abnormal.

Management

Medical

- Prokinetic drugs.

Surgical

Near-total gastrectomy and adjustment of the length of the Roux limb to a final length of 40 cm.

Clinical Pearls

- Though the delaying or reversed motility occurs in almost all patients who have undergone a Roux-en-Y anastomosis, why this is symptomatic in only a subset of people is unclear
- It is impossible to reverse the motor abnormalities in the Roux limb by any surgery once the limb has been constructed.

Prevention: "Uncut Roux" gastroenterostomy (**Fig. 11.51**)—a loop of gastrojejunostomy is made, the afferent loop is occluded by staples, which prevent the flow, but allow normal propagation

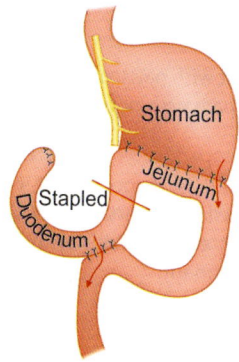

Fig. 11.51: Uncut Roux operation

of intestinal pacesetter potentials to the Roux limb. The afferent and efferent limbs are anastomosed in a side-to-side fashion (entero-enterostomy). With respect to bile flow, this functions like a conventional Roux, but the adverse effects of jejunal transection are avoided.

Gastric Remnant Carcinoma

Introduction

The pathology of this complication is not very clear, but the reflux of duodenal contents producing deconjugation of bile salts in the presence of gastric hypoacidity is suggested.

Diagnosis

Clinical Presentation

The patient may present with nausea, loss of appetite, loss of weight and upper abdominal pain with or without vomiting.

Investigations

Gastroscopy **(Fig. 11.52)** is diagnostic. It is suggested that the patients undergoing Billroth II anastomosis, should have annual or biannual endoscopic examinations with biopsies and cytologic studies of the gastric remnant.

Management

Radical excision of the gastric remnant with lymph node dissection.

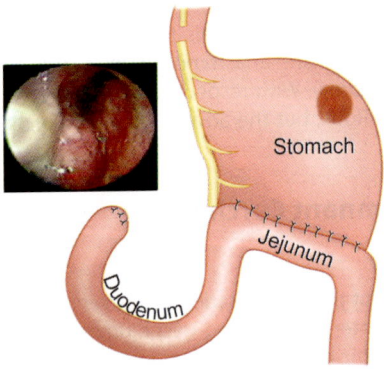

Fig. 11.52: Gastric remnant carcinoma

Clinical Pearl

- This complication is more common after Billroth II reconstruction.

Anastomotic Ulcer

Introduction

- Ulcer developing at the site of gastrojejunal anastomosis done about more than 2 years
- Can penetrate into the adjoining transverse colon to produce a gastrojejunocolic fistula.

Diagnosis

Clinical Presentation

Symptoms

- Constant, boring pain appearing in about 30 minutes of taking food. Patient describes these symptoms, especially the pain to be similar to that before previous surgery
- Vomiting is a common feature
- Hematemesis and melena are common
- History of periodicity is lost
- Gastrojejunocolic fistula causes intestinal hurry, loss of weight and infection due to regurgitation of fecal contents into the stomach.

Sign

- Patient looks emaciated.

Investigations

- *Barium enema* is diagnostic, as the barium is sucked from the colon by the peristaltic waves of the stomach
- *Upper GI endoscopy* **(Fig. 11.53)** is diagnostic.

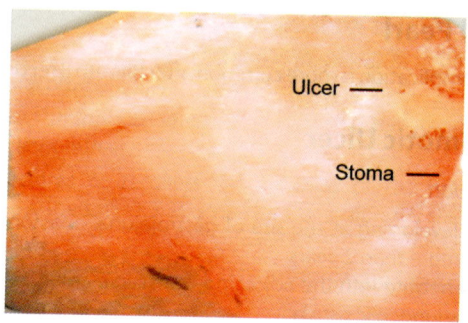

Fig. 11.53: Scopy—Anastomotic ulcer

Management

Excision of fistula and revision of anastomosis is the treatment of choice.

Recurrent Ulcer

Introduction

The ulcer can recur after a few months or years after surgery.

Etiology

The various causes of this complication are:
- Incomplete vagotomy
- Retained antrum after Billroth II reconstruction
- G-cell hyperplasia
- Gastrinoma
- Multiple endocrine neoplasia

- Long afferent loop
- Ulcerogenic drugs
- Gastric stasis.

Diagnosis

Clinical Presentation

- Upper abdominal pain relieved by food intake.

Investigation

- *Gastroduodenoscopy* is diagnostic.

Management

The surgical treatment varies according to the previous surgery, and they are:

a. If the original operation is vagotomy with a drainage procedure, and all other causes of recurrent ulcer are ruled out, and if the vagotomy is found to be incomplete, it has to be completed.

b. If the gastrectomy (Billroth I or II reconstruction) was found to be inadequate, additional gastric tissue must be excised to approximate 50% distal resection (inclusion of antrum) along with the addition of vagotomy.

c. If the original operation is vagotomy and antrectomy, the remedial operation is total gastrectomy and a Roux-en-Y reconstruction.

d. If the original operation is proximal gastric vagotomy, reoperation is rarely required, and if needed, antrectomy with Billroth I reconstruction should be done. The proximal gastric vagotomy may be converted into truncal vagotomy.

Clinical Pearls

- Recurrent ulcers may be a long-term complication following any standard operation for duodenal ulcer but unusual after the surgery for gastric ulcer
- The rate of occurrence of recurrent ulcers after Billroth I reconstruction is more when compared to after Billroth II reconstruction
- It is unusual to encounter a recurrent ulcer following vagotomy and antrectomy
- Recurrent ulcers following proximal gastric vagotomy are small and shallow and can usually be managed with drug therapy alone.

Gastrojejunocolic fistula

Introduction

A fistulous communication between the gastrojejunostomy and the overlying transverse colon (**Fig. 11.54**).

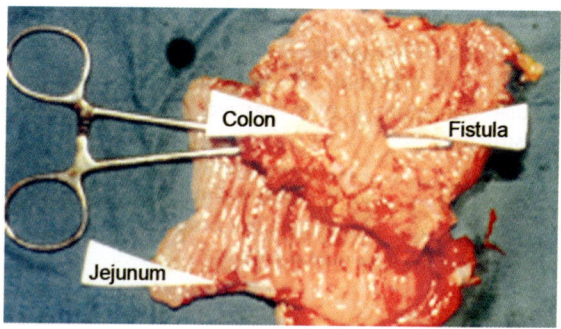

Fig. 11.54: Gastrojejunocolic fistula

Pathogenesis

Small anastomotic leaks and abscesses may open into the adjacent colon and allow the entry of colonic bacterial flora into the proximal small bowel, producing fulminant enteritis. Diversion of small bowel contents into the colon is also a contributing factor.

Diagnosis

Clinical Presentation

Marked weight loss, emaciation, diarrhea and fecal belching.

Investigations

Gastrograffin study (**Fig. 11.55**) and gastroduodenoscopy are useful in diagnosis.

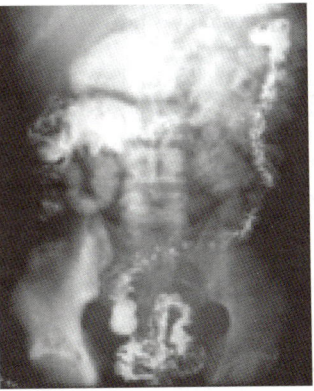

Fig. 11.55: Barium enema—Gastrojejunocolic fistula

Management

The treatment consists of vagotomy, a distal 50% gastrectomy, limited colon resection or closure of the colonic fistula. Reconstruction may be Billroth I, Billroth II or Roux-en-Y reconstruction.

Chronic Afferent Loop Obstruction

Introduction

- This complication occurs after a Billroth II reconstruction with a long afferent loop
- This complication may occur many years after the primary surgery.

Etiology and Pathogenesis

Intermittent obstruction is seen when this long redundant loop undergoes a twist, volvulus or a kink at the gastrojejunostomy site (**Fig. 11.56**). The obstruction is usually mild and corrects itself as the secretions collect in the loops. Only when the intraluminal pressure of the afferent loop becomes very high, projectile vomiting occurs.

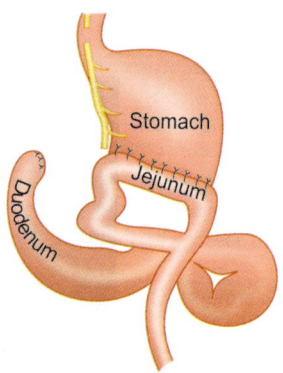

Fig. 11.56: Chronic afferent loop obstruction

Diagnosis

Clinical Presentation

- Upper abdominal pain related to consumption of meals, relieved by vomiting, which is projectile

- The vomitus is bilious and mixed with food
- It may be blood stained especially in patients with reflux gastritis.

Investigations

- ***Upper gastrointestinal endoscopy and CT scan*** are useful in diagnosis.

Management

Conversion of Billroth II to Billroth I or Roux-en-Y reconstruction is the treatment.

Chronic Efferent Loop Obstruction

Introduction

- The blockage is usually mild, intermittent and recurrent, but it may create a surgical emergency. The blockage is due to partial or total obstruction of the efferent jejunal loop (**Figs 11.57A and B**)
- An internal hernia may also account for this pathology.

Diagnosis

Clinical Presentation

The patient complains of upper abdominal discomfort with nausea. Bilious vomiting can also occur, intermittently.

Investigations

Upper gastrointestinal endoscopy and CT scan are useful in diagnosis.

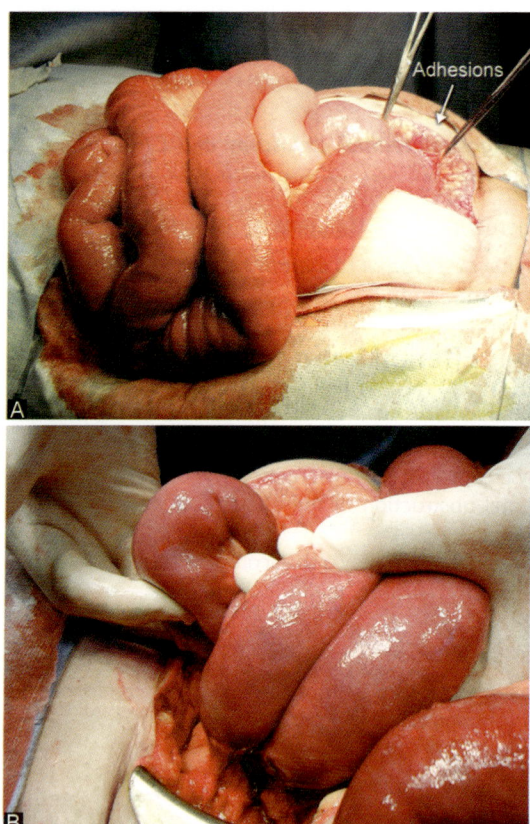

Fig. 11.57 A and B: Efferent loop obstruction
(A) Adhesions; (B) Internal herniation

Management

Simple division of the adhesive band may suffice many times. Rarely conversion of Billroth II to Billroth I or construction of Roux-en-Y may be needed.

Internal Hernia

Introduction

- Following an antecolic gastrojejunostomy, a large potential space is created through which a loop of small bowel may herniate, resulting in obstruction. The loop may be a part of afferent (when the afferent loop is long and redundant) or efferent or both **(Fig. 11.58)**
- Following a retrocolic gastrojejunostomy, two potential spaces are created, one located cephalad to the transverse mesocolon

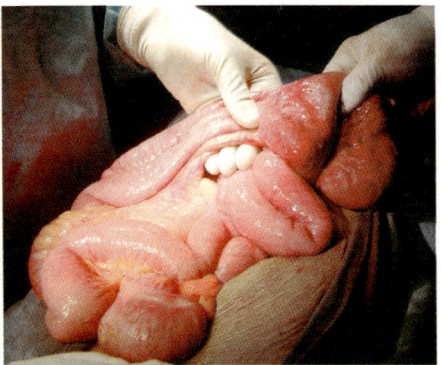

Fig. 11.58: Internal herniation of jejunum

and the other caudad to it, but the latter is prone to create complications.

Diagnosis

Clinical Presentation
- The patient presents with acute proximal small bowel obstruction, and the symptoms are less severe and may be intermittent
- The vomitus is bile stained if the efferent loop is obstructed and it does not contain bile if the afferent loop is blocked.

Investigations

Upper GI endoscopy and Barium meal studies are useful in diagnosis.

Management

At surgery, treatment consists in reduction of the herniated intestine.
- If the loop is viable, simple closure of anastomotic traps with interrupted silk sutures and suture of the afferent and efferent loops of the jejunum to the posterior parietal peritoneum may be sufficient
- If the bowel is nonviable and gangrenous, it should be resected and anastomosed
- If the gastroenterostomy itself is gangrenous, a new gastroenterostomy or a Roux-en-Y reconstruction may be made.

Clinical Pearl

- Internal herniation occurs less frequently after a retrocolic anastomosis.

Jejunogastric Intussusception

Introduction

Intussusception of the jejunal loop into the gastric remnant.

Diagnosis

Clinical Presentation

- Severe upper abdominal pain, which may be associated wth nausea or vomiting
- A firm mass may be palpable per abdomen in the epigastrium.

Investigations

- *Barium meal or Gastrograffin study* may reveal a coiled spring appearance in the gastric remnant, a sign diagnostic of intussusception
- *Gastroscopy* (**Fig. 11.59**) is diagnostic.

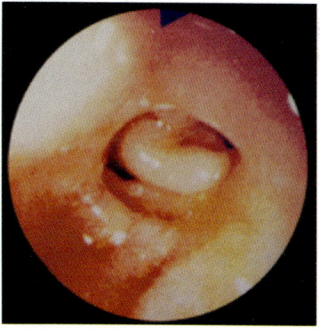

Fig. 11.59: Gastroscopy—Jejunogastric intussusception

Management

The treatment consists of reduction of the herniated small bowel and anchoring the bowel to the parietes.
- If the bowel is nonviable, resection may be required
- If the gastroenterostomy itself is gangrenous, a new gastroenterostomy or a Roux-en-Y reconstruction may be made.

Clinical Pearl

- Retrograde jejunogastric intussusception is more common than the antegrade intussusception.

Chapter 12

Small Intestine

ANATOMY

The small intestine is a tubular structure extending from the pylorus to the ileocecal junction. The length at an average is about 4–6 meters. This consists of three parts:
1. Duodenum
2. Jejunum
3. Ileum

The duodenum lies in the retroperitoneum, almost enclosing the head of pancreas, as a 'C' shaped loop, and continues as the jejunum at the duodenojejunal flexure, attached by the ligament of Treitz. The jejunum and ileum lie in the peritoneal cavity and attached to the retroperitoneum by the mesentery.

The small intestine possesses the mucosal folds called valvulae conniventes, varying in number, more in the proximal bowel than the distal bowel. The lymphoid follicles of the small bowel are called Peyer's patches.

Arterial Supply

- Duodenum—Celiac and superior mesenteric arteries
- Distal duodenum, jejunum and ileum—Superior mesenteric artery.

Venous Drainage

- Through the superior mesenteric vein.

Lymphatic Drainage

- Through the lymphatics of corresponding arteries, to the mesenteric nodes to the cisterna chili, then through the thoracic duct and ultimately into the left subclavian vein.

Nerve Supply

- Parasympathetic—Vagus
- Sympathetic—Splanchnic nerves.

Histology

The small intestine wall consists of four layers:
1. Mucosa (consists of epithelium, lamina propria, muscularis mucosae)
2. Submucosa
3. Muscularis externa
4. Serosa.

Mucosa: It is the innermost layer and the epithelium is the layer exposed to the lumen. The mucosa is organized into villi (finger like projections of epithelium and lamina propria containing blood and lymph vessels) and crypts, which contain the four varieties of cells, enterocytes, goblet cells, enteroendocrine cell and Paneth cells.

Submucosa: It consists of dense connective tissue including fibroblasts and leukocytes. It also contains extensive network of vascular and lymphatic channels, nerve fibers and ganglion cells (Meissner's plexus).

Muscularis propria: It contains outer longitudinal and inner circular smooth muscle fibers. Ganglion cells exist between these two layers (Auerbach's plexus).

Serosa: It is made up of a single layer of mesothelial cells and is a part of visceral peritoneum.

PHYSIOLOGY

Absorption and Secretion

Absorption and secretion occurs in the intestine across its epithelium. The solutes traverse the epithelium by two modes of transport. They are:
1. Active transport: Transcellular pathway (through the cell).
2. Passive transport: Paracelllular pathway (between the cells).

About 8 to 9 liters of fluid enter the small bowel daily (salivary, gastric, biliary, pancreatic and intestinal secretions), and about 7.5 liters is absorbed in the small bowel. The secretion and absorption occur through osmotic process.

- *Carbohydrates* are digested by the salivary and pancreatic amylases, to oligosaccharides and maltose. These oligosaccharides and the dietary disaccharides are hydrolyzed to monosaccharides, the absorbable form, and are absorbed through transcellular route, which ultimately enter the portal venous system
- *Proteins* are digested in the small bowel by the pancreatic peptidases to amino acids and peptides, which after absorption enter the portal venous system
- *Fats* are catalyzed by pancreatic lipase into long chain fatty acids and mono and triglycerides, which are absorbed by the intestinal epithelium, which ultimately enter the portal venous system

- ***Water-soluble vitamins*** are absorbed by translocation
- ***Fat-soluble vitamins*** are absorbed through passive diffusion
- ***Vitamin K*** is absorbed through passive diffusion and carrier mediated uptake
- ***Calcium, iron and magnesium*** are absorbed through transcellular transport and paracellular diffusion.

Motility

Motility of the intestine is maintained by coordinated contractions of the muscle layer. The outer longitudinal layer causes intestinal shortening, but inner circular layer causes luminal narrowing. The rhythmic contractions are initiated by the interstitial cells of Cajal, the intrinsic pacemaker, the contractions range from 12 per minute in the duodenum and only 7 in the distal ileum. The motility is controlled by neural and hormonal processes.

APPROACH TO THE PATIENT WITH SMALL BOWEL DISEASE

Signs and Symptoms

The most common symptoms of small intestinal diseases are:
- Abdominal pain
- Intestinal colic
- Vomiting
- Nausea
- Fullness
- Weight loss
- Early satiety

- Anorexia
- Anemia.

Signs of intestinal diseases are:
- Distension (generalized or localized)
- Tenderness
- Lump.

Investigations

- Radiologic tests
  - Plain X-rays
  - Contrast studies
  - CT scan and MRI
  - Enteroclysis
  - CT enteroclysis
  - Ultrasound
  - Capsule endoscopy/Push enteroscopy/Sonde enteroscopy/operative enteroscopy
- Urinary 5HIAA in carcinoid tumors.

Enteroclysis

A radiological method used to examine the small bowel, which involves intubation of the duodenum and the proximal jejunum, and instilling a contrast, followed by methylcellulose administration. Metoclopramide is administered to accelerate the small bowel motility. This procedure creates luminal distension of the small bowel and gives better visibility of the lesions, and has a better resolution than the barium meal followthrough procedure. CT aided enteroclysis give better information.

Enteroscopy

An endoscopic procedure to view the inside of the small bowel. There are three endoscopic methods available to view the entire small bowel.

1. *Sonde endoscopy:* A 2.75 cm dedicated instrument, which is carried down by peristalsis, but takes several hours to complete the procedure. Biopsy and therapy are not possible
2. *Push endoscopy:* This can be used to view the upper small bowel (carried forward by push technique), and biopsy and therapy are possible.
3. *Capsule endoscopy:* This is a wireless endoscopy, where a 11 x 26 mm capsule is swallowed and video images are recorded into a data recorder worn on patient's belt for approximately 8 hours. Biopsy and therapy are not possible.

SMALL BOWEL ATRESIA

Introduction

Intestinal atresias can occur anywhere from the proximal jejunum to terminal ileum. They are grouped into 5 types (**Fig. 12.1**). They are:
- *Type I*—a membrane or a web blocking the intestinal lumen
- *Type II*—proximal bulbous end is connected to the collapsed distal bowel by a short fibrous cord along the edge of the intact mesentery
- *Type IIIa*—mesenteric defect between the disconnected bulbous proximal bowel and the blind distal intestine
- *Type IIIb*—complex atresia based on the absence of a significant portion of superior mesenteric artery leading to a loss of a large amount of midgut

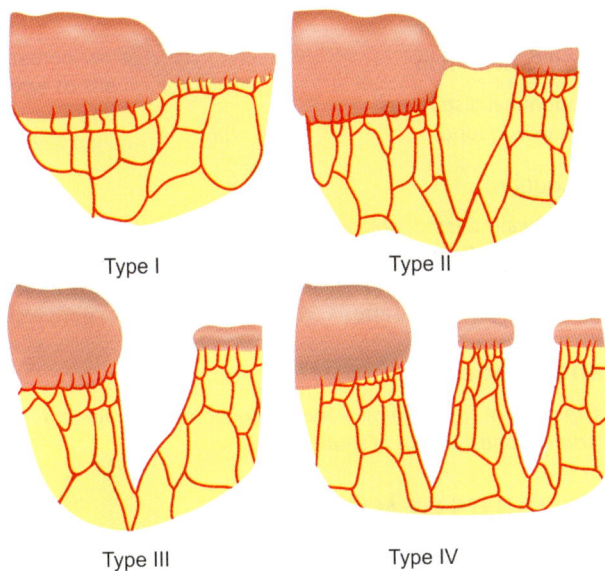

Fig. 12.1: Intestinal atresia

- *Type IV*—multiple segment atresia or a combination of type I–III (***String of sausages appearance***)—has a short bowel length and has a familial tendency and increased mortality.

Etiology and Pathogenesis

Believed to be caused by in utero vascular accident resulting in interruption of blood flow and ischemia of the affected segment.

Diagnosis

Clinical Presentation
- Abdominal distension
- Bilious vomiting.

Investigations
- ***US***—focally dilated, isolated bowel loops seen in utero
- ***Plain X-ray abdomen***—air filled loops of small bowel
- ***Double contrast enema***—failure of reflux of contrast into the ileum indicates distal atresia.

Management
- *Exploratory laparotomy + resection of atretic segments and primary anastomosis of small bowel.*

VOLVULUS OF MIDGUT

Introduction

When the process of rotation of midgut is arrested, the cecum lies in the subhepatic position, in the mid-abdomen or right hypochondrium, and the base of mesentery is foreshortened, through which the superior mesenteric vessels and lymphatic channels pass. This poses the risk of ischemia when volvulus occurs **(Figs 12.2A to C)**.

Volvulus of the bowel refers to a twisting or torsion of the intestine about its mesentery.
- *In children,* commonly before one year and rarely in neonates
- *In adults,* a loop of bowel rotates around a point of adhesion (to the abdominal wall or to an adjacent viscera).

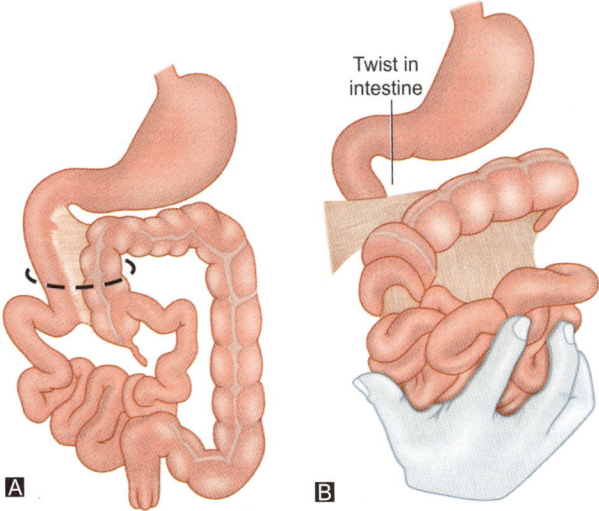

Figs 12.2A and B: Midgut volvulus

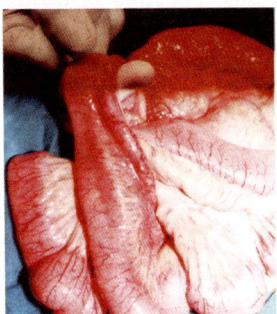

Fig. 12.2C: Torsion of midgut

Diagnosis

Symptoms and Signs

- May remain asymptomatic throughout life
- Neonates and infants:
  - Bilious vomiting, pain and shock like syndrome
  - Dark bloody stools per rectum
  - Abdominal tenderness (may indicate gangrene)
  - Abdominal distension.
- Adults
  - Intermittent or cyclical vomiting
  - Severe abdominal pain with intestinal obstruction
  - Anorexia nervosa
  - Malnutrition and failure to thrive.

Investigations

- ***Plain X-ray abdomen*** will show a dilated stomach and proximal duodenum with an air-fluid level and lack of gas in the rest of the small bowel. Gasless abdomen in a neonate is the radiological sign which is ominous
- ***Contrast study*** shows *'Cork-screw'* or *'twisted ribbon'* appearance of proximal jejunum and is indicative of volvulus
- ***US abdomen*** will show coiling of superior mesenteric vein around the artery and is highly suggestive of a volvulus. Fixed midline small bowel loops, duodenal dilatation and distal tapering are other features.

Management

Medical

- Resuscitation
- Nasogastric decompression
- Broad spectrum antibiotics.

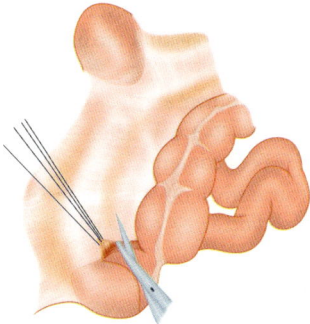
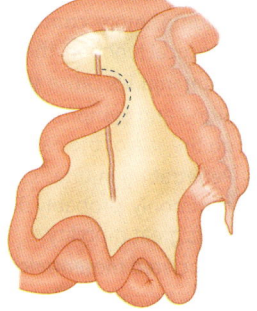

Fig. 12.3A: Division of Ladd's bands   **Fig. 12.3B:** Ladd's operation

Surgical

Emergency laparotomy (Figs 12.3A and B)—Ladd's operation— Adhesions between the cecum and ascending colon and the gallbladder and right paracolic gutter (Ladd's bands) are divided, the base of the mesentery is widened. The small bowel is placed on the right and the ascending colon in the left upper quadrant. Appendectomy is performed to avoid any confusion in future.

Clinical Pearl

- Outcome of surgery depends on the extent of resection.

INJURIES OF SMALL INTESTINE

Introduction

- Injuries to the small intestine are more common than injuries to the duodenum and large intestine, the usual mechanism

being the blunt trauma crushing the bowel against the vertebral column, more commonly the duodenojejunal flexure and the ileocecal junction, the fixed parts
- Blunt injuries cause slow necrosis of bowel and leak occurs late
- Signs and symptoms develop late—2–3 days later, depending on the size of the damage and leak of contents
- Penetrating injuries can also cause small bowel trauma, but less commonly, probably due to its sliding away from a knife because of its great mobility
- Associated mesenteric tears are common.

Diagnosis

Symptoms and Signs

- Abdominal pain, distension and vomiting
- Tenderness and guarding are pronounced around the damaged bowel and the patient may point it *(Pointing sign).*

Investigations

- *Plain X-rays* may show air under the domes of the diaphragm
- *CECT abdomen* may be useful in identifying the level of injuries
- *Paracentesis* will show bile-stained fluid.

Management

- *Simple suturing* is done for simple tears
- *Resections* are required for large tears with nonviable bowel
- *Peritoneal toileting* is mandatory under cover of antibiotics.

INTUSSUSCEPTION

Introduction

Intussusception is the invagination of a segment of bowel into the distal adjacent loop (proximal into the distal).

Etiology

In Children

- 2 per 1000 infants are affected with male preponderance, commonly affecting the age group of 3 months to 1 year
- Commonly, it is secondary to an enlarged Peyer's patch due to viral or bacterial infections (**Fig 12.4A**)

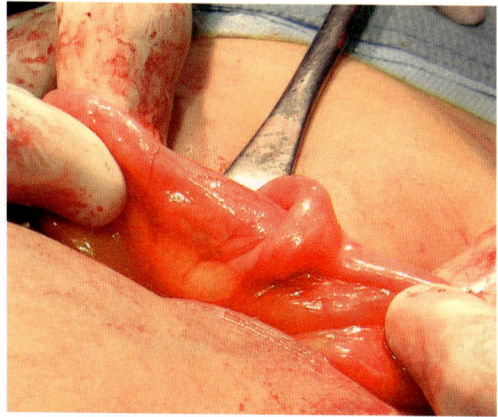

Fig. 12.4A: Ileoileal intussusception (1)

- The other less common causes are:
  - Meckel's diverticulum
  - Duplication cyst in the bowel wall
  - Polyp
  - Ectopic pancreas
  - Liposarcomas.

In Adults

Intussusception of small bowel is always secondary to a polypoid lesion, a lipoma (**Figs 12.4B and C**)

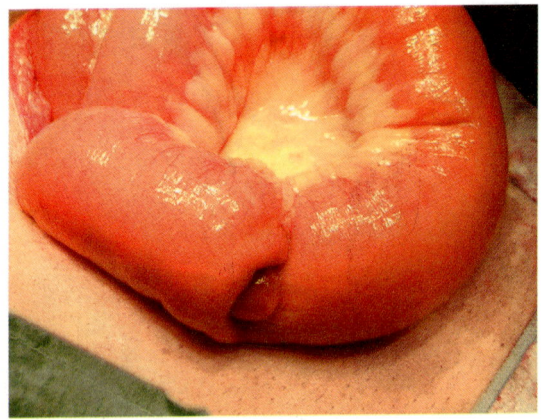

Fig. 12.4B: Ileoileal intussusception (2)

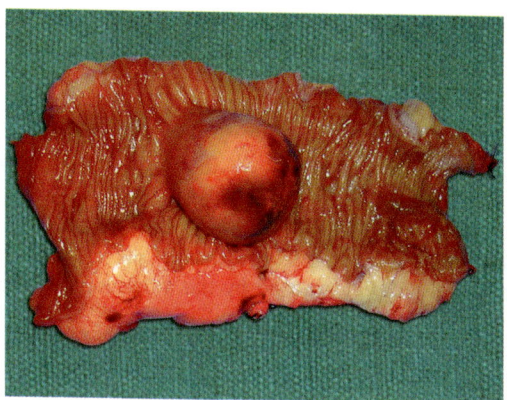

Fig. 12.4C: Lipoma the cause of ileoileal intussusception

Diagnosis

Symptoms

- In children, there may be a history of preceding gastroenteritis following a change in diet (weaning from milk to solid food)
- Severe acute colicky pain, with abdominal distension
- Passing of frequent semisolid stools with bright red blood may be predominant *(Redcurrant jelly).*

Signs

- During the attacks of pain, a sausage shaped mass may be felt, which appears during the time of colic and disappears after the colic disappears. The right iliac fossa is empty—***Sign de Dance***
- Rectal examination may reveal bloodstain on the examining finger (redcurrant jelly)

- Colorectal intussusception may be felt by the examining finger on rectal examination, or it may even present through anus, resembling a rectal prolapse.

Investigations

- *Plain X-ray abdomen*—Soft tissue shadow in the region of transverse colon with empty distal colon. Multiple air fluid levels may be seen when obstruction predominates
- *Barium enema* may show a filling defect called '*pincer shaped filling defect*' (caused by the intussusceptum with the intussuscipiens)
- *Colonoscopy* can identify, ileocolic intussusception (**Fig 12.5**)
- *US and CT* (**Fig. 12.6**) will reveal the intussuscepting mass (*target/sausage/pseudokidney appearance*).

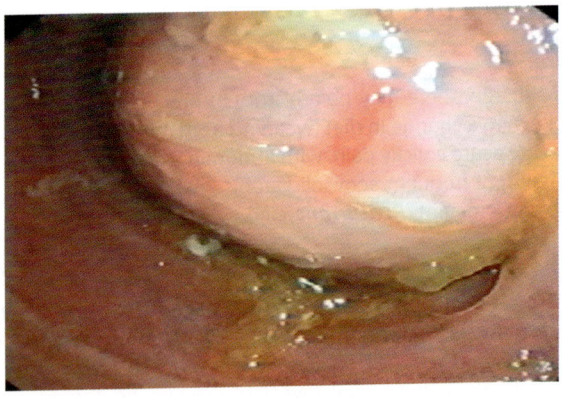

Fig. 12.5: Colonoscopy—Ileocolic intussusception

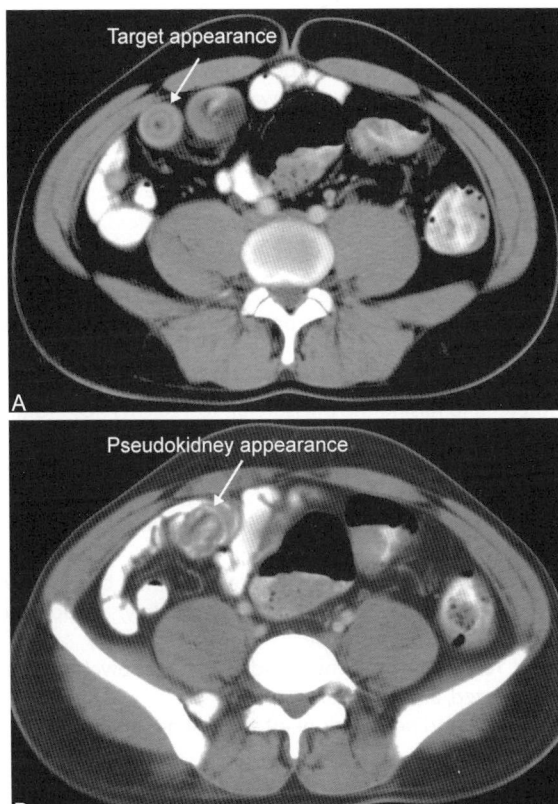

Figs 12.6A and B: CT—Intussusception

Complications

When the mesentery is drawn between the loops, it may result in venous obstruction and bowel wall edema, which may lead to arteriolar obstruction eventually resulting in:
- Strangulation
- Gangrene
- Perforation.

Management

- *Barium enema and colonoscopy*, by themselves may reduce the colonic intussusceptions
- *Air contrast enema* (air introduced through a balloon tipped catheter and raising the pressure up to 120 cm H_2O)—Glucagon may be administered to relax the colon. Free flow of contrast into the terminal ileum indicates complete reduction. 2 or 3 attempts can be made before deciding on surgery
- *Laparoscopic exploration is an excellent procedure to reduce intussusceptions*
- *Laparotomy* is required to reduce the small bowel intussusception, and treat the cause appropriately, if laparoscopic procedures are not effective
- *Bowel resections* may be needed if the bowel segment is strangulated, and non-viable
- Perforation and peritonitis need appropriate treatment.

Clinical Pearls

- Reduction by contrast enema is possible in a vast majority of cases
- When reduction fails with contrast enema, surgical (open/laparoscopic) reduction is necessary.

ABDOMINAL TUBERCULOSIS

Introduction

- Very common disease
- Affects commonly the lower socioeconomic group,
- Can affect any age and any sex
- The route of entry of the organism *Mycobacterium tuberculosis* is by ingestion or through blood and by transmigration.

Classification

Abdominal tuberculosis is of three types:
1. **Intestinal tuberculosis:**
   - *Ulcerative type:* After the swallowing of the infected sputum, the organisms reach the small bowel and get concentrated in the terminal ileum (area of excessive lymphatics), and cause mucosal ulcers, which are transverse or circular (following the pattern of the lymphatics of the bowel). Healing of these ulcers causes fibrosis and strictures. Strictures lead to obstruction of small bowel. Ulcers in the proximal distended bowel may lead to perforations and peritonitis, or internal fistulae, but rare when compared to Crohn's disease
   - *Hyperplastic type:* The bacilli reach the ileocecal region, cause solitary or multiple lesions and reside in the lymphoid follicles leading to thickening of the intestinal wall and narrowing, which may lead to intestinal obstruction.
2. **Tuberculosis of mesenteric lymph nodes:** This is common in children.
3. **Peritoneal tuberculosis:** The bacteria enter the peritoneal cavity through transmigration from the intestines, tuberculous

salpingitis or through blood (hematogenous spread) and present in two forms. They are:
- ***Moist form:*** Ascitic form
- ***Dry form:*** Ascites is absent, but forms tubercles on the peritoneum.

Diagnosis

Symptoms and Signs

Clinical features depend on the type of tuberculosis.
1. **Intestinal tuberculosis**
   - *Ulcerative type*
     - Abdominal pain, intestinal colic, loss of appetite and weight
     - Active lesions cause diarrhea and healed lesions cause constipation and features of intestinal obstruction
   - *Hyperplastic type*
     - In addition to the features of ulcerative type, the patients may present with a lump in the right iliac fossa confusing with appendicular mass, Crohn's disease, ameboma, and carcinoma.
2. **Tuberculosis of mesenteric lymph nodes**
   - Periumbilical abdominal pain is the common presentation
   - General debility, loss of appetite and weight with evening rise of temperature
   - Enlarged lymph nodes can cause kinking of the small bowel and cause intestinal obstruction.

   DD: Acute appendicitis.
3. **Peritoneal tuberculosis**
   - *Moist form:* Abdominal pain and distension due to ascites, and general malaise and weakness
   - *Dry form:* Abdominal pain without abdominal distension.

Investigations

Radiology

- *Plain X-rays of abdomen and CT without oral contrast* are useful in diagnosing obstructed bowel lesions and lymph node enlargements
- *Barium meal series (Fig. 12.7A) or CT with oral contrast (Fig. 12.7B)* is diagnostic for mucosal lesions, abscess and fistulae. Ileocecal junction is pulled up in hyperplastic type of intestinal tuberculosis.

Endoscopy

- *Colonoscopy* (Fig. 12.7C) has characteristic findings.

Serology

- *Complete analysis and PCR test for ascitic fluid, and peritoneal biopsy* are diagnostic in peritoneal type of tuberculosis.

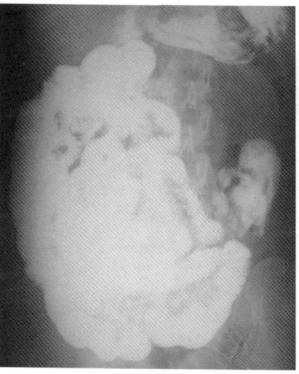

Fig. 12.7A: Barium meal series—Matted intestines of tuberculosis

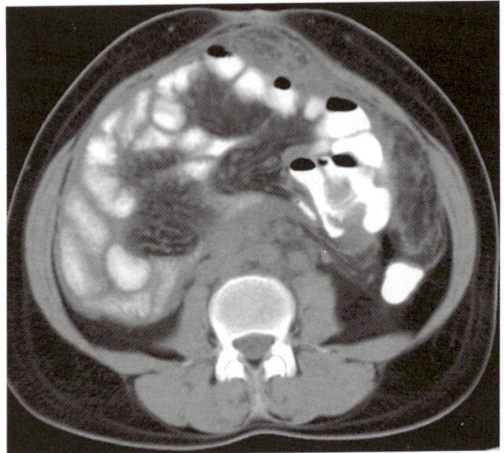

Fig. 12.7B: CT—Intestinal tuberculosis

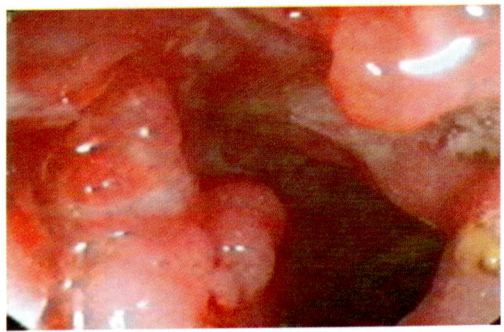

Fig. 12.7C: Colonoscopy—Ileocecal tuberculosis

Management

- *Antitubercular treatment* is curative
- *Surgical treatment* is for complications like obstructions, abscesses and fistulae.

CROHN'S DISEASE

Introduction

- An inflammatory bowel disease of uncertain etiology affecting any part of the gastrointestinal tract, commonly the small and large intestines, but rectum is characteristically spared
- It is a transmural inflammatory condition of GI tract
- Usually, a disease of young adults of the second and third decades, and rarely of the elderly
- This can present with mild, moderate or severe disease, judgment based on the intensity of diarrhea, abdominal pain, presence or absence of dehydration, anemia, malnutrition and tachycardia
- Crohn's disease affects the ileocecal junction in 50% of cases, followed by small bowel (25%), colon (20%) and upper gastrointestinal tract (5%).

Risk Factors

- Genetic predisposition (NOD-2/CARD–15 mutation in chromosome 16)
- Cigarette smoking
- Bacteria
- *M. avium* paratuberculosis.

Diagnosis

Clinical Presentation

Clinical presentation depends on the stage of the disease. Symptoms are determined by the site and stage of involvement. The most common site of involvement is ileocecal junction.

- *Inflammatory stage:* Diarrhea, pain in the right iliac fossa with a long history (contrasting with appendicular mass which has a short history) triggered by meals associated with a tender mass in the right iliac fossa. Diarrhea is usually nonbloody (diarrhea of ulcerative colitis is bloody). Fever, weight loss and extraintestinal symptoms may be associated. Perianal tags may be associated, which may resemble external hemorrhoids. Perianal fistulae and fissures are common
- *Stenosis stage:* Vomiting and constipation (features of intestinal obstruction)
- *Fistula stage:* Discharges (external fistula), recurrent infections (internal fistula).

Extraintestinal Manifestations

- *Skin:* Erythema multiforme, erythema nodosum, pyoderma gangrenosum
- *Eyes:* Iritis, uveitis, conjunctivitis
- *Joints:* Peripheral arthritis, ankylosing spondylitis
- *Blood:* Anemia, thrombocytosis, phlebothrombosis, arterial thrombosis
- *Liver:* Nonspecific triaditis, sclerosing cholangitis
- *Kidneys*: Nephrotic syndrome, amyloidosis
- *Pancreas:* Pancreatitis
- *General:* Amyloidosis.

Investigations

Radiology

- **Barium meal study** is diagnostic. It demonstrates the mucosal involvement *(cobblestone appearance)*, strictures *(string sign of Kantor)* **(Fig 12.8A)**, segmental involvement, fistulous communications to adjoining organs
- **Barium enema** demonstrates signs of inflammation in colon **(Fig 12.8B)**
- **CT with oral contrast** is more informative.

Endoscopy

- **Endoscopy** may reveal aphthoid ulcerations, rarely deep and serpiginous along the long axis of the colon. Skip areas, cobblestoning and rectal sparing are key findings.

Tissue Diagnosis

- **Biopsy** is characteristic (microscopic granulomas and transmural inflammation are pathognomonic).

Serology

- Anti-*Saccharomyces cerevisiae* antibody (ASCA) is positive and perinuclear antineutrophil cytoplasmic antibody (pANCA) is negative. [converse is true with ulcerative colitis]

Diagnosis of Crohn's disease is determined by:
- History
- Physical examination
- Endoscopy
- Biopsies
- Radiographs
- Laboratory data.

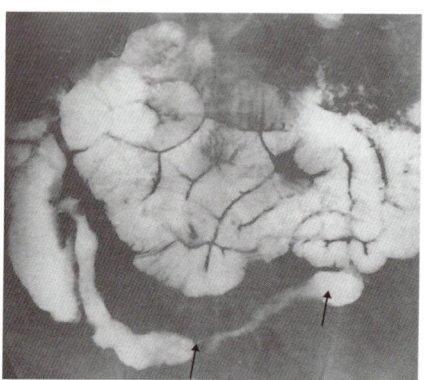

Fig. 12.8A: String sign of Kantor

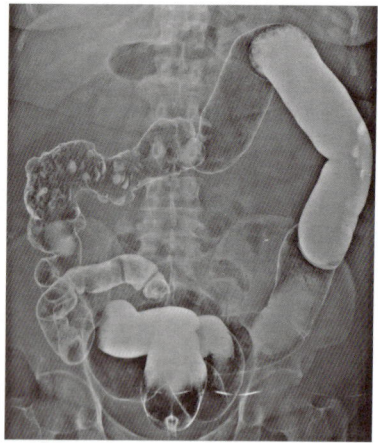

Fig. 12.8B: Barium enema—Chronic inflammatory disease of proximal colon

Classification

Crohn's disease is classified under Vienna classification **(Table 12.1)**.

Severity of Crohn's Disease

Severity of Crohn's disease can be assessed using Crohn's disease activity index (CDAI) **(Table 12.2)**. This index is a research tool used to quantify the symptoms of patients with Crohn's disease.

Harvey–Bradshaw index

The Harvey–Bradshaw index was devised in 1980 as a simpler version of the CDAI for data collection purposes. It consists of only clinical parameters:
- General wellbeing (0 = very well, 1 = slightly below average, 2 = poor, 3 = very poor, 4 = terrible)

Table 12.1: Vienna classification of Crohn's disease

	Stage	Feature	Findings
Age at diagnosis	1	< 40 years	Time of histological, surgical, radiological, or endoscopic diagnosis, no retrospective time of diagnosis
	2	> 40 years	
Location	1	Terminal ileum	Maximum extent of the lesions at any time before resection
	2	Colon	
	3	Ileocolon	Aphthous lesions or ulcerations of any size
	4	Upper GI tract	
Behavior	1	Non-stricturing, Non-penetrating	Inflammatory masses, abscesses, fistulae, perianal ulcers are defined as penetrating
	2	Stricturing	Strictures can be diagnosed radiologically, endoscopically or surgically
	3	Penetrating	Postoperative complications are excluded

Snapshots in Gastroenterology

Table 12.2: Crohn's disease activity index (CDAI)

	Variable	Weight in g factor
1.	Liquid or soft stools each day for 7 days	X2
2.	Daily abdominal pain (graded from 0–3 on severity) each day for 7 days	X5
3.	General wellbeing subjectively assessed from 0 (well) to 4 (terrible) each day for 7 days	X6
4.	Presence of complications *	X20
5.	Use of opiates for diarrhea	X30
6.	Abdominal mass (0 as none, 2 as questionable, 5 as definite)	X10
7.	47 hematocrit (males) 42 hematocrit (females)	X6
8.	Percent of body weight below standard	X1

*One point each is added for each set of complications:
- Presence of joint pains (arthralgia) or frank arthritis
- Inflammation of iris or uveitis
- Presence of erythema nodosum, pyoderma granulosum or aphthous ulcers
- Anal fissure, fistulae or abscesses
- Other fistulae
- Fever during the previous week.

Remission of disease is defined as a fall in the CDAI of less than 150. Severe disease was defined as a value of greater than 450.

- Abdominal pain (0 = none, 1 = mild, 2 = moderate, 3 = severe)
- Number of liquid stools per day
- Abdominal mass (0 = none, 1 = dubious, 2 = definite, 3 = tender)
- Complications, as above, with one point for each
- General wellbeing.

Complications

- Perforation
- Abscess
- Internal fistulae.

Differential Diagnosis

- Ulcerative colitis
- Ischemic colitis
- Diverticulitis
- Colorectal malignancy
- Viral infections
- Irritable bowel syndrome
- Lymphoma
- Celiac sprue
- Radiation enteropathy
- NSAID induced enteropathy.

The differentiating features between Crohn's disease and ulcerative colitis are given in **Table 12.3**.

Management

The disease is not curable and hence goals of therapy are to induce and maintain remission.

Table 12.3: Differentiating Crohn's disease from ulcerative colitis

Feature	Crohn's disease	Ulcerative colitis
Small bowel involvement	Yes	No
Part of colon involved	Right colon	Any part of colon
Rectal involvement	No	Yes
Fistulization	Yes	No
Perianal disease	Yes	No
Granulomas	Yes	No
pANCA	15%	75%
Antibodies to *Saccharomyces cerevisiae*	50%	Small percentage

- *Medical* (essentially symptomatic)
  - **Stop cigarette smoking**
  - **Long-term antibiotics**
  - **Sulfasalazine and 5 ASA compounds**
  - **Steroids**
  - **Immunosuppressants (azathioprine and 6-mercaptopurine, methotrexate, cyclosporine)**
  - **Biologic therapy**—Infliximab and adalimumab are recommended.
- *Surgical* treatment is warranted for patients
  - **Refractory to medical therapy**
  - **Complications**
    - *Fistulae – excision*
    - *Abscess – drainage*
    - *Strictures – stricturoplasty, excision, bypass.*

Clinical Pearls

- Patients diagnosed to have Crohn's disease must quit smoking
- Flare ups are common in smokers than non-smokers
- Intestinal infections, NSAID usage and oral contraceptives cause flare ups or recurrences of symptoms
- Inflammatory stage is more amenable to medical therapy and so also has more chances of recurrences
- Stricturing and fistulizing stages need surgical management, and fistulae almost commonly occur at the region proximal to strictures. Medical management as maintenance therapy will minimize the chance of recurrence
- Risk of malignancy is less in small bowel Crohn's disease when compared to the risk in large bowel Crohn's disease
- Risk of malignancy in Crohn's disease and ulcerative colitis seem to be similar

- In small bowel Crohn's disease, adenocarcinoma can occur. There is a small risk of lymphomas also
- Majority of patients with Crohn's disease will require surgery within 20 years of diagnosis, and 50% of them will require another operation within 10 years.

WHIPPLE'S DISEASE

Introduction

Whipple's disease is a chronic systemic illness with a variety of manifestations.

Etiology

Disease caused by a gram-positive *Actinomyces, Tropheryma whippelii*.

Diagnosis

Clinical Presentation

- Weight loss
- Diarrhea
- Joint pains.

Other manifestations are:
- ***Cardiac:*** Congestive heart failure, pericarditis, valvular heart disease
- ***Lymphatic:*** Lymphadenopathy
- ***Gastrointestinal:*** Lower GI bleeding (frank/occult)
- ***Neurologic:*** Dementia, ocular disturbances, meningoencephalitis, cerebellar symptoms.

The multisystem manifestations are shown in **Box 12.1**.

Box 12.1: Multisystem manifestations of Whipple's disease	
W–Wasting/weight loss	D–Diarrhea
H–Hyperpigmentation	I–Interstitial nephritis
I–Intestinal pain	S–Skin rashes
P–Pleurisy	E–Eye inflammation
P–Pneumonitis	A–Arthritis
L–Lymphadenopathy	S–Subcutaneous nodules
E–Encephalopathy	E–Endocarditis
S–Steatorrhea	

Investigations

- ***Small bowel and lymph node biopsy*** may show PAS positive inclusions in macrophages
- ***T. whippelii DNA concentration measurements*** (DNS sequence of the 16S-ribosomal RNA gene sequence) in synovial fluid, CSF or small bowel biopsy are the most sensitive marker.

Management

Prolonged use of antibiotics (tetracycline, penicillin, erythromycin or trimethoprim/sulfamethoxazole) for more than a year is curative. Chloramphenicol is preferred when central nervous system is involved.

Clinical Pearl

Relapses are known to occur especially when central nervous system is involved.

CELIAC DISEASE

A disease involving abnormal mucosa of small intestine that reverts to normal when treated with a gluten free diet and relapses when gluten is reintroduced in the diet. It can affect at any age.

Etiology and Pathogenesis
- Proposed to be a T-cell mediated hypersensitivity reaction to a component of gluten, may be an enterotoxin produced by a peptide corresponding to amino acids 313–49 of A-gliaden
- 10% of first degree relatives are affected.

Diagnosis

Clinical Presentation
- ***Children:*** Pallor, anorexia, abdominal distension
- ***Adults:*** Diarrhea, tiredness, weight loss, glossitis, angular stomatitis.

Investigations
- Hematocrit decrease
- Peripheral smear—target cells, Howell Jolly bodies, acanthocytes and thrombocytosis
- Low calcium, vitamin D, albumin and zinc
- IgG and IgM gliadin, IgA reticulin, IgA anti-endomysial and tissue transglutaminase antibodies (90% sensitive)
- ***Small bowel biopsy*** (4 biopsies from second part of duodenum)
- ***CT abdomen*** may show splenic atrophy and low grade lymphadenopathy.

Management
- ***Gluten free diet*** (avoid wheat, barley and oats)
- ***Steroids*** may be useful.

Clinical Pearl

About 3–4 pale, offensive loose stools is a typical finding of celiac disease.

IRRITABLE BOWEL SYNDROME

Introduction

Irritable bowel syndrome (IBS) is a functional disorder of the gastrointestinal tract characterized by chronic, recurrent abdominal pain or discomfort with disturbed bowel habits. Rome III criteria (**Box 12.2**) define that the symptoms should have been present for at least 6 months with asymptomatic intervals.

Manning criteria also helps in making the diagnosis of IBS (**Box 12.3**).

Classification

1. Diarrhea predominant IBS (IBS – D)

Box 12.2: Rome III criteria for irritable bowel syndrome

Recurrent abdominal pain or discomfort at least 3 days per month in the last 3 months (with the onset at least 6 months prior to diagnosis) associated with two or more of the following;
- Improvement with defecation
- Onset associated with a change in frequency of stool
- Onset associated with a change in form (appearance of stool)

Box 12.3: Manning criteria for IBS

- Abdominal pain relieved by defecation
- More frequent stools with onset of pain
- Looser stools with onset of pain
- Passage of mucus per rectum
- Feeling of incomplete rectal emptying
- Patient reported visible abdominal distension

2. Constipation predominant IBS (IBS-C)
3. Mixed habit with predominant symptom pattern (IBS – M)
4. Unsubtyped IBS.

Etiology and Pathogenesis

More common in women, and seen in all ages, predominantly in the third and fourth decades of life. The pathophysiology of IBS is poorly understood, and it is thought to be multifactorial **(Box 12.4)**.

Diagnosis

Symptoms
- Abdominal pain (diffuse, crampy or intermittent)
- Altered bowel habits (diarrhea, constipation or both).

Sign
- Abdominal tenderness.

Investigations
- Complete blood count
- Erythrocyte sedimentation rate
- Celiac antibody tests
- Thyroid function tests
- **Stool test** for parasites and guiac

Box 12.4: Various factors of IBS

- Visceral hypersensitivity
- Altered motility
- Immune activation
- Stress response
- Genetic component
- Colonic motility disturbances

Differential Diagnosis

- Diarrhea predominant IBS
  - Celiac disease
  - Microscopic colitis
  - Inflammatory bowel disease
  - Giardiasis
  - Lactose intolerance
  - Bacterial overgrowth
- Constipation predominant IBS
  - Chronic functional constipation
  - Drug induced constipation
  - Diverticulosis
  - Colon cancer.

Management

- Lifestyle modifications (diet, stress, exercise)
- Constipation dominant IBS
  - Laxatives
  - Lubiprostone
- Diarrhea dominant IBS
  - Opiate antidiarrheals (diphenoxylate, loperamide, codeine, tincture of opium)
  - Non-opiate antimotility drugs (hyoscyamine, clonidine)
  - Stool texture modifiers (cholestyramine, colestipol)
  - Bulking agents (psyllium, methylcellulose)
- Antispasmodics for pain
- Probiotics are useful.

Clinical Pearls

- Psychiatric disorders do not cause IBS but they can precipitate or exacerbate symptoms
- Viral or bacterial intestinal infections are known to cause IBS
- Rectal examination should be done to eliminate rectal pathology
- The diagnosis of IBS is by clinical exclusion
- Osmotic laxatives like PEG is more effective than gas producing laxatives like lactulose.

STRICTURES

Introduction

Strictures may be caused by
- Tuberculosis (healing lesions)
- Malignant lesions
- Surgery of intestines (postoperative).

Diagnosis

Clinical Presentation

- Symptoms of subacute or acute intestinal obstruction
- History of weight loss, low grade pyrexia, anemia and vague abdominal pain may be present
- Clinical examination may show a mass in the right iliac fossa (**DD**-Crohn's disease)
- Ascites may be present.

Investigations

- Barium meal studies can identify the strictures
- CT with oral contrast or enteroclysis can identify the strictures.

Management

- *Laparotomy* is needed for acute obstructions
- *Stricturoplasty (Fig 12.9) or bypass procedures or resections* are done for tubercular strictures
- *Radical resections or bypass procedures* are done for malignant strictures.

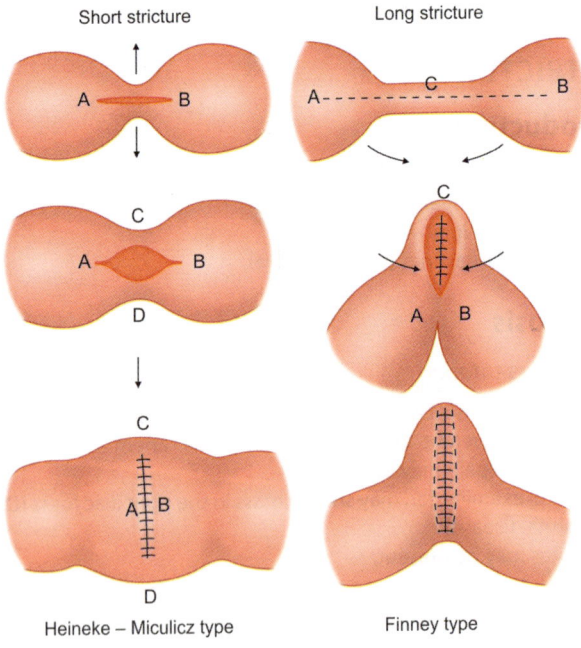

Fig. 12.9: Types of stricturoplasty

PARALYTIC ILEUS

Introduction

- Prolongation of ileus after abdominal operations beyond the third postoperative day and last for a week or more
- Usual cause being electrolyte imbalance in the postoperative period
- Retroperitoneal or intraperitoneal hemorrhage and sepsis are the other causes
- Trivial causes like an injection, application of plaster of Paris bandage and any injury anywhere, fractures, etc. (**Table 12.4**).

Table 12.4: Causes of paralytic ileus

Causes	Pathology	Mechanism
Sympathetic dysfunction	Postoperative ileus	Reflex inhibition
	Spinal injury	
	Acute renal colic	
	Trauma	Retroperitoneal hemorrhage
	Acute pancreatitis	
	Retroperitoneal malignancy	Malignant infiltration
Local causes	Peritonitis	Bacterial infection
	Advanced mechanical obstruction	Excessive distension of bowel
Pharmacological	Anticholinergics	Interference with smooth muscle contractility
	Antidiarrheals	
	Ganglion blockers	
Biochemical	Hypokalemia	
	Uremia	
	Diabetic crisis	
	Hypoxia	

Diagnosis

Clinical Presentation
- Abdominal distension without pain
- Vomiting is a predominant symptom
- On examination, the abdomen is resonant with the characteristic absence of bowel sounds.

Investigation
- *Plain radiographs of the abdomen* will show '*step ladder pattern*' of small bowel (**Fig. 12.10**) with distension of both small and large bowels.

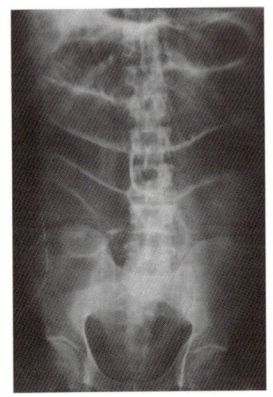

Fig. 12.10: Step ladder pattern of paralytic ileus

Management
- Correction of electrolyte imbalances
- Treatment for retroperitoneal or intraperitoneal causes like hemorrhage and sepsis.

ISCHEMIC ENTERITIS/MESENTERIC VASCULAR OBSTRUCTION

Introduction

It is usually due to the following:

Arterial Diseases
- *Occlusive diseases*
  - **Thrombosis:** Thrombosis on an atheromatous plaque (e.g. origin of superior mesenteric artery)

- **Embolism:** Embolus following atrial fibrillation/myocardial infarction/detached atheromatous plaque
- **Vasculitis:** Systemic lupus erythematosus, polyarteritis nodosa
- **Strangulation:** Volvulus, intussusception.
- *Nonocclusive diseases*
  - **Hypotension:** Hypoperfusion (cardiogenic shock, hypovolemia, sepsis)
  - **Drugs:** Vasoconstricting drugs (digoxin, noradrenaline, propranolol).

Venous Diseases

- Intra-abdominal causes
  - Acute pancreatitis
  - Intra-abdominal sepsis
  - Portal hypertension
  - Post-splenectomy
- Hypercoagulable states
  - Antithrombin III deficiency
  - Protein C deficiency
  - Protein S deficiency
  - Factor V Leiden deficiency
  - Hyperhomocystinemia
  - Oral contraceptives.

Pathogenesis

The obstruction to mesenteric blood flow causes reduced oxygen of red blood cells leading to intestinal tissue hypoxia and ischemic injury (**Fig. 12.11**).

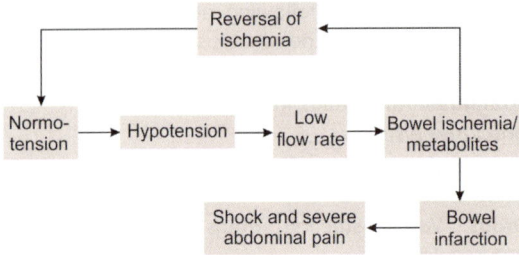

Fig. 12.11: Pathogenesis of ischemic enteritis

Classification

- Acute mesenteric ischemia
- Chronic mesenteric ischemia.

Diagnosis

Clinical Presentation

- Severe acute abdominal pain (meal induced) with copious vomiting
- Fear of vomiting (sitophobia)
- Diarrhea
- Very fast deterioration of health
- Hematemesis and melena also occur in some cases
- The clinical signs are disproportionate to the symptoms, and rarely an area of tenderness may be felt near the infarcted bowel.

Investigations

Blood Tests

- *Hematocrit*—Increased
- *White cell count*—Leukocytosis.

Radiology

- **Plain abdominal X-rays**—bowel wall thickening, loop separation, thumb printing
- **CECT**—bowel wall thickening, loop separation, thumb printing
- **Doppler US of mesenteric vessels**—decreased blood flow
- **Mesenteric angiography (MRI)**—anatomical obstructions to mesenteric blood flow.

Management

- *Conservative management to stabilize the patient*
- *Laparotomy and resection of non-viable bowel* will be necessary, if the patient is stable
- *Balloon angioplasty or bypass grafts* may be feasible in select cases.

Note: Outcome is guarded in most cases.

Clinical Pearls

- Conventional endoscopic procedures are not to be performed for the fear of complications
- Mesenteric angiography is gold standard in diagnosing mesenteric vascular occlusions.

INTESTINAL OBSTRUCTION

Introduction

- Intestinal obstructions may be dynamic or adynamic.
  - *Dynamic obstruction* is a physical or mechanical obstruction of the intestinal lumen due to various causes. They are:

1. *Intraluminal causes* (e.g. fecal impaction, worms).
2. *Mural causes* (e.g. strictures or stenosis due to tuberculosis, malignancies).
3. *Extraluminal causes* (e.g. adhesions, obstructed hernia).

– **Adynamic obstruction** of the bowel is due to its neural (autonomic) paralysis, commonly seen after abdominal surgery in the immediate postoperative period, peritonitis or any other cause like fractures, tight bandages, etc. (Paralytic ileus–See page 385).

Etiology and Pathogenesis

Causes of intestinal obstruction are different for different age groups (**Table 12.5**).

Diagnosis

Clinical Presentation

1. Sudden episodic colicky abdominal pain
2. Vomiting
3. Constipation
4. Abdominal distension.

(The symptoms vary according to the level of obstruction) (**Table 12.6**)

– *Abdominal pain:* It is sudden and squeezing, and the patient doubles up. It is felt in the umbilical region, sometimes accompanied by the appearance of a contracting loop. There may be pain free intervals. Colonic pain presents in the hypogastrium
– *Vomiting:* Vomiting is predominant in high obstructions. The vomitus consists of gastric contents, followed by the duodenal

Table 12.5: Causes of intestinal obstruction in different age groups

Newborn	Infants	Adolescents	Adults	Elderly	Rare causes
Duodenal atresia	Helminths	Bands	Post-operative adhesions	Growth	Enteroliths
Pyloric stenosis	Intussusception	Intussusception	Intussusception	Intussusception	Foreign bodies
Meconium ileus		Meckel's diverticulum	Volvulus	Obstructed or strangulated hernia	Gallstones
Hirschsprung's disease		Obstructed or strangulated hernia	Growth, obstructed or strangulated hernia		Trichobezoar Phytobezoar

Table 12.6: Signs and symptoms related to intestinal obstruction

Level of obstruction	Signs and symptoms					
	Duration of colic	Pain free interval	Vomiting	Distension of abdomen	Constipation	Dehydration
High	Short	Short	More	Minimal	Not constant	Severe
Low	Long	Long	Less	More	Late feature	Mild to moderate

and lastly the intestinal, depending on the level of obstruction. In the late stages, the vomitus becomes feculent—ominous sign. Vomiting by itself is a late sign of chronic intestinal obstruction
- **Constipation:** The patient evacuates his bowel (contents distal to obstruction) once or twice, and constipation becomes a noticeable feature after 24 hours
- **Abdominal distension:** Common feature of intestinal obstruction. Distension is:
    - *Centrally located* in small bowel obstruction (ladder pattern),
    - *More on the flanks* when distal colon is obstructed (asymmetrical)
    - *More on the left flank* in sigmoid volvulus
- **Dehydration:** When vomiting is pronounced as in high level obstructions, dehydration is a presenting feature
- **General:** Pulse rate and blood pressure are maintained at normal levels in the initial stages. As dehydration becomes prominent, tachycardia and hypotension result
- **Abdomen:** Bowel sounds are not heard as obstruction worsens.

Signs and symptoms related to intestinal obstruction are given in **Table 12.6**.

Investigation

Plain X-rays of abdomen in the erect posture will reveal multiple air fluid levels (**Fig 12.12**) and colonic obstruction may show distended colon also (**Fig 12.13**).

Management

- Management is directed towards the cause.

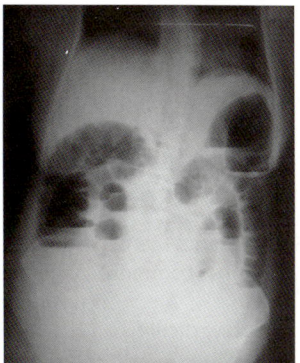 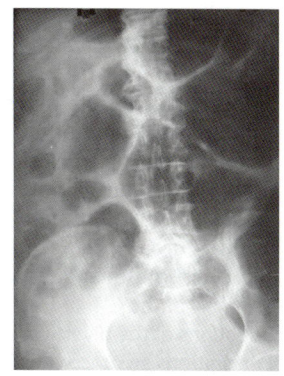

Fig. 12.12: Multiple air fluid levels of small bowel obstruction

Fig. 12.13: Distension of large bowel

Clinical Pearls

- Diarrhea can be a feature in certain situations like intussusception (redcurrant jelly stools), Richter's hernia, adynamic obstruction caused by mesenteric vascular occlusion, pelvic abscess, etc.
- Early dehydration and less abdominal distension suggests duodenal or jejunal obstruction whereas, late dehydration and more abdominal distension suggests distal ileal obstruction
- Vomiting and dehydration are usually not present in isolated acute colonic obstruction.

DIVERTICULITIS OF SMALL BOWEL

Introduction

- Diverticula occur in any portion of the small bowel, most commonly in the duodenum and jejunum (excepting Meckel's diverticulum)

- Congenital diverticula are the herniation of the entire thickness of the bowel wall, whereas the acquired diverticula consist of mucosa and serosa
- Duodenal diverticula are usually single while jejunal diverticula are multiple (**Fig 12.14**)
- Periampullary diverticula are usually found during ERCP, and make CBD cannulation difficult, and retroperitoneal perforation is seen during sphincterotomy
- Meckel's diverticulum (**Fig 12.15**) represents the persistence of the vitellointestinal duct and is the most common congenital anomaly of the GIT
- Infections of the diverticula present as diverticulitis
- Perforations are uncommon

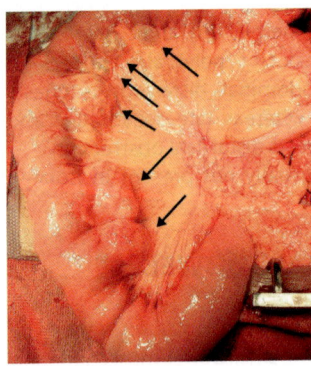
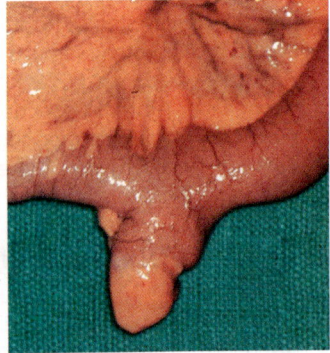

Fig. 12.14: Jejunal diverticula   **Fig. 12.15:** Meckel's diverticulum

Diagnosis

Clinical Presentation

- Lower gastrointestinal bleed with or without abdominal pain
- Stools are characteristically maroon in color

Investigations

- **Barium studies (Fig 12.16)** may show the diverticula
- **Capsule endoscopy** is useful in diagnosis.

Management

Symptomatic diverticula are removed by surgery.

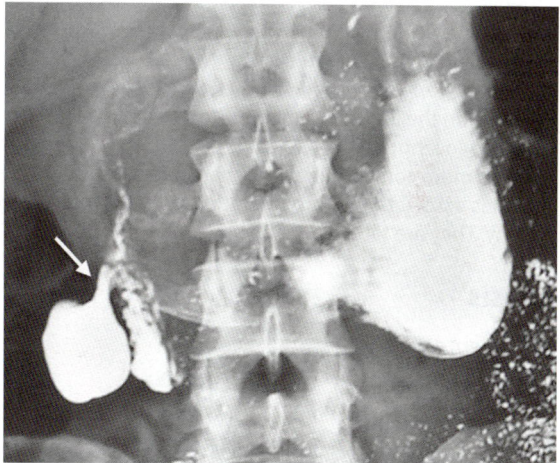

Fig. 12.16: Barium meal—Duodenal diverticulum

Meckel's Diverticulitis

Introduction

Meckel's Diverticulum

- Most prevalent congenital GI anomaly
- An embryological remnant (**see Fig. 12.15**)—a remnant of an incomplete obliteration of vitellointestinal duct, connecting the midgut and the yolk sac during embryological development. It presents as a free diverticulum with a wide mouth, about 25 to 30 cm from the ileocecal junction; may contain ectopic gastric mucosa (reason not known)
- It contains all layers of ileum and considered a true diverticulum
- Ectopic tissues can be found (e.g. gastric, pancreatic, carcinoid, duodenal, lipoma and liposarcoma tissues)
- Meckel's diverticulum has an independent blood supply
- Occurrence follows *rough rule of 2s*:
  - 2% of the population
  - 2 feet from the ileocecal junction
  - 2 inches in length
  - 2 times more common in males than in females
- Anomalies associated with obliteration of vitellointestinal duct are many. They are tabulated in **Table 12.7**.

Diagnosis

Clinical Presentation

- Right iliac fossa pain
- Fever
- Vomiting
- Abdominal tenderness.

Table 12.7: Anomalies associated with obliteration of vitellointestinal duct

Anomaly	Pathology
Umbilical vitellointestinal fistula (Fig 12.17A)	Duct not obliterated and absorbed
Meckel's diverticulum connected to umbilicus by fibrous band (Fig 12.17B)	Duct obliterated but not absorbed
Umbilical sinus (Fig 12.17C)	Duct partially obliterated but not absorbed
Umbilical cyst (Fig 12.17D)	Duct partially obliterated but not absorbed with a cyst in the mid part of fibrous cord
Fibrous cord (Fig 12.17E)	Duct completely obliterated but not absorbed

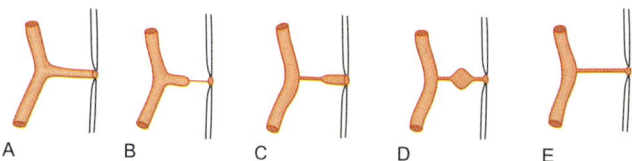

Figs 12.17A to E: Anomalies associated with vitellointestinal duct

Investigations

- *US* shows inflamed Meckel's diverticulum as a cyst like structure with thick hyperechoic internal wall and a hypoechoic outer wall, referred to as the '*gut signature*'
- *CT scan* identifies it as a blind ending structure in the right lower quadrant, with signs of inflammation and fluid collections
- *Isotope scan (Technetium 99-m pertechnetate scintigraphy)—Meckel scan* is useful in identifying the functioning ectopic tissue in the diverticulum
- *Angiography* is useful in bleeding diverticulum.

Differential Diagnosis

- Appendicitis
- Any intra-abdominal infective pathology
- Any cause of intestinal obstruction (**Refer Table 12.5**)
- Any cause of lower GI bleeding (**Refer Table 9.2**).

Complications

- Intestinal obstruction
- Rectal bleeding
- Perforation
- Peritonitis.

Uncommon Complications

- Carcinoid tumors
- Littre's hernia
- Gallstone ileus
- Parasitic impaction
- Bezoars in the diverticulum.

Management

- Acute diverticulitis warrants *diverticulectomy*
- *Ileal resection and end to end anastomosis*—for Meckel's diverticulum complicated by bleeding, perforation and tumor
- *Perforation and peritonitis need appropriate management.*

Clinical Pearls

- The vitellointestinal duct obliterates between the 7th and 8th week of gestation, and the bowel proximal to this develops into distal duodenum, jejunum and a part of ileum. The bowel distal to the duct develops into the remaining part of ileum, cecum, appendix, ascending colon and proximal 2/3 of transverse colon

- The size and shape of Meckel's diverticulum varies considerably, and the diameter is almost equal to the diameter of the small bowel
- When the diameter exceeds 5 cm, it is considered a giant Meckel's diverticulum
- Meckel's diverticulum becomes symptomatic only when it is complicated
- Bleeding from Meckel's diverticulitis can be small and chronic causing iron deficiency anemia or massive leading to hemodynamic instability, and is usually caused by ileal mucosal ulceration adjacent to acid producing ectopic gastric mucosa
- *H. pylori* does not play any role in the development of complications of Meckel's diverticulum
- Meckel's diverticulitis should be considered a possible cause for any painful intra-abdominal cause
- Appendicitis and Meckel's diverticulitis are indistinguishable clinically
- CT imaging though considered the imaging of choice, most of the time, Meckel's diverticulum is indistinguishable from normal intestinal loop
- In adults, angiography is preferred over the Meckel scan, as the ectopic gastric mucosa is not found as often as in children
- In angiography, the demonstration of bleeding from vitelline arteries is possible and diagnostic
- Prophylactic removal of Meckel's diverticulum is justified in both sexes, but the decision should be on case to case basis depending on certain risk factors like age <50 years, size >2 cm and presence of ectopic tissue and diverticular bands.

ANGIODYSPLASIA

Introduction

It is gastrointestinal vascular ectasia not associated with cutaneous lesions, systemic vascular disease or a familial syndrome.

Etiology

It may be a degenerative condition, related to chronic low-grade mucosal vein obstruction or mucosal ischemia.

Diagnosis

Clinical Presentation

- Upper or lower GI bleeding
- Occult anemia
- Acute massive hemorrhage is common in colonic lesions.

Investigations

- *Endoscopy*
- *Angiography*
- *Radionuclide scanning*
- *Intra-abdominal enteroscopy.*

Management

- *Endoscopic hemostasis*
- *Surgical resection of bowel with lesion.*

BENIGN TUMORS

Introduction

Variety of benign tumors occur in the small bowel, but they are rare.
- Adenomas
- Endocrine tumors (carcinoids)
- Stromal tumors
- Lipoma
- Vascular tumors (hemangioma)
- Neurogenic tumors
- Tumors of lymphoid tissue
- Benign polyps (Peutz-Jeghers syndrome).

Diagnosis

Clinical Presentation
- Many lesions are asymptomatic
- Presentation depends on size and location
- Large lesions are usually of villous type and present with intestinal obstruction and intussusception
- Ulcerated lesions may present with bleeding.

Investigation
- ***Enteroclysis*** is useful
- ***Double contrast radiological studies*** give adequate information
- ***CT enhanced radiological studies*** give better information
- ***Capsule endoscopy*** (Fig. 12.18) is diagnostic.

Management
- ***Excision with resection of bowel*** is the treatment for symptomatic tumors.

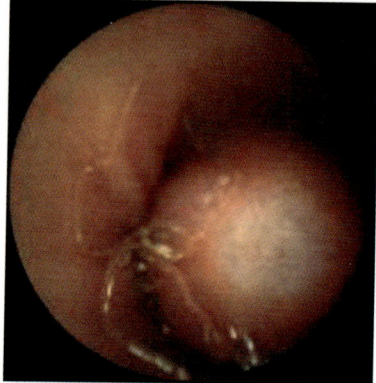

Fig. 12.18: Capsule endoscopy—Ileal lipoma

MALIGNANT TUMORS

Malignant tumors of small intestines are very rare and account for only less than 1% of all GI tumors. They are categorized as:
- *Lymphoma*
- *Adenocarcinoma*
- *Carcinoid*
- *Malignant GISTs and vascular tumors (angiosarcoma) are rare.*

Lymphoma

Introduction

- *Lymphomas* of small intestine are uncommon but account for 30% of small bowel malignancies
- Represent 5% of all GI malignancies, 2% of all extranodal lymphomas and 25% of all GI lymphomas

Small Intestine

- After the stomach, small bowel is the commonest site of GI lymphomas
- More common in the 7th decade of life with a male predominance of 2:1
- The incidence of lymphoma is in the decreasing order of ileum to jejunum to duodenum
- The subtypes vary with particular sites and ethnic groups.

Risk Factors

- α-chain disease
- Celiac disease
- Dermatitis herpetiformis
- Autoimmune disorders
- Crohn's disease
- Immunodeficiency syndromes including AIDS.

Etiology and Pathogenesis

Primary intestinal lymphoma arises from the lymphoid cells in the Peyer's patches and most commonly affects the ileocecal junction, where the lymphoid cells are in abundance.

Classification

Intestinal lymphomas belong to B cell or T (or natural killer— NK) cell lineage and various subtypes can occur. The common pathological types of lymphomas seen in the small bowel are tabulated in **Table 12.8**.

The gastrointestinal lymphomas are staged by Mushoff modification of Ann Arbor Staging (**Table 12.9**).

Table 12.8: Pathological types of small bowel lymphomas

Mature B cell lymphoma	Mature T/NK cell lymphoma	Immunodeficiency lymphoma
Diffuse large cell lymphoma	T/NK nasal type	HIV related
MALToma	Enteropathic T cell	Post-transplant lymphoma
Mantle cell lymphoma		Hodgkin's lymphoma
Burkitt lymphoma		Mixed cellularity

Table 12.9: Musshoff modification of Ann Arbor Staging of gastrointestinal lymphomas

Stage	Property
Ia	One tumor area without perforation
Ib	Multiple tumors no perforation
IIa	Gastric or mesenteric nodes involved
IIb	Perforation and adhesions
IIc	Frank peritonitis
III	Widespread thoracic/para-aortic/pelvic nodes
IV	Extralymphatic non-adjacent tissue involved

Diagnosis

Symptoms

- Chronic abdominal pain
- Nausea
- Vomiting
- Appetite loss
- Weight loss
- Fatigue
- Symptoms of obstruction (due to intussusception)
- Peritonitis (perforation)
- GI bleed.

Signs

- Abdominal mass
- Anemia
- Signs of obstruction and peritonitis.

Investigations

Radiology

- ***Barium meal*** is informative when the lesions are nodular
- ***CT*** is preferred over MRI in locating mass lesions, mesenteric and retroperitoneal lymphadenopathy and thickening of bowel wall
- ***PET scan*** may be useful but in low-grade tumors, it may not be contributory
- ***Capsule endoscopy*** (**Fig. 12.19**) is useful in identifying the lesion.

Blood Test

- ***An elevated LDH level*** may be suggestive of lymphoma.

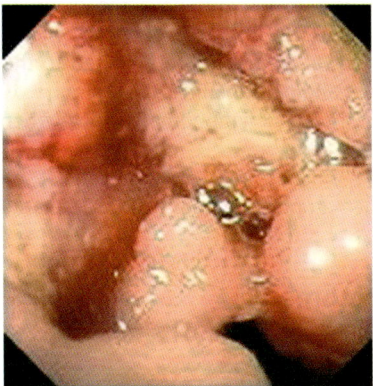

Fig. 12.19: Capsule endoscopy—Small bowel lymphoma

Histopathology

- *CT guided biopsy* may be possible if nodal involvement is present.

Management

- Bowel resection when the disease is localized
- When the disease is widespread or disseminated, multi-agent chemotherapy is the only hope
- Radiation is useful in lymphomas, in spite of complications like ileus and enteritis.

Clinical Pearls

- Burkitt's lymphoma and NK-cell lymphoma have a very dramatic course
- It is difficult to image the small intestine radiologically for a clear diagnosis
- About a quarter of patients have the diagnosis of intestinal lymphoma made only during surgery
- Most small bowel lymphomas are limited to the intestine and spread to liver and peritoneum is uncommon
- Prognosis of intestinal lymphoma is worse when compared to gastric lymphoma
- Relapses are difficult to treat and when it is disseminated, allogenic hematopoietic stem cell transplantation may be considered.

Adenocarcinoma

Introduction

- Much rarer than carcinoma of stomach and large intestine
- Periampullary region and duodenum are most common sites

- Less commonly found in jejunum and ileum
- Most cancers arise within a pre-existing adenoma (Adenoma carcinoma sequence).

Risk Factors

- Peutz-Jegher syndrome
- Familial adenomatous polyposis
- Crohn's disease
- Celiac disease
- Neurofibromatosis NF1
- Genetic predispositions (mismatch repair genes hMLH1 and hMSH2, β-catetin, E-cadherin and p53).

Diagnosis

Clinical Presentation

- Many lesions are asymptomatic
- Presentation depends on size and location
- Large lesions are usually of villous type and present with intestinal obstruction and intussusception
- Ulcerated lesions may present with bleeding and anemia.

Investigations

- ***Enteroclysis or double contrast study*** gives excellent information
- ***CT enhanced studies*** are more specific
- ***Capsule endoscopy*** is diagnostic.

Management

- ***Excision with resection of bowel*** is the treatment for symptomatic tumors.

Clinical Pearls

- Adenocarcinomas are found in the decreasing frequency in the duodenum, jejunum and ileum
- Crohn's disease is associated with increased risk of adenocarcinoma
- Enteroclysis is the best radiological investigation to study the intestines
- CT enhanced radiological studies give better results
- Operative resection is the only option available for intestinal malignancies.

Carcinoid Tumor

Introduction

- Account for about one-third of all small bowel neoplasms
- Second most common small bowel neoplasm
- More common in the 6th and 7th decades of life, with male predominance
- More common in the duodenum and ileum
- Most intestinal carcinoids are less than 2 cm in diameter
- They are slow growing and produce narrowing
- About 10% of carcinoid tumors present with carcinoid syndrome
- About 30% are multicentric and 90% metastatic.

Etiology and Pathogenesis

- Arise from the neuroendocrine Kulchitsky cells found in the base of the crypts of Lieberkuhn and a part of APUD system
- Capable of secreting multiple metabolically active hormones, the most common being the serotonin.

Small Intestine

Diagnosis

Clinical Presentation

- Many lesions are asymptomatic
- Presentation depends on size and location
- Large lesions present with intestinal obstruction and intussusception
- Ulcerated lesions may present with bleeding and anemia
- Carcinoid syndrome in about 10% of cases (stimulated by serotonin rich foods like coffee, cheese, alcohol and exercise).

Investigations

- *Enteroclysis or double contrast study* gives excellent information
- *CT enhanced studies* are more specific
- *Capsule endoscopy* is diagnostic
- *Increase in 24-hour 5-HIAA when the carcinoids secrete serotonin*
- *Somatostatin receptor scintigraphy (Octreoscan) is extremely sensitive in detecting carcinoids.*

Management

- *Radical excision with resection of bowel* is the treatment for symptomatic tumors
- *Liver metastases need cytoreductive surgery though it is palliative, as it gives better long-term survival*
- *Chemotherapy and radiotherapy give a marginal benefit.*

Clinical Pearls

- Preoperative diagnosis of intestinal carcinoids is difficult
- Small bowel carcinoids are more aggressive and have greater risk of death than carcinoids of other locations
- Wherever possible, radical resection should be carried out, as there are no additional options available
- Small bowel carcinoids have a high recurrence rate.

SURGERY OF SMALL BOWEL

Varieties of operations on small bowel **(Fig. 12.20A)**
- Resection and establishment of continuity (hand-sewn or stapled anastomosis)
- Bypass procedures (hand-sewn or stapled anastomosis) without resections
- Diversion procedures (ileostomies) **(See Chapter 16)**.

Methods of establishing continuity after resections **(Fig. 12.20B)**
- End-to-end anastomosis
- End-to-side anastomosis
- Side-to-side anastomosis.

Indications

- Obstructive lesions (strictures, tumors, intussusception)
- Strangulations with non-viable bowel

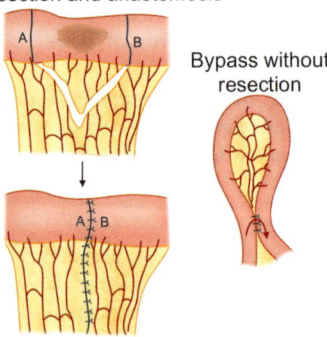

Fig. 12.20A: Varieties of surgeries

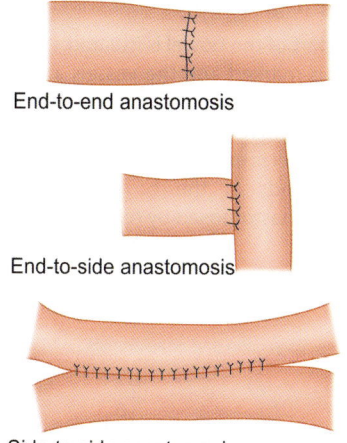

Fig. 12.20B: Types of small bowel anastomoses

Ileal resection

Incision

Midline (most popular).
Note: It has the advantage of:
- Ease
- Speed
- Versatility
- Allows access to all quadrants
- Easily extendable when needed.

Snapshots in Gastroenterology

Surgical Technique (Fig. 12.21)

- The resectable part of the bowel is isolated
- The mesentery is marked and the vessels are divided between ligatures **(Fig. 12.22A)**
- The bowels are held in noncrushing clamps **(Fig. 12.22B)**
- The resectable bowel is excised
- The two open ends of the bowel are brought together **(Fig. 12.22C)** and anastomosed by techniques given below:

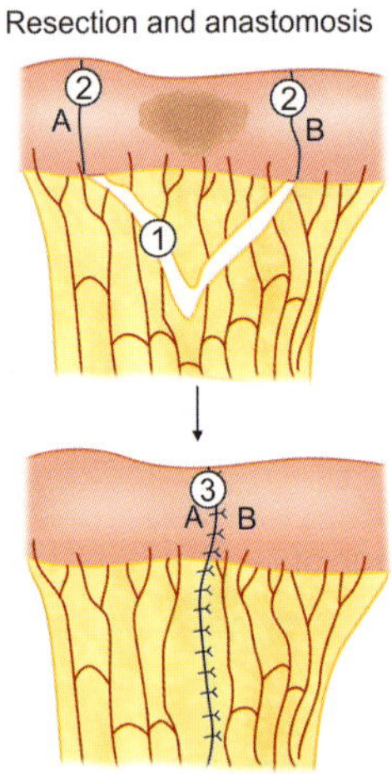

Fig. 12.21: Surgical technique. (1) Mesenteric vessels are divided; (2) Lines of resection of bowel; (3) End-to-end anastomosis

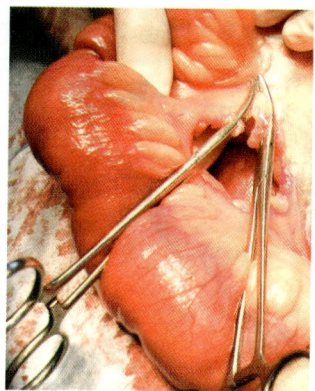

Fig. 12.22A: Division of mesenteric vessels

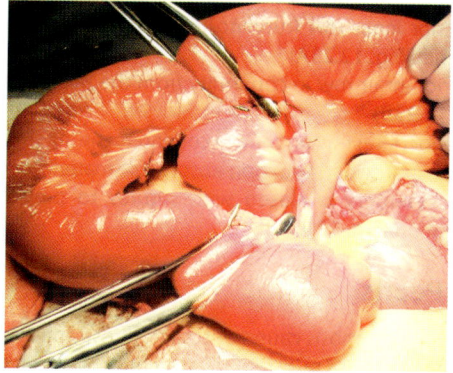

Fig. 12.22B: Bowel is held with noncrushing cramps ready for resection

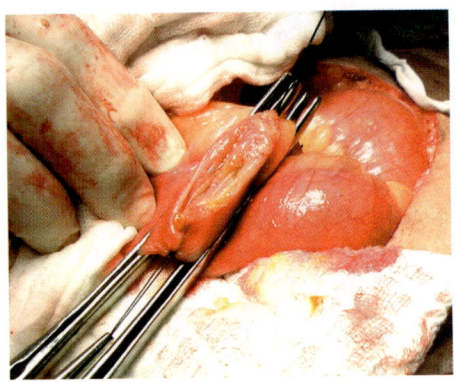

Fig. 12.22C: Cut ends of bowel are brought together

Hand-sewn Technique (Fig 12.23)

- **Double layer anastomosis**
  - Posterior inner row (running full thickness) with absorbable material **(Fig. 12.23A)**
  - Anterior inner row in continuity from the posterior inner row **(Fig. 12.23B)**
  - Posterior outer row first and in continuity the anterior outer row last (seromuscular) with non-absorbable material **(Fig. 12.23C)**
  - The mesentery is closed with sutures to prevent internal herniation **(Fig. 12.23D)**.

Clinical Pearls

- Inverting anastomosis causes serosa to serosa apposition
- Inversion of mucosa re-establishes integrity of lumen preventing leakage.

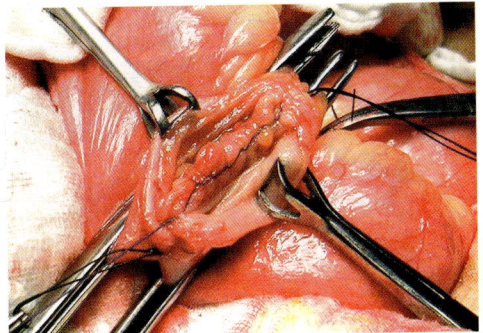

Fig. 12.23A: Suturing the inner posterior layer

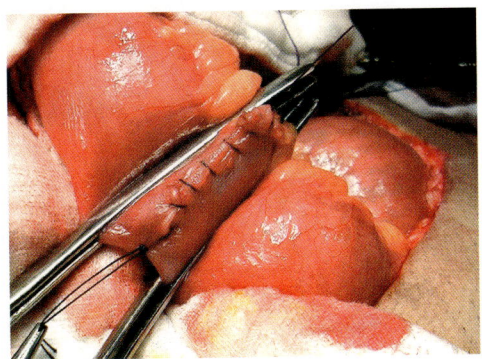

Fig. 12.23B: Suturing the inner anterior layer

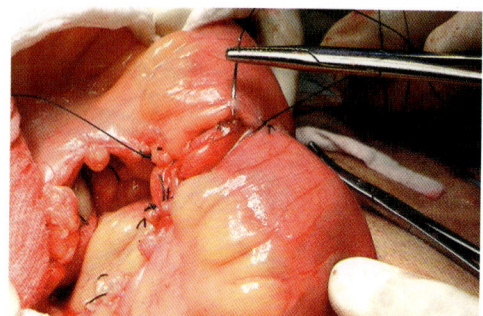

Fig. 12.23C: Suturing the outer layers

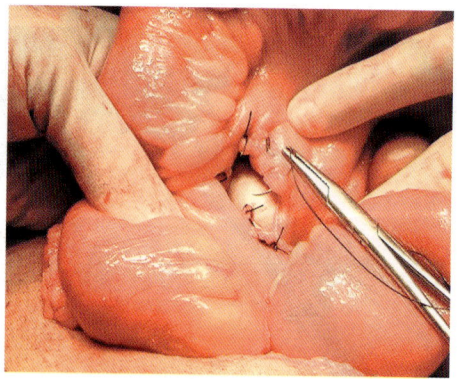

Fig. 12.23D: Closure of mesentery

End-to-end Anastomosis (Stapled) (Fig. 12.24)

- Bowel is cleared about 1 cm from the cut margin
- Gun is introduced into the proximal gut through enterotomy
- Proximal and distal ends each require a purse string suture
- The purse string sutures are snugged down over the instrument ends
- Anvil and head are brought together
- Firing is done for application of staplers
- The screw mechanism is unwound for a quarter of turn to release the bowel
- After removal of instrument, doughnuts are checked for integrity
- Enterotomy is closed with sutures or a linear stapler.

End-to-side Anastomosis (Stapled) (Fig. 12.25)

- The gun is introduced in the bowel to have end anastomosis (enterotomy)
- Purse string suture is made and snugged down over the anvil
- A small incision is made in the bowel to have side anastomosis
- The head assembly is introduced through the opening and held
- Anvil and head are brought together
- Firing is done for application of staplers
- The screw mechanism is unwound for a quarter of turn to release the bowel

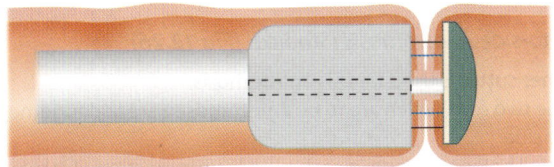

Fig. 12.24: End-to-end anastomosis (stapled technique)

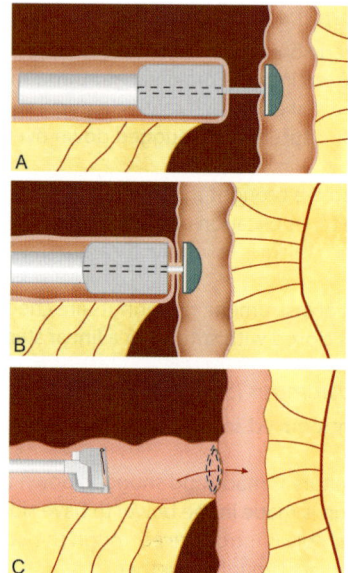

Fig. 12.25: End-to-side anastomosis (stapled technique)

- After removal of instrument, doughnuts are checked for integrity
- Enterotomy is closed with sutures or a linear stapler.

Side-to-side Anastomosis (Stapled) *(Fig 12.26)*

- Liner cutter is used for this anastomosis
- The two guts which are to be anastomosed are laid together side by side
- Small holes are made in each tube for introduction of stapler jaws
- The forks are introduced through these enterotomies

Small Intestine

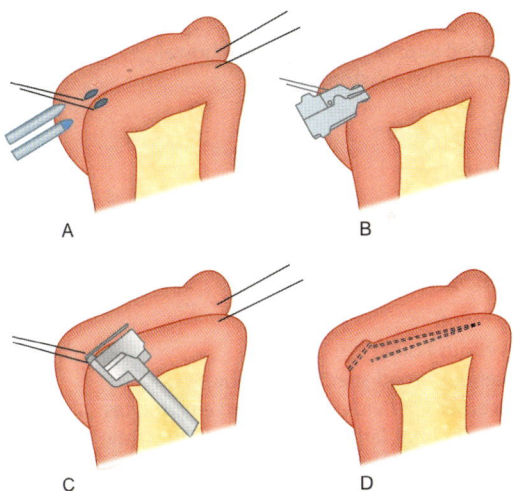

Fig. 12.26: Side-to-side anastomosis (stapled technique)

- The forks are locked together
- Stapler is activated, so that the anastomosis is made with stapling
- The forks are separated and removed
- The enterotomy openings are closed with sutures or a linear stapler.

POSTOPERATIVE COMPLICATIONS

Anastomotic Leakage

Introduction

Leakage of intestinal contents through the anastomotic line, occurs around the 2nd to 5th postoperative day due to

- Inadequate bowel preparation
- Poor blood supply to both ends of bowel
- Tension on the anastomosis.

Clinical Presentation
- Abdominal pain
- Fever
- Leakage of intestinal contents through the drain (**Fig. 12.27**).

Management
- Nil by mouth
- Intravenous fluids
- Intravenous broad spectrum antibiotics
- Replacement of fluids, calories and electrolytes
- Minor leaks heal, larger leaks take a longer time
- If fistula is formed, it may heal over a period of time
- Some may require surgery, after 6–12 weeks

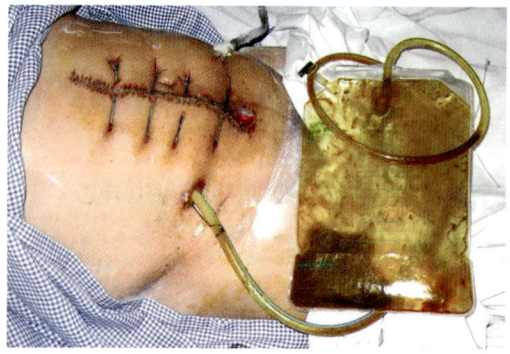

Fig. 12.27: Anastomotic leakage

Small Intestine

Intra-Abdominal Abscess

Introduction

Collection of pus in the peritoneal cavity (**Fig. 12.28**) as a residue of the spillage of bowel contents into the peritoneal cavity, around the first week of surgery.

Diagnosis

Clinical Presentation
- General malaise
- Hyperpyrexia of varying grades
- Insignificant clinical examination.

Investigations

Ultrasonography and CT are useful in localizing abscess.

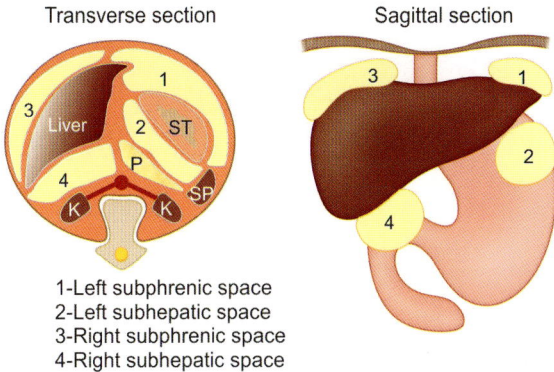

1-Left subphrenic space
2-Left subhepatic space
3-Right subphrenic space
4-Right subhepatic space

Fig. 12.28: Intra-abdominal abscesses

Management

Medical

- *Small abscesses resolve with antibiotics.*

Surgical

- *Drainage of abscess under US or CT guidance*
- *Open drainage if abscess is large and pus is thick.*

Anastomotic Stricture

Introduction

Narrowing of lumen of anastomotic area (**Fig. 12.29**), occurs as a healing process, months or years after surgery.

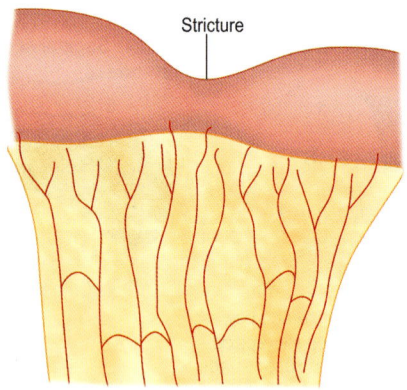

Fig. 12.29: Stricture

Diagnosis

Clinical Presentation

- Constipation
- Abdominal pain
- Vomiting
- Abdominal distension.

Investigation

- Contrast studies may be useful.

Management

- Small bowel strictures are bypassed or resection anastomosis done.

Clinical Pearl

- Strictures following stapler usage is rare, if the correct in size is chosen.

Adhesions

Introduction

Adherence of bowels between themselves or with the parietes (**Fig. 12.30**) due to:
- Postoperative fibrinous adhesions result from the healing of local inflammatory processes in the operated area
- Resolved infections of peritoneum can cause adhesions.

Snapshots in Gastroenterology

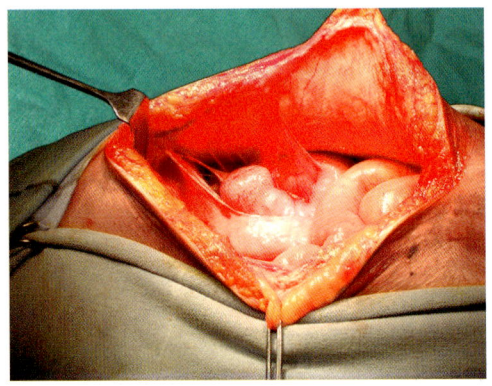

Fig. 12.30: Intra-abdominal adhesions

Diagnosis

Clinical Presentation

- Recurrent attacks of abdominal pain
- Vomiting
- Constipation
- Abdominal distension.

Investigation

- ***X-rays of abdomen*** will show distended bowel.

Management

Medical

- Nil by mouth
- Intravenous fluids and electrolytes.

Surgical

- If medical management fails, adhesiolysis by open or laparoscopic methods.

Internal Fistulae

Introduction

Communication between anastomotic line of small bowel with adjacent hollow viscera (**Fig. 12.31**) following:
- Anastomotic leak leads to collection of pus which in turn erode into the adjacent viscera
- Inflammatory bowel disease.

Diagnosis

Clinical Presentation

- Generally asymptomatic
- Recurrent urinary tract infections can occur in vesicoenteric fistulae.

Investigation

Contrast studies are useful.

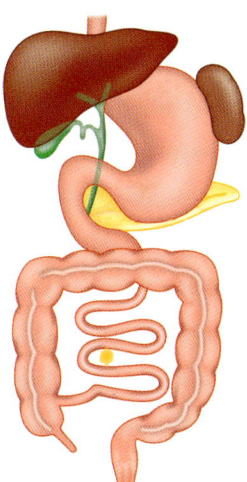

Fig. 12.31: Internal fistulae

Management

- Enteroenteric fistulae do not require any treatment
- Vesicoenteric fistulae require excision.

External Fistulae

Introduction

Leakage of intestinal contents through fistulae to the exterior when:
- Anastomotic leak leads to collection of pus which in turn drains through the drainage tube
- Intentional external drainage of collection of pus from the anastomotic leak
- Inflammatory bowel disease.

Diagnosis

Clinical Presentation

- Has had a turbulent postoperative period
- Discharging wound in the postoperative period
- Fluid and electrolyte disturbances
- Skin excoriation around the fistulous opening (**Fig. 12.32**)

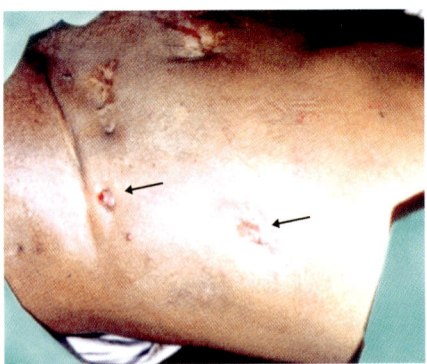

Fig. 12.32: Multiple external fistulae

- Fever
- Malnutrition, especially if large segments are lost during surgery.

Investigations

- ***Oral administration of non-absorbable marker (charcoal or Congo red)***
- ***Fistulogram* (Fig. 12.33)**
- ***US, CT with contrast or isotope scanning*** are useful.

Management

Medical

- Total parenteral nutrition.

Most lateral fistulae heal spontaneously.

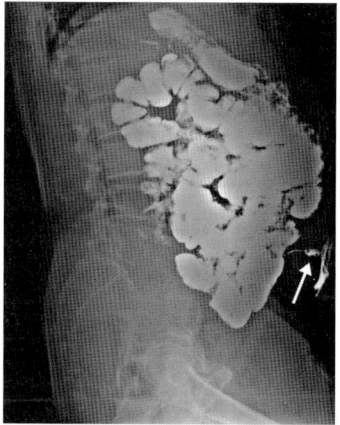

Fig. 12.33: Fistulogram—Ileocutaneous fistula

Surgical

Excision of fistula.

Nutritional Deficiencies

Introduction

Deficiency of nutritional factors secondary to surgery due to resection of large segments of bowel or essential parts of bowel (e.g. terminal ileum) **(Fig. 12.34)**. But they present clinically months or years after surgery.

Etiology and Pathogenesis
- Stagnation of intestinal contents
- Stricture

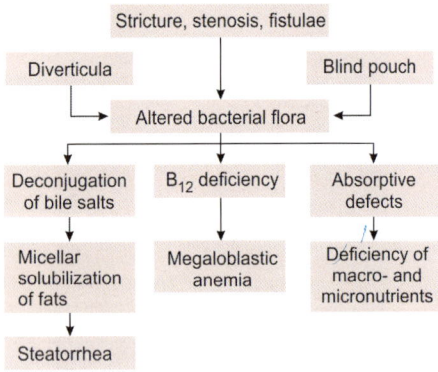

Fig. 12.34: Nutritional deficiency

- Stenosis
- Fistulae
- Blind pouch formation
- Diverticulae.

Diagnosis

Clinical Presentation

- Diarrhea
- Steatorrhea
- Anemia
- Weight loss
- Abdominal pain
- Multiple vitamin deficiency symptoms.

Investigations

- Variety of laboratory investigations may be required.

Management

Medical

- Supplement of deficient factors.

Surgical

- Stenosis, stricture and diverticulae need surgical excision.

Short Bowel Syndrome

A clinical malabsorption and malnutrition syndrome caused by extensive resection of intestine (**Fig. 12.35**). The factors, which determine the severity of short bowel syndrome (SBS), are:

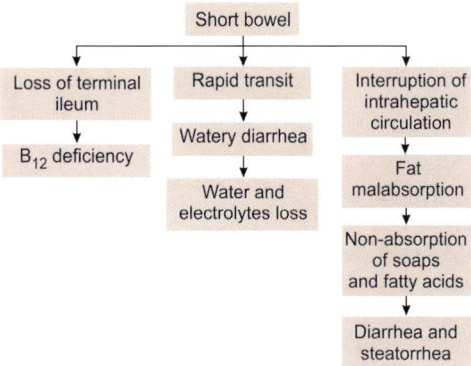

Fig. 12.35: Short bowel syndrome

- Extent and site of resection
- Any underlying intestinal disease (mesenteric vascular disease, Crohn's disease)
- Presence or absence of ileocecal valve
- Functional status of remaining GI organs
- Adaptation of the remaining intestinal remnant.

Extensive resections result in:
- Vitamin B_{12} deficiency (resection of terminal ileum)
- Water and electrolyte disturbances (resection of large segment of ileum)
- Fat malabsorption (resection of large segment of ileum).

Diagnosis

Clinical Presentation

Severe emaciation.

Investigation

Variety of laboratory investigations.

Complications

- Metabolic alkalosis and acidosis
- Symptomatic cholelithiasis
- Gastric hypersecretion
- Nephrolithiasis
- Bacterial overgrowth
- Complications of TPN.

Management

Medical

- Fat restriction
- Drugs to slow intestinal secretions and motility
- Oral bile salts (oral cholestyramine may improve bile salt binding)
- Somatostatin analogue, octreotide can improve diarrhea
- Intravenous hyperalimentation.

Surgical

- Obstructions should be relieved by non-resectional surgery (stricturoplasty) **(Refer Fig. 12.9)**
- Dilated segments of bowel encourage bacterial overgrowth, and should be eliminated (e.g. tapering surgery)
- Increasing the absorptive surface is done by increasing the length of bowel

- *Transverse procedure*—**Serial transverse enteroplasty procedure** (STEP procedure) creates a series of "v" shapes from the existing intestine, forming an accordion-like effect that increases bowel length and gives nutrients more time to be absorbed. This procedure does not require the removal of any additional intestine (**Fig. 12.36A**).
- *Longitudinal procedure*—**Bianchi procedure**—divides part of the bowel lengthwise into two narrower tubes; which are then separated and joined end to end. The result is a longer but narrower bowel (**Fig. 12.36B**).
- Procedures to decrease the intestinal transit time (artificial valves, sphincters, interpositioning reversed intestinal segments).
- Intestinal transplantation.

The treatment algorithm for the management of short bowel syndrome is given in **Fig. 12.37**.

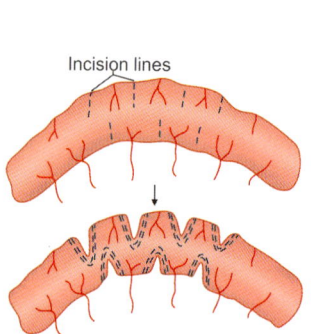

Fig. 12.36A: STEP procedure

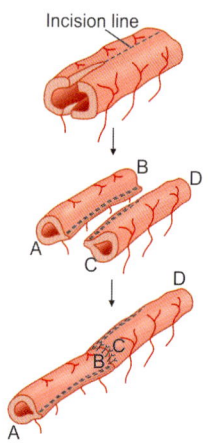

Fig. 12.36B: Bianchi procedure

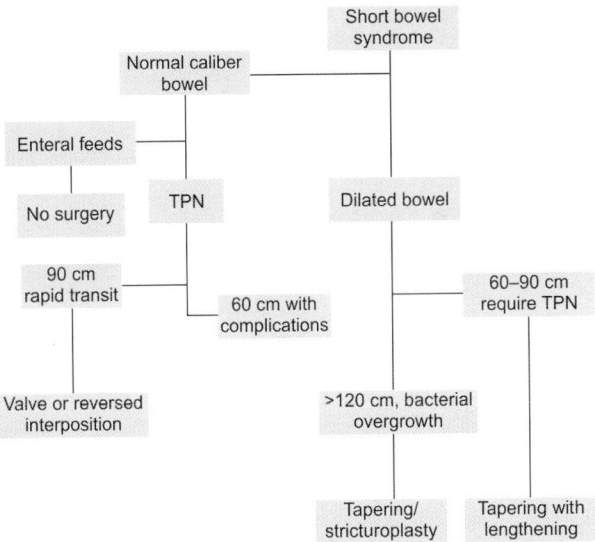

Fig. 12.37: Treatment algorithm for treatment of small bowel syndrome

Clinical Pearls

- It is better to avoid extensive resection of bowel to avoid a short bowel syndrome
- A prophylactic cholecystectomy is preferred in patients with SBS as there is increased risk of gallstones and acute biliary complications
- Medical treatment is directed to minimize intestinal secretions and controlling diarrhea, for which drugs like codeine, loperamide may be useful, due to their antisecretory and antimotility properties

- Patients with output stoma should get the intestinal motility established to improve clinically
- Many patients with SBS will require second surgery for intestinal complications, and any further resection should be avoided
- Since proximal small bowel is important to have absorptive capacity, it is necessary to have at least 100 cm of jejunum if rest of the bowel and the colon is removed, or at least 50 cm of jejunum if colon is available
- The degree of malabsorption depends on the remaining length of the small bowel.

Chapter 13

Vermiform Appendix

SURGICAL ANATOMY

In 1492, Leonardo de Vinci clearly described the appendix by an illustration, which was published in the 18th century, but in 1521 it was described by Berengario De Capri, a physician anatomist. Though debatable, the appendix in humans is considered to be a vestigial organ. This organ develops around the 8th week of fetal life, as an outpouching from the apex of the cecum. The tip takes various positions (**Fig. 13.1A**), and the most common being the retrocecal position (75%). The other positions are as follows:

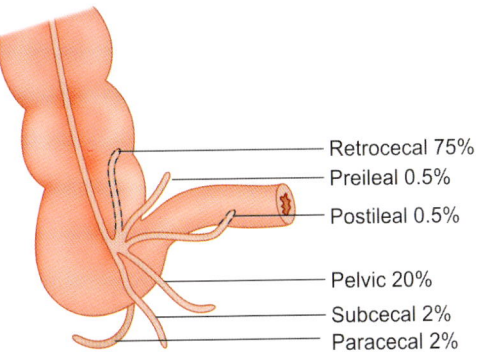

Fig. 13.1A: Various positions of appendix

- Pelvic (20%)
- Subcecal (2%)
- Paracecal (2%)
- Preileal (0.5%)
- Postileal (0.5%)

The appendix is a worm like narrow tubular structure approximately 2 cm in length (2–20 cm average being 9 cm). It is related anteriorly to the abdominal wall and posteriorly to the psoas muscle and lumbar nerve plexus.

Blood Supply

The appendiceal mesentery is a triangular fold derived from the intestinal mesentery, which envelops the appendicular vessels, lymphatics and nerves. The appendicular artery, which is a branch of ileocolic artery, is an end artery and gangrene and perforation are common when arterial thrombosis occurs.

Lymphatic Drainage

The lymphatic drainage of appendix occurs via the nodes in the mesoappendix.

Nerve Supply

The sensory innervations of the appendix are carried by the 8th, 10th and 11th thoracic nerves. The parasympathetic innervations are through the vagus nerve and the sympathetic innervation is through the celiac and superior mesenteric ganglia.

CONGENITAL ANOMALIES

Congenital anomalies of appendix are extremely rare, and duplications are reported.

They are classified into 3 types **(Fig. 13.1B)**:
- Type A: Partial duplication of appendix with a single base at the cecum
- Type B: Two completely separate appendices arising from a single cecum
  - Type B1: Two appendices attached to the cecum on either side of ileocecal valve
  - Type B2: Two appendices, one at the normal site (at the convergence point of tenia coli) and the other attached to one of the tenia coli (tenia coli type)
- Type C: Two appendices attached to two cecums.

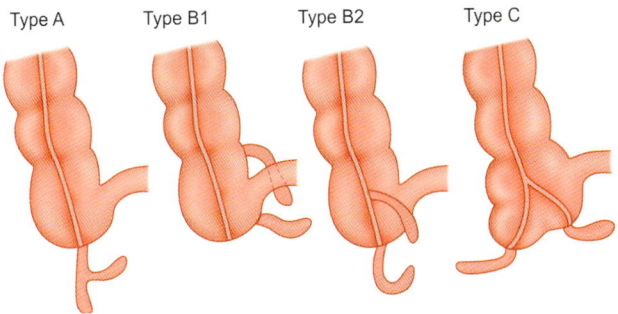

Fig. 13.1B: Congenital anomalies

ACUTE APPENDICITIS

Introduction

- Commonest acute abdominal condition, occurring at any age
- Uncommon only below the age of two
- Most commonly seen between the age of 18 and 35.

Types of Appendicitis

There are two varieties of appendicitis. They are:
1. *Catarrhal appendicitis*—occurs due to acute inflammation of the appendix (**Fig. 13.2A**), which produces edema and even gangrene due to vascular involvement in the inflammatory process. The appendix itself may be filled with pus.
2. *Obstructive appendicitis*—caused by obstruction of its lumen by worms, fecoliths (**Fig. 13.2B**) or hypertrophied lymphoid follicles.

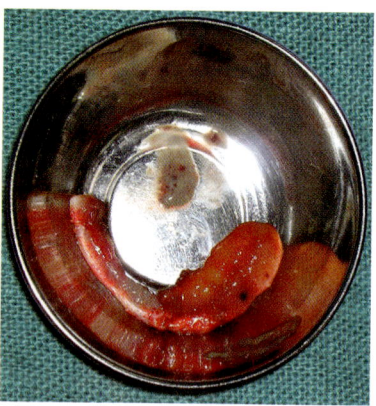

Fig. 13.2A: Acute suppurative appendicitis (note the pus in the cup)

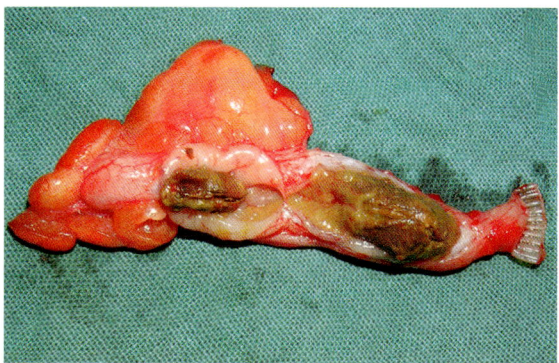

Fig. 13.2B: Appendix with fecoliths

Diagnosis

Symptoms

- Pain—a dull continuous ache starting at the umbilical region (visceral pain) and then localizing at the right iliac fossa (parietal pain)—catarrhal variety. Obstructive appendicitis presents with colicky pain (appendicular colic) in the right lower abdomen
- Nausea, vomiting and anorexia are usually present and are diagnostic
- Fever is the last to develop.

(Pain, vomiting and fever in appendicitis is called *Murphy's syndrome*).

Signs

Clinical signs and tests specific to acute appendicitis are given in **Box 13.1.**

Box 13.1: Clinical signs of acute appendicitis

- Tenderness at McBurney's point
- Rovsing's sign
- Blumberg's sign
- Cope's psoas sign
- Obturator sign
- Baldwing's sign

Tenderness at McBurney's Point

McBurney's point is the point at the junction of the lateral one thirds and medial two thirds of a line drawn between the umbilicus and the right anterior superior iliac spine (**Fig. 13.3**). Tenderness at this point is used in clinical diagnosis of Acute appendicitis.

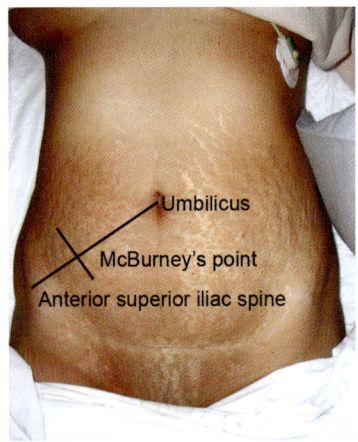

Fig. 13.3: McBurney's point

Rovsing's Sign

Application of pressure in the left iliac fossa produces pain in the right iliac fossa and this is called Rovsing's sign. This occurs due to the shift of the intestines towards the inflamed appendix (e.g. severe form of acute appendicitis) **(Fig. 13.4)**, and is used to differentiate from extra-abdominal causes of right iliac fossa pain.

Blumberg's Sign

Application of firm pressure in the right iliac fossa followed by a sudden release causes severe contraction of abdominal muscles along with the inflamed parietal peritoneum, which causes severe pain to the patient, which is called Blumberg's sign and this indicates localized peritonitis in acute appendicitis.

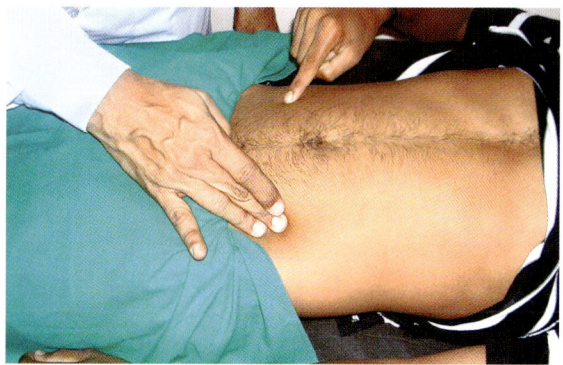

Fig. 13.4: Rovsing's sign

Cope's Psoas Test

The retrocecal appendix lies on the right psoas major muscle. By positioning the patient in the left lateral position and hyperextending the right hip joint, the patient points to the right iliac fossa for pain (**Fig. 13.5**) as this creates a stretch of the psoas major muscle, which irritates the inflamed appendix in the retrocecal position.

Obturator Sign

Internal rotation of the hip joint makes the patient point to the right iliac fossa for pain as this movement produces a stretch of this muscle and irritates the inflamed appendix in pelvic position (pelvic appendicitis), which lies in close proximity to the obturator internus muscle (**Fig. 13.6**).

Baldwing's Sign

When the patient is asked to lift the right lower limb with the knee straight, the patient points to the right iliac fossa for pain (**Fig. 13.7**),

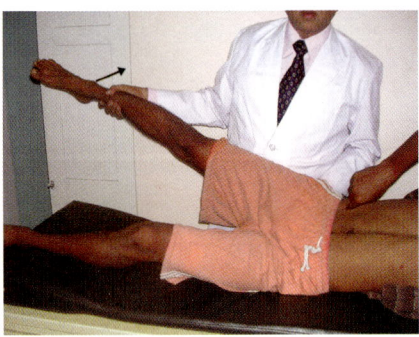

Fig. 13.5: Cope's psoas test

Vermiform Appendix

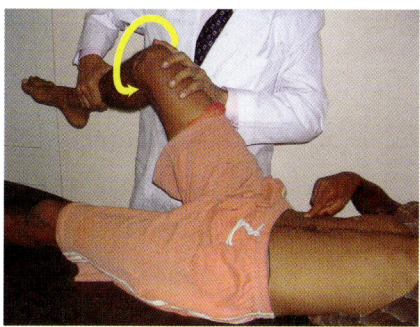

Fig. 13.6: Obturator test

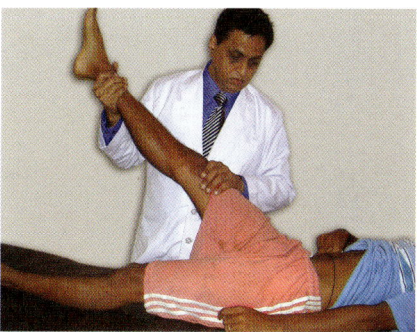

Fig. 13.7: Baldwing test

as the psoas major muscle irritates the inflamed appendix in the retrocecal position (retrocecal appendicitis). This is called Baldwing's sign.

Table 13.1: Signs and symptoms of appendicitis according to the position of the appendix

Symptoms and signs	Retrocecal and paracecal appendicitis	Pelvic and subcecal appendicitis	Pre and postileal appendicitis
Pain	Right flank and back lateral to sacrospinalis muscle	Right iliac fossa	Right iliac fossa
Diarrhea	Absent	Absent	May be present
Tenderness and guarding	Not marked	Absent	Present
Positive test	Cope's psoas test Baldwing's test	Obturator test	Nil specific
Tenderness in rectal examination	Absent	Present	May be present

- Tender mass may be felt (appendicular mass/abscess)
- Dullness on percussion (if mass already formed).

The signs and symptoms vary and depend on the position of the appendix **(Table 13.1)**

Appendicitis in Special Situations

Children

- Constitutional symptoms like fever and tachycardia are more predominant
- Percussion rebound is useful in diagnosing acute appendicitis
- Appendicular mass is rare as the omentum is small in size and does not reach the appendix.

Elderly

- Guarding and rigidity are not pronounced as the abdominal musculature is weak

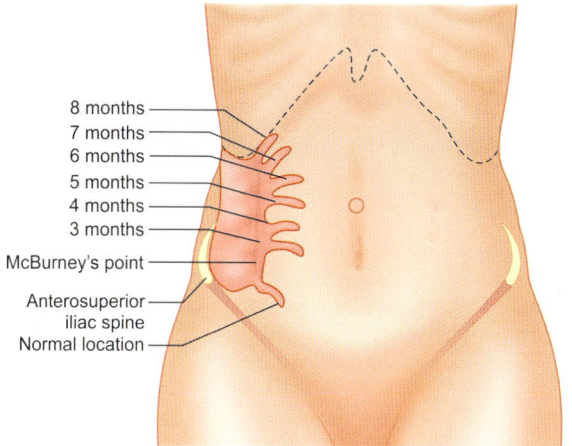

Fig. 13.8: Position of appendix in pregnant woman

- Incidence of gangrene is more as there is associated atherosclerosis
- Peritonitis supervenes early.

Pregnant Women

- The point of tenderness is shifted up, as the appendix itself is pushed up by the enlarged gravid uterus (**Fig. 13.8**)
- Pyelitis and cystitis of pregnancy add to the difficulties in diagnosis of appendicitis
- Accidental hemorrhage mimics acute appendicitis.

The cardinal signs and symptoms of acute appendicitis are given in **Box 13.2**.

Box 13.2: Cardinal signs and symptoms of acute appendicitis

- Periumbilical pain shifting to the right iliac fossa (very important)
- Association of nausea
- History of similar episodes in the past
- Tenderness at McBurney's point
- Guarding and rigidity in the right iliac fossa

Investigations

- Leukocytosis is usually present
- *US* **(Figs 13.9A and B)** may be contributory. Both transabdominal and transvaginal ultrasounds may be necessary to diagnose acute appendicitis in women especially the pregnant
    - Presence of probe tenderness indicates inflammatory process in that area
    - A thickened appendix of more than 6 mm is considered positive for diagnosis
    - Inflamed appendix may be edematous and is less compressible and may contain air in its lumen

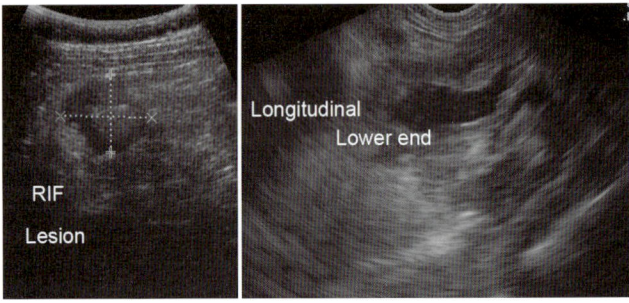

Fig. 13.9A: US—Inflamed appendix

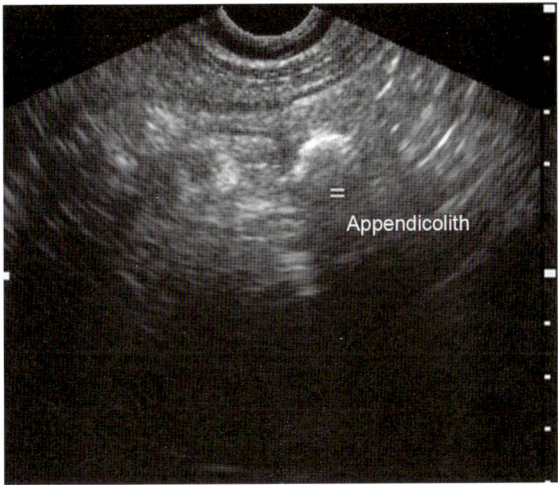

Fig. 13.9B: US—Appendicolith

- Free fluid may be present in the pelvis and particulate matter in the fluid may suggest pus
- Presence of free or localized air together with fluid indicates perforation
- A large inflammatory phlegmon indicates appendicular abscess.
- *Plain X-ray* (**Fig. 13.10**) may show the appendicolith
- *CT* is useful in identifying inflamed appendix (**Fig. 13.11**) and exhibits specific findings in acute appendicitis (**Table 13.2**)
- *MRI* is very specific and sensitive in the imaging of acute appendicitis

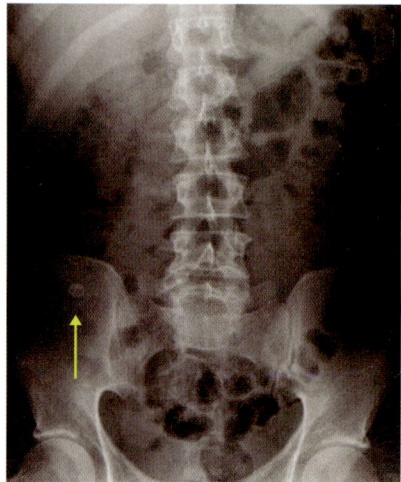

Fig. 13.10: X-ray abdomen—Appendicolith

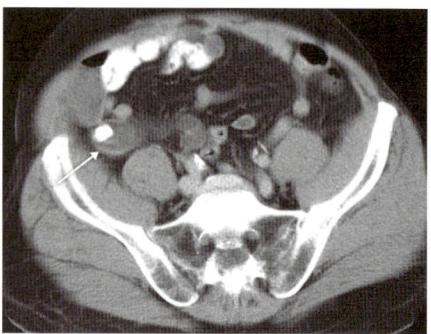

Fig. 13.11: CT—Appendicolith and dilated appendix

Table 13.2: CT findings associated with acute appendicitis

Appendiceal signs	Periappendiceal signs
Appendix >6 mm in anteroposterior diameter	Increased fat attenuation (stranding) in the right lower quadrant
Failure of appendix to fill with oral contrast or gas to its tip	Cecal wall thickening
Enhancement of appendix with IV contrast	Phlegmon in the right lower quadrant
Appendicolith	Abscess or extraluminal gas
	Fluid in the right lower quadrant or pelvis

- *Radioisotope white cell scans* may be used for diagnosis of acute appendicitis, but it is less specific and not available at many centers.

Clinical Scoring Systems

A number of scoring systems have been described to help the diagnosis of acute appendicitis. The most widely used and accepted is the Alvarado scale. This is based on three symptoms, three signs and one laboratory finding (**Box 13.3**).

- Score of 0–3, low risk for appendicitis, and the patient may be discharged with advice to return if there is no improvement
- Score of 4–6 should be admitted for observation and re-examination, and if the score remains the same after 24 hours, surgery is recommended
- Score of 7–9 should undergo appendicectomy.

Differential Diagnosis

Varieties of conditions mimic acute appendicitis clinically and need differentiation. They are tabulated in **Table 13.3**.

- Right ureteric colic (commonest)
- Right ovarian pathology in women
- Acute cholecystitis.

Box 13.3: Alvarado scale of acute appendicitis

Symptoms
- Migratory right lower quadrant pain — 1
- Anorexia — 1
- Nausea/vomiting — 1

Signs
- Tenderness right lower quadrant — 2
- Rebound tenderness — 1
- Elevated temperature — 1

Laboratory finding
- Leukocytosis — 2

Total — 9

Table 13.3: Differentiating features of acute appendicitis and right ureteric colic

Sign and symptom	Pathology	
	Acute appendicitis	**Right ureteric colic**
Pattern of pain	Periumbilical pain shifting to right iliac fossa	Loin to groin radiation on the right side
Nature of pain	Dull and continuous	Very severe and colicky with painfree intervals
Onset of pain	Slow and continuous	Sudden onset
Relationship to body movements	Aggravated	Not related to movement
Urinary symptoms	Absent	May be present
Rebound tenderness	May be present	Absent
Plain X-ray of abdomen	Nonspecific	Ureteric calculus

Vermiform Appendix

Complications

- When the adjacent tissues and omentum wall off the appendix or its perforation, it forms a mass called 'Appendicular mass'
- When there is suppuration, it forms an abscess named 'Appendicular abscess', which may burst into peritoneal cavity to produce severe peritonitis and even death.

Management

- Emergency appendicectomy (Laparoscopic or open) is the treatment of choice
- Conservative management is adopted for appendicular mass, subacute or chronic appendicitis (Oschner Scherren regime), followed by appendicectomy at a later date (interval appendicectomy).

Clinical Pearls

- Mildly swollen appendix is generally not seen in an ultrasound scan
- Leukocytosis in a patient with acute right iliac fossa pain strongly suggests acute appendicitis
- The ultrasound scan helps to eliminate other lesions like the ureteric calculus, ovarian pathology, which can be imaged by US
- The diagnosis of acute appendicitis is mostly clinical, supported by blood tests and the role of imaging is depended only when warranted.

RECURRENT APPENDICITIS

Introduction

Recurrent attacks of appendicitis caused by low-grade infections, sometimes associated with fecoliths in the appendicular lumen.

Diagnosis

Symptoms and Signs

- Patients do not present with a classic picture of appendicitis, but have vague upper abdominal discomfort (appendicular dyspepsia), with constipation, dysuria, and mild pain radiating to the right testis or thigh
- Obstructed appendix may present with recurrent colicky pain (appendicular colic). Tenderness may be felt on deep palpation.

Investigations

- *Plain X-ray abdomen* (**Refer Fig. 13.10**) may demonstrate appendicolith
- *US and Barium meal follow through* may be informative, but remain normal on many occasions
- *CT abdomen* (**Refer Fig. 13.11**) may show the appendicolith or be useful at least in eliminating other pathologies.

Management

Elective appendicectomy (laparoscopic or open).

NEOPLASMS OF APPENDIX

The neoplasms of appendix can be divided into:
- Carcinoid tumors
- Mucinous tumors.

Carcinoid Tumors

Introduction

- Carcinoid tumors are uncommon, but majority occur in the GIT
- Of the carcinoids of GIT, about 15% occur in the appendix
- In the appendix, carcinoids have an incidence of about 20% next to mucinous adenocarcinoma (incidence about 40%)
- Most carcinoids are found incidentally after appendicectomy
- Common in the age group of 40, with a female preponderance
- Most carcinoids are present in the distal third of the appendix and do not cause obstruction
- Large tumors can cause mass effect and liver metastases are not uncommon.

Etiology and Pathogenesis

These tumors secrete serotonin, prostaglandins and other physiologically active polypeptides. Serotonin is degraded into 5-HIAA, which is responsible for carcinoid syndrome. The syndrome gets prominent only when the liver metastases occur and 5-HIAA is pushed into the circulation.

Diagnosis

Symptoms
- Wheezing due to bronchoconstriction
- Flushing due to vasoconstriction

- Diarrhea due to increased GI smooth muscle constriction (increased motility and diarrhea)
- Symptoms have a rapid onset and short duration, and last for less than 30 minutes and involve the face, neck and upper part of the body
- These episodes are induced by food, alcohol, emotion, defecation and even deep palpation of the liver.

Signs
- Venous telangiectasias occur as purple colored vascular lesion on the nose, upper lip and malar areas.

Investigations

Blood Tests
- ***5 hydroxy indole acetic acid (5HIAA)***—Diagnosis of carcinoids is made by estimation of urinary 5-HIAA, which has a sensitivity of about 90%.

Serology
- ***Chromogranin A (CgA)*** is a sensitive marker but not specific to carcinoids, but has the advantage of correlation with tumor load. Other biomarkers are bradykinin, neuropeptides and substance P, but not found to be accurate or specific.

Radiology
- ***Endoscopic ultrasound, CT and MRI*** are useful. The presence of radiating strands of fibrosis and spiculation with a mass lesion is characteristic of carcinoid tumor and calcification should indicate mesenteric invasion
- ***PET scan*** is not useful as carcinoid has low metabolic activity.

Isotope Scans

- ***Octreoscan or indium–111 somatostatin analog scintigraphy*** is used to localize the octreotide receptor on the carcinoid cell surface, which has a specificity of 90% and sensitivity of 85%
- ***Bone scan*** may be useful in detecting bone metastases.

Clinical Staging *(Table 13.4)*

Management

Management is always surgical. It depends on the tumor location, its size and extent.

- Tumor less than 1 cm without invasion—appendicectomy
- Tumor of 1–2 cm without mesoappendicular invasion—appendicectomy

Table 13.4: TNM staging of appendicular carcinoids

T status	N status	M status
T_0-No evidence of tumor	N_0–No regional lymph node metastases	M_0–No distant metastases
T_1-Tumor <2 cm	N_1–Regional lymph node metastases	M_1–Distant metastases
T_2-Tumor 2–4 cm/ extension to cecum		
T_3-Tumor >4 cm/extension to ileum		
T_4-Invades adjacent structures		
Stage grouping		
Stage I	$T_1 \, N_0 \, M_0$	
Stage II	$T_{2-3} \, N_0 \, M_0$	
Stage III	$T_4 \, N_0 \, M_0$/Any T $N_1 \, M_0$	
Stage IV	Any T any N M_1	

- Tumor of 1–2 cm with mesoappendicular invasion—right hemicolectomy
- Tumor of >2 cm with or without mesoappendicular invasion—right hemicolectomy.

Clinical Pearl

Sometimes, fibrous tissue deposits can occur on the endocardium of valvular cusps, chambers of heart and pulmonary arteries predominantly on the right side (due to release of serotonin into the venous blood from the liver metastases), which is called carcinoid heart disease.

Mucinous Tumors

Introduction

- The appendix has a greater density of mucus cell than the rest of the large intestine and the mucinous tumors present as mucoceles
- Mucocele is a pathological term, which indicates a benign or malignant appendicular tumor with a ruptured or intact appendix
- It is defined as abnormal accumulation of mucus causing distension of the appendiceal lumen, irrespective of the underlying cause
- Appendiceal mucocele is a rare clinical entity with a prevalence of 0.2–0.3% in appendectomy specimens.

Classification

They are pathologically divided into:
1. Retention mucocele (appendix lined by normal mucosa or inflammatory granulation).
2. Mucocele due to mucosal hyperplasia.

3. Mucinous cystadenoma-mucocele with neoplastic epithelium similar to villous adenomas or adenomatous polyps of colon.
4. Mucinous cystadenocarcinoma—mucocele with neoplastic epithelium similar to colonic adenocarcinomas.

Pathogenesis

- Retention mucocele is very rare and occurs due to occlusion of appendicular lumen from postinflammatory scarring, age related atrophy, congenital obstruction of Gerlach's valve ultimately leading to atrophic mucosa
- The neoplasia related mucoceles account for 62–76% of all cases, majority of them due to cystadenomas. Calcifications are thought to be a dystrophic response to chronic inflammatory process incited by mucus in the appendiceal wall, ultimately leading to the development of porcelain appendix. When the mucus gets conglomerated, it appears as translucent globules or as cluster of eggs, called 'myxoglobulosis' or 'caviar appendix' with an incidence of 0.35–0.8%.

Diagnosis

Symptoms and Signs

- Usually asymptomatic and diagnosed incidentally at surgery
- Rarely, they produce symptoms like vague abdominal pain, chronic or intermittent colicky pain, right iliac fossa mass, gastrointestinal bleeding and urinary symptoms
- Other presentations include acute appendicitis, intussusception and small bowel obstruction.

Investigations

Radiology

- ***Plain radiograph*** may reveal a soft tissue shadow or specks of calcification in the lower abdomen

- ***Ultrasonography*** shows an echo-poor mass, due to mucin, with an indistinct cyst wall–***"Onion skin sign"***. Wall thickening of > 6 mm favors acute appendicitis which is absent in mucocele
- ***CECT of abdomen***, the most specific investigation, demonstrates a well encapsulated mass with smooth regular wall. The degree of attenuation depends on the amount of mucin. The presence of punctate calcification or curvilinear calcification in the right lower quadrant strongly suggests appendiceal mucocele (**Fig. 13.12**)
- ***MRI*** has less specificity than CT especially when calcified.

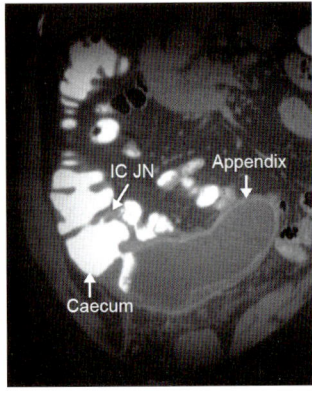

Fig. 13.12: CT—Calcified mucocele

Endoscopy

- ***Colonoscopy*** shows an erythematous soft mass with a central crater from which mucus discharges—***"Volcano sign"***.

Differential Diagnosis

- Mesenteric cyst and duplication cyst.
- Right ovarian cyst or hydrosalpinx (in women).

Complications

The worst complication is pseudomyxoma peritonei or peritoneal dissemination caused by spontaneous or iatrogenic perforation of the appendix.

Management

Treatment for appendiceal mucocele is surgical.

- Appendicectomy is enough for benign lesions **(Fig. 13.13)**
- If malignancy is suspected, or demonstrated by signs like local invasion into the cecum or ileum, right hemicolectomy is preferred.

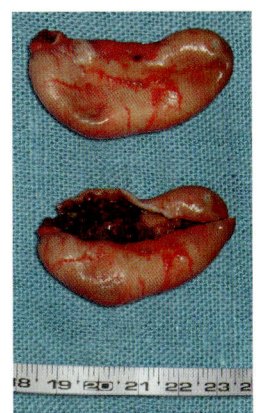

Fig. 13.13: Appendicectomy for mucocele

Clinical Pearls

- Majority of mucoceles are benign and they present as acute appendicitis.
- Preoperative diagnosis of appendiceal mucocele becomes essential to avoid iatrogenic trauma to appendix and the resultant pseudomyxoma peritonei
- During laparotomy, the abdomen should be carefully explored for other coexisting tumors of the ovaries or gastrointestinal tract. All apparent mucinous tissue should be aggressively debulked, if generalized pseudomyxoma peritonei is found
- Intraoperative histologic examination is not always definitive
- Laparoscopic surgery carries the risk of appendicular rupture and diffuse peritoneal carcinomatosis
- An appendiceal mucinous tumor encountered at laparoscopy requires absolutely atraumatic appendectomy, to avoid spillage, and conversion to open method should be considered without hesitation.

SURGERY OF APPENDIX

Appendicectomy is the only operation for appendicular pathologies.

Indications

- Acute appendicitis
- Chronic or recurrent appendicitis
- Tumors of appendix.

Appendicectomy

Incisions for open appendicectomy (**Fig. 13.14**):
- McBurney's incision (Most popular)—an oblique 2-inch incision made at McBurney's point—devised by Charles McBurney of USA in 1889
- Lanz incision—A 2-inch transverse incision made at McBurney's point—devised by Otto Lanz of Amsterdam in 1908
- Right lower paramedian incision.

Surgical Technique

Essential Steps *(Fig. 13.15A)*

1. Dividing the appendicular artery between ligatures/clips.
2. Dividing the appendix at its base.
3. Burying the appendicular stump in the cecum.

Open Appendicectomy

- Position: supine
- The abdominal cavity is entered through the muscle splitting incision

Vermiform Appendix

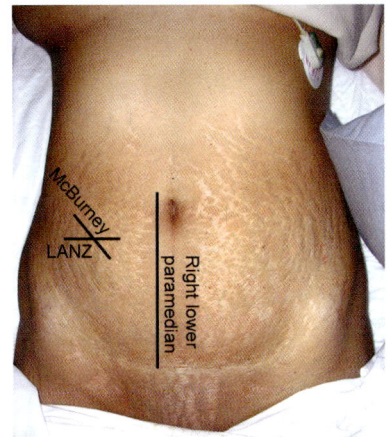

Fig. 13.14: Incisions for appendicectomy

- The appendix is identified and held with Babcock's forceps and brought out of the wound (**Fig. 13.15B1**)
- Appendicular artery identified in the mesoappendix (**Fig. 13.15B2**)
- Appendicular artery divided between clamps or ligatures (**Fig. 13.15B3**)
- Appendix is crushed at its base (**Fig. 13.15B4**)
- Clamp applied at the crushed site, and advanced distally
- Ligature applied at the crushed site with absorbable material (**Fig. 13.15B5**)
- Appendix is divided between the suture and the clamp, and removed
- Purse string suture applied on the cecum and appendicular stump buried.

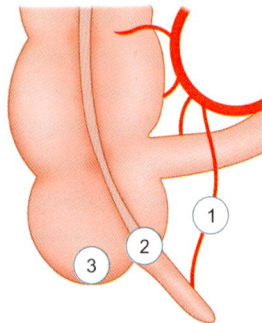

Fig. 13.15A: Appendicectomy surgery. (1) Dividing the appendicular artery between ligatures/clips, (2) Dividing the appendix at its base, (3) Burying the appendicular stump in the cecum

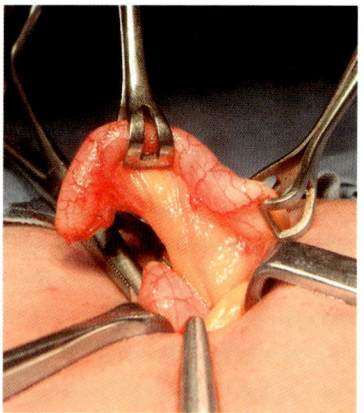

Fig. 13.15B1: Appendix exposure

Vermiform Appendix

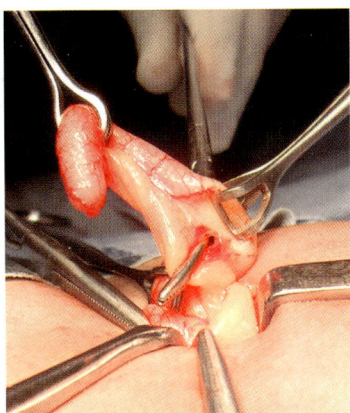

Fig. 13.15B2: Mesoappendix clamping

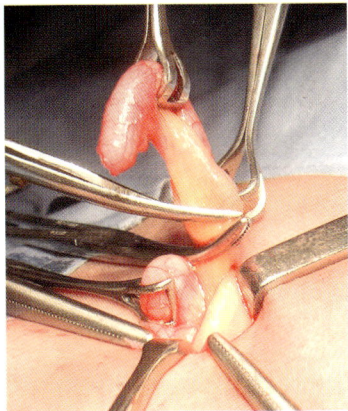

Fig. 13.15B3: Mesoappendix division

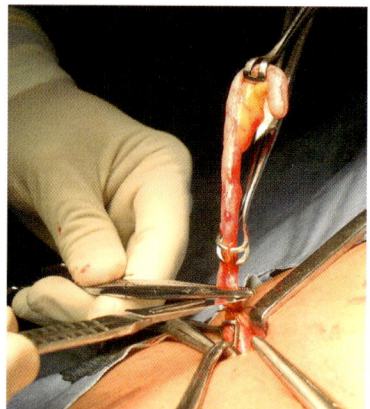

Fig. 13.15B4: Appendix crushing

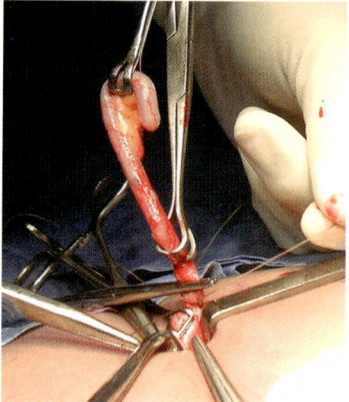

Fig. 13.15B5: Appendix ligation

Laparoscopic Appendicectomy

Three port technique:

- Surgeon and camera assistant take appropriate positions (**Fig. 13.16A**)
- Camera port at the umbilicus
- CO_2 pneumoperitoneum is created
- Additional 5 mm port entries are made at the suprapubic region and right iliac fossa (**Fig. 13.16B**)
- Exploration and intraperitoneal fluid is aspirated
- Appendix is identified
- Mesoappendix is dissected free with diathermy or stapled or clipped at its base (**Fig. 13.16C1**)
- Base of the appendix is ligated with double endoloops proximally and one ligature distally leaving adequate space to cut (**Fig. 13.16C2**)
- Appendix is divided between ligatures (**Fig. 13.16C3**)
- Appendix is retrieved (**Fig. 13.16C4**)
- Camera port facial closure done with non-absorbable sutures.

Clinical Pearls

Laparoscopic procedure may not be possible when there are gross adhesions, perforation and gross contamination and conversion to midline laparotomy may be justified.

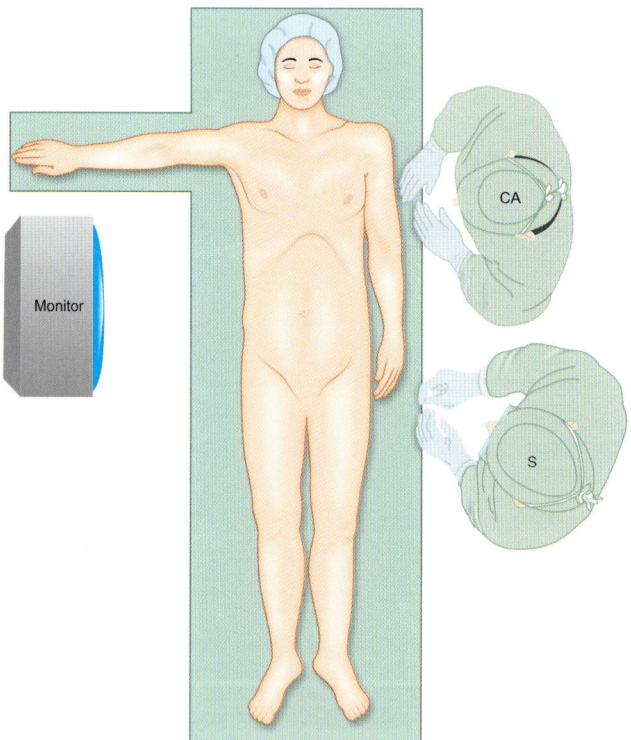

Fig. 13.16A: Positions of surgeon and camera assistant

Vermiform Appendix

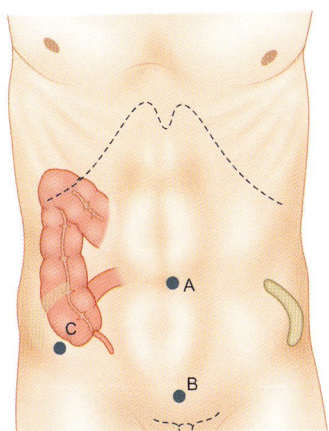

Fig. 13.16B: Port positions

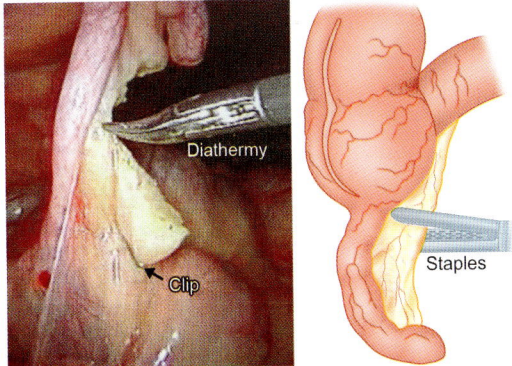

Fig. 13.16C1: Division of mesoappendix

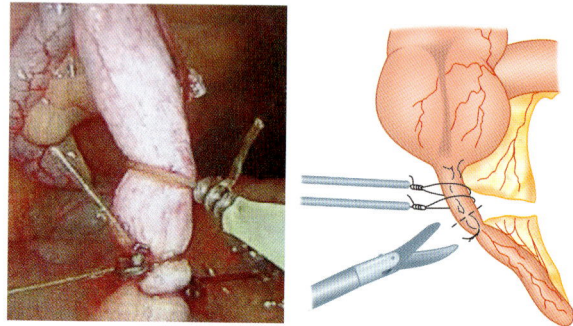

Fig. 13.16C2: Application of endoloops

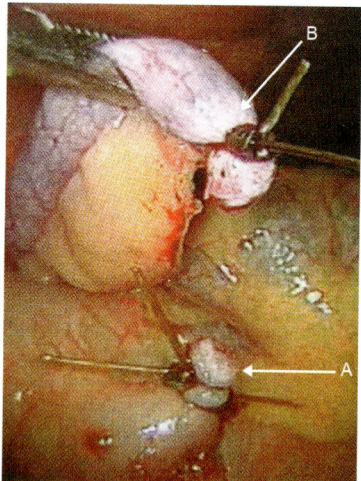

Fig. 13.16C3: Division of appendix

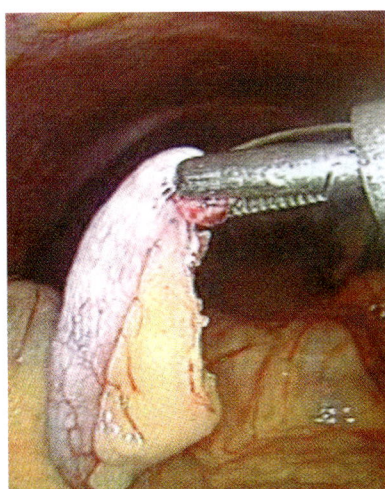

Fig. 13.16C4: Extraction of appendix

COMPLICATIONS OF APPENDICECTOMY

Hemorrhage from Appendicular Stump

Introduction

Bleeding in the abdominal cavity expected around 2nd to 3rd postoperative days.

Etiology

- Leakage of blood from the appendicular stump
- Slipped ligature of the appendicular artery.

Diagnosis

Clinical Presentation
- Severe lower abdominal pain
- Guarding in right iliac fossa.

Investigations
- ***US and CT*** may be contributory.

Management
Exploration of abdomen and ligation of mesoappendix.

Paralytic Ileus

Introduction
Delayed recovery of intestinal movements.

Etiology and Pathogenesis
- Peritonitis
- Electrolyte disturbances (hypokalemia).

Diagnosis

Clinical Presentation
- Vomiting
- Abdominal distension
- Constipation

Investigations

X-ray abdomen shows distended loops of small bowel (***Step ladder pattern***) **(Refer Fig. 12.10)**.

Management
- Correction of electrolytes
- Nasogastric aspiration.

Wound Infection after Appendicectomy

Introduction

Occurs around 2nd to 5th postoperative days, due to:
- Spillage of infected appendicular contents
- Extension of infection from appendix to abdominal wall.

Diagnosis

Clinical Presentation
- Fever
- Discharge from wound **(Fig. 13.17)**
- Pain in the wound.

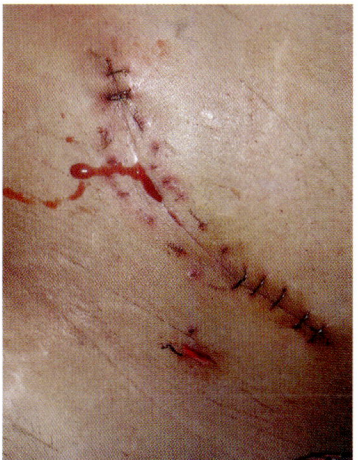

Fig. 13.17: Wound infection (appendicectomy)

Investigations

Pus culture to identify the incriminating organisms.

Management

- Drainage of collection of abscess
- Appropriate antibiotics
- Wound care.

Pelvic/Paracolic Abscess

Introduction

Collection of pus in the region adjacent to cecum or pelvic cavity around 5th to 7th postoperative days due to:

- Spillage of appendicular contents
- Incomplete resolution of generalized peritonitis.

Diagnosis

Clinical Presentation

- Abdominal pain
- High grade fever
- Constipation.

Investigations

US and CT (**Fig. 13.18**) are diagnostic.

Management

- Drainage under US or CT guidance or open method
- Appropriate antibiotics.

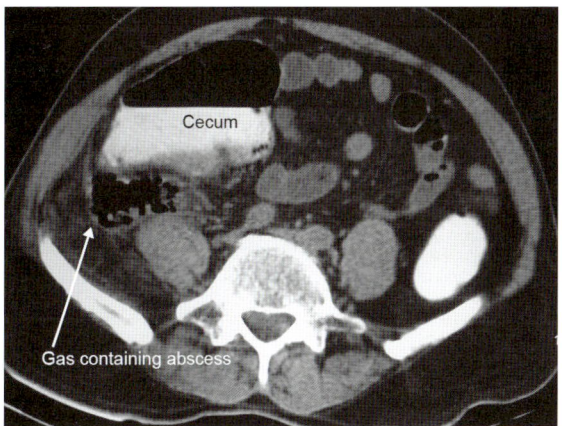

Fig. 13.18: CT—Paracolic abscess

Rupture of Stump

Introduction

Dehiscence of appendicular stump around 3rd to 5th postoperative days due to:
- Sloughing of appendicular stump
- Administration of enema in the operative period.

Diagnosis

Clinical Presentation

- Right lower quadrant pain
- Vomiting
- Tenderness at the operated area
- Constipation.

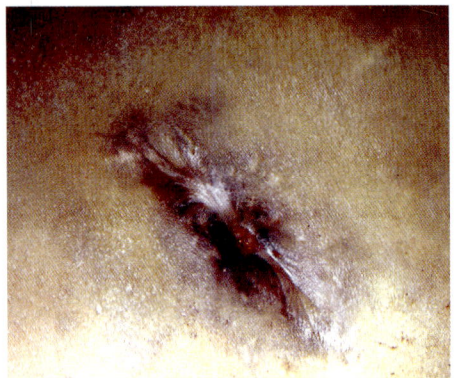

Fig. 13.19: Appendicocutaneous fistula

Investigations

US may be useful in localizing abscess.

Management

Medical
- Antibiotics
- Drainage of collection (appendicocutaneous fistula may result) **(Fig. 13.19)**.

Surgical
- Cecostomy will prevent further spillage.

Hernia (Postappendicectomy)

Introduction

Prolapse of intra-abdominal contents at the appendicectomy scar due to:

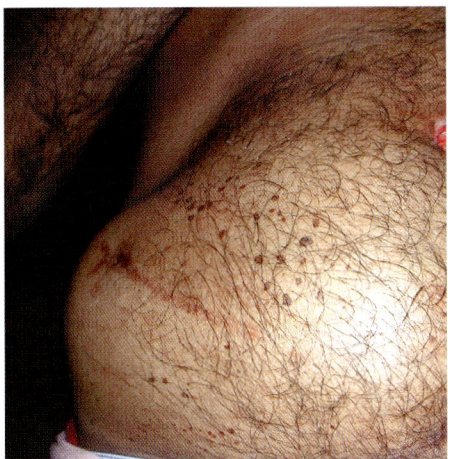

Fig. 13.20: Ventral hernia (postappendicectomy)

Weakness of muscles due to:
- Postoperative infection
- Chronic cough
- Chronic sneeze
- Chronic constipation.

Diagnosis
Clinical Presentation
- Swelling of the abdomen around the operated area (**Fig. 13.20**)
- Pain if obstruction occurs.

Management
Surgical repair with a mesh.

Intestinal Obstruction

Introduction
Mechanical obstruction of small bowel months or years after surgery due to postoperative adhesions in the ileocecal area.

Diagnosis

Clinical Presentation
- Recurrent attacks abdominal pain
- Associated vomiting and constipation.

Investigations
- Plain X-ray (**Refer Fig. 12.12**) may be useful
- Contrast studies are useful
- Laparoscopy is diagnostic.

Management

Medical
Conservative management.

Surgical
Release of adhesions (laparoscopic or open).

Chapter 14

Large Intestine

ANATOMY

The large intestine extends from the ileocecal junction to the anus. It is divided into colon, rectum and anal canal. The colon is divided into cecum and ascending colon, transverse colon, descending colon and sigmoid colon. The ascending and descending colons are located in the retroperitoneum, but the transverse colon and sigmoid colon are intraperitoneal. The hepatic flexure marks the transition of ascending colon to transverse colon, and the splenic flexure marks the transition of transverse colon to descending colon. Cecum is the widest part of the colon, and the sigmoid is the narrowest part of the colon. The sigmoid is a very redundant colon, with mobility.

Histology

The wall of the colon consists of five layers;
1. Mucosa
2. Submucosa
3. Inner circular muscle
4. Outer longitudinal muscle
5. Serosa

The outer longitudinal muscle layer is separated into three tenia coli, which converge proximally at the appendix and distally at the rectum. The inner circular muscle converges to form internal anal sphincter. The mid and lower rectum lack serosal layer.

Arterial Supply

- *Cecum, appendix*—ileocolic artery (branch of superior mesenteric artery)
- *Ascending colon*—right colic artery (branch of superior mesenteric artery)
- *Transverse colon*—right branch of middle colic artery (branch of superior mesenteric artery)
- *Descending colon*—left colic artery (branch of inferior mesenteric artery)
- *Sigmoid colon*—sigmoidal arteries (branch of inferior mesenteric artery).

Venous Drainage

Venous drainage corresponds to the arteries and carry the same terminology.

Lymphatic Drainage

Lymphatic drainage originates at the network of lymphatics in the muscularis, and the lymphatics follow the arteries. Lymph nodes are found on the colonic wall (epicolic nodes), along the margins of colon (paracolic nodes), around the mesenteric vessels (intermediate nodes) and at origin of superior and inferior mesenteric arteries.

Nerve Supply

- Sympathetic—T6–T12 and L1–L3 segments
- Parasympathetic—vagus nerves.

PHYSIOLOGY

About 90% of water contained in the ileal fluid is absorbed in the colon. This amounts to about 1–2 liters per day. A large amount of sodium (up to 400 mEq/day) is absorbed in the colon, through Na-K ATPase.

Colon contains microorganisms, predominantly the anaerobes (*Bacteroides species*) and aerobes (*E. coli*). This forms about 30% of fecal dry weight. Colonic bacteria breakdown the carbohydrates, and proteins and participate in the bilirubin, bile acids, estrogen and cholesterol metabolism. They are also necessary for production of vitamin K.

Intestinal gas is from swallowed air, diffusion from blood and intraluminal production. Intestinal gas contains nitrogen, oxygen, carbon dioxide, hydrogen and methane. Nitrogen and oxygen are from swallowed air, carbon dioxide is from digestion of triglycerides and fatty acids, whereas the hydrogen and methane are produced by colonic bacteria.

VOLVULUS

Introduction

- Volvulus is defined as a twist of the bowel around its mesenteric axis
- It is more common in the large bowel (commonly the sigmoid colon) than in the small bowel, but may involve any segment of colon
- In the colon, volvulus is more common in the sigmoid than in the cecum, rarely in the transverse colon and splenic flexure
- Rotation of more than 180° may result in strangulation.

Risk Factors

- Long and mobile mesentery with a narrow base
- Chronic constipation
- Megacolon
- Neurologic diseases
- Adhesions
- Hirschsprung's disease
- Ileus
- Pregnancy

Sigmoid Volvulus

Etiology and Pathogenesis

- Disease of the middle aged and elderly
- Rotation of the sigmoid around its axis occurs when the sigmoid is mobile and its mesentery is unusually long with a relatively narrow mesenteric attachment (the sites of fixation are relatively close to each other) **(Fig. 14.1)**
- The rotation may be either clockwise or counterclockwise
- Gross features of the sigmoid volvulus include progressive widening and eventual loss of tenia coli, absence of appendices epiploicae and a thickened narrowed fibrous mesentery

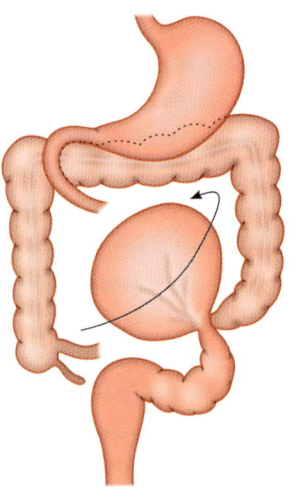

Fig. 14.1: Sigmoid volvulus

- Once the rotation reaches 360°, a closed loop obstruction develops
- Hyperperistalsis and fluid secretion into the closed loop add to increased pressure and tension
- As blood flow is compromised, ischemia and necrosis develop

Diagnosis

Symptoms and Signs
- Sudden severe pain, frequently when straining to pass stool. The patient retches and develops hiccoughs
- The patient may give history of attacks of abdominal pain with constipation, relieved by passing watery stools and large volumes of flatus in the past
- Abdomen rapidly distends, disproportionate to the duration of pain, and the distension is confined more to the left flank
- Rectum is empty on examination.

Investigations
- ***Plain radiograph of the abdomen*** will reveal a massively distended sigmoid, giving the characteristic ***'omega' or 'inverted coffee bean', 'bent inner tube' sign or Freeman Dahl sign*** (**Fig. 14.2**) (Convergence of three white lines towards the base of the pedicle)
- ***Barium enema*** will show the obstruction at the rectosigmoid junction, with the classical ***'bird's beak'*** appearance

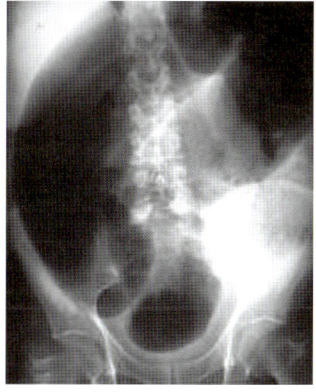

Fig. 14.2: X-ray—Sigmoid volvulus

- **CT abdomen** shows *'whirl pattern'* of the dilated sigmoid loop around the mesocolon and the affected segments giving the 'bird's beak' appearance.

Differential Diagnosis

All causes of colonic obstruction
- Mechanical causes
  - Diverticulitis
  - Inflammatory bowel disease
- Non-mechanical causes
  - Colonic pseudo-obstruction (Ogilvie's syndrome).

Management

Noninvasive
- *Detorsion may be attempted using colonoscope/blind passage of a rectal tube/administration of barium* when there is no evidence of gangrene. Recurrence is common.

Surgical
- *Untwisting of the volvulus, and fixing the colon to parietal peritoneum* to prevent recurrence
- *Mesosigmoidoplasty (Fig. 14.3)* to create a shortened broad mesentery precluding future bowel rotation
- *Sigmoidectomy with primary anastomosis* is the treatment of choice for long redundant or gangrenous sigmoid colon.

Clinical Pearls

- If ischemia is suspected or visualized, the detorsion attempts should be abandoned and surgical intervention should be undertaken immediately

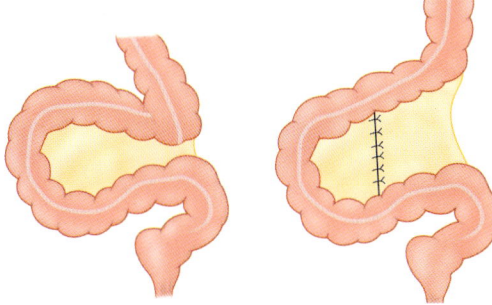

Fig. 14.3: Mesosigmoidoplasty

- Detorsion attempted in an ischemic colon may lead to perforation
- In the elderly frail patients, perforation and peritonitis is uniformly fatal
- Non-resectional procedures without fixation carry a high incidence of recurrence.

Cecal Volvulus

Introduction

- True cecal volvulus is an axial torsion of the cecum, terminal ileum and ascending colon about its mesentery (**Fig. 14.4A**)
- This occurs in those whose entire right colon has a mesentery continuous with that of the small bowel, and the cecum does not lie in the right iliac fossa.

Etiology and Pathogenesis

- Prior abdominal surgery with colonic mobilization
- Recent surgical manipulation

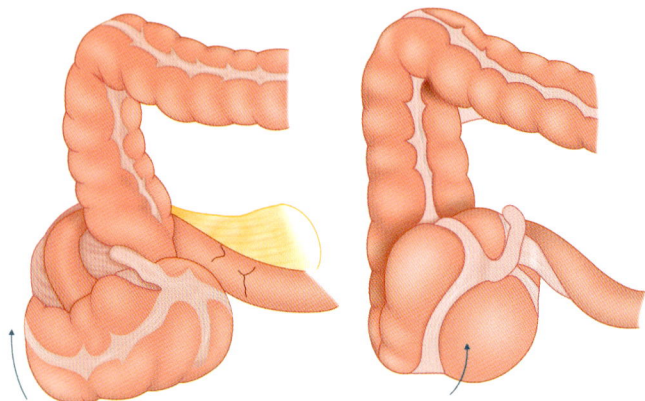

Fig. 14.4A: Cecal volvulus   **Fig. 14.4B:** Cecal bascule

- Adhesions and bands
- Distal colonic obstruction
- Hyperperistalsis.

Cecal Bascule

It is a variant of cecal volvulus, and occurs when the cecum folds anteriorly over the ascending colon without an axial twist (**Fig. 14.4B**). This represents about 10% of cases of cecal volvulus.

Diagnosis

Symptoms and Signs

- Symptoms and signs of small bowel obstruction
- A distended, tense palpable resonant mass in the umbilical region, with an empty right iliac fossa

- Acute volvulus results in a closed loop obstruction and distal small bowel obstruction, which may progress to a more fulminant presentation when ischemia and gangrene develop.

Investigations

- *Plain radiograph of the abdomen* is diagnostic (coffee bean deformity directed toward the left upper quadrant)
- *Barium enema* may reveal a 'bird's beak' or 'colon cut off sign' in the right colon.

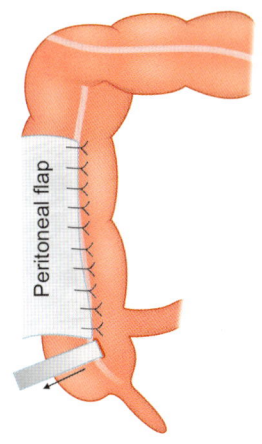

Fig. 14.5: Colopexy and cecostomy

Management

Surgical

- *Untwisting of the volvulus with or without resection of the segment of the bowel and cecopexy (entire lateral peritoneal flap is elevated along the ascending colon and sutured to the ascending colon so that the cecum and ascending colon becomes partially retroperitoneal) (Fig. 14.5) and cecostomy (to serve as a vent and also to fix the cecum to the anterior abdominal wall)* is required
- *Right hemicolectomy* gives best results
- *Gangrenous bowel requires resection.*

Clinical Pearls

- Cecal volvulus is much less common than the sigmoid volvulus

- Clinical diagnosis of cecal volvulus is difficult and requires high index of suspicion, and the diagnosis is usually made at laparotomy
- Distension of abdomen of cecal volvulus is much less than the distension of sigmoid volvulus.

Transverse Colon Volvulus

Introduction
- Volvulus of the transverse colon is extremely rare
- It is seen more in the young with a female preponderance

Etiology and Pathogenesis

More commonly in those who have:
- Chronic constipation and use laxatives liberally
- Undergone abdominal surgery
- Usage of high fiber diet
- Recurrent distal colonic obstruction
- Long redundant transverse colon
- Long transverse mesocolon with narrow attachments of the flexures

Diagnosis

Symptoms and Signs
- Symptoms of large bowel obstruction.

Investigations
- *Plain X-ray* shows distended proximal colon with decompressed distal colon with distinct air-fluid levels representing two limbs of volvulized transverse colon. This gives the appearance of bent inner tube appearance with the apex pointing inferiorly

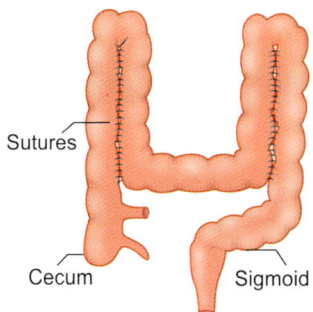

Fig. 14.6: Mortensen's U-shaped colopexy

- ***Barium enema*** will show a bird's beak deformity of distal transverse colon.

Management

Surgical Treatment
- ***Detorsion with or without colopexy and resection***
- ***Mortensen's U-shaped colopexy*** (**Fig. 14.6**) is useful.

Clinical Pearl
- Clinical diagnosis of transverse colon volvulus is difficult.

Ileosigmoid Knotting

Introduction
- It is also called a compound volvulus
- A rare form of voluvlus, in which the long small bowel winds round the redundant sigmoid colon or the redundant sigmoid colon can wind round a long loop of small bowel

- Seen in population who consume single large meal in a day, and also in those who consume large quantities of bulky, carbohydrates and liquid containing diet.

Etiology and Pathogenesis

Association of abnormally long small bowel mesentery with a long narrow pedicled sigmoid mesentery, allow abnormal mobility of the bowels, which is exaggerated by the heavy bulk of food and liquid.

Diagnosis

Symptoms and Signs
- Acute abdominal pain
- Features of small bowel obstruction

Investigations
- ***Plain X-ray*** will show features of small bowel obstruction
- ***CT without contrast*** may be useful

Differential Diagnosis
- All causes of distal small bowel obstruction.

Management
- Emergency laparotomy is necessary, as the incidence of gangrene of bowel is very high
- En bloc removal of both segments of bowel without attempts to untwist them, with ileocolic anastomosis.

Clinical Pearl
- This condition carries a very high mortality both by its presentation (as gangrene), and also by the magnitude of surgery (short bowel syndrome).

INJURIES OF LARGE INTESTINE

Introduction

- Large bowel injuries can be caused by penetrating and non-penetrating injuries
- Ruptures may be:
    - ***Extraperitoneal*** for ascending and descending colon injuries, whereas
    - ***Intraperitoneal,*** when the injuries are of transverse and sigmoid colons
- Patient develops septic complications quickly as the large fluid leak is fecal and infected
- Delayed presentation is not uncommon as in small bowel injuries.

Diagnosis

Symptoms and Signs

- Abdominal pain, vomiting and distension
- High grade fever occurs due to fecal contamination
- Clinical examination will show signs of peritonitis.

Investigations

- *Plain X-rays* may show air under the domes of the diaphragm (intraperitoneal rupture)
- *Paracentesis* will show feculent fluid.

Management

- *Early laparotomy* is required
- *Closure of tears with proximal diversion* is necessary
- *Peritoneal toileting* is mandatory under cover of broad spectrum antibiotics.

ULCERATIVE COLITIS

Introduction

A chronic mucosal and submucosal inflammatory disease of colon and rectum with remissions and exacerbations.

Etiology and Pathogenesis

- Etiology is uncertain
- Occurs equally in both sexes
- Occurs in both sexes between the age of 20 and 40, but rarely in the sixties
- Involves rectum alone in 40%, left colon in 40% and entire colon in 20%
- Inflammation is said to occur due to:
  - Altered mucosal metabolism
  - Defective mucosal barrier
  - Immune deficiencies
- Pathology involves mucosa and submucosa of the bowel, starting at the rectum proceeding upwards to affect the entire colon.

Risk Factors

- Genetic
- Infections
- Low fat diet
- Psychological stress.

Diagnosis

Symptoms and Signs

- Acute inflammation is one of its clinical presentations

Large Intestine

- Incessant diarrhea, mixed with blood, mucus and pus with constitutional symptoms
- Abdominal discomfort and crampy pain
- Raised body temperature in acute or fulminant attacks
- Muscle wasting, emaciation and anemia due to chronic blood loss
- Abdominal distension due to supervening **toxic megacolon** (acute dilatation)
- Systemic signs (anorexia, malaise and weight loss) are useful in assessing the severity of disease.

Extraintestinal Manifestations

- Peripheral arthritis
- Synovitis
- Primary sclerosing cholangitis
- Eye inflammations (iritis, episcleritis, anterior uveitis)
- Skin lesions (pyoderma gangrenosum).

Investigations

- ***Low hematocrit, leukocytosis and thrombocytosis*** indicate severe disease
- ***Microscopy and culture of stools*** are required to eliminate infections
- ***Plain X-ray abdomen*** (**Fig. 14.7A**) evaluates the colonic caliber (diameter > 6 cm) and rules out perforation
- ***Barium enema*** is diagnostic (**Fig. 14.7B**). It shows a dilated colon with loss of haustrations and mucosal ulcerations. Pseudopolyps are seen as filling defects
- ***CT abdomen with contrast*** gives clearer pictures (**Fig. 14.7C**)
- ***Sigmoidoscopy and colonoscopy*** (**Fig. 14.7D**) show findings of hyperemia of colonic mucosa, diffuse hemorrhagic areas and ulcerations, a granular appearance, extending proximally from the anal verge (rectum is spared in Crohn's disease). Pseudopolyps (**Fig. 14.7E**) may be seen

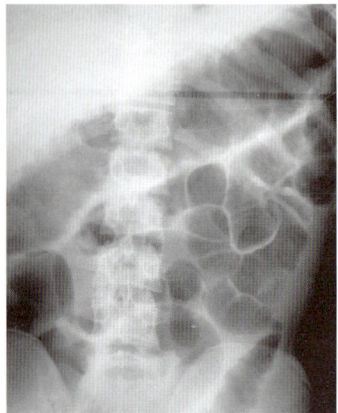

Fig. 14.7A: Toxic megacolon

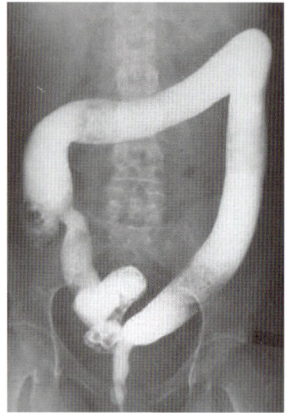

Fig. 14.7B: Barium enema—Ulcerative colitis (Loss of haustrations)

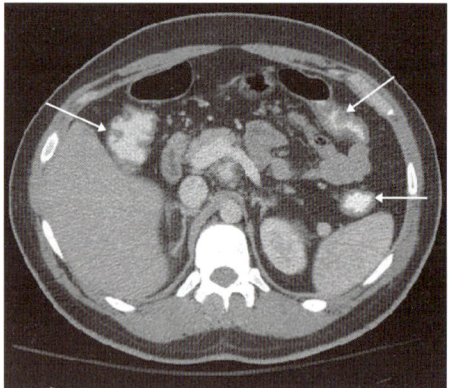

Fig. 14.7C: CT—Thickened mucosa of ulcerative colitis

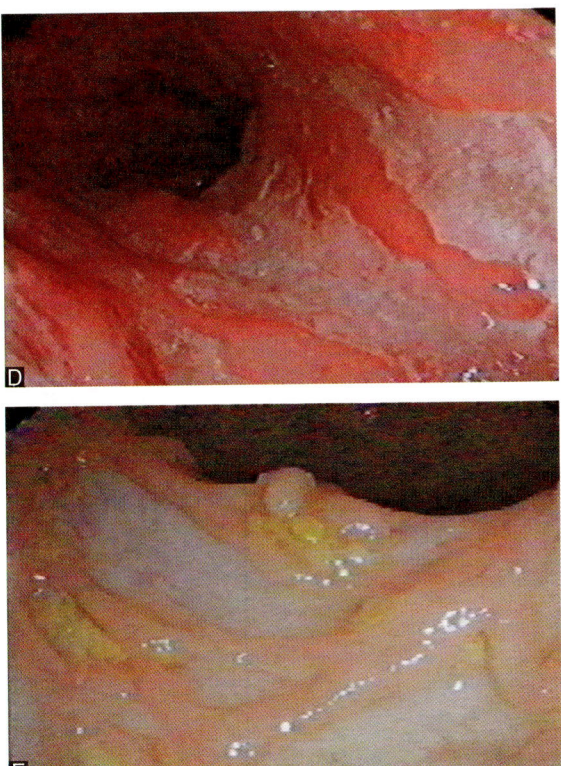

Figs 14.7D and E: Colonoscopy—Ulcerative colitis

Table 14.1: Truelove and Witts classification of severity of ulcerative colitis

	Mild	Moderate	Severe	Fulminant
Stools per day	<4	4–6	>6	>10
Rectal bleeding	Infrequent	Intermediate	Frequent	Continuous
Temperature (°C)	<37.5	Intermediate	>37.5	>37.5
Heart rate (b/mt)	<90	Intermediate	>90	>90
Hemoglobin (G%)	>10	Intermediate	<10	Requires transfusion
ESR (mm/1 hr)	<30	Intermediate	>30	>30

- *Histology* reveals mucosal inflammation, muscularis propria and serosa remain unaffected except in fulminant disease. Inflammatory cells are seen within the crypts and along the dilated vessels of the lamina propria. Crypt abscesses can occur.

The severity of ulcerative colitis is classified according to Truelove and Witts **(Table 14.1)**.

Differential Diagnosis

- Infectious colitis
  - Viral
  - Bacterial
  - Protozoal
- Noninfectious colitis
  - Drug induced
  - Diverticulitis
  - Ischemic colitis
  - Radiation colitis
  - Microscopic colitis.

Complications

- *Gastrointestinal*
  - Stricture
  - Perforation and paracolic abscess
  - Carcinoma
  - Pseudopolyps
  - Ischiorectal abscess
  - Fistula in ano
  - Cirrhosis of liver
- *Non-gastrointestinal*
  - ***Skin:*** Erythema nodosum, pyoderma gangrenosum
  - ***Eye:*** Iritis, episcleritis
  - ***Joints:*** Ankylosing spondylitis, rheumatoid type arthritis
  - ***Kidneys:*** Glomerulonephritis, secondary amyloidosis
  - ***Pulmonary:*** Pulmonary embolism.

Management

Medical

- Symptomatic
- **Oral:** Aminosalicylates. Mesalazine (4 g/day), steroids–prednisolone 5 mg/day
- **Rectal:** Mesalazine suppositories or enemas
- When adequate response is not reached in 2 weeks, oral prednisolone can be raised to 20 mg/day and gradually tapered over a month, and mesalazine is given as maintenance therapy. Two-year therapy is suggested for left-sided disease and indefinite therapy for pancolitis
- Patients who relapse after steroid therapy are treated with azathioprine or 6-mercaptopurine

- Refractory cases may be treated with cyclosporine (intravenous followed by oral) or infliximab (0, 2, and 6 weeks followed by 8 weekly infusions).

Surgical treatment: It is warranted for complications (failure of medical treatment, stricture, perforation and peritonitis, malignancy).
- *Total proctocolectomy with Brook ileostomy/continent ileostomy*
- *Subtotal colectomy with ileorectal anastomosis*
- *Total colectomy with ileal pouch–anal anastomosis.*

Clinical Pearls

- Colonoscopy is suggested for patients with long-standing ulcerative colitis
- Appendicectomy seems to reduce the incidence of ulcerative colitis
- Patients with a relapse of ulcerative colitis should be managed by aggressive medical treatment but with conservative surgical treatment
- 5ASA compounds have a good response rate and reduced relapse rates
- Flares are treated with oral prednisolone (40 mg daily)
- Hospitalization and parenteral steroids are required for patients with severe disease
- Patients on high dose intravenous steroids and stools >8/day and patients with stools 3–8/day with a CRP of >45 mg/L will require colectomy
- When emergency operation is required, a subtotal colectomy and end ileostomy should be performed, and a long sigmoid stump is left within the subcutaneous tissues at the lower pole of the wound, to be resected later after stabilizing the patient. Ileal pouch anal anastomosis should be avoided

- Incomplete endoscopic excision of any dysplastic colonic lesion within an area of colitis is an indication for proctocolectomy
- Subtotal colectomy with ileorectal anastomosis is a compromised procedure as the rectum is retained and total colectomy with ileal pouch–anal anastomosis is the standard surgery for ulcerative colitis
- Ileal pouch–anal anastomosis should be positioned 2–3 cm above the anal margin.

PSEUODMEMBRANOUS COLITIS

Introduction

Inflammation of colon precipitated by the overgrowth of *Clostridium difficile*, an anaerobic, gram–positive, spore forming, toxin producing bacteria. The overgrowth occurs when broad spectrum antibiotics are used, which disrupt the normal fecal flora. Many of them remain asymptomatic, but a few can progress to a situation of ileus and toxic megacolon, warranting surgical management and can even result in death.

Etiology and Pathogenesis

Disruption of the normal flora of the colon, is primarily caused by the antibiotics. The entry of organism is through oral fecal route, and the ingested spores survive the acidic milieu of the stomach, and germinate and overgrow in the colon and produces toxins. The *C. difficile* overgrowth produces two toxins, A and B, of which toxin B is more toxic than toxin A. The toxins produce mucosal damage and inflammation of the colon by disrupting the actin cytoskeleton in the epithelial cells of the intestine while triggering an inflammatory cascade. Strains which produce toxin B exclusively (not producing toxin A) cause pseudomembranous colitis, by entering the damaged mucosa.
- Proximal colon is affected in about 10% of patients

Risk Factors

- Antibiotic exposure (clindamycin, 3rd generation cephalosporins)
- Advanced age
- Renal failure
- Cancer chemotherapy
- Immunocompromised status
- Uremia
- Enteral feeding.

Diagnosis

Symptoms and Signs

- Abdominal pain and cramps
- Fever
- **Watery stools *(severe cases)***
- Shock (very severe cases).

Investigations

- **Leukocytosis** (>30000/cmm in severe cases)
- **Hypoalbuminemia**
- Stool culture for *C. difficile* (highly sensitive but does not distinguish the pathogenic and non-pathogenic strains)
- **Tissue cytotoxin B assay**—highly sensitive and is gold standard, but it takes 48 hours to get the result
- **Enzyme immunoassays for toxins A and B**–most widely used and the result is available in a short time, but expensive
- **Sigmoidoscopy/colonoscopy** is reserved for situations where there is a need to rule out another disease, and stool sample cannot be obtained. In mild cases, colonoscopy is normal. In severe disease, the colonic mucosa has creamy-white-yellow plaques (pseudomembranes), which arise from a point of

superficial ulceration, with acute and chronic inflammation of lamina propria. The pseudomembrane consists of fibrin, mucin, debris of sloughed mucosal epithelial cells and polymorphonuclear cells
- *Histopathology* shows patchy epithelial necrosis and fibrin exudates.

Differential Diagnosis

- Staphylococcal enterocolitis

Management

Medical

- Stop the implicated antibiotics
- Oral metronidazole 500 mg thrice daily for 5 days, or vancomycin 250 mg thrice daily for 5 days
- In severe cases, parenteral metronidazole is preferred

Surgical

- **Emergency surgery (*Total colectomy with end ileostomy and Hartmann's pouch*)** for situations like cecal perforation and toxic megacolon with secondary sepsis.

Clinical Pearls

- Clostridia which do not produce toxins are nonpathogenic
- Symptoms usually appear within 1–2 weeks of antibiotic treatment, but it can occur between 1 day to 6 weeks of therapy
- *C. difficile* spores survive in the environment for years and common in places where infected individuals have stayed, commonly the hospitals

- Among the silent carriers of *C. difficile* spores, only a third become symptomatic
- Diarrhea is the presenting symptom of pseudomembranous colitis
- Any antibiotic even a single dose can precipitate pseudomembranous colitis, and is not associated with duration or dose of treatment
- The hallmarks of pseudomembranous colitis are fever, hypoalbuminemia, shock and high levels of C-reactive protein
- Antidiarrheals are not to be used in the treatment of *C. difficile* colitis, as the toxins may not get cleared easily
- Due to increased risk of perforation, endoscopy should be avoided and performed as a last resort
- In about a quarter of patients, diarrhea resolves spontaneously
- Metronidazole is the first drug of choice as vancomycin resistance is known
- Recurrence of symptoms occur in a sizeable population of patients, which warrant higher doses of vancomycin with probiotics (*Saccharomyces boulardii* or *Lactobacillus*)
- Segmental colonic resections/simple diverting ileostomy without colonic resections are not useful.

RADIATION COLITIS

Introduction

Radiation to the adjoining organs of the colon can cause inflammation of the colon. Radiation to rectal, cervical, uterine, prostatic and urinary bladder carcinoma cause colonic inflammation, especially the most fixed part, the rectosigmoid. Tumors, which require higher doses of radiation, are associated with greater risk or damage to the colon. Adjoining small bowel is protected by its peristaltic movement, and has a very low risk of radiation injury.

Diagnosis

Symptoms and Signs
- Nausea and vomiting
- Diarrhea
- Tenesmus
- Bleeding (rare).

Investigation
- **Colonoscopy** may be normal or may show telangiectasia (**Fig. 14.8**) or friable mucosa. Presence of atypical fibroblasts is typical. Chronic ischemia can lead to strictures and bleeding.

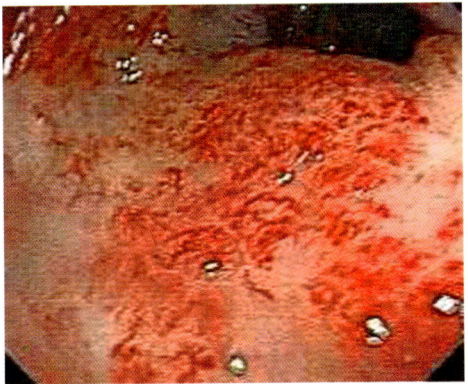

Fig. 14.8: Colonoscopy—Telangiectasia of rdiation colitis

Management

Medical

- Oral and topical sucralfate
- Oral and topical steroids
- 5 ASA compounds
- Sulfasalazine
- Metronidazole.

Endoscopic

- Argon laser photocoagulation
- Heater probe
- Bipolar cautery

Surgical

- Surgical treatment may be required when strictures cause obstruction and perforation

ISCHEMIC COLITIS

Introduction

- A disease of the elderly population, with embolus or thrombosis of mesenteric artery, as part of a generalized vascular disease
- Ischemia can be isolated to the colon
- Any region of the colon can be affected, but has a tendency for segmental distribution
- Ischemic colitis is the commonest form of vascular injury to the GI tract
- Mesenteric vascular ischemia is another cause, the exact pathogenesis of which is not clear

- Usually affects the watershed areas between the arterial distributions of SMA and IMA
  - Rectosigmoid
  - Descending colon
  - Splenic flexure
  - All the above in combination
- Right colon and rectum are rarely involved
- It is of two varieties:
  1. Acute fulminant colitis
  2. Subacute ischemic colitis.

Etiology

The etiologic factors are given in **Table 14.2**.

Diagnosis

Symptoms and Signs

- Usually nonspecific
- High index of suspicion especially in patients with risk factors
- Acute fulminant colitis presents with acute severe lower abdominal pain and massive rectal bleeding

Table 14.2: Etiologic factors of ischemic colitis

Non-occlusive factors	Occlusive factors
Idiopathic	Arterial (embolus, thrombosis, trauma, vasculitis)
Shock (septic, hemorrhagic, cardiogenic, hypovolemic)	Venous (hypercoagulable status, pancreatitis)
Drugs (catecholamines, diuretics, digitalis, NSAIDs, cocaine)	
Colon obstruction (colon cancer, fecal impaction)	

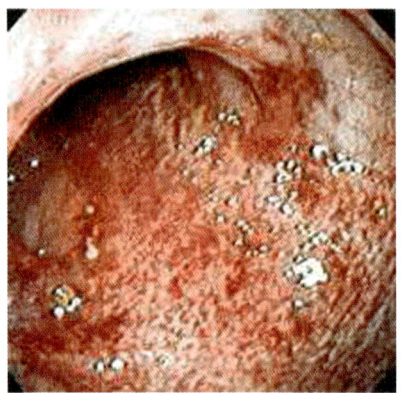

Fig. 14.9: Colonoscopy—Ischemic colitis

- Urge to defecate
- Subacute variety presents with lesser degree of symptoms.

Investigations

- ***Colonoscopy*** within the first 3 days of symptoms is the best diagnostic method **(Fig. 14.9)**
- ***Plain abdominal X-rays**—'Thumbprinting'* due to subdepithelial edema and hemorrhage
- ***Arteriography*** is diagnostic, when there is obstruction
- ***Barium enema*** is contributory (Thumbprinting), but should not be done in acute fulminant variety for the fear of perforation.

Differential Diagnosis

- Infectious colitis
- Diverticulitis
- Inflammatory bowel disease.

Complications

- Toxic megacolon
- Gangrene
- Perforation
- Pericolic abscess
- Stricture

Management

- **Vasodilators** form the mainstay of medical treatment
- **Surgery** is indicated for perforations, abscesses, stricture formation and gangrene (segmental resection of ischemic colon with proximal diverting colostomy).

Indications for Surgery

- **Acute**
  - Peritonitis
  - Massive lower GI bleeding
  - Fulminant colitis.
- **Subacute**
  - Segmental colitis with persistent symptoms
  - Protein losing colopathy
  - Recurrent sepsis attributable to ischemic colitis
- **Chronic**
  - Symptomatic stricture
  - Symptomatic segmental ischemic colitis

Clinical Pearls

- In non-occlusive disease, no investigation is useful
- Ischemic colitis is reversible in majority of patients whose symptoms subside within 48 hours

- High index of suspicion is necessary for the diagnosis of ischemic colitis
- Repeated examination and evaluation is necessary while patients are on conservative management
- When irreversible changes occur, toxic megacolon, gangrene and perforation can occur.

OGILVIE'S SYNDROME

Introduction

- Acute pseudo-obstruction localized to the colon, due to *nonmechanical factors*
- Reported by Leithauser and Sir H Ogilvie simultaneously in 1948, but referred to as Ogilvie's syndrome
- The patients with pseudo-obstruction are clinically ill, as they are in the recovery phase of a major surgery or trauma.

Etiology

This dilatation of colon is precipitated by various causes. They are shown in **Box 14.1**. The precise cause is not known.

Pathogenesis

The pathogenesis is not fully understood, but an imbalance in the autonomic regulation of the colon is suggested. The vagus supplies the colon up to the splenic flexure, and the distal colon is supplied by the spinal segments S2–S4 (sacral parasympathetic nerves). The parasympathetic nervous system stimulates the motility of colon, while sympathetic nerves inhibit contraction of smooth muscles. Decreased activity of the parasympathetic nervous system and increased activity of sympathetic nervous system is implicated in the pathology of this functional obstruction.

> **Box 14.1:** Etiological factors of Ogilvie's syndrome
>
> **Postoperative**
> - Laparotomy
> - Orthopedic
> - Gynecological
> - Urological
> - Neurological
>
> **Trauma**
> - Spinal cord injuries
> - Burns
> - Retroperitoneal injuries
>
> **Systemic diseases**
> - Sepsis (e.g. septicemia)
> - Cardiopulmonary diseases (e.g. heart failure)
> - Renal insufficiency
> - Gastrointestinal (e.g. pancreatitis)
> - Endocrine disorders (e.g. hypothyroidism)
> - CNS and peripheral nervous system disorders (e.g. Parkinsonism, Guillain-Barre syndrome)
>
> **Drugs**
> - Narcotics
> - Anticholinergics
> - Digitalis
> - Alcohol

Diagnosis

Symptoms and Signs

- Painless distension of abdomen
- Constipation
- Diarrhea (rare)
- Nausea and vomiting

- Non-tender distension of abdomen
- Absent bowel sounds
- Peritoneal signs indicate ischemia or perforation.

Investigations

- **Plain X-ray abdomen** reveals distended proximal colon with the descending and sigmoid colon of normal caliber and is diagnostic
- **Barium enema** is required to rule out mechanical cause.

Complications

- **Ischemia** can occur probably due to increased intramural pressure
- **Perforation** of cecum caused by overdistension as the cecal wall is thinnest.

Management

Medical

- Nil by mouth, nasogastric aspiration, fluid and electrolyte replacements
- Decompression of colon by flatus tube (questionable as it does not reach the proximal colon)
- Stoppage of drugs which interfere with GI motility (e.g. opiates, anticholinergics)
- Persistence of symptoms for >48 hours and a cecal diameter of >13 cm requires therapy
- Neostigmine 2.5 mg IV bolus over 3 minutes (or as an infusion for 30–60 min) is useful, response is seen within about 20 minutes, the same treatment can be tried three times, and has a success rate of about 90%, but the response is sustained in about 75%. Atropine should be administered for bradycardia if it occurs
- Plain X-ray films should be obtained every 12 hours to evaluate the colonic diameter

Endoscopic

Colonoscopic decompression and catheter placement at the right colon, are tried if the medical therapy fails. This procedure has a success rate of about 75%

Surgical

When cecal diameter is >13 cm and refractory to medical treatment, tube cecostomy may be necessary for sick patients, and right hemicolectomy may be the ultimate

The treatment algorithm is given in **Figure 14.10**.

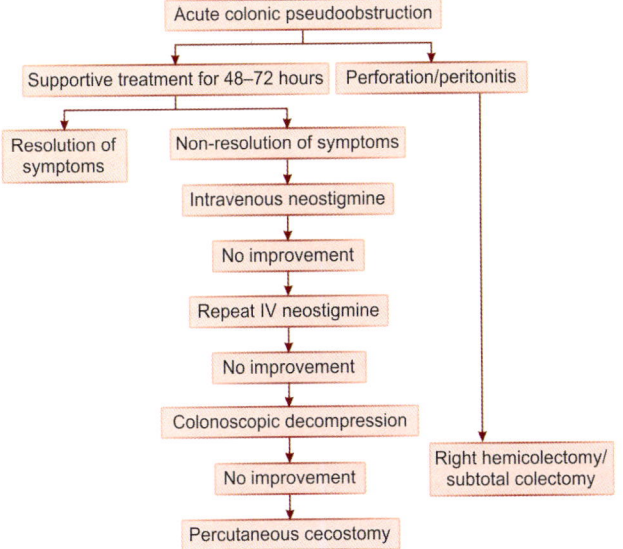

Fig. 14.10: Treatment algorithm of colonic pseudo-obstruction

Clinical Pearls

- Though the abdominal distension is reported to be painless, 80% have mild pain
- Severe abdominal pain may indicate complications like ischemia and perforation
- When the cecal diameter exceeds 13 cm, the risk of perforation increases considerably
- It is necessary to establish that there is no perforation or bowel ischemia before initiating any interventional treatment
- Neostigmine inhibits acetylcholinesterase, the enzyme which hydrolyzes acetylcholine at the neuromuscular junction, and its use in pseudo-obstruction, causes relative increase in acetylcholine, which enhances cholinergic transmission and smooth muscle contraction
- Side effects of neostigmine administration include bradycardia, salivation, sweating, restlessness, nausea, abdominal pain, bronchoconstriction and hypotension. Bradycardia (<60/min), hypotension (<90 mm Hg), recent myocardial infarction, acidosis and serum creatinine of >3 mg% are relative contraindications to neostigmine therapy
- Intravenous infusion of neostigmine has lower risk of bradycardia when compared to the bolus dose
- Surgical treatment is the last resort to treat acute pseudo-obstruction as it carries a very high mortality
- Contrast enema rules out mechanical obstruction, may itself decompress the colon, but when there is a doubt about ischemia or perforation, the study itself is contraindicated.

DIVERTICULITIS

Introduction

A diverticulum is a pouch or sac which can occur either naturally or by herniation of the mucous membrane through a defect in the muscular layer of a tubular organ. Those occurring in the colon are called colonic diverticula. They are of two types **(Fig. 14.11)**:
- *Congenital* (rare)—these diverticula contain all the layers of colon, and said to be true diverticula
- *Acquired* (common)—these diverticula are considered false or pulsion diverticula, and they contain serosa covered outpouchings of mucosa through gaps in muscularis caused by increased intracolonic pressure.

Etiology and Pathogenesis

- Rare under the age of 35, but the incidence increases with age, to 50% of diverticula are found in the age of 80–90
- Commonly affects the left sided colon (95%), more especially the sigmoid colon (70%)

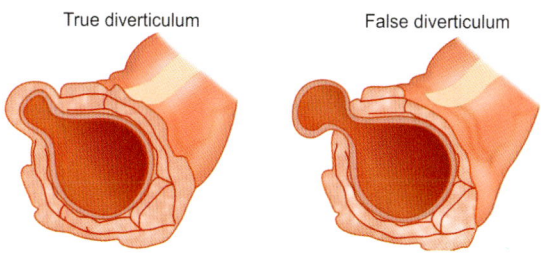

Fig. 14.11: Types of diverticula

- Generalized diverticulosis is seen in only about 5% of population
- Consumption of low fiber diet is a common factor associated with diverticular disease of colon. This decreases the stool volume and increases segmentation during peristalsis. Exaggerated segmentation causes herniation of mucosa through the muscular layer at a point where vasa recta penetrate the circular muscular layer. Diverticula appear in rows between the mesenteric and lateral tenia coli, more commonly in the sigmoid colon following LaPlace's law.
- People with diverticulosis, commonly have thickening of circular and longitudinal muscular layers of colon, which result in shortening of teniae and narrowing of colonic lumen, which exaggerates the process of segmentation, giving a concertina effect. This is called *myochosis (Fig. 14.12).*
- There are of two stages:
    - ***Diverticulosis stage:*** Diverticula without inflammation
    - ***Diverticulitis stage:*** The neck of the diverticulum is narrow and its obstruction causes collection of fecal material inside the diverticulum, encouraging bacterial overgrowth, combined with microperforation caused by 'impacted' inspissated

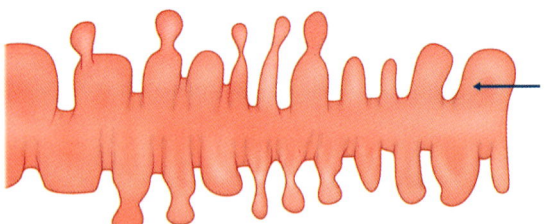

Fig. 14.12: Concertina effect of myochosis

fecal matter, causing diverticulitis. Resulting distension of diverticula may cause focal ischemia, which may be a precursor to perforation.
- The diverticulitis can be divided into
  - *Acute* (symptoms with acute inflammation)
    - *Simple* (localized)
    - *Complicated* (with perforation)
  - *Chronic* (persistent, low grade inflammation)
    - *Atypical* (symptoms without signs)
    - *Recurring* (symptoms with systemic signs)
  - *Complex* (with fistula, stricture, obstruction)
  - *Malignant* (severe, fibrosing).

Risk Factors

- Advanced age
- Mechanical factors
- Environmental factors
- Lifestyle factors
- Low dietary fiber

Diagnosis

Symptoms

- *Diverticulosis stage*—asymptomatic
- *Diverticulitis stage*
  - Left lower abdominal pain
  - Irregular bowel habits
  - Episodic diarrhea or constipation
  - Feeling of incomplete evacuation
  - Rectal bleeding (rarely due to associated malignancy)
  - Fever may be present

- Pneumaturia, fecaluria, or passage of feces and gas through vagina may indicate colovesical or colovaginal fistula

Signs

- Mild tenderness over the descending colon
- Acute episodes of diverticulitis cause acute abdominal pain mainly in the left side of abdomen, may be associated with diarrhea and bleeding per rectum
- Abdominal mass due to localized abscess and phlegmon
- Generalized abdominal tenderness may represent gross perforation causing fecal or purulent peritonitis. Guarding and rigidity may be present.

Hinchey's classification (**Fig. 14.13**) of complicated acute diverticulitis:

- *Stage I*—pericolic or mesenteric abscess
- *Stage II*—walled off pelvic abscess
- *Stage III*—generalized purulent peritonitis
- *Stage IV*—generalized fecal peritonitis

Investigations

- **ESR** may be elevated during acute diverticulitis stage
- *Plain X-ray* may show air under the diaphragm when the diverticulum perforates
- *Barium enema* is diagnostic [Diverticula—pouch like projections (**Fig. 14.14A**), diverticultis—*'Saw tooth' appearance* (**Fig. 14.14B**)]. Reflux of contrast may be seen in internal fistulae but is seen in a minority of patients
- *CECT abdomen* is the test of choice for simple and uncomplicated diverticulitis with very high sensitivity, can distinguish complicated and uncomplicated varieties, extracolonic pathology (**Fig. 14.14C**)

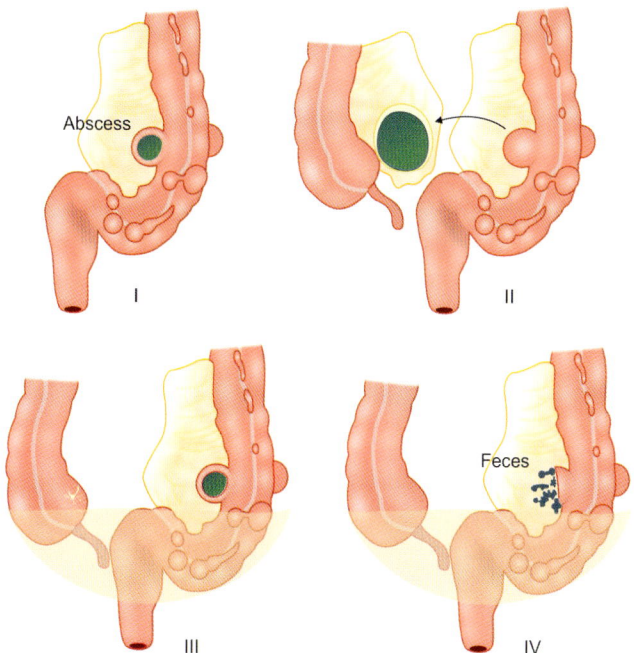

Fig. 14.13: Hinchey's classification of diverticulitis

- ***MRI** has high correlation with CT*
- ***US abdomen*** has a specificity of about 80%
- ***Colonoscopy*** **(Figs 14.14D and E)** is specific and should be performed only when the disease is quiet without complications, which has the advantage of diagnosing malignancies.

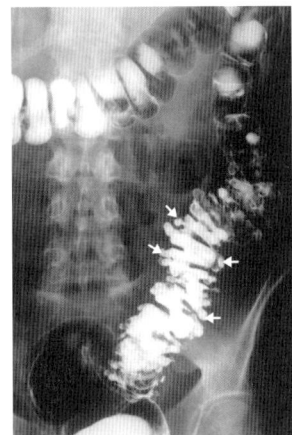

Fig. 14.14A: Barium enema—Colonic diverticulosis

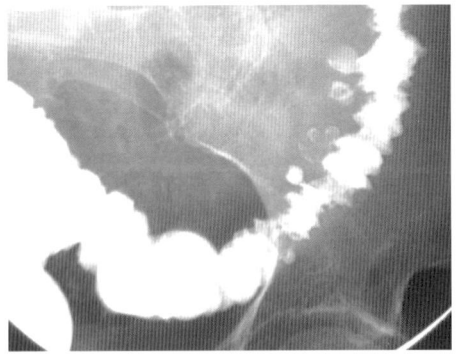

Fig. 14.14B: Barium enema—Diverticulitis

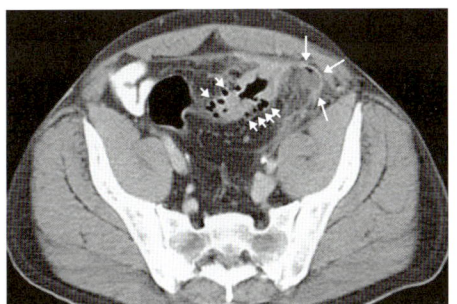

Fig. 14.14C: CT—Colonic diverticulitis

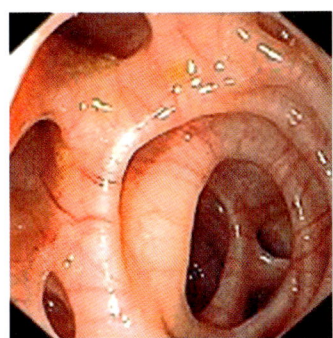

Fig. 14.14D: Colonoscopy— Diverticulosis

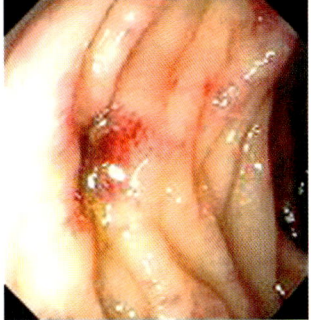

Fig. 14.14E: Colonoscopy— Diverticulitis

Table 14.3: Diseases which mimic symptoms of diverticulitis

Elderly	Middle age and young	Others
Ischemic bowel disease	Appendicitis	Infectious colitis
Malignancy	Inflammatory bowel disease	Amebic colitis
Volvulus	Penetrating ulcer	Irritable bowel syndrome
Obstruction	Urinary infection	
Penetrating ulcer	Pancreatitis	
	Salpingitis	

Differential Diagnosis

Many diseases mimic diverticulitis but it can be listed according to the prevalence in various age groups (**Table 14.3**).

Complications

- Perforation
- Pericolic abscess or intra-abdominal abscess
- Peritonitis
- Internal fistulae (colovesical and colovaginal fistulae)
- Strictures

Management

- *Diverticulosis* needs no treatment
- *Diverticulitis* can be managed conservatively
    - *High fiber low residue diet* to increase the bulkiness to increase the lumen size, decrease transit time and intraluminal pressure, which will ultimately decrease segmentation
    - *Antispasmodics* to reduce pain
    - *Antibiotics to cover gram-negative and anaerobic bacteria*

- *Surgical management* is for patients with
  - Failure of management for severe and extensive colitis,
    - Sigmoid colectomy with anastomosis with or without proximal diversion
    - Subtotal colectomy
  - Complications
    - ***Perforations***—Diversion with oversewing of the perforation site with proximal diversion, subtotal colectomy, peritoneal lavage
    - ***Small paracolic abscess of less than 1 cm diameter resolve by antibiotic therapy***
    - ***Large abscess may require CT guided percutaneous drainage, and rarely open drainage.***

Indications

- Failure to respond to conservative management
- Perforation with peritonitis
- Obstruction that does not resolve with conservative therapy.

Clinical Pearls

- Segmentation is a motility process in which the colon is separated into two chambers by the proximal and distal segmental muscular contractions
- Development of diverticula follow the La Place's law, which states that colonic wall pressure is proportional to the wall tension and inversely proportional to the colonic radius, explaining the increased incidence of diverticula in the sigmoid colon
- Diverticulitis occurs in about 10–20% of patients with diverticulosis of colon
- Patients with hemorrhage, perforations and peritonitis are febrile and present as acute emergency

- Symptoms of acute diverticulitis correspond to the location of inflamed diverticula, e.g. transverse colon diverticulitis pain mimics peptic ulcer disease and right colon diverticulitis pain mimics acute appendicitis
- Diverticulitis of redundant sigmoid colon will present with right iliac fossa pain mimicking appendicitis
- About a third of patients with diverticulosis remain asymptomatic, a third have episodes of discomfort and a third have recurrent episodes of symptoms with increased morbidity and mortality due to complications
- Corticosteroids and NSAIDs are known to exacerbate diverticulitis, and high dose steroids are known to mask the symptoms of diverticulitis related complications
- The colovesical fistula is the commonest complication of diverticulitis; colovaginal fistula follows in occurrence. Other fistulae are colocolic, ureterocolic, colouterine, colosalpingeal, coloperineal and others
- Usually, the perforation is small forming a microabscess, a phlegmon which becomes a large abscess. Free perforation is rare but fistulization is relatively frequent
- Giant diverticula of colon are rare but associated with sigmoid diverticular disease
- In general, most Hinchey class I and some class II cases can be managed with a one stage procedure and Hinchey class III and IV cases can be managed with a two stage procedure
- ***Saint's triad:*** Association of diverticulosis, cholelithiasis and hiatus hernia.

CECAL DIVERTICULITIS

Introduction

- Solitary diverticulum is common in the cecum

- Inflammation of the diverticulum presents like acute appendicitis and mislead the examiner.

Classification

- **Grade I:** Easily recognizable projecting inflamed cecal diverticulum
- **Grade II:** Inflamed cecal mass
- **Grade III:** Localized abscess or fistula
- **Grade IV:** Free perforation or ruptured abscess with diffuse peritonitis.

Diagnosis

Symptoms and Signs

- Pain in the right iliac fossa (similar to acute appendicitis)
- A lump may be felt in the right iliac fossa.

Investigations

- *US and CT* may be useful
- *Colonoscopy* is diagnostic.

Management

When discovered accidentally during laparotomy, many options are available:
- *Appendicectomy, nonresection of diverticulum*
- *Appendicectomy, diverticulectomy for Grade I and II diseases*
- *Right hemicolectomy for Grade III and IV diseases.*

Clinical Pearls

- Cecal diverticulitis is diagnosed correctly preoperatively only in a small percentage of time

- Appendicectomy should always be done when diverticulectomy is not contemplated, but the base of appendix is not inflamed, to avoid a diagnostic confusion at a later date.

COLORECTAL POLYPS

Introduction

- A true polyp is defined as a protrusion above the mucosal surface into the lumen. A pseudopolyp is defined as the normal mucosa which appears like a protrusion when the surrounding mucosa is depressed by ulcerations (**Fig. 14. 15A**)
- More common in males
- Uncommon before the age of forty
- Most colorectal polyps are benign adenomas
- Adenomas may be solitary or multiple
- All polyps have the potential for malignant change
- They are either pedunculated or sessile.

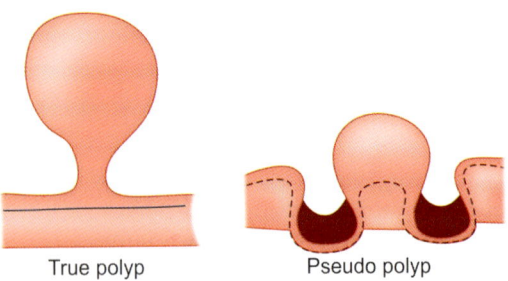

Fig. 14.15A: Differentiating true and pseudopolyps

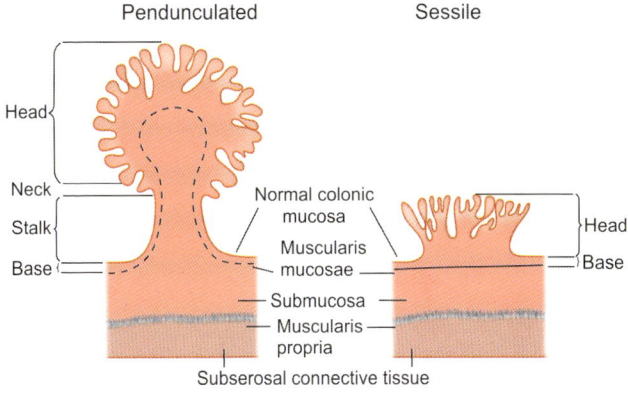

Fig. 14.15B: Anatomy of polyps

Anatomy (Fig. 14.15B)

Pedunculated Polyp

- A polyp has the following regions:
  - **Base:** Area of colon on which the stalk is attached
  - **Stalk:** A longitudinal stem arising from the base, covered by normal mucosa and has a central core of submucosa
  - **Neck:** The line at which the normal and adenomatous epithelium join, which is the line of transition between the stalk and the head of polyp
  - **Head:** Area of adenomatous epithelium.

Sessile Polyp

A sessile polyp does not have a stalk and a neck. Adenomatous epithelium directly sits on the normal colonic mucosa.

Classification

- Polyps mat be classified into:
  - **Neoplastic**
    - **Epithelial**—adenomas, adenocarcinoma, carcinoid
    - **Nonepithelial**—lipoma, leiomyoma, lymphomatous polyps
  - **Non-neoplastic**—hyperplastic polyps, hamartomas, inflammatory polyps.

Neoplastic Polyps

- Clinical presentation divides the colorectal polyps into
  - Sporadic
  - Hereditary
- Histologically they are of three types:
  1. Tubular
  2. Villous
  3. Tubulovillous (20% tubular and 80% villous)
- Multiple colonic polyps occur in some syndromes
  - Peutz-Jeghers syndrome
  - Gardner's syndrome
  - Familial adenomatous polyposis
  - Cowden syndrome
  - Turcot's syndrome
  - Cronkhite-Canada syndrome.

Adenomas

- Adenomas are the most important and the most common colorectal polyps
- They may be single or multiple
- They are dysplastic and premalignant.

Etiology and Pathogenesis

Polyps result due to disordered and persistent cell replication coupled with retarded cell maturation. There are many factors, which play a role in the development of colonic polyps. They are:

- **Genetic factors:** Aneuploidy, tetraploidy, DNA hypomethylation. Altered expression of oncogenes *fos, myc, ras*. Mutations in APC, DCC, p53 hare been reported.
- **Environmental factors**: Diet.
- **Drugs:** NSAIDs.

Diagnosis

Symptoms and Signs

- Polyps remain generally asymptomatic
- Symptomatic polyps present with rectal bleeding, sometimes leading to iron deficiency anemia by occult blood loss
- Distal lesions may cause tenesmus and may prolapse through the anus.

Investigations

- *Barium enema* (**Fig. 14.16A**) reveals most polyps of significant size
- *CT colonography* can diagnose colonic polyps
- *Total colonoscopy* (**Figs 14.16B to E**) is diagnostic. Malignancy should be suspected when the surface of the polyp is irregular, ulcerated, friable, firm or hard in consistency, thick stalk and non-lifting with submucosal saline injection
- *Histopathology* exhibits the dysplastic and malignant changes.

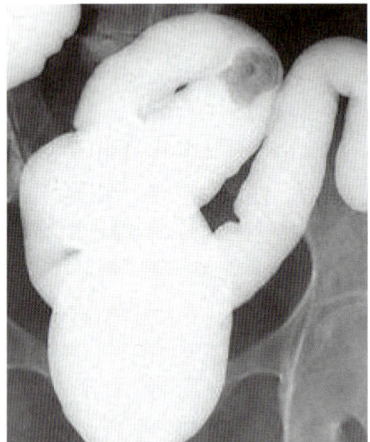

Fig. 14.16A: Barium enema—Sigmoid colon polyp

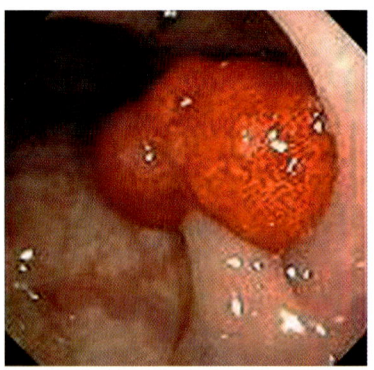

Fig. 14.16B: Colonoscopy—Bleeding colonic polyp

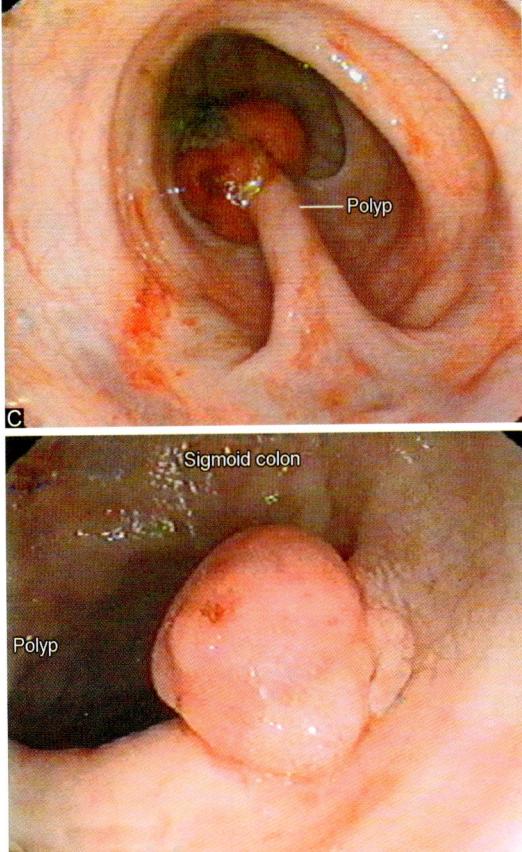

Figs 14.16C and D: Colonoscopy—Pedunculated colonic polyp

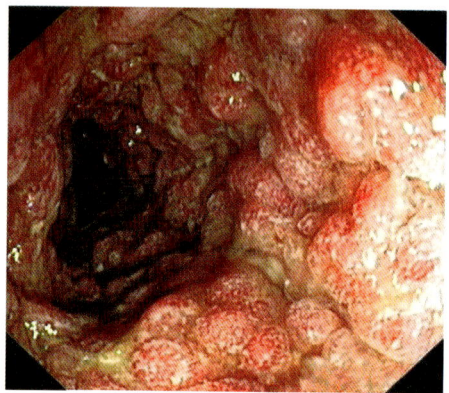

Fig. 14.16E: Colonoscopy—Multiple polyps

Differential Diagnosis

- Non-neoplastic polyps
  - Hyperplastic polyps (<5 mm, multiple, usually not premalignant)
  - Inflammatory polyps (Pseudopolyps—islands of residual mucosa amongs the ulcerated mucosa of ulcerative colitis, Crohn's disease)
  - Hamartomatous polyps (mucosal projections consisting of excess lamina propria and dilated cystic glands, regress spontaneously)
- Connective tissue tumors (lipomas, fibromas, leiomyomas)
- Pneumatosis
- Angiomas
- Benign lymphoid nodules
- Metastatic lesions
- Carcinoids.

Complications

Malignant Transformation

Risk Factors

- **Size**—adenoma of >2 cm
- **Histology**—tubular, villous or tubulovillous
- **Type**—sessile.

Malignant Polyps

- A malignant polyp is defined as a polyp with cancer cells invading the muscularis mucosa
- They account for about 10% in polypectomy series
- Based on the level of invasion, they are classified *(Haggitt's classification)* **(Fig. 14.17)**:
  - *Level 0*—Noninvasive (severe dysplasia)

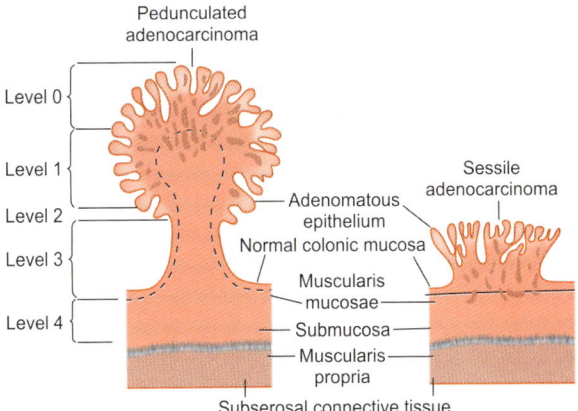

Fig. 14.17: Haggitt's classification

- *Level 1*—Cancer invading through the muscularis mucosa but limited to the head of a pedunculated polyp
- *Level 2*—Cancer invading the neck of pedunculated polyp
- *Level 3*—Cancer invading the stalk of a pedunculated polyp
- *Level 4*—Cancer invading the submucosa of the bowel below the stalk of a pedunculated polyp. All sessile polyps with invasive cancer at level 4.

- Kudo's classification considers the depth of submucosal invasion into three levels **(Fig. 14.18)**:
  - *Level Sm_1*—Invasion into upper third of submucosa
  - *Level Sm_2*—Invasion into the middle third of submucosa
  - *Level Sm_3*—Invasion into the lower third of submucosa

(Haggitt levels 1, 2, and 3 are Kudo Sm_1, Haggitt level 4 may be Sm_1, Sm_2, or Sm_3).

Management

- *Colonic polyps have to be removed by colonoscopic snare polypectomy (Fig. 14.19A)*
- *If polypectomy is done for a suspiciously malignant polyp, the removed site should be marked by tattooing the bowel wall with a dye*
- Large polyps may require snaring in several pieces. Histopathology examination is essential for diagnosis and for

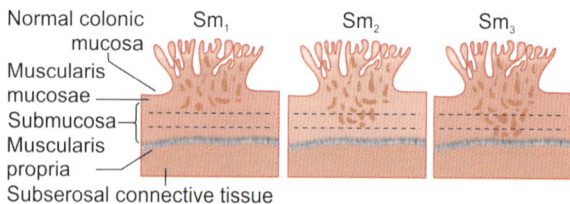

Fig. 14.18: Kudo's classification

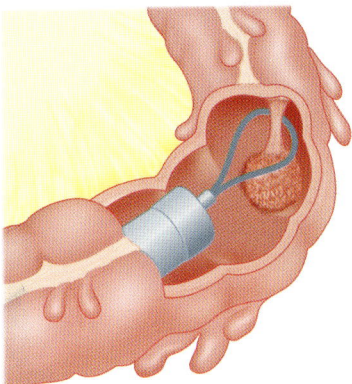

Fig. 14.19A: Colonoscopic polypectomy

determining the completeness of excision. Incomplete removal of malignant polyps requires bowel resection. Patients who have undergone snaring should have colonoscopy the next year and then every 3–5 years
- Large sessile polyps of >3 cm have a high risk of recurrence and should be followed by colonoscopies done every 3–6 months in the first year, every 6–12 months in the second year and yearly till the 5th year
- Large number of polyps at close intervals and with suspicious features of malignancy, will have to be treated by colectomy in a conventional manner
- A clear margin of 2 mm beyond the deepest level of invasion is needed to consider the margin clear and a positive margin after polypectomy should be taken as inadequate treatment. This rule applies to both pedunculated and sessile polyps

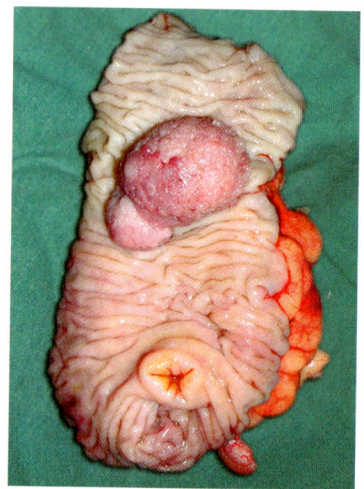

Fig. 14.19B: Colectomy for polyp with dysplasia

- Colonic resections **(Fig 14.19B)** are necessary when:
  - A pedunculated polyp belongs to Haggitt level 4 with invasion to distal third of submucosa, or with lymphovascular invasion
  - Polypectomy with margin < 2 mm
  - Sessile lesions removed piecemeal
  - Sessile lesion with depth of invasion into distal third of submucosa (Sm_3).

Clinical Pearls

- *Flat or depressed adenomas:* Not elevated above the surface (not true polyps), identified only by chemoendoscopy, have high risk for cancer, requires excision (endoscopic or open)

- **Serrated adenomas:** Adenomas described as hyperplastic polyps containing adenomatous features. Carries the same risk of adenomatous types.

Non-neoplastic Polyps

Hyperplastic Polyps

Most common polyps found during colonoscopy. They are small, <3–5 mm, common in the rectosigmoid region and asymptomatic. They occur due to a failure of programmed cell death. The main cellular components are mature goblet cells, reduced in number when compared to adenomatous polyps. When associated with hereditary syndromes, carry a high risk for malignancy.

Hamartomas

These are localized overgrowth of normal mature cells, and they are juvenile polyps. They appear round, pink, smooth and pedunculated and rarely sessile. Muscularis mucosa does not take part in its formation. They are known to twist on their own and autoamputate and wither off. Clinical presentation is rectal bleeding, mucus discharge, diarrhea and abdominal pain, intussusception and prolapse through the anus. Treatment is snare polypectomy.

Inflammatory Polyps

These are islands of normal or minimally inflamed mucosa, between the ulcers (e.g. inflammatory bowel disease). By the surrounding ulcers, they appear elevated and are also called pseudopolyps. Treatment is towards the underlying disease.

Lymphoid Polyps

These are benign lymphoid follicle enlargements and they have a normal overlying mucosa. They are multiple and the cause is not known. Histologically, the lymphoid tissue is in the mucosa and submucosa not invading the muscularis propria.

Clinical Pearls

- Colonic polyps are seen more commonly in patients with colonic cancer, and a third of colon cancer patients have a polyp elsewhere in the large bowel
- Size has an influence on malignant transformation in colonic polyps, larger the polyp higher the incidence of malignancy
- Histology also has significance in the malignant transformation of polyps, villous adenomas have more malignant potential than the tubular adenomas.

POLYPOSIS SYNDROMES

Introduction

- These syndromes are associated with colorectal and other cancers with increased risk
- They have diffuse GI polyposis and are premalignant.

Diagnosis

The inheritance pattern and clinical manifestations vary (**Table 14.4**).

Symptoms and Signs

- Usually they are asymptomatic
- GI bleeding is common.

Investigations

- Classical FAP is diagnosed when more than 100 polyps are found (when <100 polyps are found, it is called attenuated FAP).

Table 14.4: Polyposis syndromes

Disorder	Inheritance	Features	Malignancy risk
Peutz–Jeghers syndrome (PJS)	Autosomal dominant, caused by mutation of LKB1 on chromosome 19p13.3 which encodes a serine-threonine kinase	Diffuse GI polyposis (small bowel 70%, stomach 40%, colon 40%, rectum 30%), mucocutaneous pigmentation of lips, gums, genitalia	High
MYH associated polyposis (MAP)	Autosomal recessive, caused by bi-allelic mutation in MYH gene	Colorectal adenomas, with osteomas, CHRPE, no desmoids	High risk
Familial adenomatous polyposis (FAP)	Autosomal dominant, by mutation of APC gene	Multiple polyps of stomach, small and large bowel, duodenal cancer and desmoids disease are the extracolonic manifestations	100% risk
Juvenile polyposis	Autosomal dominant, with incomplete penetrance SMAD4 and BMPR1A genes are implicated	>5 juvenile polyps in the colon and rectum, and other parts of GIT	High
Gardner's syndrome	Autosomal dominant, caused by mutation in the APC gene located in chromosome 5q21 (band q21 on chromosome 5)	Multiple polyps in the colon together with tumors outside the colon. The extracolonic tumors may include osteomas of the skull, thyroid cancer, epidermoid cysts, fibromas and sebaceous cysts	Unclear

Contd...

Contd...

Disorder	Inheritance	Features	Malignancy risk
Cowden syndrome	Autosomal dominant, mutation of PTEN gene	GI polyposis, multiple hamartomas, macrocephaly, trichilemmomas, neoplasms of thyroid, breast, uterus and skin	Unclear
Bannayan-Riley-Ruvalcaba syndrome	Autosomal dominant, mutation of PTEN gene	GI polyposis, multiple hamartomas, macro-cephaly, trichilemmomas, neoplasms of thyroid, breast, uterus and skin	Unclear
Turcot's syndrome		Glioblastomas or medulloblastomas, multiple colonic polyps	Premalignant
Cronkhite-Canada syndrome	No evidence of inheritance. Considered acquired	GI hamartomatous polyposis, alopecia, atrophy of nails, pigmentation, watery diarrhea, multiple colonic polyps	Unclear

Management

- *Prophylactic colectomy* before the age of 20
- In juvenile polyposis, endoscopic polypectomy (in whichever part of GIT), and gastrectomy, bowel resection or colectomy if dysplastic changes are seen.

Surveillance

- *In PJS*, upper and lower GI endoscopy, barium study of small bowel every 2–3 years
- In juvenile polyposis, surveillance should be done every year.

Clinical Pearls

- Patients with familial polyposis, have a high potential to develop colonic cancer
- Desmoid tumor and duodenal cancer are important causes of death in patients with FAP who have undergone colectomy
- The predictive testing should start around the age of 14
- When there is no family history in FAP, the cause is new mutation
- Small bowel polyps, family history and pigmental macules on the buccal mucosa and lips are diagnostic features of PJS
- In PJS, polyps can occur in extraintestinal sites like kidneys, ureters, gallbladder and nasal passages
- Prophylactic proctocolectomy with ileo-anal pouch anastomosis is preferred to total colectomy and ileorectal anastomosis by some, keeping the rectal cancer in mind.

COLONIC MALIGNANCY

Introduction

- Rare before the age of 50 (except in familial adenomatous polyposis)
- The incidence of colonic malignancy varies anatomically (**Fig. 14.20**).

Risk Factors

- Advanced age
- Diet
- First degree relatives of colonic cancer patients have a very high preponderance
- Adenomas
- Three or more polyps at initial colonoscopy

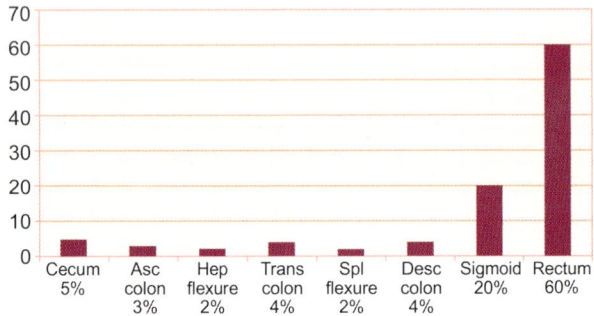

Fig. 14.20: Incidence of colonic malignancy

- Familial adenomatous polyposis (FAP)
- Hereditary non-polyposis colon cancer (HNPCC) accounts for about 20% cases
- Peutz-Jeghers syndrome
- Turcot's syndrome
- Inflammatory bowel disease.

Etiology and Pathogenesis

Carcinomas develop from an adenoma and this transition takes a period of about 5–10 years.

There are two steps in the carcinogenesis of colon:

1. *Tumor initiation:* This involves the formation of an adenoma, which is thought to arise from an initial loss of APC gene function. Acquired somatic mutations of both alleles give rise to sporadic adenomas and these polyps occur later in life. This deactivation allows further mutations to occur in the oncogenes, targeting K-ras, DD and p53. Whereas, in familial adenomatous polyposis (FAP) one allele is inherited in a mutant form, the other

is acquired but in a lesser time, hence its occurrence in a younger age.
2. *Tumor promotion:* This involves progression of adenomas to carcinoma. This involves mutations or deletions in tumor suppressor genes located on chromosome 17 (p53) and 18. This stage goes uncontrolled in HNPCC, and progression is very rapid.

Macroscopically the tumors are:
- Polypoid (exophytic and protrude into the lumen)
- Ulcerative
- Annular
- A combination of the above.

Malignant Polyps

- A malignant polyp is defined as a polyp with cancer cells invading the muscularis mucosa
- They account for about 10% in polypectomy series
- Based on the level of invasion, they are classified

Haggitt's and Kudo's Classifications—(**See Pages 529–30 and Refer Figs 14.17 and 14.18**).

Duke's Classification

Microscopically, they are adenocarcinomas of varying differentiations and is staged conventionally by **Duke's classification (Fig 14.21A)**
- *Stage A:* Neoplastic cells confined to the mucosa
- *Stage B:* Tumor extension into all layers of colon without lymph node involvement
- *Stage C:* Tumor extension into all layers of colon with lymph node involvement
  - *C1:* Local lymph nodes only
  - *C2:* Proximal lymph nodes.

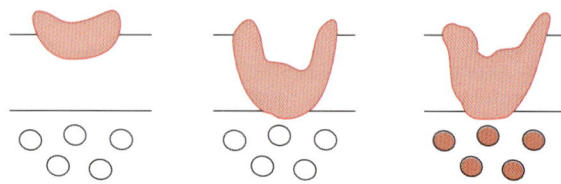

Fig. 14.21A: Duke's classification

Spread of Colonic Malignancy

- Colonic carcinomas spread by:
    - *Direct extension* to the wall extending into the serosa and neighboring structures (sacral plexus posteriorly, ureters laterally and bladder in the males and uterus in the females anteriorly)
    - *Lymphatic spread* first to mesocolic nodes and then to para-aortic nodes
    - *Hematogenous spread* reaches first to liver and uncommonly to the lungs and bones
    - *Transcelomic spread* occurs by implantation into the peritoneal cavity to produce ascites and also on the ovaries
    - *Direct implantation* occurs when the exfoliated cells implant on a breached mucosa.

Synchronous Lesions

- Synchronous polyps and cancers are possible in colon
- Synchronous cancers should raise the suspicion of HNPCC.

TNM Classification

It is given in **Table 14.5**.

Table 14.5: TNM classification of colonic malignancy

	Tumor status
T_X	Primary tumor cannot be assessed
T_0	No evidence of primary tumor
T_{is}	Carcinoma in situ: intraepithelial or invading lamina propria
T_1	Tumor invading submucosa
T_2	Tumor invading muscularis propria
T_3	Tumor invades through the muscularis propria into pericolorectal tissues
T_{4a}	Tumor penetrates to the surface of the visceral peritoneum
T_{4b}	Tumor directly invades or is adherent to other organs or structures

	Lymph node status
N_X	Regional lymph nodes cannot be assessed
N_0	No regional node metastasis
N_1	Metastasis in 1 to 3 regional nodes
N_{1a}	Metastasis in one regional lymph node
N_{1b}	Metastasis in 2–3 regional lymph nodes
N_{1c}	Tumor deposit(s) in the subserosa, mesentery, or nonperitonealized pericolic or perirectal tissues without regional nodal metastasis
N_2	Metastasis in 4 or more regional lymph nodes
N_{2a}	Metastasis in 4–6 regional lymph nodes
N_{2b}	Metastasis in 7 or more regional lymph nodes

	Metastatic status
M_0	No distant metastasis
M_1	Distant metastasis
M_{1a}	Metastasis confined to one organ or site (for example, liver, lung, ovary, nonregional node)
M_{1b}	Metastases in more than one organ/site or the peritoneum

Contd...

Contd...

Stage grouping					
Stage	T	N	M	Duke's	MAC
0	T_{is}	N_0	M_0		
I	T_1/T_2	N_0	M_0	A	A / B1
II A	T_3	N_0	M_0	B	B2
II B	T_{4a}	N_0	M_0	B	B2
II C	T_{4b}	N_0	M_0	B	B_3
III A	T_1	N_{2a}	M_0	C	C1
III B	T_3-T_{4a}	N_1/N_{1c}	M_0	C	C1
	T_2, T_3	N_{2a}	M_0	C	C1/C2
	T_1-T_2	N_{2b}	M_0	C	C1
III C	T_{4a}	N_{2a}	M_0	C	C2
	T_3, T_{4a}	N_{2b}	M_0	C	C2
	T_{4b}	$N1, N_2$	M_0	C	C3
IV A	Any T	Any N	M_{1a}		
IV B	Any T	Any N	M_{1b}		

Diagnosis

Symptoms and Signs

Malignancies of the colon on the right and left side have different clinical presentations. This is due to two factors:

1. Right colon is capacious and its fecal matter is liquid or semisolid in consistency, whereas, the left colon is narrow in caliber and fecal matter is more solid.
2. Clinical features of colonic malignancy are shown in **Table 14.6**.
   - The common clinical presentation is bleeding per rectum. The character of blood and its mixing with the stools depends on

Table 14.6: Clinical features of colonic malignancies

Feature	Malignancy	
	Right colon	**Left colon**
Type of lesion	Cauliflower like exophytic growth	Annular or sclerosing type
Obstructive symptoms	Late feature	Early feature
Associated symptoms	Anemia, malaise, abdominal pain	
	Altered bowel habits usually absent	Constipation, diarrhea or alternating constipation and diarrhea
Clinical presentation	Lump in the right iliac fossa or right flank	Lump in the left lower abdomen with distended colon with fecal matter
	Hepatomegaly, if liver is involved	
	Ascites due to peritoneal metastases	

the level of the lesion, which determines the consistency of the fecal mass.
- Constipation is the symptom of tumors of the left colon, due to relatively smaller diameter of colon.
- Stenosed lesions and perforations with pericolic abscess present as acute abdomen.
- Malignant polypoid growths (**Fig. 14.21B**) can cause colocolic intussusception, and present with colonic obstruction (**Fig. 14.21C**).

Investigations

Blood Tests
- *Low hematocrit* is usually present
- *Fecal occult blood* may be positive

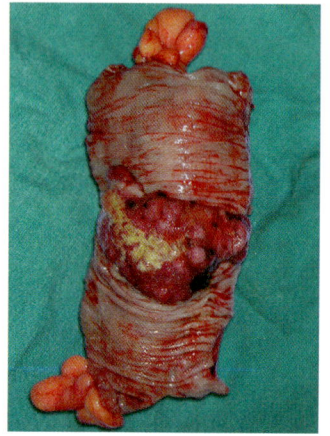 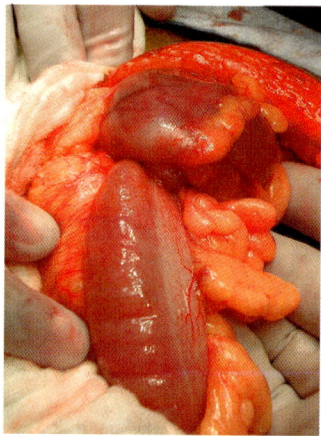

Fig. 14.21B: Malignancy of colon   **Fig. 14.21C:** Colocolic intussusception

- *Serum CEA level* is usually elevated and is a useful tumor marker for follow-up.

Radiology

- *Barium enema* is diagnostic "*Apple core sign*" (**Figs 14.22A and B**)
- *CT abdomen* is useful in assessing local invasion (**Figs 14.22C and D**), lymph nodal and hepatic metastases
- *PET scans* when metastatic disease is suspected.

Endoscopy

- *Colonoscopy* (**Fig. 14.22E**) has the added advantage of getting tissue for histopathology.

Tissue Diagnosis

- *Histopathology* is conclusive.

Large Intestine 545

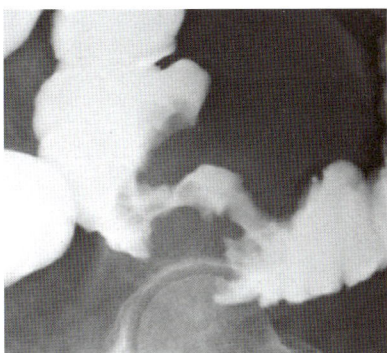

Fig. 14.22A: Barium enema—Malignant growth colon—Apple core appearance

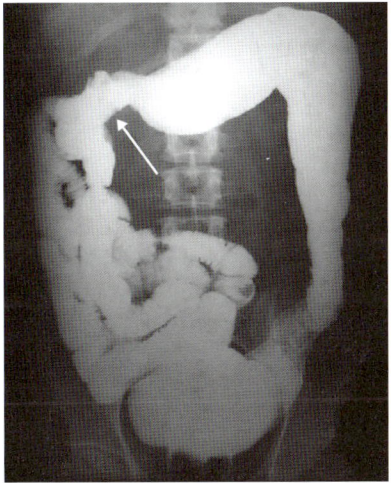

Fig. 14.22B: Barium enema—Malignant growth with ulcerative colitis

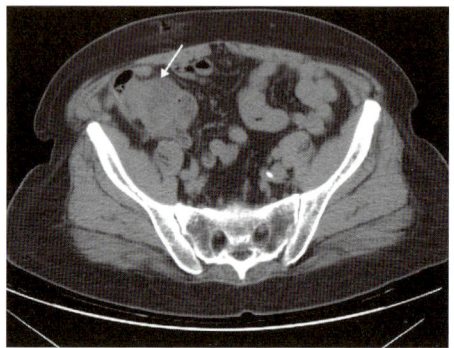

Fig. 14.22C: CT—Carcinoma cecum

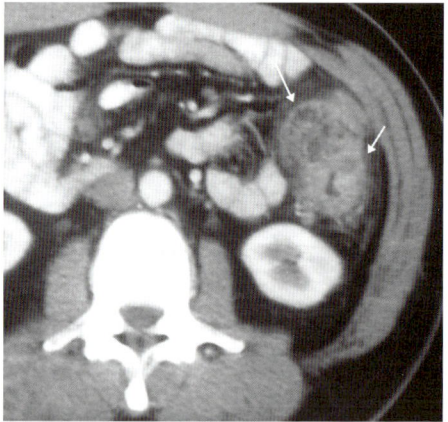

Fig. 14.22D: CT—Malignancy of descending colon

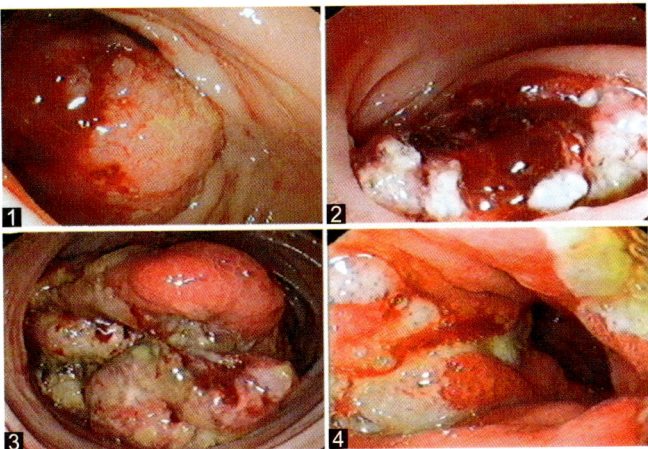

Fig. 14.22E: Colonoscopy—Malignancy colon

Germ Line Mutation Tests for Hereditary Colonic Cancers

- Genome sequencing (95% sensitive)
- Protein truncation (80% sensitive)
- Strand gel electrophoresis and protein truncation tests (80% sensitive)
- Linkage analysis (99% sensitive).

Management

Curative

- *Radical excision of tumor-bearing colon (Radical colectomies) (Fig. 14.23)*
- *Postoperative chemotherapy and radiotherapy* are administered in majority of cases.

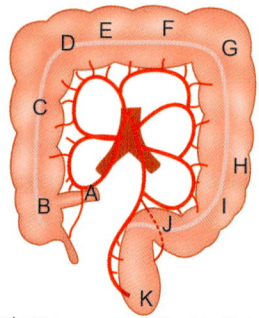

A⇒C = Ileocecectomy
A⇒E = Right hemicolectomy
A⇒F = Extended right hemicolectomy
D⇒G = Transverse colectomy
F⇒H = Left hemicolectomy
E⇒H = Extended left hemicolectomy
H⇒J = Sigmoid colectomy
A⇒J = Total colectomy
A⇒K = Total proctocolectomy

Fig. 14.23: Varieties of colon resections

Palliative

- ***Defunctioning colostomy*** for non-resectable, advanced and obstructed malignancies
- ***Surgical excision (wedge resection to hepatectomy)*** of metastases limited to a lobe of liver
- ***Chemotherapy*** for multiple diffuse metastases.

Screening for Colonic Cancers

All patients with average age of risk and those with adenomatous polyps at age of 50 years should be screened. The methods available are:

- Fecal occult blood test
- Flexible colonoscopy.

The schedule for colonoscopy in patients with the history of adenomatous polyps is:

- One or two tubular adenomas—next colonoscopy at 5 years
- Large sessile adenoma (>2 cm)—next colonoscopy at 3–6 months
- Large adenomas (>1 cm) with dysplastic changes—next colonoscopy at 3 years.

Clinical Pearls

- If the preoperative colonoscopy clears all colonic polyps, it is enough to screen the patients every 3–5 years. When preoperative colonoscopy is not total, it is necessary to perform the colonoscopy between 1–3 years
- It is suggested that it takes about 3 years for an adenoma of <5 mm to grow to a size of 1 cm, and another 5 years for the 1 cm adenoma to turn into cancer
- Signet cell tumors have a worse prognosis when compared to non-signet cell tumors
- Tumors with lymph nodal, venous and perineural invasions have a poor prognosis
- When a constricting lesion is encountered, the examination of proximal colon is difficult to find a synchronous lesion, and alternate methods like contrast study, virtual colonoscopy or intraoperative colonoscopy should be used
- PET scans are used only when metastatic disease is suspected, and not for primary staging of colonic malignancy.

HEREDITARY NON-POLYPOSIS COLORECTAL CANCER (HNPCC)

Introduction

An autosomal dominant condition, malignancy occurs in discrete adenomas but polyposis does not occur. Majority are caused by germline mutations in genes involved in repair of DNA damaged during replication. These genes are called mismatch repair genes and include hMSH2 on chromosome 2 and hMLH1 on chromosome 3.

Criteria for HNPCC

At least three relatives with HNPCC associated cancer plus all of the following:
1. One affected patient is a first-degree relative of the other two.
2. Two or more successive generations affected.
3. One or more cases of colon cancer diagnosed before age 50
4. FAP excluded.
5. Tumors verified by pathological examination.

Diagnosis

Diagnosis is made on clinical grounds.

Investigation

- Genetic testing.

Management

Radical excision.

Clinical Pearls

- Patients with known or suspected HNPCC should have surveillance colonoscopy every 2 years, from the age of 20, and annually after 35
- In women patients with HNPCC, periodic vacuum curettage should be done from the age of 25, supported by ultrasound of the pelvis and CA-125 levels
- In women patients with HNPCC, abdominal total colectomy with ileorectal anastomosis should be combined with hysterectomy and bilateral oophorectomy
- Annual colonoscopy with removal of benign polyps decrease the incidence of cancer
- Villous nature of the polyps has an influence on the development of cancer.

SURGERIES OF COLON

Varieties of Operations on Large Bowel

- Resection and establishment of continuity (hand sewn or stapled anastomosis)
- Bypass procedures (hand sewn or stapled anastomosis) without resections
- Diversion procedures (colostomies).

Types of Large Bowel Resections (Refer Fig. 14.23)

- Right hemicolectomy
- Extended right hemicolectomy
- Transverse colectomy
- Left hemicolectomy
- Extended left hemicolectomy
- Sigmoid colectomy
- Total colectomy with ileorectal/ileal pouch anal anastomosis

Varieties of Reconstructions of Large Bowel (Refer Fig. 12.20B)

- End-to-end anastomosis
- End-to-side anastomosis
- Side-to-side anastomosis

Note:
- Hand-sewn anastomosis can be made in single layer or double layers (similar to small bowel anastomosis)
- Anastomosis between the terminal ileum and transverse colon (ileotransverse colostomy) or rectum and anus (ileorectal anastomosis/ileal anal pouch anal anastomosis) can be made similarly
- Intestinal staplers can be used for any type of anastomosis.

Indications

- Obstructive lesions (strictures, tumors, intussusception)
- Strangulations with non-viable bowel
- Inflammatory bowel disease (ulcerative colitis)
- Extensive diverticulitis

All Colonic Resections Need Optimization
Optimization for Colonic Surgeries

- Mechanical bowel preparation
- Prophylactic antibiotics
- Thromboembolism prophylaxis

Incisions

- Midline (most popular)
- Left lower paramedian for left colon
- Right lower paramedian for right colon.

Note: Midline incision has the advantage of:
- Ease
- Speed
- Versatility
- Allows access to all quadrants
- Easily extendable when needed.

Colonic Resections

Essential Steps *(Fig. 14.24)*
- Isolation of resectable part of colon
- Vascular control of the resectable part of colon

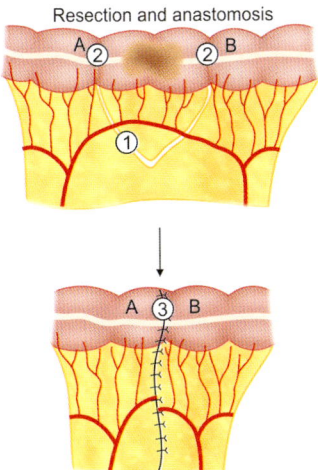

Fig. 14.24: Resection of colon. (1) Division of vessels in mesocolon; (2) Lines of resection of bowel; (3) End to end anastomosis

- Resection of colon with clear healthy margins
- Establishing the continuity by anastomosis.

Hand-sewn Technique (Fig. 14.25)

- Adequate mobilization (**Fig. 14.25A**)
- Vascular control (division of vessels between ligatures) (**Fig. 14.25B**)
- Marking the lines of resection
- Division of bowel
- Anastomosis of the bowel ends (single or double layer)
- *Single layer anastomosis*
    - Alignment of bowel ends (**Fig. 14.25C**)
    - Application of full thickness sutures (outside in and inside out)
    - Knotting on the outside
- *Double layer anastomosis (Refer Figs 12.23A to D)*
    - Posterior inner row (running full thickness) with absorbable material (**Fig. 14.25D**)
    - Anterior inner row in continuity from the posterior inner row (**Fig. 14.25E**)
    - Posterior outer row first (seromuscular) with non-absorbable material (**Fig. 14.25F**)
    - Anterior outer row last (seromuscular) with non-absorbable material (**Fig. 14.25G**)
    - The anastomosis is complete (**Fig. 14.25H**)

Clinical Pearls

- Inverting anastomosis causes serosa to serosa apposition
- Inversion of mucosa reestablishes integrity of lumen preventing leakage

Large Intestine

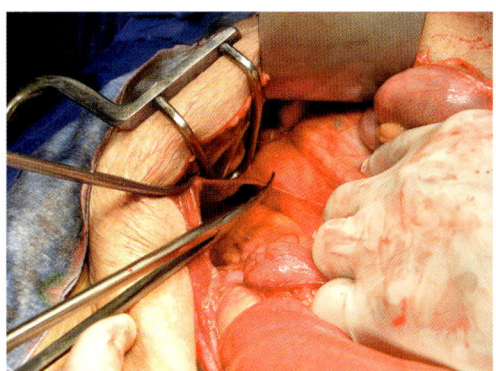

Fig. 14.25A: Mobilization of ascending colon

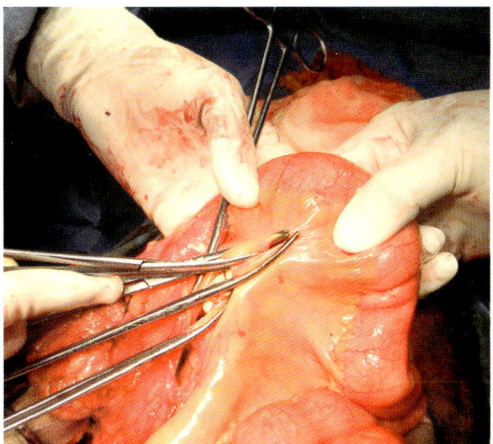

Fig. 14.25B: Division of mesocolic vessels

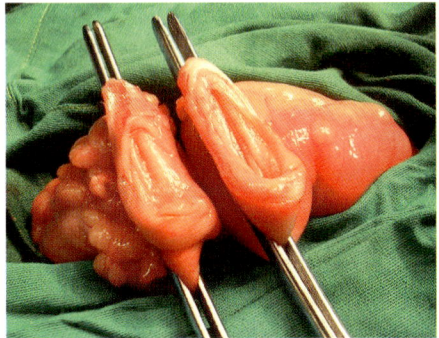

Fig. 14.25C: Alignment of cut ends of bowel

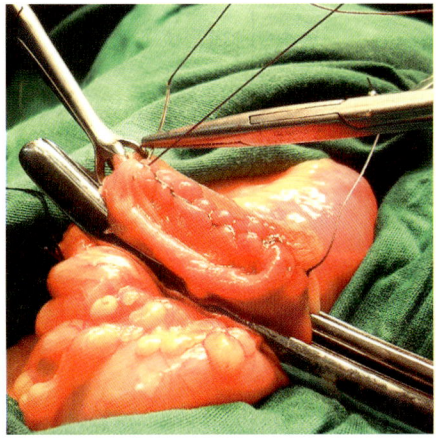

Fig. 14.25D: First layer anastomosis

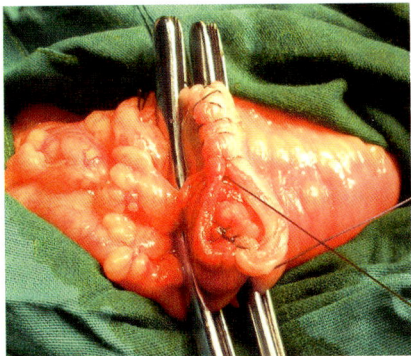

Fig. 14.25E: Second layer anastomosis

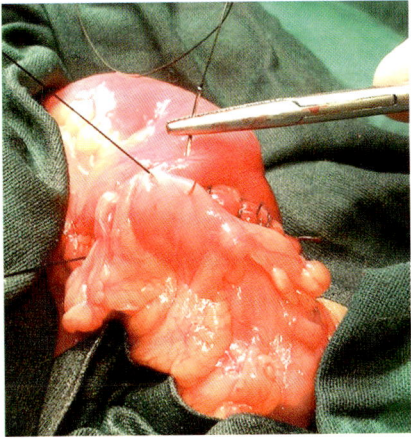

Fig. 14.25F: Third layer anastomosis

558 Snapshots in Gastroenterology

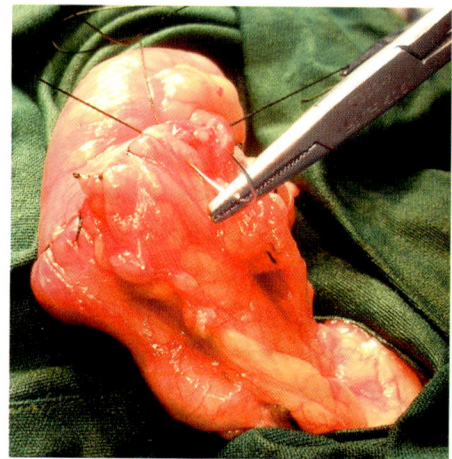

Fig. 14.25G: Fourth layer anastomosis

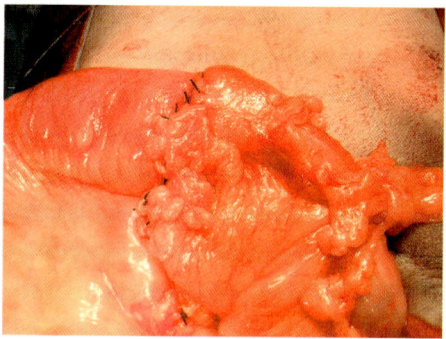

Fig. 14.25H: Completed ileotransverse colostomy

Large Intestine

- The ureter should be safeguarded while performing the colonic resections, as they lie close to the colonic mesentery

Stapled Anastomosis

- The terminal ileum and ascending colon are isolated well **(Fig. 14.26A)**
- The terminal ileum is divided using a linear cutter **(Fig. 14.26B)**
- The proximal transverse colon is divided using a linear cutter **(Fig. 14.26C)**
- Side to side ileotransverse colostomy performed using a linear cutter **(Fig 14.26D)**.

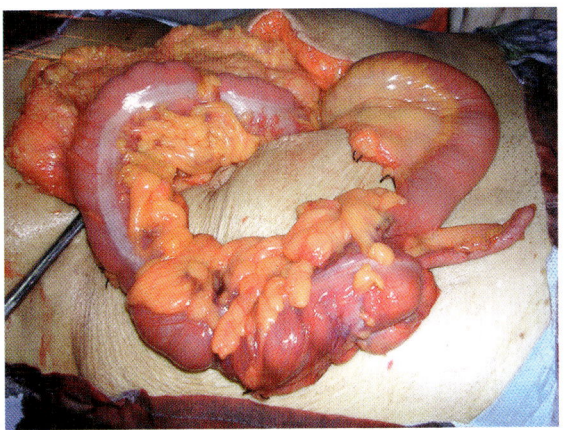

Fig. 14.26A: Isolated terminal ileum and ascending colon

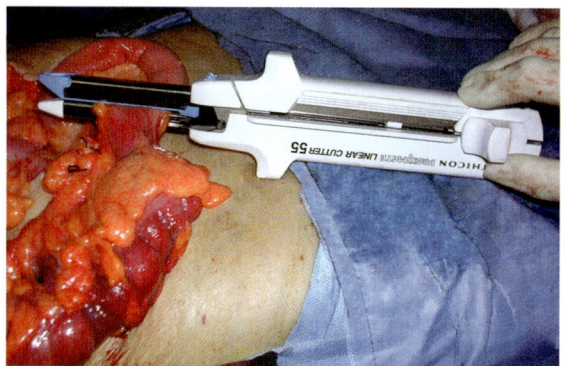

Fig. 14.26B: Division of terminal ileum with linear cutter

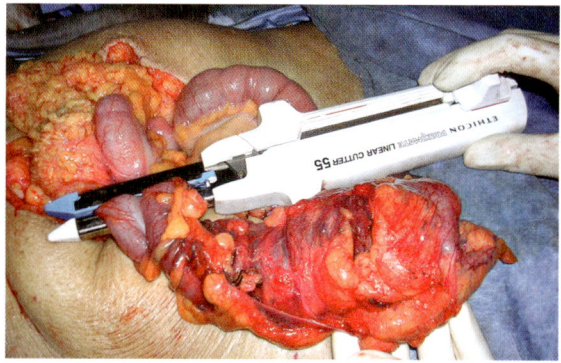

Fig. 14.26C: Division of proximal transverse colon using a linear cutter

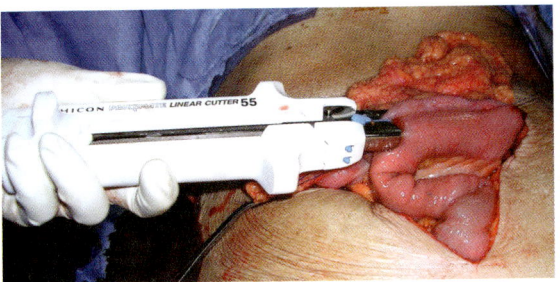

Fig. 14.26D: Iloetransverse colostomy using a linear cutter

ILEORECTAL/ILEOANAL ANASTOMOSIS

The ileum can directly be anastomosed to the rectum or anus. The disadvantages are:
- Variable frequency of defecation
- Nocturnal defecation
- Risk of cancer in the rectum
- Rectal inflammation

ILEAL POUCH–ANAL ANASTOMOSIS

Since the direct anastomosis between the ileum and rectum results in continuous anal discharge of fluid, pouch creation of terminal ileum following a near total proctocolectomy, and ileal pouch-anal anastomosis came into practice. The pouch can be in many forms **(Fig. 14.27)**:
- J pouch
- S pouch
- W pouch

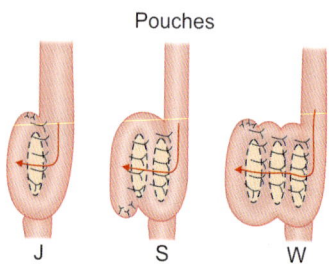

Fig. 14.27: Various pouches

The pouch causes retention of intestinal contents and improves the consistency of the contents. This with the patent anal sphincter, helps in improved continence. However, antidiarrheal drugs may be needed to reduce the number of stools and also to improve the consistency of stools.

A temporary loop ileostomy is needed as an adjunct procedure, which can be closed after 6–12 weeks.

Sphincter strengthening exercises should be taught and encouraged to improve functional results.

Complications

- Cuff abscesses
- Anastomotic leak
- Stenosis of pouch anal anastomosis
- Pouchitis
- Pelvic sepsis
- Recurrent intestinal obstruction due to adhesions
- Pouch vaginal fistula.

COMPLICATIONS OF COLONIC SURGERY
WOUND INFECTION AFTER COLONIC SURGERY

It is a common complication after colonic surgery due to the spillage of infected colonic contents. This is encountered around the 2nd to 5th postoperative day, as pus discharge from the wound. The treatment consists of antibiotics and drainage of pus if present.

Anastomotic Leakage

Leakage of intestinal contents through the anastomotic line (**Fig. 14.28**) which may occur due to:
- Inadequate bowel preparation
- Poor blood supply to both ends of bowel
- Tension on the anastomosis.

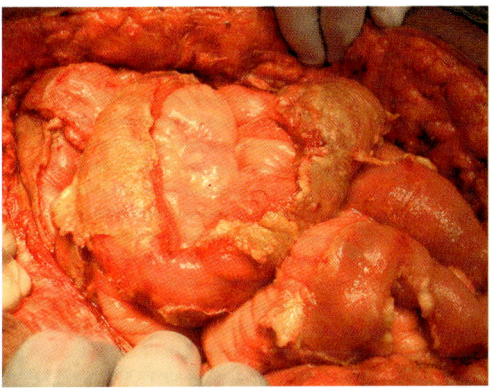

Fig. 14.28: Anastomotic leakage producing fecal peritonitis

This clinically presents around the 2nd to 5th postoperative days with:
- Abdominal pain
- Fever
- Leakage of intestinal contents through the drain.

Complications
- Shock syndrome
- Intra-abdominal abscesses
- Anastomotic stricture
- Adhesions

Management
- *Nil by mouth*
- Intravenous fluids
- Intravenous broad spectrum antibiotics
- Replacement of fluids, calories and electrolytes
- Minor leaks heal, larger leaks which produce fecal peritonitis need laparotomy (**Fig. 14.28**) (exteriorization of bowel/peritoneal toileting)
- If fistula is formed, it may heal over a period of time, and may require surgery, after 6–12 weeks.

Anastomotic Stricture After Colonic Anastomosis

Narrowing of lumen of anastomotic area (**Fig. 14.29**) due to the healing process of a circular anastomosis, but occurs months or years after surgery. It presents as:

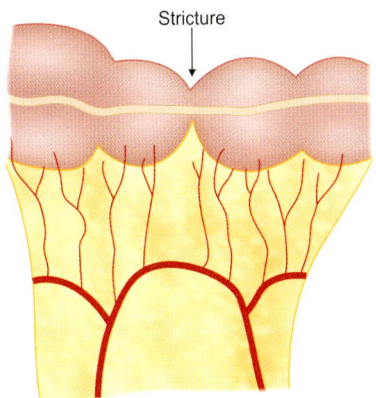

Fig. 14.29: Anastomotic stricture

- Constipation
- Abdominal pain
- Vomiting
- Abdominal distension.

Investigations

Contrast studies may be useful.

Management

Local resections or stricturoplasties are necessary.

Clinical Pearl

Strictures following stapler usage is rare, if the correct is size is chosen.

Adhesions

Adherence of bowels between themselves or with the parietes due to:
- Postoperative fibrinous adhesions result from the healing of local inflammatory processes in the operated area
- Resolved infections of peritoneum can cause adhesions.

It clinically present months–years after surgery, with
- Recurrent attacks of abdominal pain
- Vomiting
- Constipation
- Abdominal distension.

Management

Medical
- Nil by mouth
- Intravenous fluids and electrolytes.

Surgical
- If medical management fails
- Adhesiolysis by open or laparoscopic methods.

External Urinary Fistulae After Colonic Surgery

Fistulous communication between the ureter and exterior can happen due to inadvertent clamping, cutting or damage to the ureter, which occurs as a late complication, and presents with a discharge of straw-colored clear fluid. Contrast studies are useful. The management consists of:

- Ureteric fistulae due to
  - Partial injury—ureteric catheterization and spontaneous healing
  - Complete injury—resection and anastomosis (uretero-ureterostomy, ureteroneocystostomy).

External Colonic Fistulae

Leakage of colonic contents through fistulae to the exterior due to:
- Anastomotic leak lead to collection of pus which in turn drain through the drainage tube
- Intentional external drainage of collection of pus from the anastomotic leak.

Clinically if shows up months after surgery.

It presents clinically as:
- Has had a turbulent postoperative period
- Discharging wound in the postoperative period **(Fig. 14.30)**
- Fluid and electrolyte disturbances
- Skin excoriation around the fistulous opening
- Fever.

Investigations

- Oral administration of non-absorbable marker (charcoal or Congo red)
- Fistulogram
- US, CT with contrast or isotope scanning are useful.

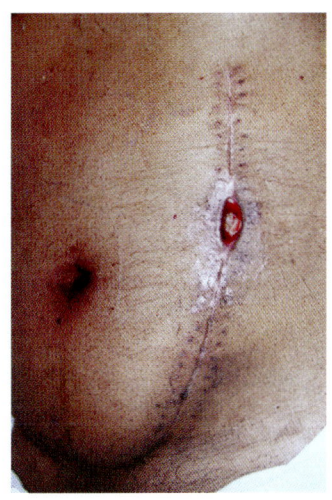

Fig. 14.30: External colonic fistula

Management

Most lateral fistulae heal spontaneously.

Surgical

Excision of fistula.
Indicated when there is:
- Evidence of obstruction
- Active disease
- Interruption of bowel continuity
- Closure not occurred by 6 weeks

Chapter 15

Rectum and Anal Canal

ANATOMY

The rectum is about 12–15 cm long and extends from the rectosigmoid junction (marked by the convergence of tenia coli) to the anal canal, marked by the passage into the pelvic floor muscles. The rectum lies anterior to the sacrum, and forms three curves, creating folds called valves of Houston. The intraperitoneal rectum gradually becomes extraperitoneal at about 12–15 cm from the anus and becomes extraperitoneal completely at about 6–8 cm from the anus. The rectum is fixed posteriorly by Waldeyer's fascia, laterally by the lateral ligaments and anteriorly by Denonvillier's fascia.

The anal canal starts at the dentate line (the junction of the glandular mucosa of the rectum and the squamous lining of the anal canal and perianal skin) and ends at the anus. The anus is a collapsed anteroposterior slit 3–4 cm long, supported by anal sphincters (internal and external anal sphincters). The internal sphincter is a continuation of circular muscles of rectum, which is involuntary. The external sphincter, a voluntary muscle extends proximally into the puborectalis and levator ani muscles.

Histology

The rectal wall is composed of:
- Mucosa
- Submucosa

- Circular and longitudinal muscles
- Serosa (proximal rectum only)

Arterial Supply

- ***Proximal rectum:*** Superior rectal artery (terminal branch of inferior mesenteric artery)
- ***Mid-rectum:*** Middle rectal artery (branch of internal iliac artery)
- ***Distal rectum:*** Inferior rectal artery (branch of internal pudendal artery).

Venous Drainage

- Venous drainage corresponds to the arteries and carry the same terminology.

Lymphatic Drainage

Lymphatic drainage parallels the vascular supply.

- ***Upper and mid-rectum:*** Inferior mesenteric nodes
- ***Lower rectum:*** Inferior mesenteric nodes and internal iliac nodes
- ***Anal canal above dentate line:*** Inferior mesenteric nodes and internal iliac nodes
- ***Anal canal below dentate line:*** Inguinal lymph nodes (also inferior mesenteric nodes and internal iliac nodes)

Nerve Supply

- Sympathetic: L1–L3 segments from the inferior mesenteric plexus
- Parasympathetic: Nervi erigentes (originate from S2–S4).

Internal anal sphincter: It is innervated by sympathetic and parasympathetic fibers, which are inhibitory and keep the sphincter in a state of contraction constantly.

External anal sphincter and puborectalis muscles: They are innervated by inferior rectal branch of internal pudendal nerve.

PHYSIOLOGY

The normal function consists of storage and release of intestinal waste. The normal volume of rectum is about 1 liter.

APPROACH TO THE PATIENT WITH ANORECTAL DISEASE

Signs and Symptoms

The common symptoms of anorectal diseases are:
- Constipation
- Incontinence
- Bleeding per rectum
- Anal pain
- Weight loss
- Anorexia
- Fullness of abdomen
- Anemia

Signs of anorectal diseases are:
- Mass per rectum
- Anal discharge
- Tenderness

Investigations

- **Endoscopy**
  - Anoscopy

- Proctoscopy
- Sigmoidoscopy/colonoscopy
- Capsule endoscopy
- **Radiology**
  - Plain X-rays
  - Contrast studies
  - Computed tomography
  - Virtual colonoscopy
  - Magnetic resonance imaging
  - Positron emission tomography
  - Angiography
  - Endorectal and endoanal ultrasound
- **Pelvic floor investigations**
  - Manometry
  - Rectal evacuation studies
- **Laboratory studies**
  - Stool studies
  - Serum tests
  - Tumor markers
  - Genetic testing

HIRSCHSPRUNG'S DISEASE

Introduction

- An important cause of congenital megacolon
- Affects 1 in 5,000 childbirths, caused by an aganglionic segment in the rectum, affects 80% male children
- A number of abnormal genes have been identified in families with Hirschsprung's disease
- Autosomal dominant or recessive inheritance with low penetration.

Etiology

Absence of ganglionic cells from myenteric and submucosal plexuses, extending proximally from internal anal sphincter. This leads to failure of colonic relaxation and proximal dilatation of proximal normal ganglionic large intestine.

Diagnosis

Symptoms and Signs

- Presents at birth or within few days
- Usually the baby is unable to pass the meconium, which can be helped out by a finger or a tube. Slowly abdominal distension develops with visible peristalsis. Enterocolitis may supervene
- Rectal examination reveals a contracted empty rectum and a normal anus. After the examination, usually the meconium and flatus are passed.

Investigations

- *Plain X-ray abdomen*—may show the aganglionic segment with proximal dilated normal colon
- *Barium enema* is diagnostic, which shows a dilated normal rectosigmoid proximal to a narrow distal aganglionic rectal segment (**Fig. 15.1**)
- *Rectal biopsy* confirms diagnosis
- *Anorectal manometry* may show resting internal anal sphincter pressure to be normal or elevated and rectal distension response to contraction of internal sphincter instead of relaxation.

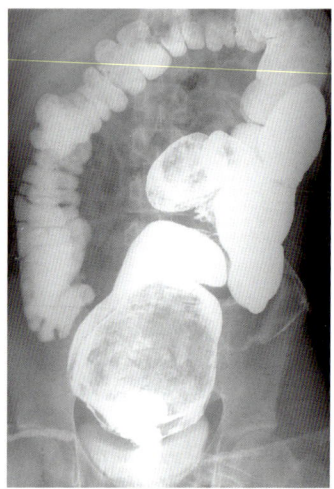

Fig. 15.1: Barium enema—Hirschsprung's disease

Management

Needs surgical correction, primary rectal pull through operation (with a defunctioning stoma at the level of ganglion cell—leveling colostomy).

Clinical Pearl

Children with total Hirschsprung's disease will require an ileostomy.

ANORECTAL MALFORMATIONS

Introduction

- Imperforate anus or anorectal malformations (ARMs) are birth defects in which the rectum is malformed, with a spectrum of different congenital anomalies, varying from fairly minor lesions, to complex anomalies
- It has an estimated incidence of 1 in 5,000 births
- It affects boys and girls with similar frequency. However, imperforate anus will present as the low version 90% of the time in females and 50% of the time in males.

Etiology and Pathogenesis

The terminal part of hindgut enters into the cloaca, an endoderm-lined cavity in direct contact with surface ectoderm. The urorectal septum arises as a transverse ridge in the angle between allantois and hindgut, and grows caudally dividing the cloaca into an anterior primitive urogenital sinus and a posterior anorectal canal. The cloacal membrane gets divided into anterior urogenital membrane and posterior anal membrane (**Fig. 15.2**).

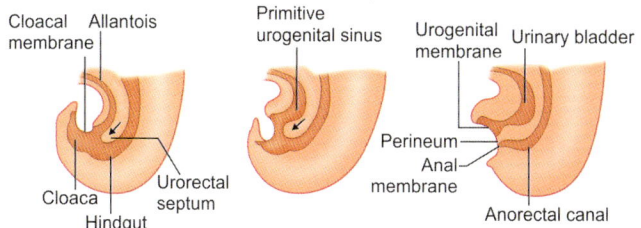

Fig. 15.2: Development of rectum and anus

- During this course, the anal membrane is surrounded by mesenchymal swelling and by about the eighth week it is located at the bottom of the ectodermal depression known as anal pit or proctodeum and by the ninth week, anal membrane ruptures to form the anal opening. Any abnormality in the above process leads to the various anorectal malformations
- The cause of ARMs is unknown; the genetic basis of these anomalies is very complex because of their anatomical variability; in an 8% of patients, genetic factors are clearly associated with ARM.
- Anorectal malformation in Currarino syndrome represents the only association for which the gene HLXB9 has been identified.

Classification

Anorectal malformations (ARMs) are generally classified using Wingspread classification **(Table 15.1)**.

Table 15.1: Wingspread classification of ARMs

Level	Male	Female
High	Anorectal agenesis	Anorectal agenesis
	• With rectoprostatic fistula	• With rectovaginal fistula
	• Without fistula	• Without fistula
	Rectal atresia	Rectal atresia
Intermediate	Rectobulbar urethral fistula	Rectovestibular fistula
	Anal agenesis without a fistula	Anal agenesis without a fistula
Low	Anocutaneous fistula	Anocutaneous fistula
	Anal stenosis	Anal stenosis
		Anovestibular fistula
		Cloacal malformations
	Rare malformations	Rare malformations

Table 15.2: International classification

Major clinical groups	Rare/regional variants
• Perineal fistula	• Pouch colon
• Rectourethral fistula	• Rectal atresia/stenosis
• Prostatic	• Rectovaginal fistula
• Bulbar	• H fistula
• Rectovesical fistula	• Others
• Vestibular fistula	
• Cloaca	
• No fistula	
• Anal stenosis	

- Imperforate anus is usually present along with other birth defects—spinal problems, heart problems, tracheoesophageal fistula, esophageal atresia, renal anomalies, and limb anomalies are among the possibilities
- The new international classification (**Table 15.2**) enables the different operative procedures to be more comparable to each other than with the Wingspread classification.

Diagnosis

Symptoms and Signs

- A very obvious defect, probing will confirm the non-patency
- Associated anomalies should be assessed.

Investigations

- ***US*** can determine the type of the anomaly
- ***Plain X-ray*** (***Wangensteen-Rice invertogram***)—X-ray of the child in inverted position 12–24 hours after birth, when swallowed air

has reached rectum and can act as a natural contrast and will show the level of obstruction by cessation of air level
- *MRI* is a better method to assess the level of the atretic rectal cul-de-sac with respect to the pubococcygeal line (the radiological landmark for the upper border or the levator ani muscle)
- *Contrast studies* will confirm the level of obstruction precisely.

Management

- Imperforate anus usually requires immediate surgery to open a passage for feces unless a fistula can be relied on until corrective surgery takes place. Depending on the severity of the imperforate, it is treated with *a posterior sagittal anorectoplasty (PSARP) with or without a colostomy*
- Complete rectal reconstruction is required where the anorectal system is linked by fistulae into the urinary tract
- Sometimes surgical treatment involves relocating the anal and rectal area into their normal positions.

Clinical Pearls

- The decision to open a colostomy is usually taken within the first 24 hours of birth
- With a high lesion, many children have problems controlling bowel function and most also become constipated. With a low lesion, children generally have good bowel control, but they may still become constipated
- For children who have a poor outcome for continence and constipation from the initial surgery, further surgery to better establish the angle between the anus and the rectum may improve continence and, for those with a large rectum, surgery to remove that dilated segment may significantly improve the bowel control for the patient. An antegrade enema mechanism can be

established by joining the appendix to the skin (Malone stoma); however, establishing more normal anatomy is the priority.

INJURIES OF RECTUM

Introduction

The injuries of the anus and rectum can be:
- Self-inflicted
- By erotic sex (anal sex)
- Following trauma (accidental sitting on sharp objects, or part of road traffic accidents)
- A part of injuries inflicted by others (consequence of a fight or shooting incident).

Diagnosis

Symptoms and Signs
- Painful bleeding per rectum, with a preceding history of trauma
- Rectal examination by finger will be diagnostic. The examining finger may feel the rent or it may get stained by frank blood
- Proctoscopy is necessary for assessment of anal and low rectal injuries.

Investigations
- ***Variety of investigations like barium enema*** are useful
- ***US*** may be needed depending upon the seriousness of the injury.

Management

Primary repair of the injuries may be needed ***with or without defunctioning colostomies***, as per the situation.

HEMORRHOIDS

Introduction

- Hemorrhoids (Piles) are the varicosities of the hemorrhoidal plexus of veins, as cushions of specialized vascular tissue in the submucosal space of the anal canal. When there is no obvious cause found, it is called *'primary hemorrhoids'*
- Hemorrhoids may occur in the late middle age or elderly, secondary to rectal growths infiltrating or compressing the hemorrhoidal veins, called *'secondary hemorrhoids'*.

Etiology

Hemorrhoids are caused by:
- Chronic constipation
- Prolonged straining
- Irregular bowel habits
- Purgation
- Pregnancy
- Heredity
- Erect posture
- Malignancies

Pathogenesis

- Hemorrhoidal cushions are thickened mucosa containing elastic tissue, connective tissue, smooth muscle and arteriovenous channels
- The subepithelial vessels and sinusoids (veins lack muscular lining) constitute the hemorrhoidal plexuses. The plexus above the dentate line, the internal hemorrhoidal plexus, drains through

the middle rectal veins, whereas the external hemorrhoidal plexus, which is below the dentate line drains into the inferior rectal veins and also into the middle rectal veins. Ultimately, the rectal veins drain into the internal iliac veins
- External piles are covered by skin and the internal piles are covered by mucosa
- The arteriovenous channels control the size of the anal cushions and take care of continence to liquids and gases, by computing to the actions of internal sphincters and prevent a complete closure of the anus, which aids in fecal incontinence, especially when the patient strains like coughing, sneezing, etc.
- Such vascular cushions are located at three places of the anal canal, one in the left lateral, right anterior and right posterior positions (**Fig. 15.3A**). These positions are fairly constant, at any age. These topographic positions are described conventionally

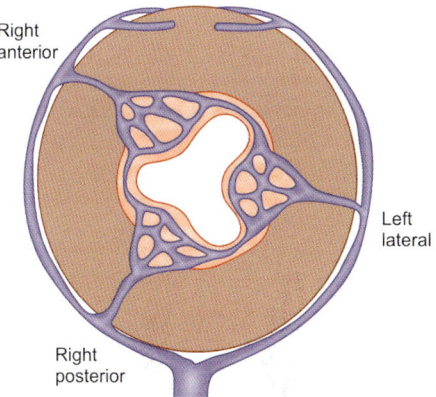

Fig. 15.3A: Position of hemorrhoids

by numbers on the face of a clock, in a supinely lying patient (3, 7 and 11 o'clock position).

Theories of Development of Hemorrhoids
- The cushions are thought to slide downward to cause hemorrhoids (sliding anal cushion theory)
- The supporting tissues in the anal canal are thought to undergo repeated stretching, and lose the support and allow the vascular cushions to prolapse. Constipation and straining to pass stools may make the displacement worse.

Classification

Hemorrhoids are divided into three types.
1. **External hemorrhoids:** Hemorrhoids located in distal one-third of the anal canal distal to the dentate line, and are covered by anoderm or skin (squamous epithelium without skin appendages) **(Fig. 15.3B)**. The overlying skin is somatically innervated and is sensitive to touch, pain, stretch and temperature.
2. **Internal hemorrhoids:** Hemorrhoids located in the anal canal proximal to the dentate line, and are covered by anal mucosa (columnar or transitional epithelium) **(Fig. 15.3B)**. They are viscerally innervated and is not sensitive to touch, pain or temperature.
3. **Interoexternal hemorrhoids (Mixed hemorrhoids):** Combination of internal and external hemorrhoids **(Fig. 15.3B)**.

    Internal hemorrhoids are further classified into four degrees, by their appearances **(Fig. 15.3C)**. Their clinical presentations and pathogenesis are shown in **Table 15.3**.

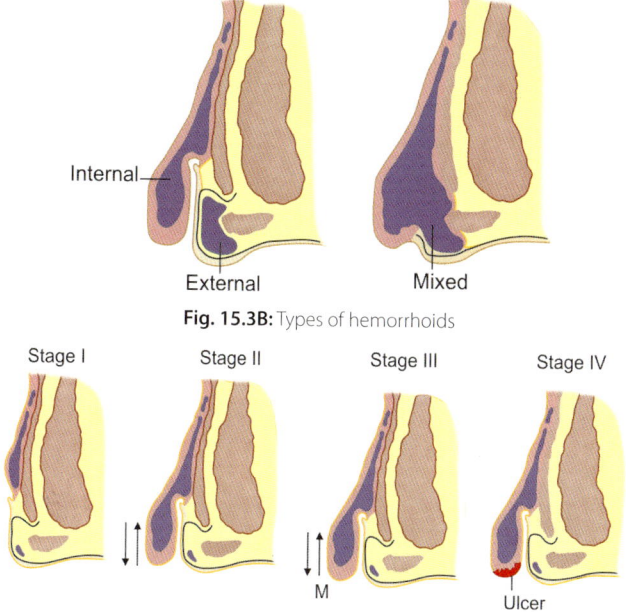

Fig. 15.3B: Types of hemorrhoids

Fig. 15.3C: Degrees of internal hemorrhoids

Diagnosis

Symptoms and Signs

- *Painless bleeding is the presenting symptom of hemorrhoids* (bleeding is from the presinusoidal arterioles which communicate with the venous sinusoids, and hence it is bright red in color)

Table 15.3: Classification of internal hemorrhoids

Degree	Clinical appearance	Pathogenesis
First	Diffuse bulge into the lumen, often bleed, without a prolapse	Circulatory disturbances within the anal cushions leading to engorgement and swelling of the hemorrhoidal tissues
Second	Masses prolapse on straining and reduce spontaneously when straining ceases (**Fig. 15.4A**)	Partial rupture of suspensory ligaments of Parks allows the slide of hemorrhoidal tissues downwards during straining, the residual contractile power of intact fibers cause spontaneous reduction
Third	Masses prolapse on straining and need manual reduction (**Fig. 15.4B**)	Complete rupture of suspensory ligaments of Parks, which allows the slide and also does not allow spontaneous reduction due to complete loss of contractile power
Fourth	Masses stay prolapsed at all times and not reducible (**Fig. 15.4C**)	Chronic prolapse of hemorrhoidal tissues leads to a permanent prolapse and no reduction possible

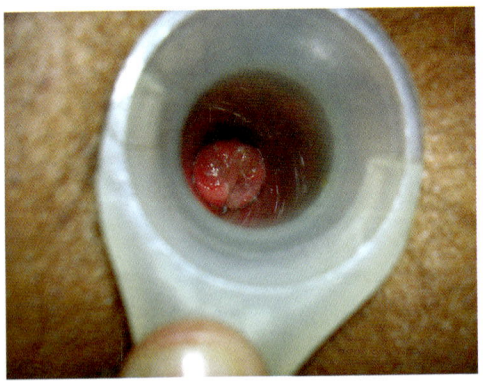

Fig. 15.4A: Second degree hemorrhoids

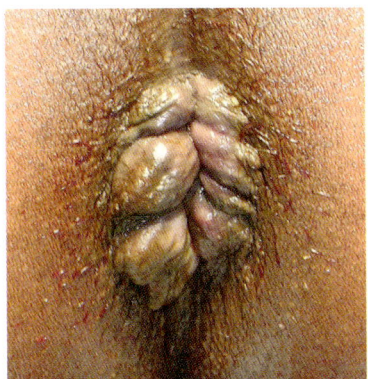

Fig. 15.4B: Third degree hemorrhoids

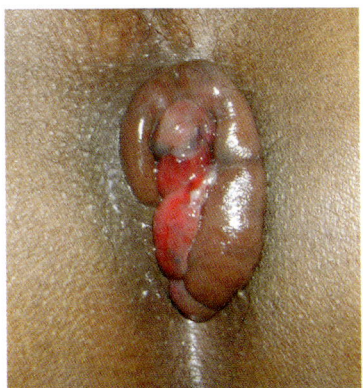

Fig. 15.4C: Prolapsed hemorrhoids

- Mucous leakage, fecal leakage and pruritus can occur in the 2nd, 3rd and 4th degree hemorrhoids
- Constipation is a common accompaniment
- Pain is felt when the pile masses are thrombosed and strangulated.

Signs

- Inspection may reveal
  - Fourth degree hemorrhoids with or without complications
  - Complicated hemorrhoids may show signs of bleeding
  - Skin tags may be seen, which are end result of resolved thrombosed hemorrhoids
- ***Digital examination*** to rule out associated sphincter spasms and tumors
- ***Anoscopy/Proctoscopy*** is diagnostic.

Investigations

No special investigation is required unless other pathologies like malignancies are suspected.

Differential Diagnosis

- **Painless bleeding:** Polyps, cancer
- **Painful bleeding**
  - **Acute pain:** Acute fissure, proctitis, fistula
  - **Chronic pain:** Chronic fissure, fistula, anal crohn's disease
- **Purulent discharge**
  - **With pain:** Abscess
- **Pruritus and discharge:** Any anorectal pathology
- **Mass:** Abscess, skin tags, polyps, ano rectal cancer, anal crohn's disease, prolapsed anal papilla, rectal prolapse.

Complications

- Profuse hemorrhage
- Prolapse
- Strangulation
- Infection (**Fig. 15.5A**)
- Thrombosis (**Fig. 15.5B**)
- Ulceration (**Fig. 15.5B**)
- Gangrene
- Fibrosis.

Management

Treatments are classified into three categories:
1. *Medical treatment*
   - Dietary and lifestyle modifications

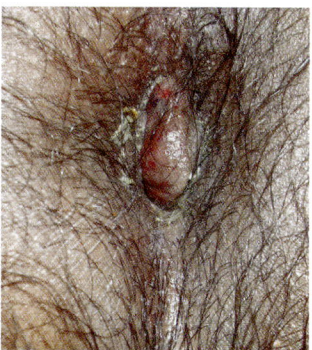

Fig. 15.5A: Inflamed hemorrhoids

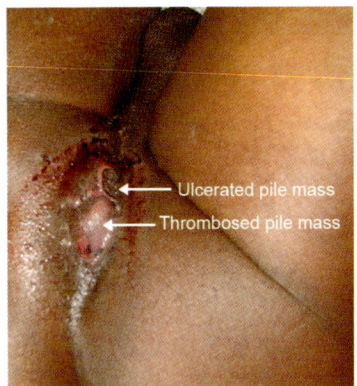

Fig. 15.5B: Thrombosed and ulcerated pile masses

- Vasotopic drugs
- Topical applications.
2. *Invasive treatment*
    - Nonoperative/office procedures.
3. *Surgical treatment*
    - Operative hemorrhoidectomy.

Medical Treatment for Hemorrhoids

Dietary and Lifestyle Modifications

- Efforts to minimize straining during passing stool
- Increased fluid and fiber (> 25–30 g/day) intake, exercise, laxatives.

Vasotopic Drugs

- ***Trihydroxyethylrutosides and Calcium dobesilate*** reduce the blood viscosity
- ***Micronized purified flavonidic fraction (MPFF Daflon 500)*** enhances the venous tone.

Topical Applications

- Topical anesthetics and steroids give symptomatic relief, though they cannot reduce the size of hemorrhoids.

Invasive Treatment

Nonoperative/Office Procedures

The nonoperative treatment which is invasive, is aimed to prevent the prolapse of tissues by fixation to the underlying muscular coat by creating submucous fibrosis or through ulceration, which prevents or minimizes prolapse of cushions through or into the anal canal during defecation. These can be done as office or outpatient procedures.

Sclerotherapy

Indications: 1st and 2nd degree hemorrhoids.

Materials Required

- Lubricant
- Proctoscope (Illuminated)
- Gabriel glass syringe/phenol denatured plastic syringe
- Needle with beveled buffer
- Luer-Lok device for the needle

- 5% phenol in almond oil or Arachis oil/Quinuride solution containing 2.4% of anhydrous quinine-urea, with pH adjusted to 2.6.

Procedure

- Position of the patient: Left lateral/knee chest
- Preparation of bowel: Oral or rectal cathartic may be used
- Technique (**Fig. 15.6A**):
    - Proctoscopy is done in conventional manner

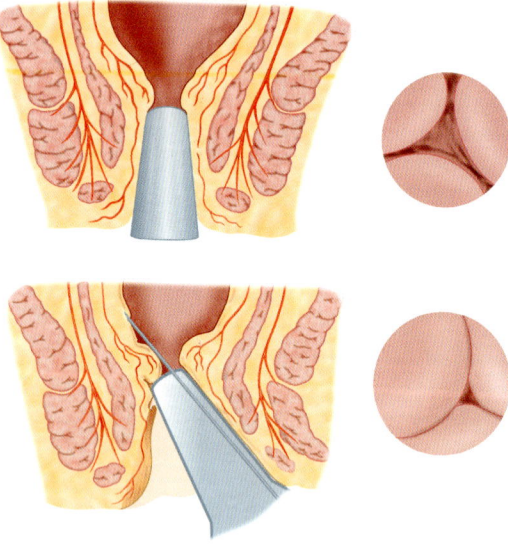

Fig. 15.6A: Sclerotherapy of hemorrhoids

- The vascular cushions are identified
- Injection of 3 mL sclerosant is made at the base of the cushion 1 cm deep (beveled buffer is useful)
- Blanching occurs indicating a successful injection
- Process repeated at all the cushion bases.

Complications

- Pain
- Submucous infiltration may cause a bleb which will necrose to form an ulcer
- Injection into prostate and seminal vesicles may occur when anterior mass is injected, which may cause immense pain, hematuria, hemospermia
- Adjoining areas of necrotic areas conglomerate to form a circular fibrotic ring causing obstruction to fecal flow.

Infrared Photocoagulation

Indications: 1st, 2nd and 3rd degree hemorrhoids.

Principle

Infrared rays cause an area of protein coagulation, which is used to arrest bleeding from hemorrhoidal mass. This coagulation is expected to obliterate and scar the area, which eventually produce fixation of the hemorrhoidal tissue. This procedure creates a 1.5s pulse of infrared irradiation to give a tissue temperature of 100°C, which produces an area of coagulated protein 3 mm in diameter and 3 mm in depth. After 14 days, the dead tissue separates leaving a granulation-lined ulcer. The rate of re-epithelialization varies with the size of the ulcer but is usually complete in 4 weeks.

Snapshots in Gastroenterology

Materials Required

Source of infrared irradiation is a 15V Wolfram halogen lamp with a gold plated reflector that focuses the rays through a quartz light shaft to the side of mucosa through a proctoscope. The tip is covered by a polymer cap, which prevents adherence of the probe to the tissues. This unit has a timing device, which allows a variable duration of radiation (**Fig. 15.6B**).

Procedure

- The probe tip is pressed directly on to the mucosa and trigger pulled
- Pulse of irradiation is automatically timed
- Precaution: The contact of the probe tip with the mucosa should be total, or else the intervening mucus or bowel contents will get burnt and adhere to the polymer tip
- The time of contact is usually 30 seconds
- Up to 6 coagulations can be made at the base in one sitting.

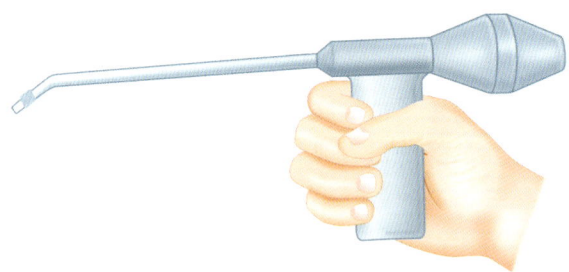

Fig. 15.6B: Infrared coagulator

Complications

- Severe pain
- Bleeding.

Rubber Band Ligation

Indications: 2nd and 3rd degree hemorrhoids.

Principle

The rubber band produces ischemic necrosis of the hemorrhoidal mass, due to constriction of the neck. Necrosis causes the mass to fall out.

Materials Required

- Lubricant
- Proctoscope (Illuminated)
- Rubber band ligator (Barron) (**Fig. 15.6C**)

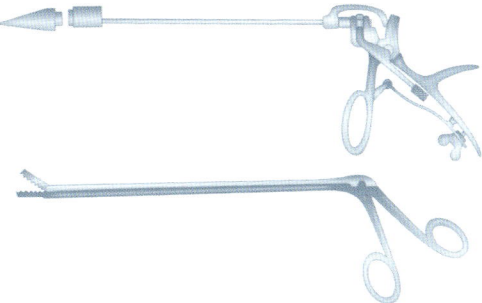

Fig. 15.6C: Barron ligator

- This comprises of a long shaft to introduce the instrument through the proctoscope. It contains within it, a rod that activates the inner of the two connecting cylinders at the inner end of the instrument. Proximally, the handle when squeezed activates or moves the outer drum to release the rubber ring loaded on the inner ring
- Rubber bands.

Procedure

- A rubber band is loaded on the inner cylinder of the Barron's hemorrhoidal ligator with the help of the conical loader provided **(Fig. 15.6D)**
- The proctoscopy is done and the pile masses are identified
- The proctoscope is stabilized at this place by an assistant
- A long grasper is introduced through the cylinders and the entire setting is introduced into the rectum
- The pile mass is held with the long grasper and pulled
- The pile mass is now inside the inner drum

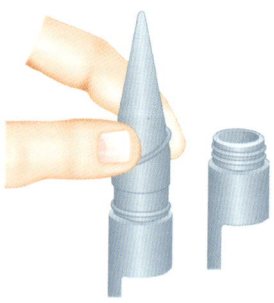

Fig. 15.6D: Loading of rubber bands

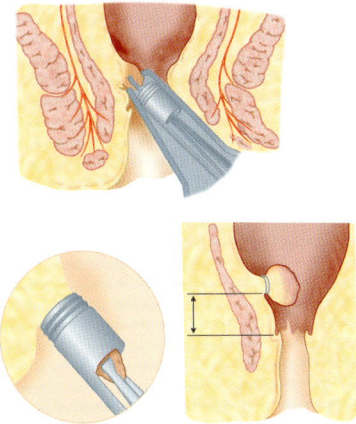

Fig. 15.6E: Barron rubber banding

- The handle is squeezed, which activates or pushes the rubber band, which on release holds and squeezes the neck of hemorrhoidal mass (**Fig. 15.6E**)
- Hemorrhoidal mass so ligated changes color showing effective ligation
- The grasper is now removed and the hemorrhoidal mass inspected for color change and the position of rubber band
- Satisfied with the procedure, the rubber band ligator is removed followed by the proctoscope.

Complications

- Immense pain (usually the procedure is painless)
- Slippage of rubber band
- Bleeding

- Infection
- Life-threatening pelvic and perineal sepsis.

Bipolar Diathermy and Direct Current Electrotherapy

- Bipolar diathermy is essentially cautery in which the heat does not penetrate as deeply as in monopolar coagulation, and this treatment is preferred for first to third degree hemorrhoids
- Direct current electrotherapy is applied through a probe placed via the proctoscope onto the mucosa at the apex of the hemorrhoidal mass.

Surgical Treatment

Only about 5–10% of patients need surgical hemorrhoidectomy.

Principle

Totally excise the prolapsing hemorrhoidal mass.

Indications

- Excessive bleeding
- Uncontrolled by rubber band
- Severe prolapse
- Pain.

Relative Contraindications

- Crohn's disease
- Portal hypertension
- Leukemia
- Lymphoma
- Bleeding disorders.

Open Hemorrhoidectomy (Milligan and Morgan)

Procedure

- Position of the patient: Lithotomy
- Anesthesia: General/regional
- Preparation of bowel: oral or rectal cathartic may be used
- Technique (**Fig. 15.7A**):
    - Proctoscopy is done in conventional manner
    - The vascular cushions are identified
    - The hemorrhoidal mass is held with artery forceps
    - The anoderm is incised with scissors and the hemorrhoid is undermined
    - Dissection is continued proximally up to above the anorectal ring

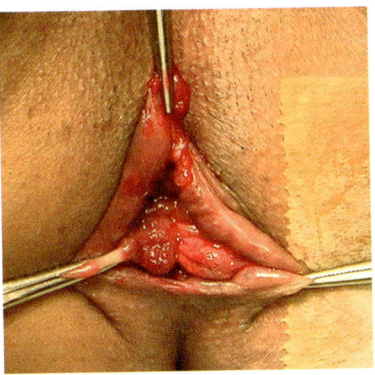

Fig. 15.7A1: Holding of hemorrhoidal mass

Snapshots in Gastroenterology

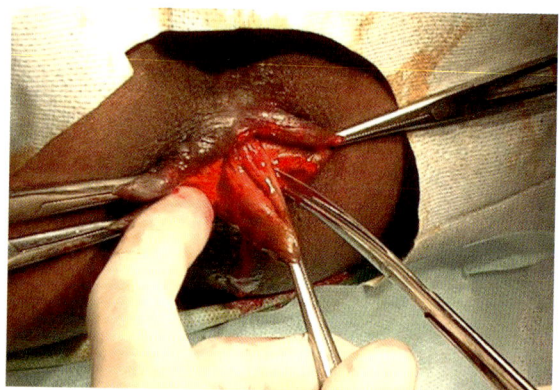

Fig. 15.7A2: Dissection of hemorrhoid

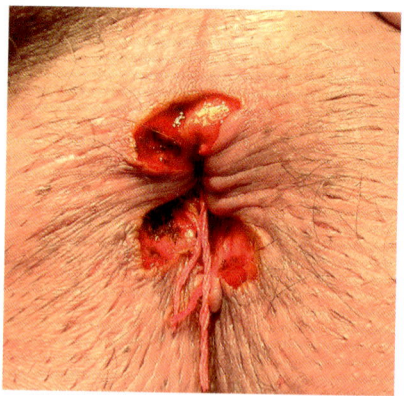

Fig. 15.7A3: Final result after open hemorrhoidectomy

Rectum and Anal Canal

- The pedicle is transfixed and ligated with thick non absorbable suture
- The cut ends of the suture are left long, which will fall off in a week's time
- The pedicle is cut below the sutures and allowed to retract after establishing it is not bleeding
- Same steps are repeated for each pile mass
- The cut mucosal edges are inspected for bleeding and if there is any coagulated
- These wounds are allowed to heal by secondary intention
- Since skin wounds by healing have the potential to cause anal stenosis, islands of normal skin are allowed to be present so that this complication is prevented.

Closed Hemorrhoidectomy (Ferguson and Heaton)

Principle

Totally excise the prolapsing hemorrhoidal mass, with added advantages like:
- Removal of entire vascular tissue with sacrificing on the anorectum
- Reduced secretions due to primary suturing
- Primary suturing prevents anal stenosis.

Procedure

Same steps as in open hemorrhoidectomy, and these wounds are approximated with sutures (**Fig. 15.7B**) to allow them to heal by primary intention.

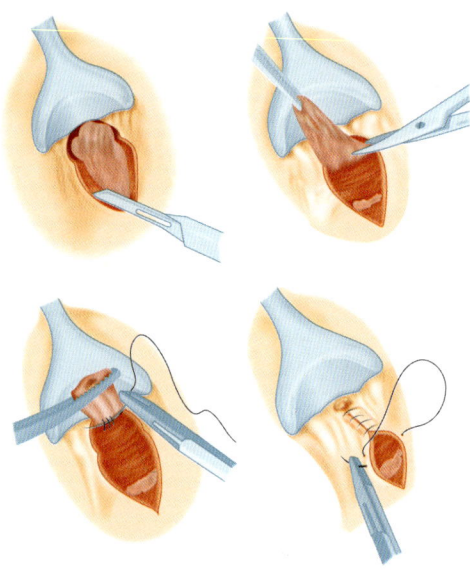

Fig. 15.7B: Closed hemorrhoidectomy

Laser Hemorrhoidectomy

The Laser (NdYAG/Oxygen) destroys the hemorrhoidal tissue to aid in the dissection of hemorrhoid as part of open/closed hemorrhoidectomy.

Stapled Hemorrhoidectomy

Principle

Reduces the mucosal and hemorrhoidal prolapse by excision of transverse band of the prolapsed anal mucosa between the distal rectal ampulla and proximal anal canal.

- It has the advantage of restoring the topographic relationship between the anal mucosa and anal sphincter improving the venous outflow. This also reduces the chances of incontinence and obstruction
- The mucosa-mucosa anastomosis reduces the postoperative pain

Materials Required (Fig. 15.8)

- 33 mm head circular stapler (HCS 33)
- Suture threader (ST 100)
- Circular anal dilator (CAD 33)
- Purse string suturing anoscope (PSA 33).

Procedure

- **Position of the patient:** Lithotomy or Jackknife
- **Anesthesia:** General/regional
- **Preparation of bowel:** Oral or rectal cathartic may be used

Technique

- Proctoscopy is done in conventional manner
- CAD33 is introduced in the anal canal, to reduce the prolapse and parts of anal mucosa (**Fig. 15.9A**)
- It is fixed to the perianal skin with silk (6 and 12 o'clock points)
- Once the obturator is removed, dentate line is visualized

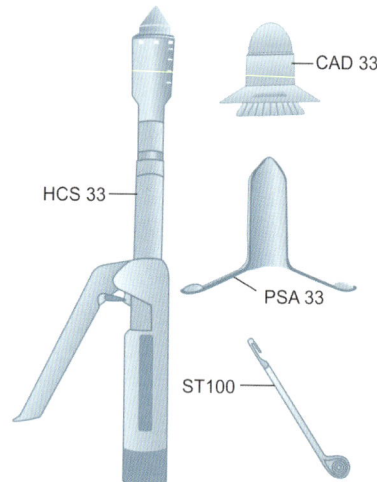

Fig. 15.8: Stapler for hemorrhoidectomy

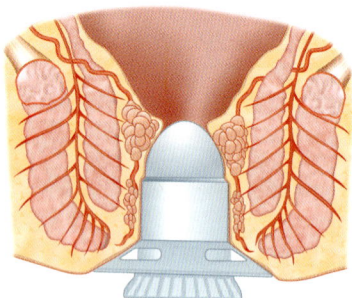

Fig. 15.9A: Introduction of CAD 33

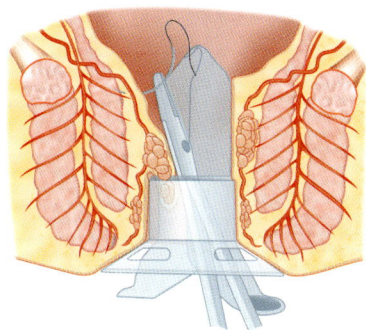

Fig. 15.9B: Application of sutures

- PSA33 is introduced through the CAD33 (**Fig. 15.9B**)
- This will move the mucosal prolapse along the rectal wall through a 270° circumference, while the mucosa which protrudes through PSA 33 can be easily contained in a suture that only includes the mucous membrane
- A bite is taken in the mucous membrane 5 cm proximal to the dentate line (**Fig. 15.9B**)
- The PSA 33 is rotated to carry out the purse string and the entire anal canal circumference
- PSA 33 is removed
- HCS 33 is opened to its maximum position
- The opened HCS 33 head is introduced proximal to purse string which is then tied (**Fig. 15.9C**)
- With the help of ST 100, the ends of the thread are pulled through lateral holes of HCS 33

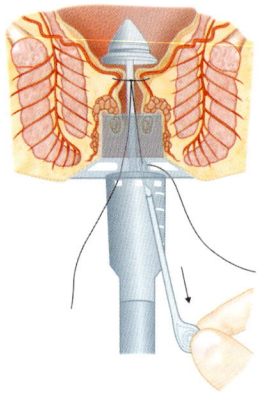

Fig. 15.9C: Introduction of HCS 33

- The ends of the thread are knotted externally and fixed using forceps
- With moderate traction on the purse string, the prolapsed mucosa is brought into the casing of HCS33 and tightened and left in position for 20 seconds allowing to settle and improve hemostasis **(Fig. 15.9D)**
- Gun is fired and held in that position for 20 seconds **(Fig. 15.9E)**
- Gun is completely opened to release the tissues and removed along with CAD 33
- Suture line is inspected using PSA33 **(Fig. 15.9F)**.

Postoperative Complications

- Pain
- Reactionary and secondary hemorrhage (1–5%)

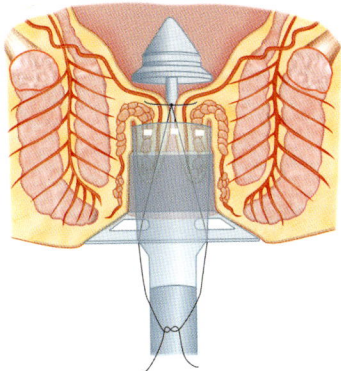
Fig. 15.9D: Tightening the sutures

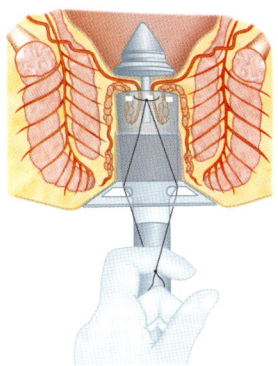
Fig. 15.9E: Firing the gun

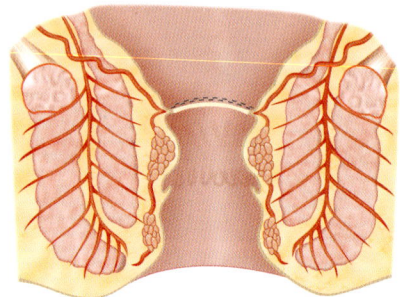

Fig. 15.9F: End result of staper hemorrhoidectomy

- Urinary retention (5–35%)
- Infection (1–5%)
- Anal fissure/unhealed wound
- Abscess/fistula
- Skin tags
- Epidermal cysts
- Pseudopolyps
- Incontinence (2–10%)
- Anal stenosis (1–5%).

Management of Postoperative Complications

- *Pain:* Injectable NSAIDs and opioids are very effective in controlling pain. Topical metronidazole is said to decrease the post-hemorrhoidal pain
- *Reactionary and secondary hemorrhage*
- *Infection*
- *Anal fissure/unhealed wound*
- *Abscess*

- *Fistula in ano*
- *Skin tags (4–6%)*
- *Epidermal cysts*
  - *Pseudopolyps*
  - *Incontinence:* May last for 6 weeks to 2 months, and majority will recover
  - *Anal stenosis*
    - Excision of eschar and sphincterotomy
    - Island flap **(Fig. 15.10A)**

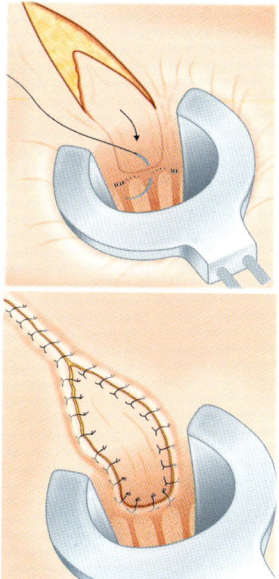

Fig. 15.10A: Island flap repair for anal stenosis

- Rotation flap (**Fig. 15.10B**)
- Advancement flap
- Y–V flap
- Anoplasty (**Fig. 15.10C**).

Clinical Pearls

- Uncomplicated hemorrhoids are not felt by the examining finger
- Thrombosed piles masses are firm to feel and visible on inspection, and present with gross edema and ulcerations
- Mucous leakage, fecal leakage and pruritus can occur in the 2nd, 3rd and 4th degree hemorrhoids

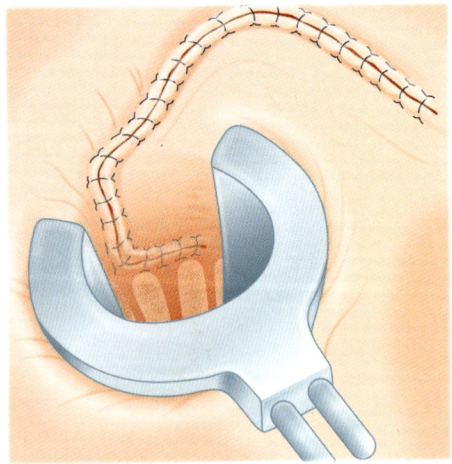

Fig. 15.10B: Rotation flap repair for anal stenosis

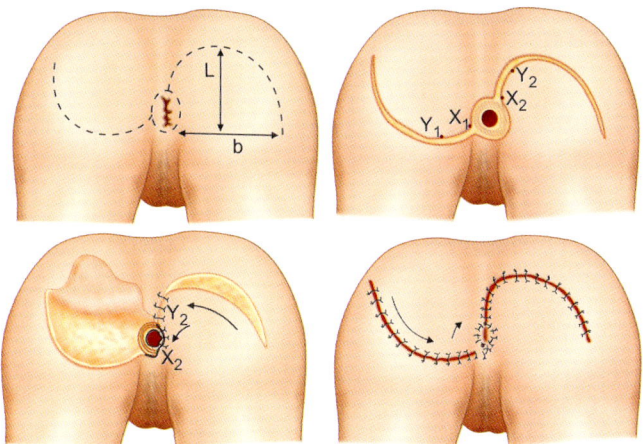

Fig. 15.10C: S-anoplasty for anal stenosis

- 3rd and 4th degree hemorrhoids are prone to complications, and profuse hemorrhage can be a complication of hemorrhoids of any degree, more commonly in patients with deranged coagulation mechanism or on anticoagulants
- Hemorrhoids are rarely a cause of anemia, and to rule out a cause, a total colonoscopy is necessary. If the colonoscopy is normal, upper GI endoscopy is necessary
- Older patients of >50 years of age especially with a positive family history of colonic malignancy should be subjected to total colonoscopy
- Small first degree hemorrhoids with recurrent bleeding may require treatment, whereas, fourth degree hemorrhoids without

symptoms do not require treatment. Immaterial of the degree, only symptomatic hemorrhoids need treatment
- In general, cases with minor symptoms like minor bleeding can be treated by simple measures like dietary modification, change in defecatory habits or nonoperative procedures
- Barron's rubber band ligator requires the help of an assistant to hold the proctoscope in position
- McGown and Pembroke piles ligators are suction ligators and require no assistant during procedure, but has the disadvantage of drawing less tissue for banding due to small inner barrel
- O'Regan disposable banding system has a disposable syringe like ligator, which simplifies the procedure
- Sclerotherapy should not be performed when anorectal infection is present or for prolapsed hemorrhoids
- Sclerotherapy should not be repeated too often, as this may result in severe scarring and stricture formation
- Sclerotherapy is reserved for first and second degree hemorrhoids
- Patients at risk should be given antibiotics during sclerotherapy
- About 90% of patients of hemorrhoids can be managed without surgery.
- Hemorrhoids with more symptoms like the third and fourth degree hemorrhoids are more likely to be treated by surgical methods
- In the jackknife position, since the right posterior pile is always difficult to access, it should be injected first, whereas in lithotomy position, the anterior pile should be injected first, for the same reason
- Stapled hemorrhoidopexy is as effective as operative treatment for hemorrhoids.

PERIANAL HEMATOMA

Introduction

- It is sometimes called as *'thrombosed piles'*, but it is not related to hemorrhoids
- The cause is not exactly known
- Occurs due to thrombosis of a subcutaneous vein below the transitional zone.

Diagnosis

Symptoms and Signs

- A discrete painful swelling (**Fig. 15.11**)
- On examination, it is tender and lies external to the anal canal.

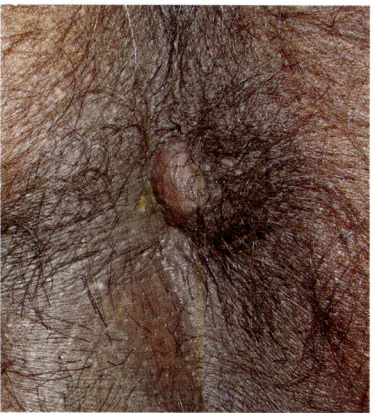

Fig. 15.11: Perianal hematoma

Management

- *No treatment,* as most of them resolve
- *Incision and curettage* gives quick relief from painful swellings
- *Since it opens up a vein, bleeding may be troublesome.*

ANAL FISSURES

Introduction

- It is a longitudinal tear in the anal skin, distal to the dentate line, following a bout of constipation and passage of a large hard stool
- They can occur at any age, but common in young and middle aged adults
- They are usually found in the 6 o'clock (posterior midline)— 90% or 12 o'clock positions (anterior midline)—10%
- The anterior fissures are more common in women
- Posterior fissures are common than the anterior due to following reasons:
  - Impact of trauma of passage of hard stool is maximum at the posterior midline
  - Presence of sustained resting rectal hypertonia in patients with anal fissures
  - Anal canal is posteriorly angulated
  - Anal orifice is elliptical in shape
  - Posterior part of the anus is not supported by the muscles
  - Local ischemia.

Classification

Anal fissures are of two types. They are:
1. *Acute fissures:* Acute tear in the anal skin due to forceful expulsion of hard fecal matter

2. **Chronic fissures:** Non-healing of acute fissure due to repeated trauma caused by hard fecal matter.

Pathologies Associated with Recurrent Anal Fissures

- Crohn's disease
- Ulcerative colitis
- Syphilis
- Tuberculosis
- Leukemia
- HIV infection.

Diagnosis

Symptoms and Signs

- *Acute fissure* is a very painful condition associated with fresh bleeding (streak of blood on the hard fecal matter), presenting with a linear tear in the anal skin (**Fig. 15.12A**)

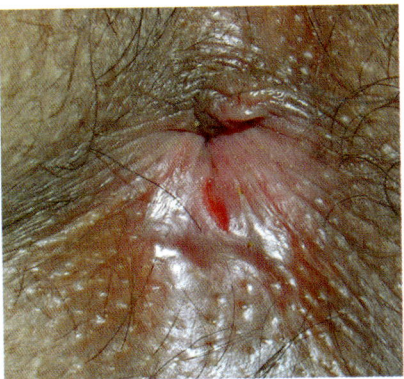

Fig. 15.12A: Acute fissure in ano—6 o'clock position

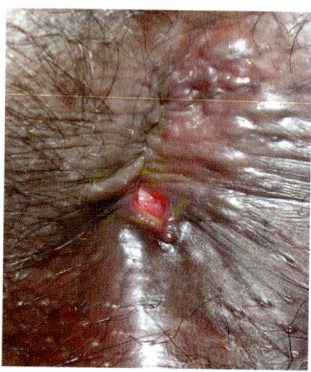

Fig. 15.12B: Chronic fissure in ano—6 o'clock position

- *Chronic fissure* has a tear with swollen skin exhibiting inflammatory changes at its lowest part called *'sentinel pile'* or a hypertrophied anal papilla in the proximal part of the fissure in the anal canal. The internal anal sphincter may be seen at the fissure base (**Fig. 15.12B**).

Management

Acute Fissure

- *Laxatives to relieve constipation will help healing*
- *Analgesics and Sitz bath* are useful.

Chronic Fissures

- *Excision or lateral internal sphincterotomy*
- *Sphincter relaxants* are expected to reduce the maximum resting anal pressure without permanently damaging the sphincter tone (chemical sphincterotomy)

- Topical nitrate formulations (glyceryl trinitrate, nitroglycerin)
- Oral and topical calcium channel blockers—nifedipine
- Adrenergic antagonists
- Topical muscarinic agonists (bethanechol)
- Botulinum toxin.

Secondary fissures require appropriate management.

Clinical Pearls

- Most fissures are easily seen by simple spreading of the buttocks
- Most patients with fissure do not allow digital or proctoscopy examinations for it is acutely painful
- Anal fissures secondary to disease processes occur at lateral positions and are usually multiple
- Most acute fissures heal with conservative measures.

Operative Procedures for Fissures

Lateral Internal Anal Sphincterotomy (Fig. 15.13A)

Position of patient: Supine lithotomy.

Procedure

- With the help of an anal speculum, a radial skin incision is made in the anal canal distal to the dentate line
- The intersphincteric groove gets exposed and also the internal anal sphincter
- The sphincter is elevated and divided
- The skin wound is closed with sutures.

Closed Internal Anal Sphincterotomy (Fig. 15.13B)

Position of patient: Supine lithotomy.

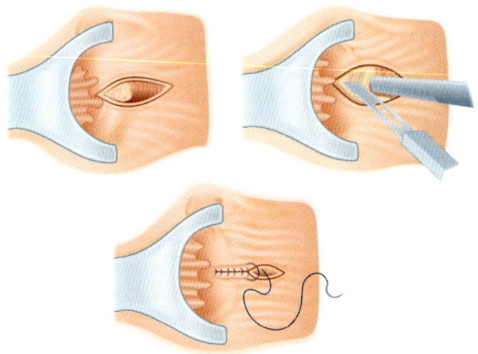

Fig. 15.13A: Open sphincterotomy

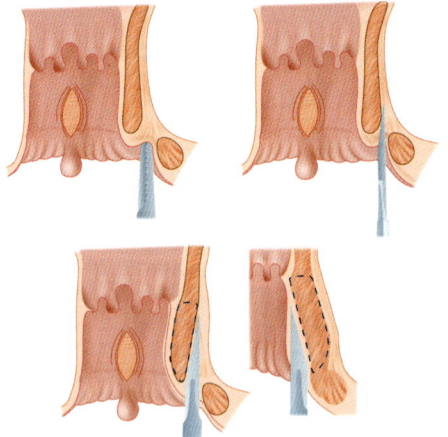

Fig. 15.13B: Closed internal sphincterotomy

Procedure

- The intersphincteric groove is located in the perianal area
- A small stab incision is made in the perianal skin
- The blade is advanced in the intersphincteric plane and a blind lateral subcutaneous internal anal sphincterotomy is done.

ANORECTAL ABSCESSES

Introduction

- Acute infections of the anal intersphincteric glands caused by aerobic and anaerobic organisms
- They are of four types (**Fig. 15.14**):
  1. Pelvirectal abscess
  2. Submucous abscess

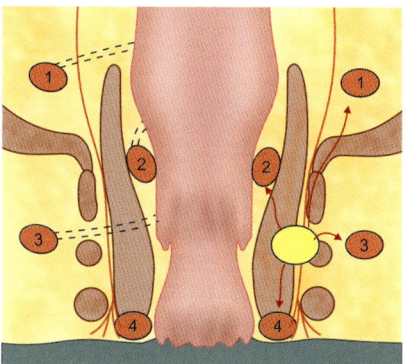

1. Pelvirectal abscess
2. Submucous abscess
3. Ischiorectal abcess
4. Perianal abscess

Fig. 15.14: Anorectal abscesses

3. Ischiorectal abscess
4. Perianal abscess.

Etiology

Nonspecific

- Cryptoglandular infection.

Specific

- Inflammatory bowel disease
- Ulcerative colitis
- Tuberculosis
- Actinomycosis
- Lymphogranuloma venereum
- Foreign body
- Episiotomy
- Hemorrhoidectomy
- Malignancy
- Lymphoma
- Radiation.

Pathogenesis

Obstruction of a duct may result in stasis, infection and formation of an abscess.

- The infection originating in the intersphincteric space may spread in four directions
    1. Upwards
    2. Downwards
    3. Horizontally and
    4. Circumferentially.

Rectum and Anal Canal

- When the anal gland epithelium persists in the tract between the crypt and blocked part of the duct and when infection spreads in the vertical direction, that is upwards and downwards, and opens at two places, forming an internal opening in the rectum and an external opening on the perianal skin, it results in a *fistula*.

Diagnosis

Symptoms

- A painful lump in the perianal region, associated with fever
- Signs of acute inflammation in the perianal region
- Supralevator or intersphincteric abscesses may cause severe rectal pain accompanied by urinary symptoms such as dysuria, retention, etc.

Signs

- Inspection may reveal an erythematous swelling
- Fluctuation is difficult to demonstrate due to pain
- Digital examination may be difficult, but if done will demonstrate a tender mass
- Supralevator abscess can be palpated by vaginal examination
- Proctoscopy is inappropriate in an acute situation.

Investigations

- ***No special investigation*** is necessary
- ***Transrectal ultrasound*** is useful
- ***Rarely CT or MRI*** may be useful
- ***Diagnostic aspiration*** is an useful investigation.

Management

- *Incision and drainage* of painful abscess under general anesthesia, under cover of antibiotics
- *Large ischiorectal or horseshoe abscesses* require counter incisions over each ischiorectal fossa to allow drainage of anterior extensions of the abscess *(Hanley procedure)* (**Fig. 15.15A**)
- *Pelvirectal abscesses* need special attention (**Fig. 15.15B**)
- *Appropriate antibiotics* are necessary based on culture examination of pus, after drainage.

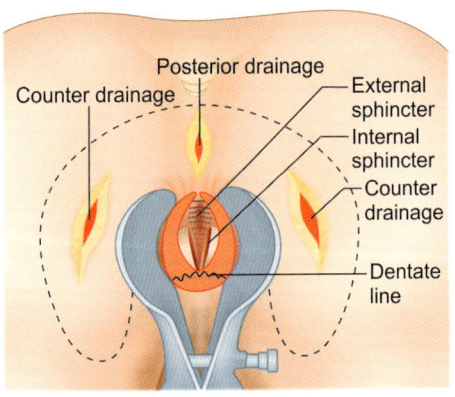

Fig. 15.15A: Drainage of horseshoe abscess

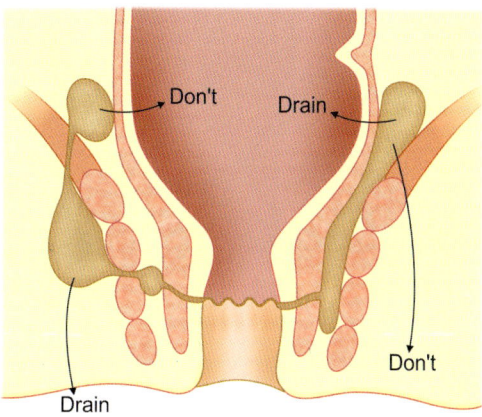

Fig. 15.15B: Drainage of pelvirectal abscess

FISTULA IN ANO

Introduction

A tract lined by epithelium or granulation tissue, with two openings one at the outside on the skin and the other inside the anal canal. Most of them are end results of cryptoglandular infections or anorectal abscesses.

Classification

- When the internal opening is
  - **Above the anorectal ring** it is called *'high fistula'*
  - **Below the anorectal ring** it is called *'low fistula'*

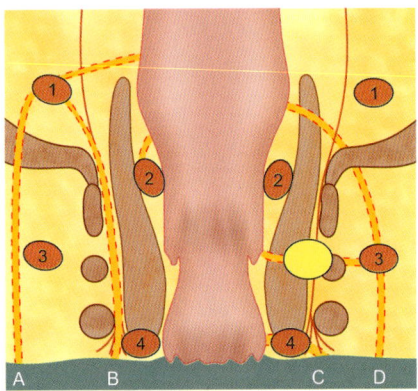

A. Suprasphincteric fistula   B. Intersphincteric fistula
C. Extrasphincteric fistula   D. Transsphincteric fistula

Fig. 15.16: Anal fistulae

- Anal fistulae are classified **(Fig. 15.16)** in relation to the anal musculature (sphincters) *(Park's classification)*. They are:
  1. *Transsphincteric:* Primary tract is across the external sphincter with the internal opening above (high fistula) or below the levator ani muscle (low fistula).
  2. *Intersphincteric:* The primary tract is between the sphincters (usually high fistula).
  3. *Suprasphincteric:* Primary tract with the internal opening above the levator ani (high fistula).
  4. *Extrasphincteric:* Low fistula away from the anal sphincters.

Etiology

- This is the end product of anorectal cryptoglandular sepsis

- Recurrent and multiple fistulae are caused by infections like:
  - Tuberculosis
  - Crohn's disease
  - Ulcerative colitis
  - Colloid carcinoma.

Diagnosis

Symptoms

- Intermittent anal discharge, purulent or blood stained
- Pain may be present during discharge-free intervals.

Signs

- A discharging opening in the perianal skin (**Figs 15.17A and B**)
- Digital examination of rectum may show the tract as an indurated tissue
- The internal opening may be felt as an indurated nodule or a depression, seen at proctoscopy
- Tuberculosis and Crohn's disease may present with multiple external fistulous openings, associated with bowel symptoms

Goodsall's Rule

- When the external fistulous opening lies **anterior to transverse anal line** (an imaginary line connecting both the ischial tuberosities), and is
  - **More than 3 cm away from the anal orifice**, it takes a curved course to open at posterior midline internally at 6 o'clock position, whereas
  - **Within 3 cm from the anal orifice**, it takes a direct course to open at its corresponding position running radially

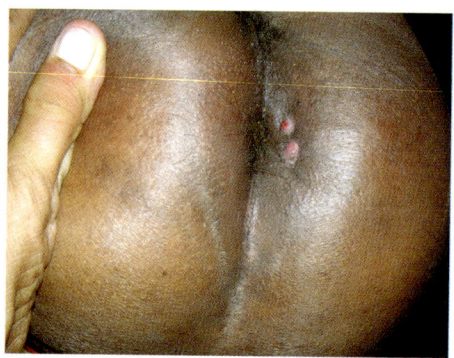

Fig. 15.17A: Fistula in ano

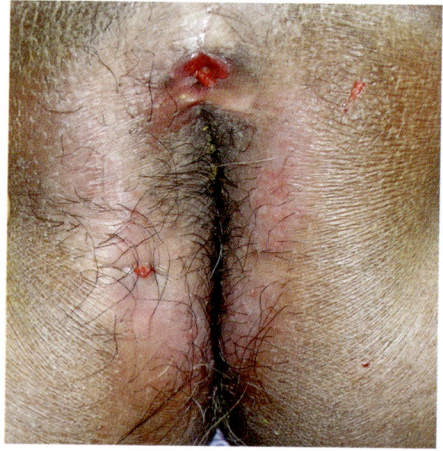

Fig. 15.17B: Multiple anal fistulae

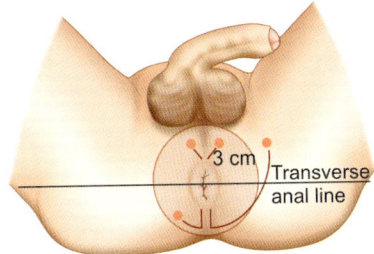

Fig. 15.18: Goodsall's rule

- When the external fistulous opening lies ***posterior to transverse anal line***, whatever distance it is away from the anal orifice, takes a curved course and opens at the posterior midline internally (Fig. 15.18).

Investigations

Special investigations are necessary in recurrent fistulae.

- ***Fistulogram*** (Fig. 15.19) is useful for treatment planning
- ***CT or MR fistulogram*** delineates the fistula and also defines the surrounding structures
- ***Endoanal ultrasound*** may be useful in complex fistulae.

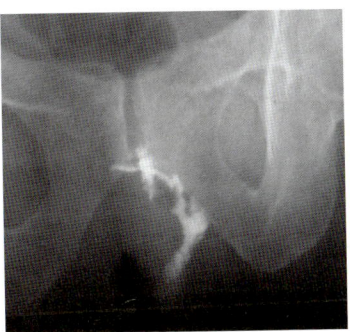

Fig. 15.19: Anal fistulogram

Management

The management of anal fistula is always surgical.
- *Lay-open technique (Fistulotomy) (Fig. 15.20A)*
- *Seton (Fig. 15.20B)*
- *Anorectal advancement flap (Fig. 15.20C)*
- *Fistulectomy*
- *Appropriate medical treatment* is for recurrent fistulae caused by infections like tuberculosis and Crohn's disease.

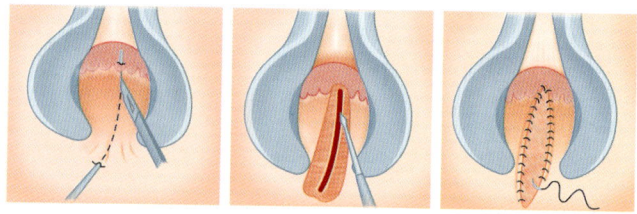

Fig. 15.20A: Lay-open technique (Fistulotomy)

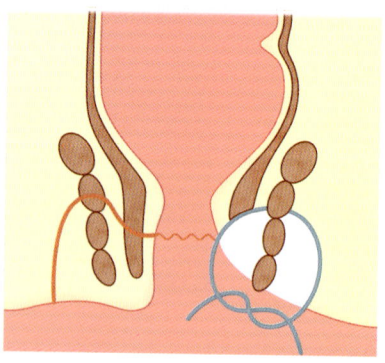

Fig. 15.20B: Seton

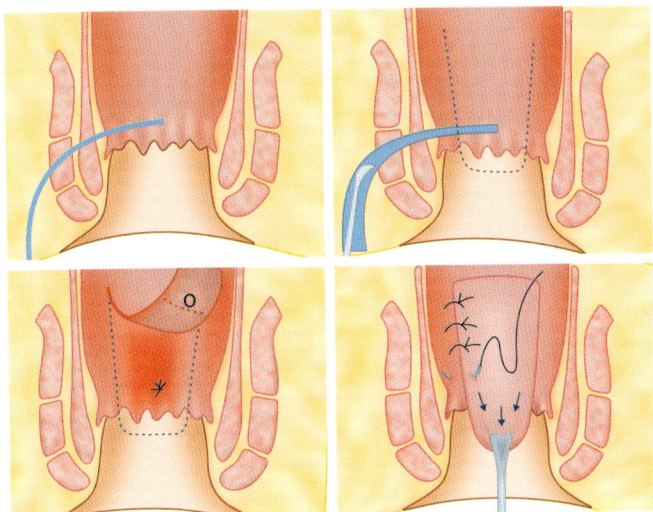

Fig. 15.20C: Anorectal advancement flap for anal fistula

Clinical Pearls

- Often, the patient will recount a history of an abscess drained surgically or spontaneously in the past
- Majority of the times, the internal opening is not apparent on examination
- Goodsall's rule is generally accurate with regard to posterior fistulae, but not with anterior fistulae
- It is not necessary to explore quiescent fistulae.

Surgical Treatment of Anal Fistulae

All surgical procedures are performed in supine lithotomy position.

Principle

The principle of surgical treatment of anal fistula is to:
- Eliminate the fistula
- Prevent recurrence
- Preserve sphincter function.

Preoperative Preparation

- Mild laxative the previous night will keep the rectum empty
- Glycerin suppositories or disposable enemas on the day of the surgery will be useful.

Anesthesia

General/spinal/epidural
- When the fistula is very superficial or marked by a seton, fistulotomy is feasible under local anesthesia and is safe.

Lay-open Technique (Fistulotomy) (Fig. 15.20A)

- A malleable probe is inserted into the external opening and brought out through the internal opening. The overlying tissue is incised, the fistula is opened longitudinally. The granulation tissue lining the fistula is curetted and sent for histopathology
- The edges of the wound can be sutured to the edges of the incision with a continuous locking sutures (marsupialization)
- By this technique, if the fistula is of a high variety, incontinence may result due to the division of the sphincter.

Seton (Fig. 15.20B)

- Seton is any foreign substance (e.g. non-absorbable suture material, rubber bands, silastic catheters) that can inserted into the fistulous tract through the external opening and brought out through the internal opening. When this is tightened in a phased manner, the sphincter though gets divided, will heal by stimulating fibrosis as the next step of division (by tightening the seton) is done. This process of fistulotomy is expected to conserve the sphincter tone.

Procedure

- The external opening is identified and the suture is inserted into the fistula tract
- The suture is brought out of the internal opening
- The ends are tied with multiple knots to create a handle for manipulation
- This is called cutting seton, which is tightened at regular intervals to slowly cut through the sphincter, which allows the tract to become more superficial, converting a high fistula into a low fistula
- The proximal fistulotomy usually heals by fibrosis establishing the continuity of the anorectal ring to prevent separation of sphincter muscle

Seton usage is encouraged in the following special circumstances:

- To identify and promote fibrosis around a complex fistula in ano that encircles most or all of the sphincter mechanisms
- When anatomical landmarks are obscured as in transsphincteric fistula with massive sepsis, seton can be used to mark the site of fistula
- In high anterior transsphincteric fistulae, especially in women, seton is useful as puborectalis is absent and also fistulotomy may result in incontinence
- In transsphincteric fistulae with doubtful healing as in AIDS patients, seton can be used
- To prevent premature skin closure and formation of recurrent abscesses as in Crohn's disease, seton can be used to promote epithelialization

- In patients who have undergone various surgeries for fistula in ano.

Anorectal Advancement Flap (Fig. 15.20C)

Indications

- Anterior fistulae in women
- Previous fistula surgeries
- High fistulae
- Multiple and complex fistulae.

Procedure

- The external fistulous opening is dilated and the granulation tissue curetted
- The internal opening is identified with a color dye
- A mucous flap is created with a pedicle above the internal opening
- The flap is mobilized downwards towards the anus and sutured to the anal mucosa
- The flap will cover the internal opening.

Advantages

- Reduction of healing time
- Reduction of discomfort
- Lack of deformity to the anal canal
- Spares the sphincter muscles.

Fistulectomy

The excision of fistula is no longer performed by many surgeons, as the resultant wounds are large and have a prolonged healing time. There is a high incidence of sphincter damage and incontinence.

Procedure

- **Position of the patient:** Supine and lithotomy
- **Anesthesia:** General/spinal/caudal/epidural
- **Preparation of bowel:** NBM for 6 hours, Mild laxatives previous night
- **Technique:**
  - The fistula can be delineated with a color dye, which will also show intercommunicating or horseshoe fistulae. The dye is injected through the external opening using a fine feeding catheter
  - A malleable probe is passed through the external opening and tried to be brought out through the internal opening without undue pressure
  - A circumscribed incision is made around the entire fistula and it is dissected well and excised in toto
  - While safeguarding the internal sphincter, all tissues stained by the dye should be excised
  - Wound is left open and allowed to heal by secondary intention.

Clinical Pearls

- Fistulectomy causes larger wounds to heal, which takes more time to heal
- Fistulectomy causes greater separation of sphincter muscles, which may lead to incontinence.

Postoperative Care

- Normal diet, bulk agents and analgesics
- Frequent Sitz baths are advised to keep the area clean
- The wound should be intentionally conical, so that the defect granulates well and heals from within outwards, thereby preventing the pocketing of pus

- Cavities may be filled with loose dressing
- The wound should be inspected periodically at 2 weekly intervals and ensured that wounds are clean and granulating satisfactorily and that there is no pocketing of pus or skin bridging.

Complications

- Urinary retention
- Hemorrhage
- Fecal impaction
- Fecal incontinence
- Recurrence.

Incontinence

Minor incontinence is common in about 20–50% patients, which disappears in due course of time, but permanent and major fecal incontinence is seen in about 6–7% of patients.

- The risk of permanent incontinence is high is patients with complicated fistulae, high openings, posterior openings and wide extensions
- Seton usage does not prevent or reduce the incidence of incontinence.

Recurrence

Recurrence rates vary from 0% to 20%

- Failure to identify the internal opening and lateral and upward extensions cause recurrence.

Fibrin Glue

Injecting fibrin glue is effective in a small percentage of patients. The treatment failures occur due to inadequate curettage of granulation tissue and presence of a cavity.

Recent Advances

Bioprosthetic Fistula Plug

- A biosynthetic plug made from lyophilized porcine intestinal submucosa is used for complex fistulae
- The plug is rehydrated in sterile saline and tied to a Vicryl suture which is advanced through the primary opening to exit at the secondary opening. Excess plug is trimmed and sutured to the internal opening with a figure of 8 suture. An advancement flap may be placed over the plug for more security. The excess plug at the secondary opening is excised and left open to allow drainage.

Clinical Pearls

- Special situations like high fistulae, suprasphincteric fistulae, horseshoe fistulae, rectovaginal fistulae require meticulous and thoughtful surgery
- *Crohn's disease and anal fistulae*
    - Anal fistulae in Crohn's disease are most difficult to manage, as they are complex in nature
    - Anal fistulae constitute the most common perianal manifestation in Crohn's disease
    - In Crohn's disease, about a third of cases of anal fistulae heal on conservative management
    - Incontinence is common after surgical treatment in patients with Crohn's disease
    - Multiple unsuccessful repairs require a covering stoma for better healing.

AMEBIC PROCTITIS AND ULCERS

Introduction

- Infection of the rectum and colon caused by *Entamoba histolytica*
- The cysts are consumed through contaminated food or water.

Diagnosis

Symptoms and Signs

- Chronic or, mild to fulminant acute dysentery
- Proctoscopy or sigmoidoscopy will be conclusive.

Investigations

- **Identification of the organisms in stool**
- **Endoscopic (Fig. 15.21) biopsy of the ulcer**
- **Serologic tests** are conclusive.

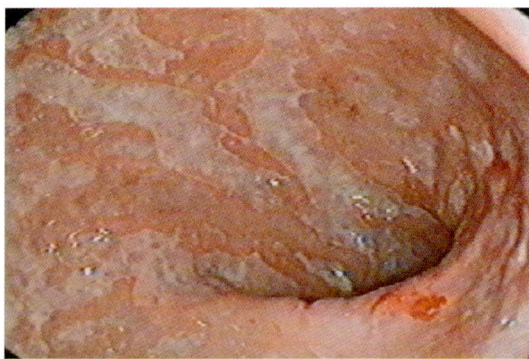

Fig. 15.21: Sigmoidoscopy—Multiple amebic ulcers of rectum

Rectum and Anal Canal

Management

Antiamebic treatment (metronidazole, tinidazole or ornidazole) is curative.

RECTAL POLYPS

Introduction

- Polyps of rectum are common, may be associated with those of the colon (familial polyposis)
- Juvenile polyps occur in infants and children
- They have a strong malignant potential.

Diagnosis

Symptoms and Signs

- Rectal bleed
- On examination, they can be felt as sessile or pedunculated growths.

Investigation

Total colonoscopy (Fig. 15.22) is necessary to rule out familial varieties (Familial adenomatous polyposis).

Management

- *Excision of polyps by colonoscopy* is the treatment of choice
- *Total colectomy with ileostomy or ileoanal anastomosis with pouch construction* is done for familial polyposis and multiple polyposis.

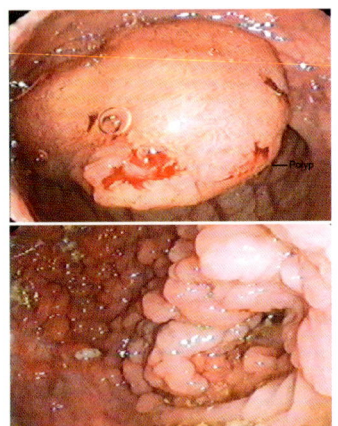

Fig. 15.22: Sigmoidoscopy—Rectal polyps

RECTAL MALIGNANCY

Introduction

- Malignancies of the rectum include:
  - Adenocarcinoma (commonest)
  - Squamous cell carcinoma
  - Lymphoma.

Diagnosis

Symptoms and Signs

- Most patients present with rectal bleed, recent change in bowel habit like constipation or overflow diarrhea, mucus in nature

- Sense of incomplete evacuation and tenesmus are also possible symptoms
- Constant anal pain may suggest invasion of the anal sphincters or the pelvic floor
- Digital examination and proctoscopy confirm the clinical diagnosis in low rectal tumors
- Examination of the abdomen for hepatomegaly is essential in case of rectal malignancies (The commonest spread is to the liver).

Investigations

Blood Test

- ***Increased CEA levels*** are suggestive.

Endoscopy

- ***Proctoscopy or Sigmoidoscopy* (Fig. 15.23)** is diagnostic
- ***Total colonoscopy is necessary to look for synchronous lesions.***

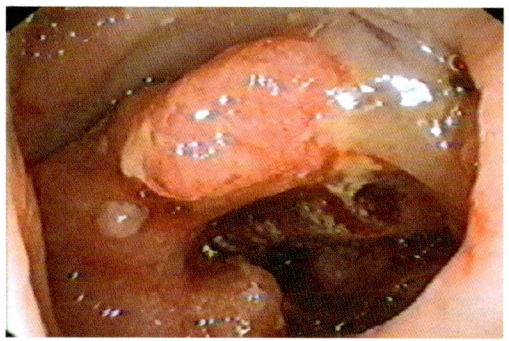

Fig. 15.23: Sigmoidoscopy—Malignant growth

Tissue Diagnosis

- **Punch biopsy and histopathology** are conclusive.

Radiology

- **CT/MRI imaging of abdomen** is necessary to evaluate the metastases, and the depth of invasion and lymph nodal involvement
- **Endoluminal US** is highly useful in assessing the depth of invasion.

Management

- *Adenocarcinoma:*
  - **Appropriate radical surgery (abdominoperineal resection or low anterior resection of rectum) with adjuvant chemoradiation** is the treatment of choice
  - **Preoperative chemoradiation** is useful in locally advanced tumors
- *Squamous cell carcinoma:* Chemoradiation, and surgery for obstructive lesions
- *Lymphoma:* Chemoradiation is useful.

Note: Pretherapy defunctioning colostomy may be needed for obstructive tumors, and the same may be performed as a complementary procedure when anastomosis during surgery is thought to be compromised.

Clinical Pearls

- Though multimodality therapy is available for the treatment of rectal cancer, surgery is the mainstay, to achieve cure

- Since the rectum is fixed, and lacks a serous covering and is surrounded by perirectal fat, its cancer has the propensity to spread directly to the contiguous structures, whereas, the colonic cancers spread by lymphatic and hematogenous route commonly
- Though a clear margin of at least 5 cm is required to get a clearance in colonic cancers, it is enough to have a clear margin of 2 cm in the distal rectal tumors.

Surgical Treatment for Rectal Cancer

The options are:
1. Local excision (for T1 and T2 lesions)
2. Sphincter saving low anterior resection (LAR)
3. Abdominoperineal resection (APR).

Margins

Distal intramural spread of rectal cancer is only to about 2 cm (excepting in poorly differentiated cancers).

Total Mesorectal Excision (Fig. 15.24)

This procedure involves precise sharp dissection and removal of the entire rectal mesentery, including that distal to the tumor, as en bloc specimen. This is done under direct vision to preserve autonomic nerves, have complete hemostasis and avoid the disturbance of mesorectal envelope. This is based on the principle that the rectal tumor spread is limited by this envelope and its total removal would make it complete.

Clinical Pearls

Each patient with rectal cancer should be individually evaluated, and surgery is planned. Mentally unstable patients may find it

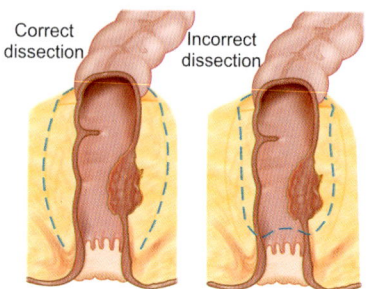

Fig. 15.24: Total mesorectal excision

difficult to manage a colostomy, and an LAR is the best option. In multiparous obese women, when LAR may be technically difficult, APR would be the best option.

Abdominoperineal Resection (Fig. 15.25)

Incisions

- Lower midline (most convenient)
- Lower left paramedian.

Surgical Technique

Position of patient: ***Lithotomy Trendelenburg position.***

- ***Abdominal dissection***
  - Lower midline incision
  - Release of sigmoid colon (**Fig. 15.26A**)
  - Identification and preservation of left ureter (**Fig. 15.26B**)
  - Release of sigmoid colon from the right side (**Fig. 15.26C**)
  - Both incisions are joined anteriorly in the rectovesical or rectouterine pouch

Rectum and Anal Canal

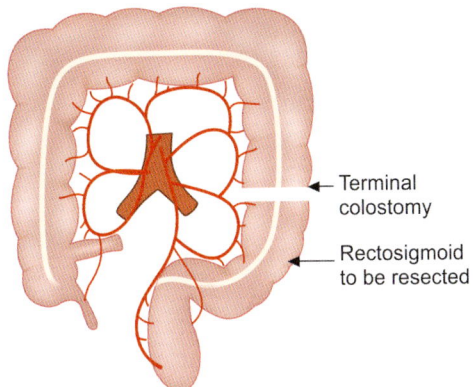

Fig. 15.25: Abdominoperineal resection

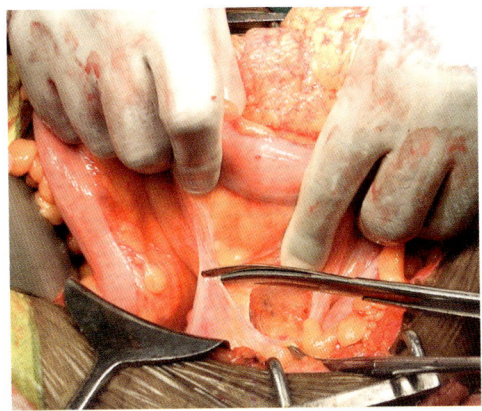

Fig. 15.26A: Mobilization of sigmoid colon

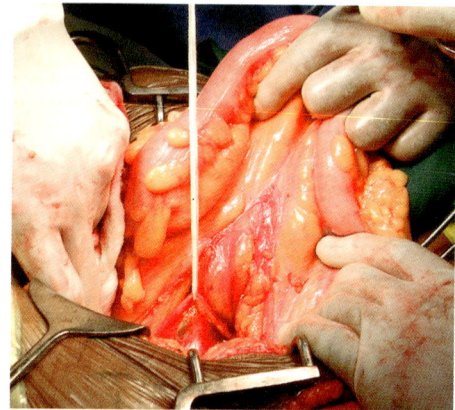

Fig. 15.26B: Identification of left ureter

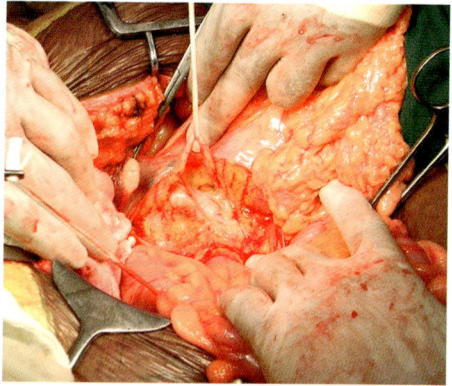

Fig. 15.26C: Identification of right ureter

- Rectum dissected and separated from the urinary bladder and prostate
- Rectum is separated fully in the presacral space as far down as possible
- Rectum separated fully on both the lateral sides dividing lateral ligaments (**Fig. 15.26D**) containing the middle rectal vessels
- Inferior mesenteric vessels flush ligated.
- *Perineal dissection*
  - Elliptical incision around the anus
  - Rectum is separated on all sides and dissection carried proximally to meet the abdominal surgeon (**Fig. 15.26E**)
- *Completion of operation*
  - The colon is divided and the specimen removed through the perineal wound (**Fig. 15.26F**)
  - Terminal colostomy created (**Figs. 15.26G and H**).

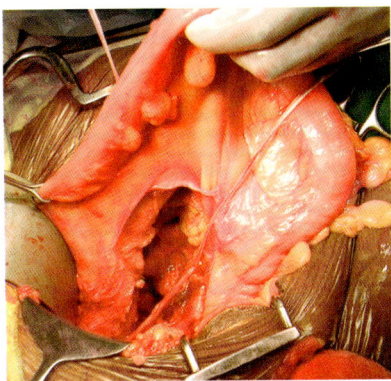

Fig. 15.26D: Fully mobilized sigmoid colon

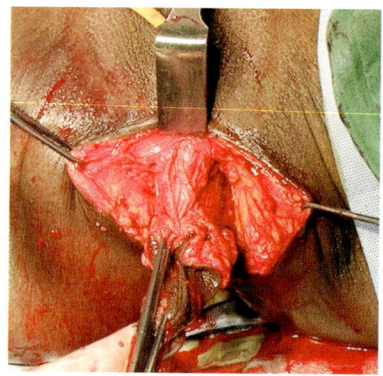

Fig. 15.26E: Dissection through the perineal wound

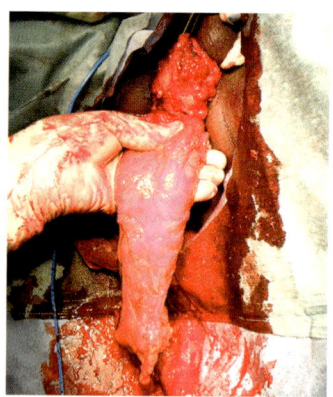

Fig. 15.26F: Removing the colon through the perineal wound

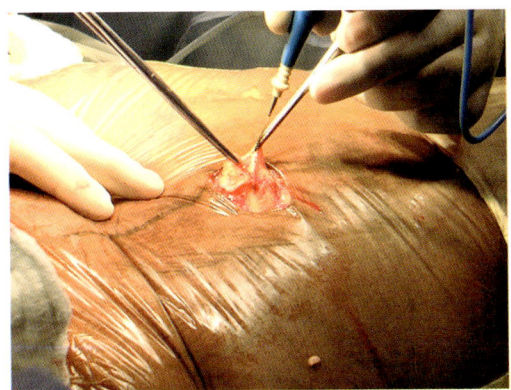

Fig. 15.26G: Creation of end colostomy

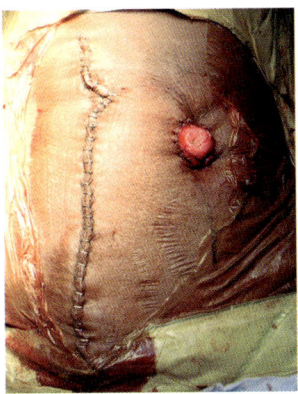

Fig. 15.26H: Created terminal colostomy

Complications

- ***Hemorrhage and shock:*** Bleeding is visible through the perineal wound, which occurs around the 2nd postoperative day, and may present with shock. Minor bleeds may be treated with blood transfusions and larger ones need re-exploration
- ***Rupture of pelvic peritoneum:*** The pelvic peritoneum may give way partially or completely allowing the prolapse of the intestines in the perineum. If viable, the bowel needs to be pulled into the abdominal cavity by laparotomy. Gangrenous bowel has to be resected
- ***Perineal hernia:*** Slow prolapse of intestines can lead to a swelling in the perineum, which needs surgical correction
- ***Infection of perineal wound*** to be treated by antibiotics and secondary suturing if necessary
- ***Internal hernia:*** Possible when small bowel herniates in the paracolic gutter. This needs surgical correction, non-viable bowel needs resection.

Low Anterior Resection (Fig. 15.27)

Surgical Technique

- **Position of patient**
  - Lithotomy Trendelenburg position.
- ***Abdominal dissection***
  - The steps are same as in APR
  - Rectum stapled and transected low (using linear stapler)
  - Colon transected at mid-sigmoid level
  - The specimen is removed.
- ***Stapler anastomosis (Figs 15.28A to D)***
  - Circular stapler introduced into the distal rectal stump through the anus
  - Anvil is introduced into the proximal colon

Rectum and Anal Canal

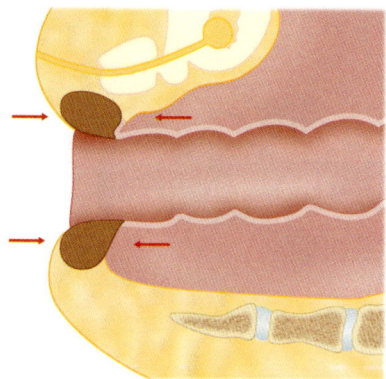

Fig. 15.27: Low anterior resection

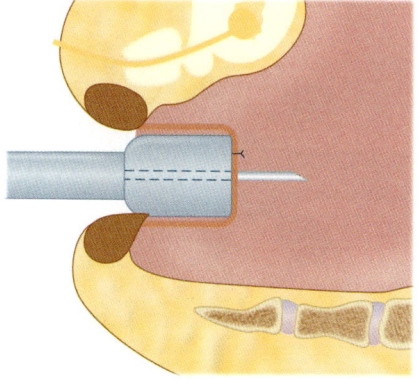

Fig. 15.28A: Stapler anastomosis-1

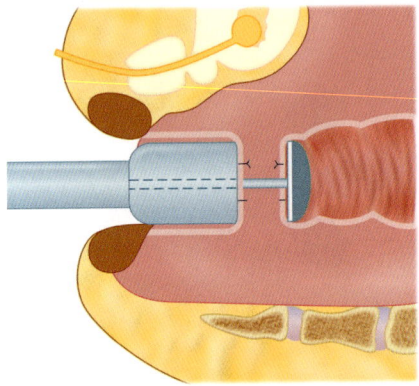

Fig. 15.28B: Stapler anastomosis-2

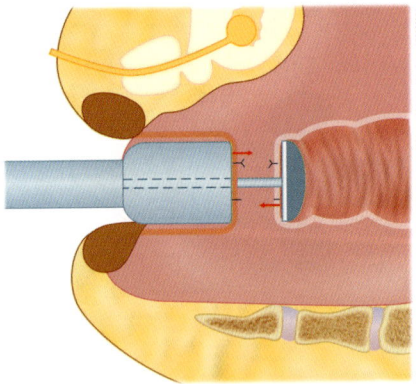

Fig. 15.28C: Stapler anastomosis-3

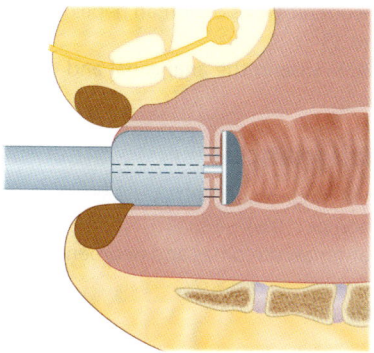

Fig. 15.28D: Stapler anastomosis-4

- Proximal and distal guts are approximated
- The gun is fired to throw the staples
- Stapler is opened a little and gut released
- Stapler is removed.
- ***Testing the integrity of anastomosis***
  - Checking the doughnuts
  - By filling the pelvis with saline and injecting air in the bowel and check for the air leak
  - By filling the rectum with dilute povidone iodine solution and check for the solution leak.

ANAL MALIGNANCY

Introduction

- Anal malignancies are rare
- Affects the elderly more in women

- Linked to oncogenic types of human papilloma virus (HPV) types 16, 18, 32 and 33
- More than 80% arise in the anal canal and the reminder in the anal margin.

Types of Malignancies

- Squamous cell carcinomas (>80%)
- Adenocarcinomas (10%)
- Others (melanomas, sarcomas and neuroendocrine tumors).

Risk Factors

- Genital warts
- Homosexuality (receptive anal sex)
- Human papilloma virus type 16
- HIV infection
- Tobacco smoking
- Chronic fistulae
- Pelvic radiation.
- Anal intraepithelial hyperplasia.

Macroscopic and Microscopic Appearances

- *Macroscopically*, it appears as a
  - Nodule
  - Polyp
  - Ulcer with everted edges
- *Microscopically*, they are
  - Squamous cell carcinoma (90%)
  - Adenocarcinoma from mucous glands (10%)
  - Basal cell carcinoma (rare)
  - Malignant melanoma (rare).

Spread of Anal Canal Malignancy

The tumor spreads
- *Circumferentially and longitudinally* within the anus and rectum and invade perianal skin distally
- *Laterally* to sphincters, ischiorectal fossae, *anteriorly* to vagina (anovaginal fistula) and urethra
- *Lymphatically* to inguinal nodes, iliac nodes
- *Hematogenously* to liver, lungs and skeleton (very rare).

Diagnosis

Symptoms

- Bright rectal bleeding (60%)
- Perianal pain (60%)
- Mass (30%)
- Discharge (30%)
- Irritation/discomfort
- Bleeding
- Tenesmus.

Signs

- Distal anal tumors are evident on inspection, as warty growths with ulcerations **(Fig. 15.29)**
- Fixity to surrounding structures
- Inguinal lymph nodes may be palpable.

Investigations

- *Endoanal US* is very informative
- *Punch biopsy and histopathology* is conclusive
- *Sentinel node biopsy* is useful

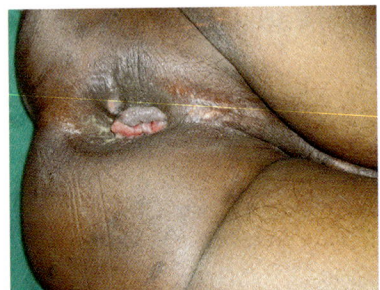

Fig. 15.29: Anal canal malignancy

- ***MRI of pelvis*** (to assess local invasion and pelvic/inguinal lymphadenopathy)
- ***CT abdomen and thorax*** (to assess distant metastases).

Differential Diagnosis

- Melanomas
- Bowen's disease (intraepithelial neoplasia)
- Paget's disease (intraepithelial mucinous adenocarcinoma from dermal apocrine sweat glands.

Management

Curative

- ***Radiotherapy with or without chemotherapy*** is the treatment of choice
- ***Surgery*** is reserved for some tumors
- ***Prophylactic groin irradiation*** is known to reduce the incidence of nodal metastases.

Palliative

- **Defunctioning colostomy for inoperable tumors**
- **Radiotherapy**
- **Abdominal perineal resection** for persistent or recurrent disease.

Clinical Pearls

- More than 80% of anal canal cancers are squamous cell carcinomas
- Delay and misdiagnosis is more common in anal cancer as the symptoms resemble benign anorectal conditions
- If clear resection margins cannot be obtained, radical surgery should not be chosen as the survival benefit is minimal.

RECTAL PROLAPSE

Introduction

- Generally caused by chronic constipation and straining at stool and when the pelvic floor is weak
- Occurs at extremes of age.

Diagnosis

Symptoms

- The rectum presents as a prolapsed mucosa, varying from partial to full thickness (**Fig. 15.30**), appearing more during the act of defecation
- It can reduce spontaneously or may need manual reduction
- There may be associated mucous discharge, bleeding, pain and incontinence

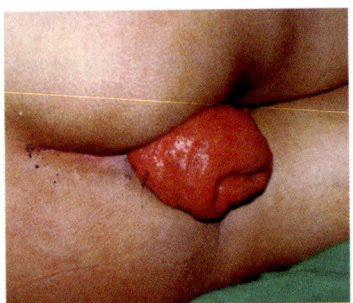

Fig. 15.30: Prolapse rectum

- Patient may have to strain to make it prolapse for clinical examination, in most cases.

Signs
- Prolapse up to 5 cm is considered to be partial and more than that is considered complete
- They can be differentiated by feeling the wall with the thumb and the index finger.

Differential Diagnosis

- Hemorrhoids
- Intussusception.

Management

The surgeon should decide between the various operations based on the extent of operation, potential morbidity, rate of recurrence and impact on fecal continence. Various operations have been described for the management of rectal prolapse. The abdominal operations have the risk of sexual dysfunction.

Abdominal Procedures

- *Repair of pelvic floor*
- *Suspension—fixation procedures*
  - *Sigmoidopexy (Pemberton–Stalker)*
  - *Presacral rectopexy*
  - *Lateral strip rectopexy (Orr-Loygue)*
  - *Anterior sling rectopexy (Ripstein procedure) (Fig. 15.31A)*
  - *Posterior sling (Ivalon sponge) rectopexy (Wells operation) (Fig. 15.31B)*
  - *Puborectalis sling (Wells)*
- *Resection procedures*
  - *Abdominal rectopexy +/− sigmoid colectomy (Fig. 15.31C)*
  - *Anterior resection.*

Perineal Procedures

- *Perineal rectosigmoidectomy (Altemeier operation) (Fig. 15.32A)*
- *Mucosal sleeve resection (Delorme operation) (Fig. 15.32B)*
- *Anal encirclement (Thiersch procedure) (Fig. 15.32C)*
- *Perineal suspension fixation (Wyatt operation).*

Clinical Pearls

- Surgical management is aimed at restoring physiology by correcting the prolapse and improving continence and constipation, whereas in patients with concurrent genital and rectal prolapse, an interdisciplinary surgical approach is required.

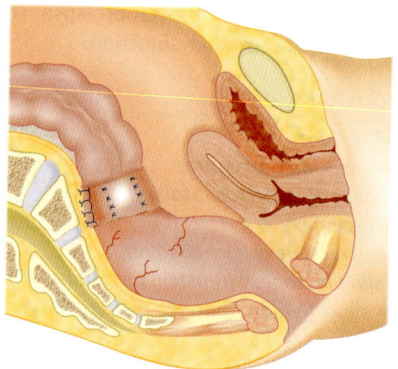

Fig. 15.31A: Mesh rectopexy (Ripstein's procedure)

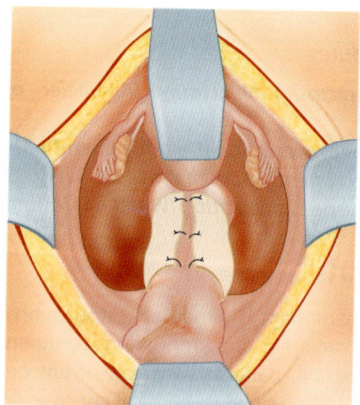

Fig. 15.31B: Wells Ivalon sponge rectopexy

Rectum and Anal Canal

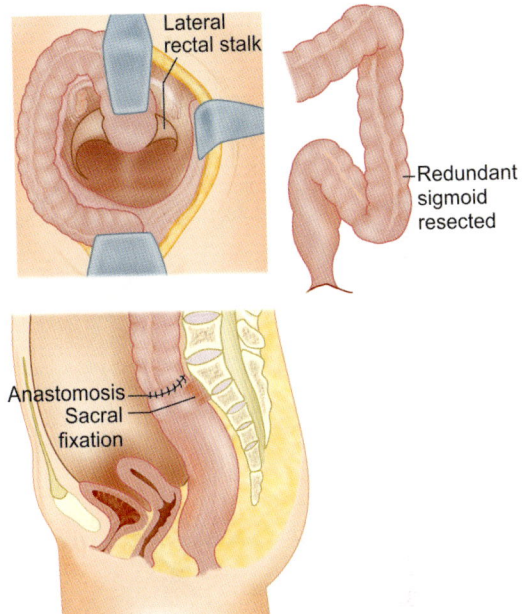

Fig. 15.31C: Abdominal rectopexy and sigmoidectomy

- Operation should be reserved for those patients in whom medical treatment has failed, and it may be expected to relieve symptoms.
- Numerous surgical procedures have been suggested to treat rectal prolapse. They are generally classified as abdominal or perineal according to the route of access. However, the

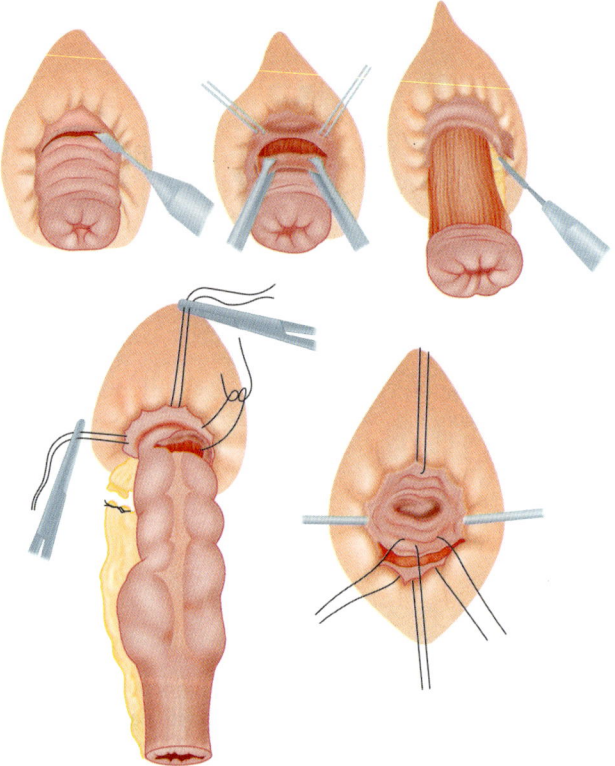

Fig. 15.32A: Altemeier operation

Rectum and Anal Canal

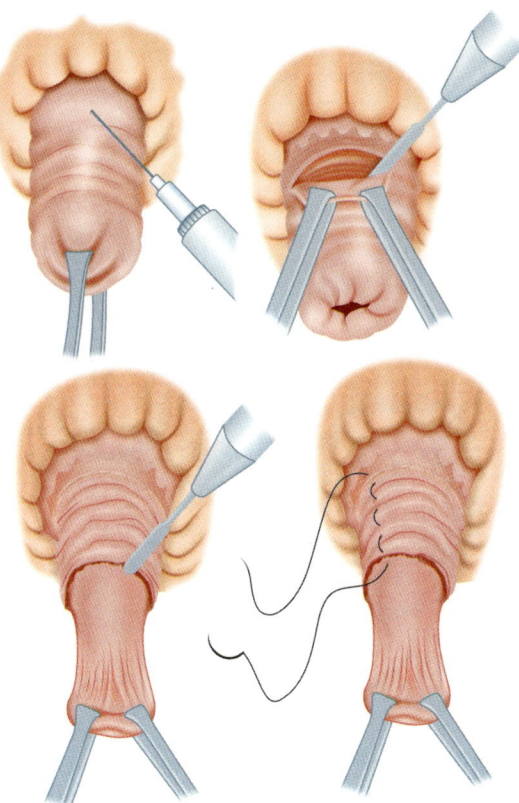

Fig. 15.32B: Delorme's operation

Snapshots in Gastroenterology

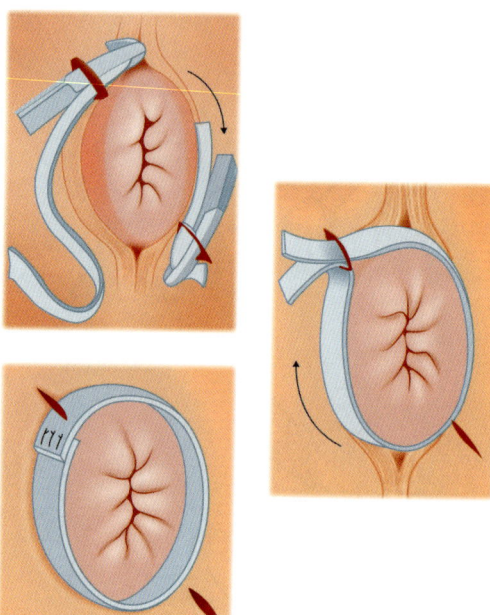

Fig. 15.32C: Thiersch operation

controversy as to which operation is appropriate cannot be answered definitively, as the extent of a standardized diagnostic assessment and the types of surgical procedures have not been identified in published series.

SOLITARY RECTAL ULCER

Introduction

This occurs in patients who strain to pass stools, producing an internal intussusception occasionally a prolapse, resulting in a solitary ulcer in the rectum

Diagnosis

Symptoms and Signs
- Rectal bleed associated with mucus
- Proctoscopy reveals a solitary ulcer usually on the anterior rectum just above the anal canal with a 'punched out' appearance with a gray-white base
- The ulcer may be polypoid or elevated.

Investigations
- ***Proctoscopy or sigmoidoscopy*** (Fig. 15.33) is diagnostic
- ***Histopathology*** is conclusive.

Differential Diagnosis

- Colitis cystica profunda
- Polyps
- Endometriosis
- Inflammatory granuloma
- Infectious disorders
- Drug-induced colitis
- Mucus-producing adenocarcinoma.

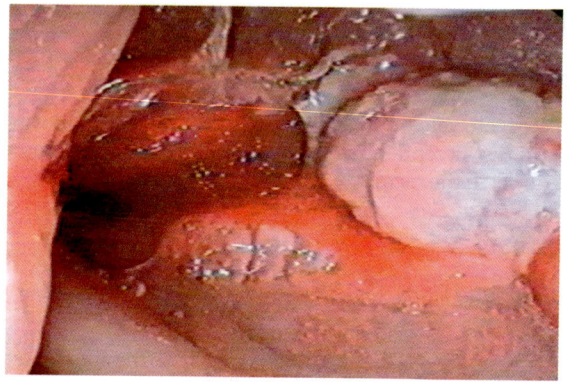

Fig. 15.33: Sigmoidoscopy—Solitary rectal ulcer

Management

- *High fiber diet*
- *Bowel modifying measures*
- *Localized resection in selected patients*
- *Treatment of prolapse if associated.*

Chapter 16

Intestinal Stomas

INTRODUCTION

- A stoma is a surgically created opening between a hollow organ and the body surface (e.g. colostomy) or between two hollow organs (e.g. gastrojejunostomy)
- It is a Greek word for mouth
- Ostomy is named by the organ involved (e.g. ileostomy– opening from the ileum, colostomy—opening from colon)
- Stomas which are utilized for administering food or drugs are called input stomas (e.g. feeding gastrostomy, feeding jejunostomy), and those which are used to decompress or divert the outflowing contents are called output stomas (e.g. ileostomy, colostomy).

INPUT STOMAS

Artificial enteric nutritional support is vital in the management of subjects who are unable to maintain oral nutrition during or following conditions such as upper gastrointestinal malignancy, surgical resection, cerebrovascular disease, or dysmotility. The intestinal tract can be accessed through two routes, the stomach and jejunum. For this purpose, a stoma can be created for feeding purposes and they are called the input stomas.

Snapshots in Gastroenterology

The common input stomas are:
- Feeding gastrostomy
- Feeding jejunostomy.

Gastrostomy (Fig. 16.1)

Indications

- Obstructive lesions of esophagus
- Anastomosis involving the esophagus (e.g. esophagogastrostomy)
- Neuromuscular disorders (e.g. stroke, motor neuron disease)
- Used for feeding purposes.

Open Surgical Gastrostomy

Stamm's Gastrostomy
- Incision—upper midline

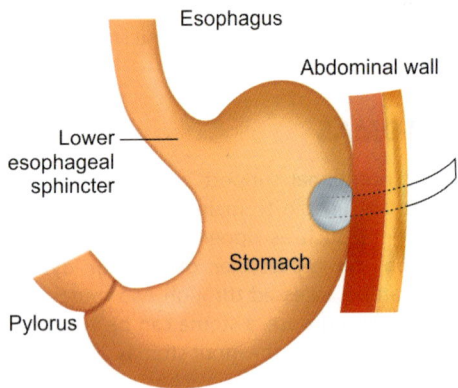

Fig. 16.1: Gastrostomy surgery

Intestinal Stomas

- Anterior wall of stomach is picked up with Babcock forceps (**Fig. 16.2A**)
- Stab wound is created in the anterior wall
- Malecot's catheter is inserted through the stab wound (**Fig. 16.2B**)

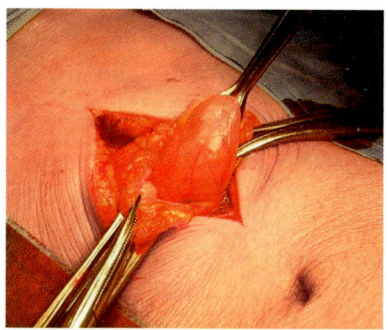

Fig. 16.2A: Picking up the anterior wall of stomach

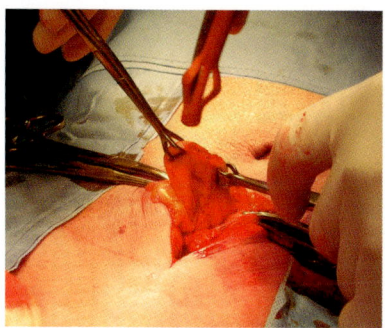

Fig. 16.2B: Introducing a catheter through a stab incision

- The catheter is fixed with a purse-string suture with absorbable material and invert the stomach (**Fig. 16.2C**)
- The stomach is fixed to the parietal peritoneum with absorbable sutures (**Fig. 16.2D**)
- Incision is closed in layers.

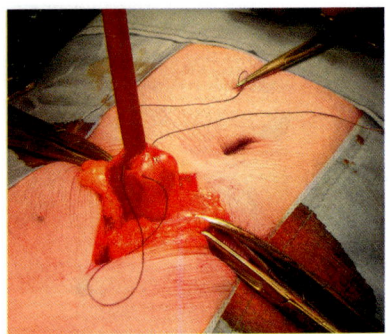

Fig. 16.2C: Application of purse-string suture

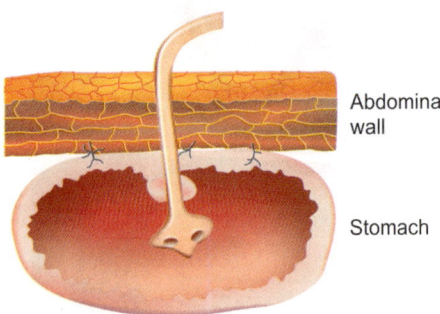

Fig. 16.2D: Final result of Stamm's gastrostomy

Witzel's Gastrostomy

- Incision—upper midline
- Anterior wall of stomach is picked up with Babcock forceps
- Stab wound is created in the anterior wall
- A Malecot's catheter is inserted through the stab wound
- The catheter is fixed with a purse-string suture with absorbable material and invert the stomach
- The anterior surface of stomach is tunneled over the catheter **(Fig. 16.3)**
- The stomach is fixed to the parietal peritoneum with absorbable sutures
- Incision is closed in layers.

Janeway's Gastrostomy *(Fig. 16.4)*

- Incision—upper midline

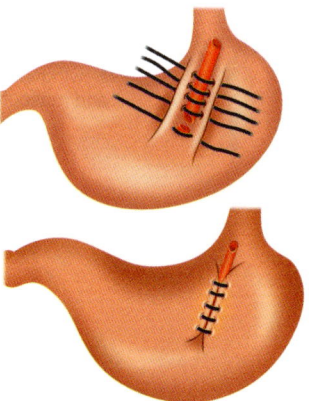

Fig. 16.3: Witzel's gastrostomy

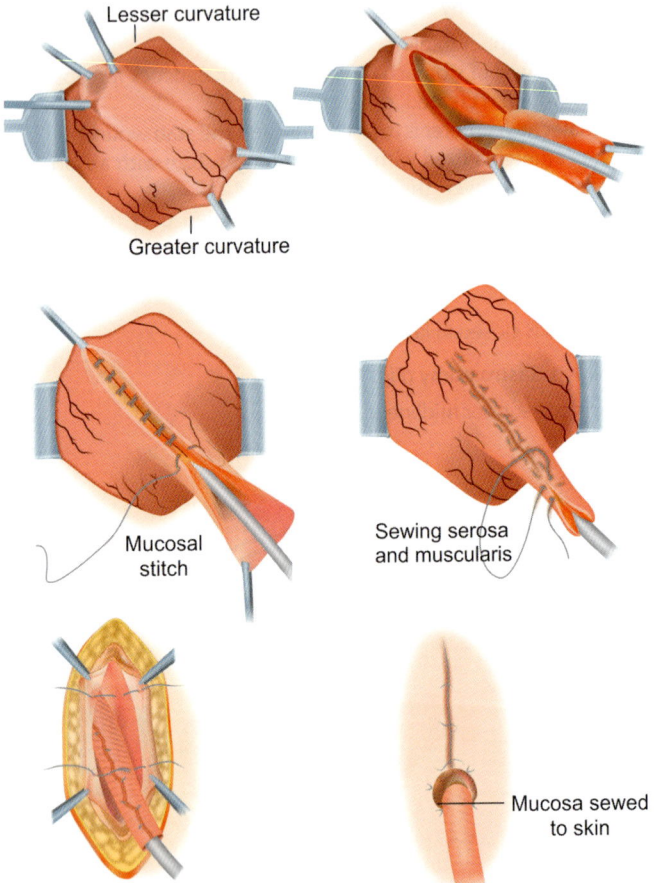

Fig. 16.4: Janeway gastrostomy

Intestinal Stomas

- A flap is created in the anterior wall of the stomach with the base towards the greater curvature
- The flap is sutured so as to enclose the catheter to form a tube
- The mucosa of the tube is fixed to the skin with non-absorbable sutures
- Incision is closed in layers.

Percutaneous Endoscopic Gastrostomy (PEG)

Procedure Steps *(Fig. 16.5A)*

- Gastroscopy is done to exclude lesions in the stomach
- The anterior wall of stomach is identified, and illuminated by the gastroscope (1)
- The skin is prepared on the illuminated area, and infiltrated with local anesthetic
- The needle followed by the guidewire is introduced into the stomach (2)
- The guidewire is grasped by the snare of the gastroscope and pulled out of the mouth as the endoscope is withdrawn (3)
- The feeding tube is attached to the guidewire and pulled out of the external bumper on the skin (4 and 5)
- The button (internal bumper) on the PEG tube keeps it impacted against the gastric wall (**Fig. 16.5B**)
- The tube is attached to the feeding source
- Preoperative antibiotic may be necessary to avoid infection of the stoma site.

An Exclusive Kit is Available for PEG Procedure (Fig. 16.6)

Contraindications to PEG

- GI tract obstruction
- Malignant infiltration of stomach
- Gastric varices

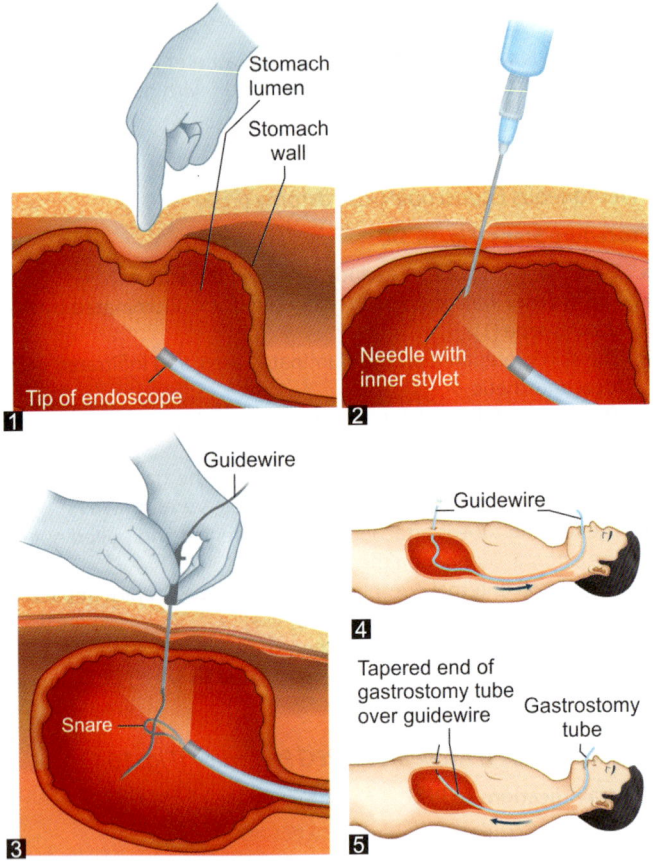

Fig. 16.5A: Percutaneous endoscopic gastrostomy procedure

Intestinal Stomas

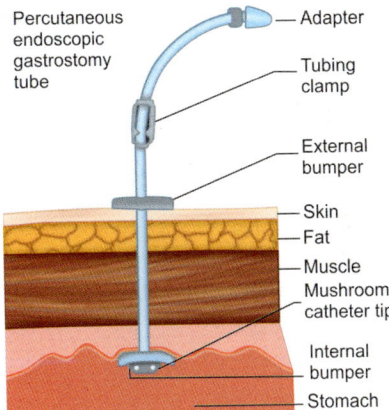

Fig. 16.5B: Positioning of PEG tube

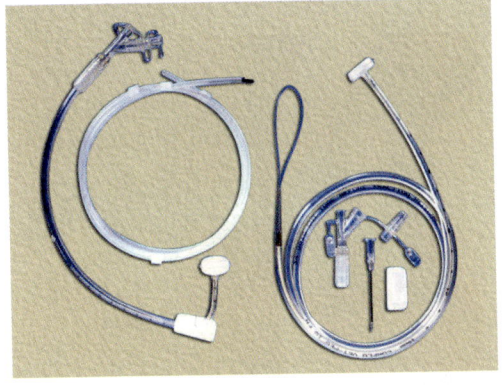

Fig. 16.6: Percutaneous endoscopic gastrostomy kit

- Uncorrectable coagulopathy
- Operated stomach which precludes the ability to appose the anterior abdominal wall and the anterior stomach wall.

JEJUNOSTOMY (FIG. 16.7)

For the delivery of postpyloric feeding, the jejunum is accessed by two methods.
1. Open surgical jejunostomy
2. Percutaneous endoscopic jejunostomy (PEJ)
   - Direct percutaneous endoscopic jejunostomy (DPEJ)
   - Percutaneous endoscopic gastrostomy with jejunal extension (PEG–J).

Indications

- Obstructive lesions of esophagus and stomach
- Anastomosis of esophagus and stomach.

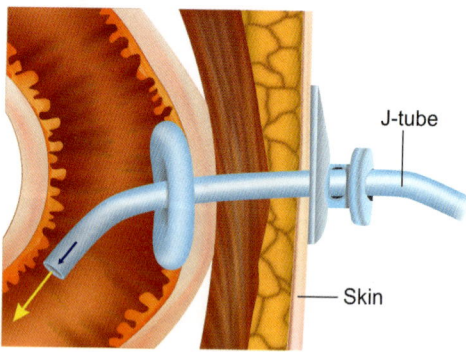

Fig. 16.7: Jejunostomy

Open Surgical Jejunostomy (Witzel's Type) (Figs 16.8A to D)

Surgery Steps

- Incision—midline (when done separately)
- The proximal jejunum is identified
- Jejunostomy site is marked and a purse-string suture is taken
- A stab wound is made with a diathermy at the marked site **(Fig. 16.8A)**, and a feeding tube is inserted into the jejunum directed isoperistaltically **(Fig. 16.8B)**

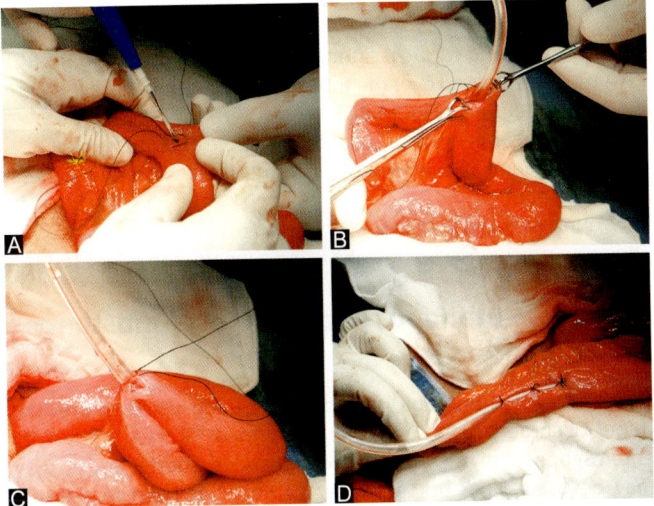

Figs 16.8A to D: Witzel's open surgical jejunostomy

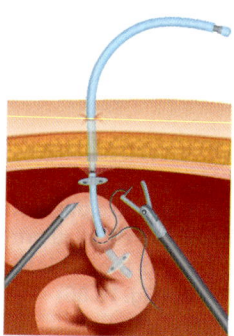

Fig. 16.9: Feeding jejunostomy by laparoscopy

- The purse-sting suture is tightened around the tube (**Fig. 16.8C**)
- A tunnel is created over the tube for a distance of about 8–10 cm using the sutures (**Fig. 16.8D**)
- The jejunostomy tube is brought out of the abdomen
- The jejunum at the jejunostomy site is fixed to the parietal peritoneum
- Wound is closed in layers.

The same procedure can be done using a laparoscope (**Fig. 16.9**).

Direct Percutaneous Endoscopic Jejunostomy (Figs 16.10A to H)

The choice of endoscope used depends upon whether previous upper GI surgery has been done; if the upper GI tract is intact, an enteroscope (with overtube) is usually needed; shorter endoscopes may be used if part of the upper GI tract has been resected or anastomosed.

Intestinal Stomas

- The endoscope is advanced into the first loop of jejunum; with experience, this loop is usually readily identifiable. The endoscope position can usually be confirmed by finger indentation in the left upper quadrant or with fluoroscopy (if a gastrojejunostomy has been done then the endoscope position is more variable). Transillumination may also be seen here
- The abdominal wall is then cleansed.
- The illuminated site is infiltrated with a local anesthetic, and a 21G pilot needle (4 cm long) is advanced and is used to search for the jejunal lumen. At this point, intermittent fluoroscopy can be used to help guide the needle into the gut lumen immediately in front of the endoscope tip

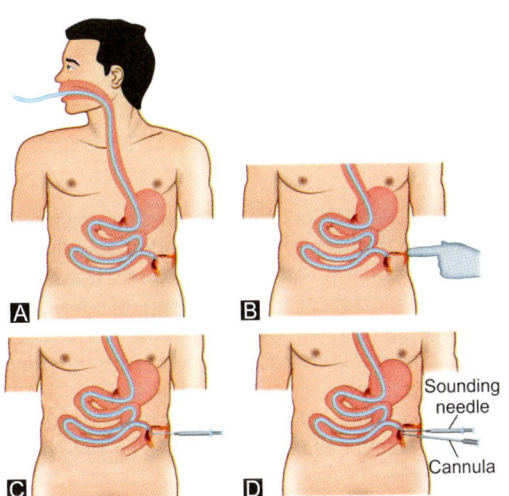

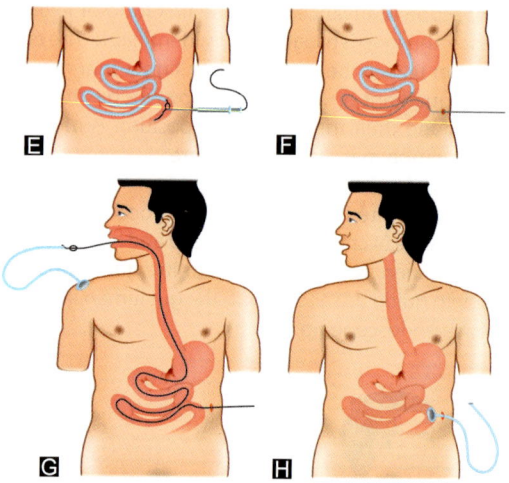

Figs 16.10A to H: Direct percutaneous endoscopic jejunostomy

- Continuous aspiration on the pilot needle is maintained; when air is aspirated the needle should be endoscopically visible at the same time to confirm entry into the correct bowel loop and to help exclude puncture of interposed loops of bowel. If the needle is not visible after aspirating air then it may be in a superimposed loop of gut, and the endoscope may need to be moved into a different loop to achieve a safe puncture site
- After an appropriate puncture site has been identified, a trocar or drainage access needle is advanced alongside or in place of the 21 G needle

- Once the gut has been successfully punctured, the trocar or needle is then snared, and the procedure can be completed as for a conventional PEG insertion
- Fresenius 15 Fr PEG kit is available for these procedures.

Percutaneous Endoscopic Gastrostomy with Jejunal Extension (PEG–J) (Fig. 16.11)

- The procedure is to do a PEG as described above
- Once the gastric part of the tube is in place, the jejunal part of the tube is threaded down the inside of the gastric tube
- The tip of the jejunostomy tube is taken beyond the duodenum under fluoroscopy or by using an enteroscope.

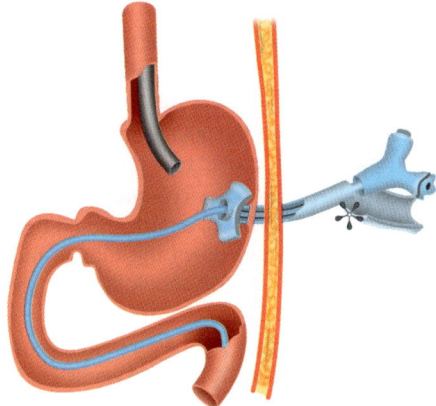

Fig. 16.11: Percutaneous endoscopic gastrostomy with jejunal extension

Clinical Pearls

- Catheters commonly used for radiologic enteral access include Cope loop catheters, balloon catheters, and mushroom (or bumper) catheters. Interventional radiologists most commonly use the first two types of above-mentioned catheters
- No catheter is ideal in all situations, and the choice of catheter frequently depends on the physician's preference and individual patient considerations
- Low profile balloon retained transgastric-jejunal feeding tube (MIC-J) is a good alternative.

Postoperative Management

Caring for the PEG-J Tube

- Unlike gastrostomy tubes, transgastric jejunal tubes must not be rotated. This is because the rotation of the tube would cause a twist (kink) to occur in the jejunal tube
- To prevent blocking, both the jejunal and gastric tubes need to be flushed regularly with cooled boiled water
- Flushes should take place before a continuous feed is started and when it is stopped. In addition, a flush should be given before and after a medicine is put down the tube. If more than one medicine is being given, a flush should also be given between each medicine
- If the gastric access ports are not being routinely used, it should be flushed every 24 hours with 10 mL of water
- If the jejunal access port is not being routinely used, it should be flushed every 6–12 hours with 5–10 mL of sterile water.

COMPLICATIONS OF INPUT STOMAS

Intraperitoneal Leak

By not fixing or improperly fixing the stomach/jejunum around the ostomy to the parietes, the enteric contents and the feeds administered through the ostomy tube, may leak into the general peritoneal cavity and result in peritonitis.

Diagnosis

Clinical Presentation

Patient presents with fever and signs of peritonitis.

Investigation

Ultrasonography will reveal the leak and collection of purulent material in the abdominal cavity.

Management

It is wise to open the abdomen and do a thorough peritoneal toileting and refashion the gastrostomy.

Excoriation and Infection of Stoma

The acidic secretions of the stomach along with the food administered through the gastrostomy tube, may regurgitate through the stoma peritubally, and create excoriation of the skin. The skin losing its integrity gets secondarily infected and creates painful discharge of seropurulent material.

Diagnosis

Clinical Presentation

The patient presents with pain and seropurulent discharge around the gastrostomy stoma (**Fig. 16.12**).

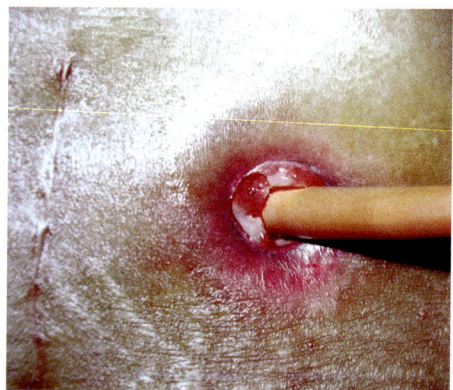

Fig. 16.12: Discharge and excoriation around gastrostomy stoma

Investigations

No special investigation is required, as the diagnosis is evident.

Management

Local care of the peritubal area with frequent wiping using wet cotton and administration of appropriate antibiotics should suffice. The patency of the tube has to be established. If the tube has not been changed for a longtime, it is better to replace the tube.

OUTPUT STOMAS

Introduction

- Ileostomy and colostomy are output intestinal stomas
- This can be a temporary procedure either as an end ostomy in the acute setting for a later planned takedown and anastomosis

or as a proximal loop diversion to protect a distal anastomosis. A permanent end colostomy is performed as an adjunct to abdominoperineal resection
- A permanent ostomy may be warranted after resection of distal bowel (e.g. resection of rectum) or to manage incurable fecal incontinence or injuries to the distal bowel (e.g. trauma or rectourethral fistula).

Physiology

Output
- Loss of continence is the primary disadvantage of a stoma
- Ostomy output is directly related to the location of the bowel opening. Sigmoid colostomy produces well-formed stools equal to the consistency of normal stools.
- Right sided colostomies produce high volume fecal output with bad odor due to the effects of colonic bacteria
- Ileostomy discharges watery content, though over a period of time, it becomes thicker.

Volume
- Though initially the volume is high from an ileostomy, the average volume rests at about 500 mL/day
- The ileostomy discharges almost continuously immaterial of the food intake, but food intake as such may increase the intestinal hurry.

Nutrition
- Loss of terminal ileum and the following ileostomy results in loss of absorption of bile acids, fats and fat-soluble vitamins
- Loss of absorption of vitamin B_{12} will result in pernicious or macrocytic anemias and will require monthly vitamin B_{12} replacement

- Fluid and sodium loss are the consequences of ileostomy, leading to chronic dehydration, which may lead to acidic urine and renal stones
- Colostomies do not disturb the nutritional status of the patient, as the function of the colon is only water absorption.

Preoperative Evaluation and Considerations

- Patient counseling is important
- Planning the stoma site and it should consider the following:
    - Occupation
    - Dressing style (especially the belt line)
    - Body stature
    - Flexibility
    - Abdominal wall contour (while sitting and standing)
    - Physical disabilities
    - Prior abdominal surgery
    - Abdominal girth
    - Stability of the appliance during patient movements.

Standard Stoma Sites

- Ostomy site is usually sited on either side of the midline overlying the rectus abdominis muscle
- It should be about 5 cm away from prior incisions, bony prominences, the umbilicus and patient's belt line
- The stoma should be planned and marked while the patient is sitting as the management of the stoma can also be done while sitting
- If the abdominal wall is pendulous, it becomes difficult to manage the stoma by the patient, and in such a situation, the supraumbilical stoma is meaningful and logical

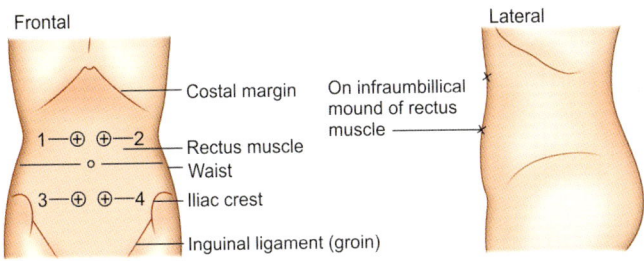

Fig. 16.13: Sites for creating a stoma

- Most left colon end stomas are placed in the left lower quadrant exiting through the rectus muscle, and the end ileostomies are placed in the right lower quadrant
- The stoma must be visible to the patient for care and if below the umbilicus, it must be sited on the summit of the infraumbilical mound. Effectively there are four suitable sites for stoma over the flat surface of the rectus above or below the umbilicus **(Fig. 16.13)**.

ILEOSTOMY

There are four types of ileostomies **(Fig. 16.14A)**. They are:
1. End ileostomy (Brooke's ileostomy)
2. Loop ileostomy (the bowel is not divided)
3. Loop end ileostomy (the bowel is divided).
   – When the bowel loop is divided, the distal segment is allowed to be open, it discharges mucus, hence called mucous fistula
4. Koch's continent ileostomy: Brooke's end ileostomy is not continent, and a first continent ileostomy was reported by Nils

Koch in 1969. It is a reservoir made from the terminal ileum with a nipple valve, but has the disadvantage of complications of stasis **(Fig. 16.14B)**. It is rarely performed today.

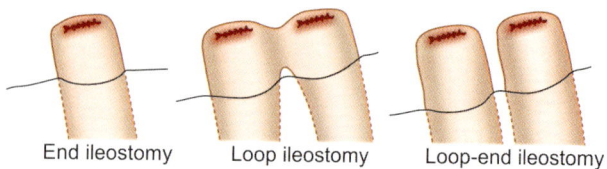

Fig. 16.14A: Types of ileostomies

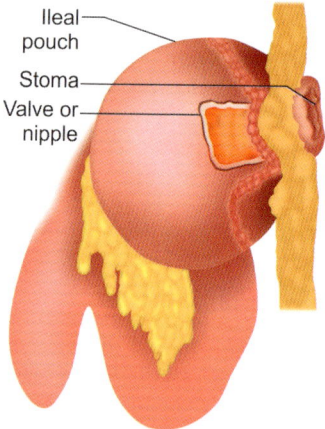

Fig. 16.14B: Koch's continent ileostomy

COLOSTOMY

There are five types of colostomies (**Fig. 16.15**). They are:
1. Loop colostomy
2. End colostomy (usually associated with excision of distal segment).
3. End colostomy with the distal segment closed (Hartmann's procedure).
4. Double barreled colostomy (Bloch-Paul-Mikulicz operation).
5. Divided colostomy (Devine)—colostomy with a skin island.

Preoperative bowel preparation of bowel is useful while creating a colostomy, but during emergency situation, and while creating an ileostomy, this may not be possible.

Diverting Stomas

- These stomas are expected to prevent fecal matter from reaching the area of potential leak (difficult anastomosis) or to treat a leak following traumatic injury, perforation or anastomotic leak
- The diverting stomas can be loop ostomy or an end loop ostomy, and both have the advantage of not requiring a laparotomy for takedown
- Loop ostomies are usually expected to be temporary
- Loop ostomies are created without dividing the mesenteric vessels, reducing the incidence of ischemia to virtually nil
- Between the loop ileostomy and loop transverse colostomy, the former is a better choice, as the advantage of the effluent less malodorous and is easier to pouch and manage.

Loop ostomies need closure, but this process can be done after a period of about 3 months, when the inflammation subsides and the purpose of diversion is achieved.

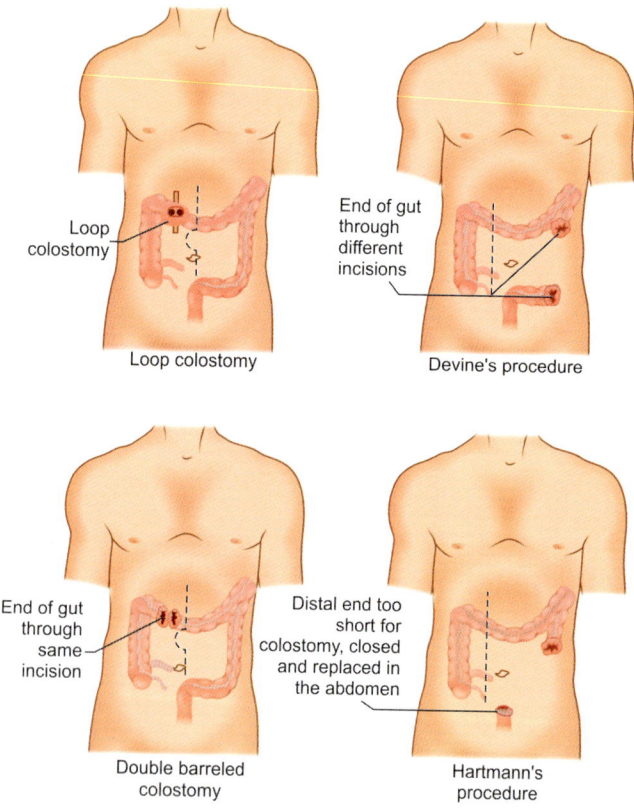

Fig. 16.15: Types of colostomy

Creation of Stomas

End Ostomy

Surgery Steps (Figs 16.16A and B)

- A circular opening of 5 cm diameter is made in the abdominal wall at the proposed site of ostomy
- A loop of intestine (colon) is selected, and divided between clamps
- The proximal intestine is brought out through the opening
- The bowel is fixed to the parietal peritoneum by sutures to prevent retraction
- The free end of the bowel is inverted and the mucosal edge is stitched to the skin edge with interrupted sutures at 1 cm intervals, with absorbable material.

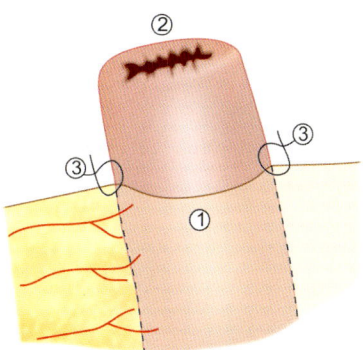

Fig. 16.16A: Surgical procedure

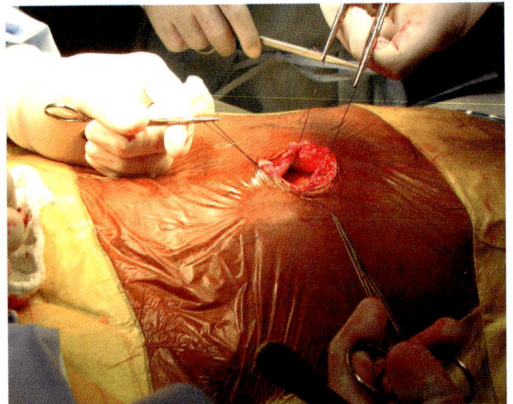

Fig. 16.16B1: Creating the hole for the stoma

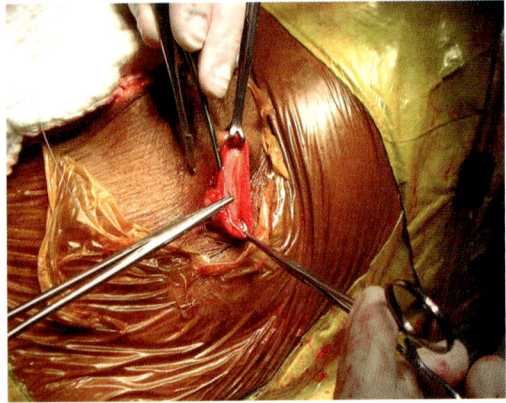

Fig. 16.16B2: Mucocutaneous suturing to create the stoma

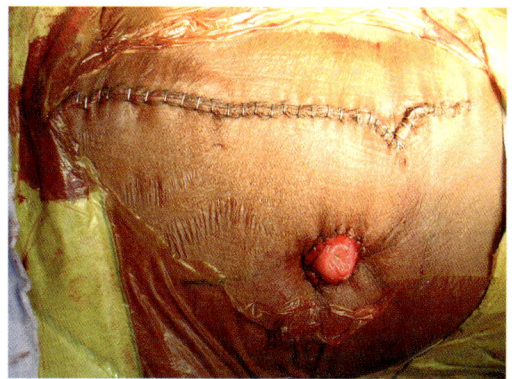

Fig. 16.16B3: End colostomy

Loop Ostomy (Figs 16.17A to D)

- A transverse incision is made at the chosen site, and the abdominal cavity reached
- A loop of bowel is picked up
- The bowel is kept stable using a rigid plastic tube, by inserting the tube through the mesentery in the avascular area
- The bowel is fixed to the parietal peritoneum with sutures
- The bowel is opened longitudinally
- The mucosal edge is stitched to the skin edge with interrupted sutures at 1 cm levels, with absorbable material.

End Loop Ostomy

The procedure is the same as for loop ostomy, but the loop is divided and the afferent and efferent loops are separated, and the end result is like two-end ostomies, *without a skin bridge*. It is also called 'double

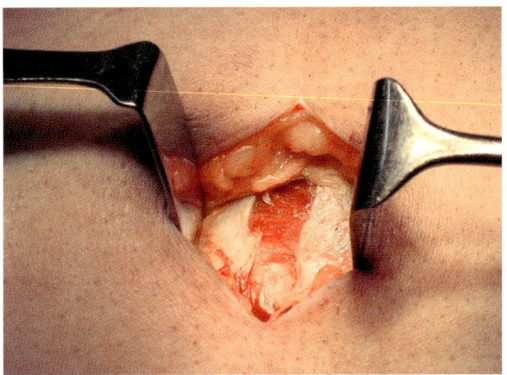

Fig. 16.17A: Opening the abdomen

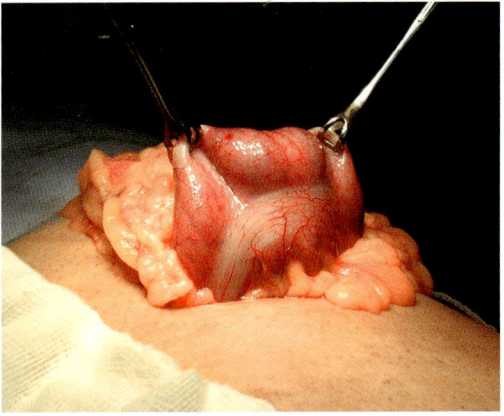

Fig. 16.17B: Picking the transverse colon loop

Intestinal Stomas

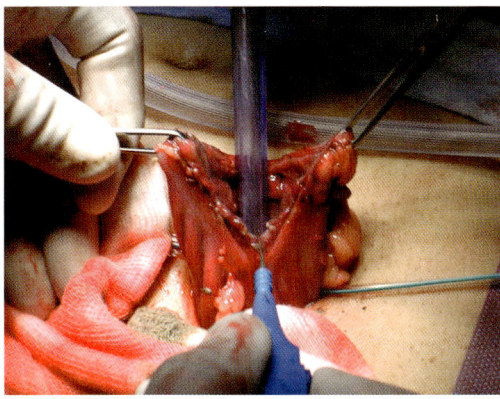

Fig. 16.17C: Opening the loop of the colon

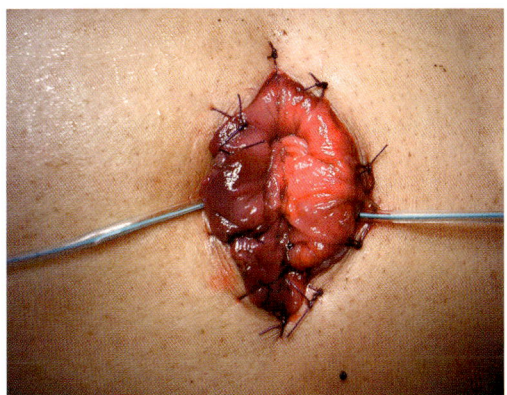

Fig. 16.17D: Mucocutaneous suturing to create the stoma

barreled colostomy'. The proximal bowel discharges the feces and the distal bowel secretes only mucus, hence called *'mucous fistula'*.

Divided Colostomy

The procedure is the same as for loop ostomy, but the loop is divided and the afferent and efferent loops are separated far away (or an intervening segment of bowel is excised) *with a skin bridge* and the end result is like two-end ostomies, *with a skin bridge*.

Hartmann's Operation

The procedure is like divided colostomy, but the distal bowel is closed with sutures or staples.

Clinical Pearls

- Maturation technique of the ostomies differ because of the effluent and the size of the lumen
- Due to the solid consistency of the colonic effluent, it is enough if the stoma is flat or with small protrusion, whereas for an ileostomy, the effluent is liquid, the stoma is expected to project 2 cm above the abdominal wall surface so that the effluent falls directly into the bag without excoriating the skin
- The mucocutaneous suturing is always advocated to prevent the indrawing of the stoma
- Occasionally, stoma may have to be created at unusual sites, but management of such stomata may be extremely difficult
- Hartmann's procedure is not indicated in distal obstructive lesions, as it may result in a closed loop and the pent-up secretions will cause rupture and peritonitis.

Postoperative Management of Ostomy

- Usually, the ostomy bag may be applied in the operation theater soon after the stoma is created
- Usually, the colostomy discharges feces by the second or third day; if not, there is no concern, so long as the patient is able to tolerate oral feeds. It is useful to insert a lubricated finger in the stoma to make sure that the stoma is not blocked by hard stools or a constriction. Sometimes, withdrawal of the finger is followed by a gush of feces. Insertion of bisacodyl suppositories may help to clear the distal bowel.

Long-term Management of Colostomy

An ostomy is a sphincterless opening. It takes about 3 months for the bowel to adapt, but it is never the same as the preoperative status. The regularity with which the colostomy functions may vary from one or two actions per day to an almost continuous discharge.

The colostomy can be controlled by two methods:

1. **Natural method**
   – A high fiber diet and a judicious use of laxatives can help in the restoration of normalcy.
2. **Irrigation**
   – The principle of irrigation is to keep the distal colon empty, as it displays a few mass peristaltic motions each day and that these can be stimulated by distension of intestine. A cone tip that fits into the stoma enough to provide a seal, is inserted into the stoma and about 500–1,000 mL of water is introduced. A drainage bag is applied, and the patient can proceed with morning chores. Once contractions are induced, the contents are evacuated through a spout or a large bore tube in the toilet. Many such irrigations can be made to empty the distal colon (**Figs 16.18A to D**).

Snapshots in Gastroenterology

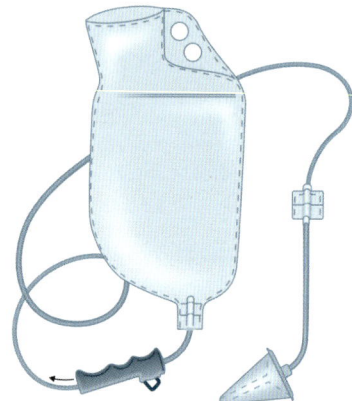

Fig. 16.18A: Irrigation bag

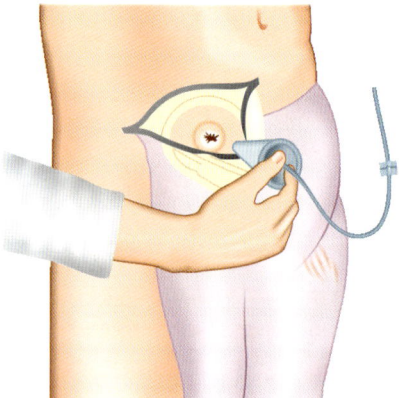

Fig. 16.18B: Introduction of spout for irrigation

Intestinal Stomas

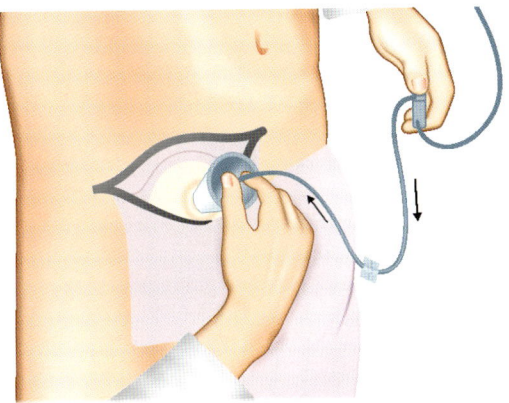

Fig. 16.18C: Irrigation in progress

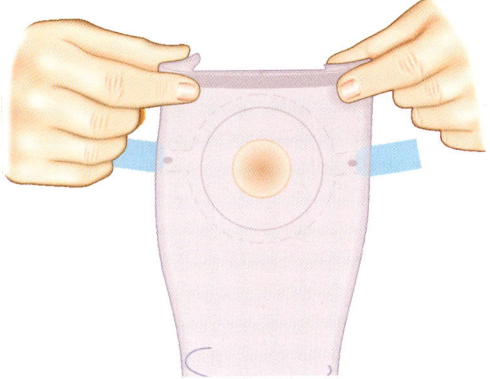

Fig. 16.18D: Application of bag after irrigation

The advantages of irrigation are:
- Reduction in the need for wearing the appliance at all times
- Provision of a more regulated lifestyle
- Reduced passage of uncontrolled gas
- Less leakage of stool between irrigations
- General feeling of comfort.

APPLIANCES

A variety of appliances are available in the market, and the patient should be made aware of them. There may be initial difficulties in the first few weeks in managing the appliance, but with practice, the patients develop skill and confidence in the management of appliances. The appliances are either,
- Adhesive or non-adhesive
- Disposable or non-disposable (reusable)
- Drainable or non-drainable.

Adhesive or Non-adhesive Appliance

Adhesive appliances are preferred to non-adhesive type, as they provide security from leakage and odor. The components are available either as a single piece or multiple components (flange and bag separately) (**Figs 16.19, and 16.20A and B**).

Disposable or Non-disposable (Reusable)

Disposable bags are made of thin plastic material, which can be either clear or opaque and may be decorated. They require to be changed daily. They are usually available as a single piece appliance. *Non-disposable bags* are usually of white or black carbonated

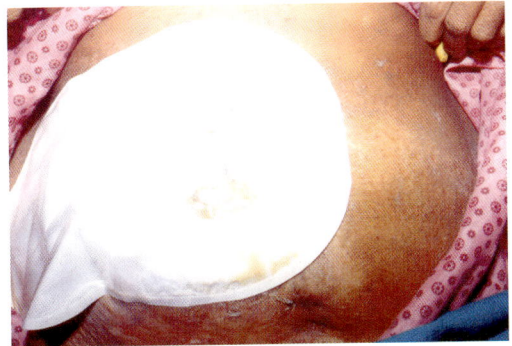

Fig. 16.19: One piece pouch

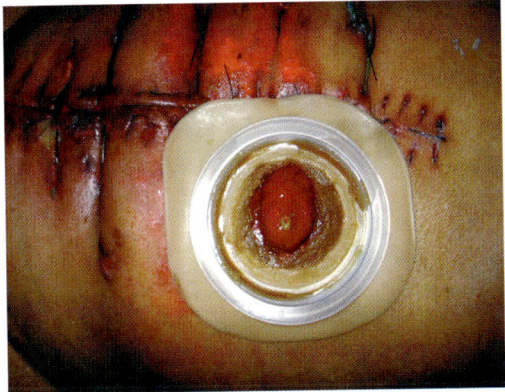

Fig. 16.20A: Flange of two piece appliance

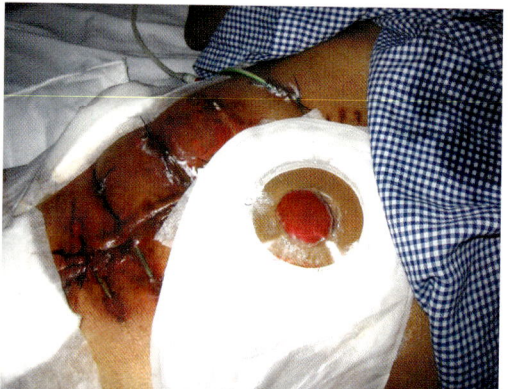

Fig. 16.20B: Drainage bag applied to the flange

rubber and require to be washed daily with soap and water, dried thoroughly and dusted with talcum powder, and they last for a month or two.

Drainable or Non-drainable

Drainable bags can be emptied, without being detached, by means of clip at the lower end of the bag. ***Non-drainable bags*** are usually single piece equipment, and are disposable.

Fitting the One Piece Appliance (Figs 16.21A and D):
- The stoma opening in the flange is cut to size of the stoma
- The flange is stuck to the dry skin after applying an adhesive like tincture benzoin

Intestinal Stomas

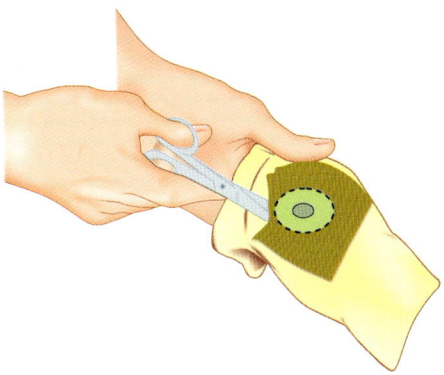

Fig. 16.21A: Cutting the flange to the size of stoma

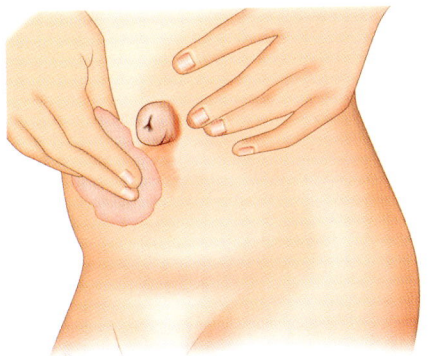

Fig. 16.21B: Preparation of skin

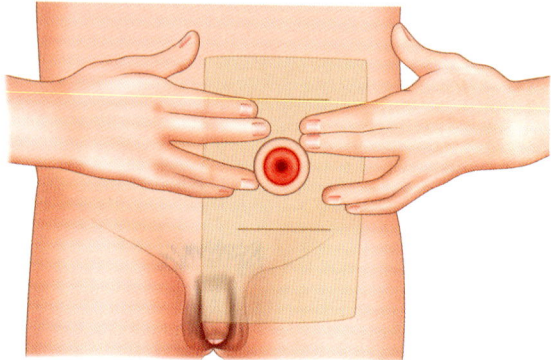

Fig. 16.21C: Sticking the bag

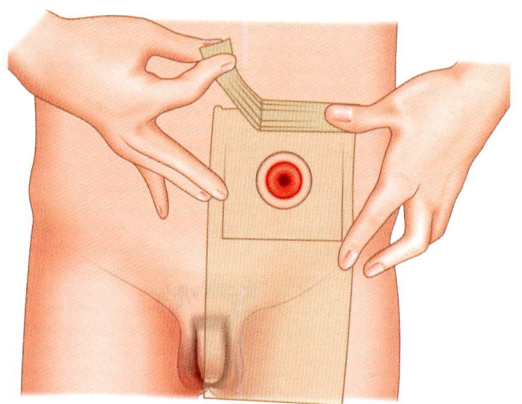

Fig. 16.21D: Application of plaster

- Hypoallergenic plaster is applied to the edges of the flange for extra protection.

Fitting the Two Piece Appliance (Fig. 16.22A to F)

- The stoma opening in the flange is cut to size of the stoma
- The flange is stuck to the dry skin after applying an adhesive like tincture benzoin
- The exposed skin in the space between the stoma and the flange is protected by zinc cream to prevent excoriation
- The bag is clipped to the flange
- Clip is applied to the outlet
- Belt in the flange may be tied around the abdomen for extra-protection.

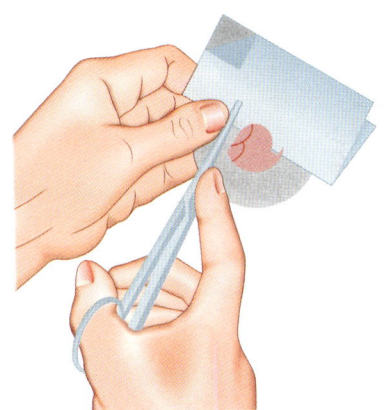

Fig. 16.22A: Cutting the flange to the size of stoma

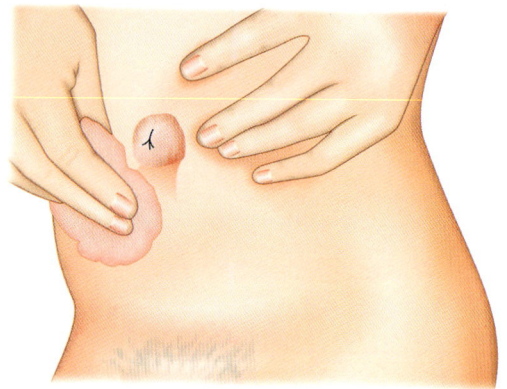

Fig. 16.22B: Preparation of skin

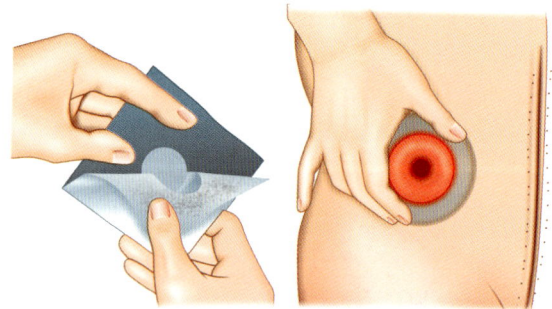

Fig. 16.22C: Sticking the flange

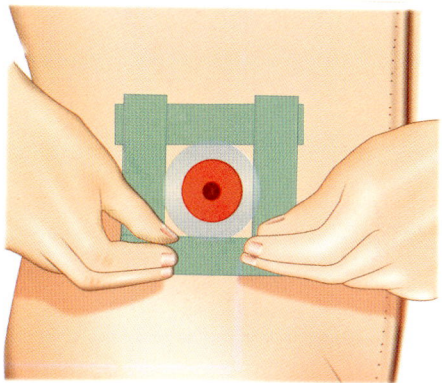

Fig. 16.22D: Reinforcing the flange

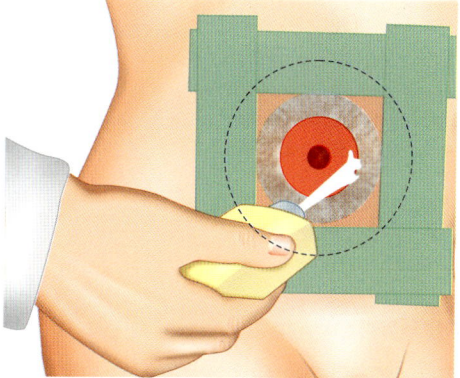

Fig. 16.22E: Application of skin protection cream

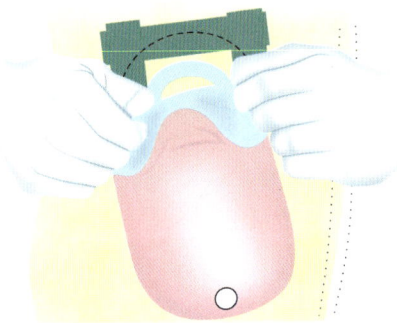

Fig. 16.22F: Application of bag to the flange

Emptying or Changing the Bag

The time at which the patient chooses to empty or change the bag will vary depending on the appliance used, frequency of the colostomy actions and his personal preference. It is not necessary to empty the bag as soon as the motion occurs, but many patients prefer to empty the bag, as a heavily loaded bag may snap from the abdominal wall and cause leakage. Removal of the flange is fairly easy by peeling it from the skin. If there is difficulty, it is better to ease the plaster with methylated ether.

Cleaning the Bag

It applies to the nondisposable bag, which can be done by regular washing with soap and water, and drying.

PROBLEMS

Problems of the Appliance

Odor

Most bags are odor free and appearance of bad odor indicates:
- Leakage
- An appliance left too long
- An old bag
- Incorrect fitting of the appliance.

Odor is not a problem for ileostomates, but is possible in some colostomates.

Management
- Consuming odor free diet
- Deodorizing sprays in the room
- Keeping deodorizing tablets in the bag
- Consuming deodorizing tablets like charcoal, bismuth subgallate before each meal or four times daily.

Leakage

Leakage occurs due to:
- Manufacturing defects in the bag
- Improperly applied clip to the drainage bag.

Management
- Proper preparation of bag for application
- Emptying it before it is full.

Detachment of Bag

The bag may get detached from the skin due to:
- Bag becoming full and heavy with the effluent
- Sudden twisting due to exercise

- Catching the bag between the thigh and bed on turning over in bed
- Consuming large meals in late evenings.

Management

- Emptying the bag before it is full
- Emptying the bag before severe exercise and retiring to bed
- Avoiding large meals in the evening.

Problems of the Adhesive

The principal problems with adhesive are due to:
- Inefficient and improper application
- Moist and unclean skin
  - Wrinkles in the plaster
  - Folds in the skin.

Management

- Cleaning and drying the skin before application of flange
- Application of adhesive additionally to the flange edges.

Problems of the Skin

Skin problems are much more common in ileostomates than in colostomates, as the effluent is more fluid and contains chemical irritants and digestive enzymes, which rapidly damage the skin. In all cases, skin lesions are largely preventable.

Trauma

Trauma is usually caused by frequent changing of bag and adhesive plaster.

Management

- Thorough drying of skin before application of adhesive
- Less frequent changes of adhesive plasters.

Skin irritation

This is very common in ileostomates, due to the liquid nature of effluent rich in enzymes.

Management

- Close fitting faceplate prevents the exposure of skin around the stoma
- Skin protective creams may be applied on the exposed skin to prevent skin irritation, but due care is to be taken that the cream should not interfere with the adherence of the faceplate.

Allergy

Allergic dermatitis secondary to wafer is not rare and is also associated with zinc oxide adhesive plaster.

Management

- Use of hypoallergenic adhesive plasters
- Topical corticosteroid creams
- Oral prednisolone.

COMPLICATIONS OF OSTOMY

Necrosis

The stoma may necrose due to inadequate blood supply, secondary to compression of the stoma by a tight opening. It presents with a color change and darkening of stoma occurs (**Fig. 16.23A**). Early recognition is important and release of tight opening may be

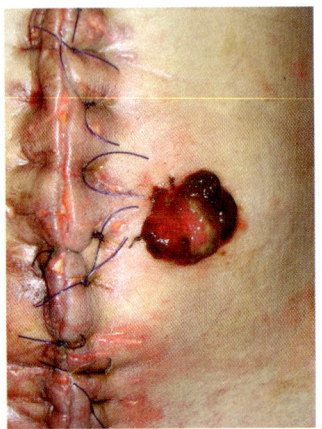 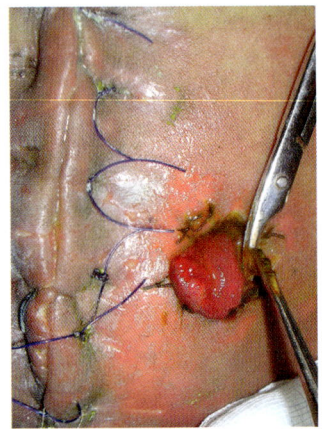

Fig. 16.23A: Mucosal slough of ileostomy

Fig. 16.23B: Excision of mucosal slough

necessary if expectant treatment fails. The necrosed edges may have to be excised (**Fig. 16.23B**).

Mucocutaneous Infection

The mucocutaneous margin may get infected due to fecal contamination, which is recognized by purulent discharge. It is managed by antibiotics, and dressings. This injury heals by secondary intention.

Separation of Ostomy

When the mucocutaneous junction heals after infection, the skin edges may separate from the stoma (**Fig. 16.24**). Expectant treatment with antibiotics is sufficient.

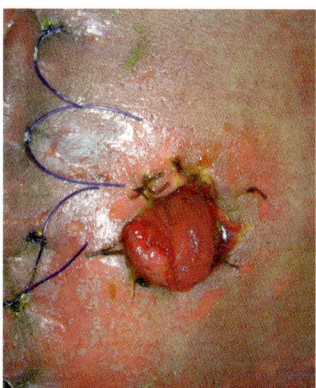

Fig. 16.24: Separation of ostomy

Stricture, Stenosis and Retraction

Following the infection of mucocutaneous junction, healing occurs by secondary intention. This healing process leads to circumferential stricture, constricting the stoma, resulting in stricture or stenosis (long segment stricture). The stenosed stoma may also retract below the skin surface (**Fig. 16.25A**). Patient presents with constipation and passes feces through the stoma with difficulty (**Fig. 16.25B**). This may be treated by dilatation using a lubricated finger or a dilator (**Fig. 16.25C**). If this is not beneficial, the stoma is detached fully, and the stoma is reconstructed at the same site or a little away (**Fig. 16.25D**).

Prolapse

When the healing occurs, and the adhesions do not occur between the stoma edge and skin edge, the stoma remains unsupported

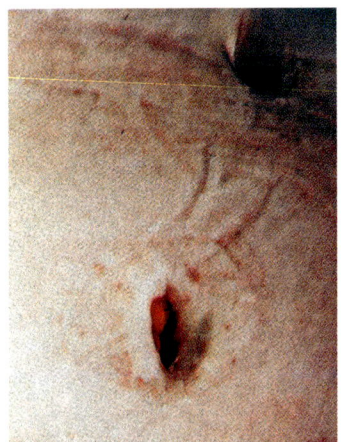

Fig. 16.25A: Stenosis of ileostomy

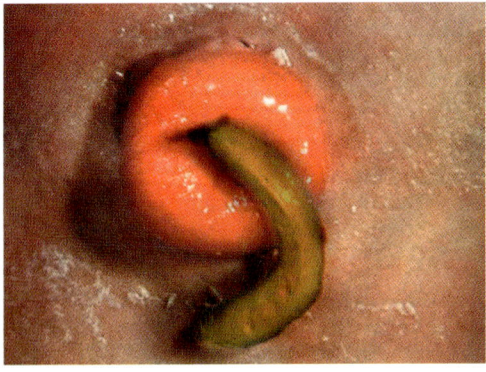

Fig. 16.25B: Passage of thin fecal matter

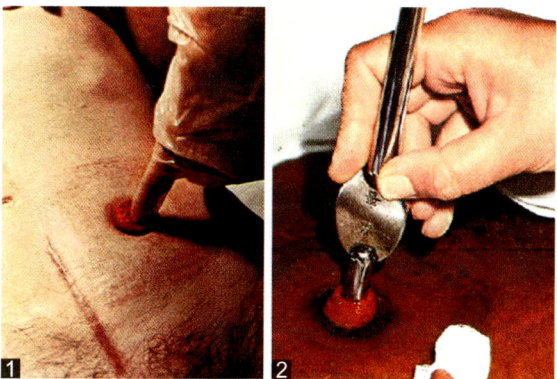

Fig. 16.25C: Dilatation of stenosis of stoma with (1) Finger; (2) Dilator

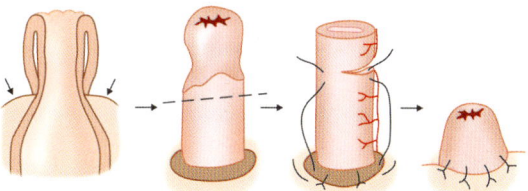

Fig. 16.25D: Operative treatment of ileostomy stenosis

and it may prolapse (**Fig. 16.26A**). This can occur if the colostomy is constructed when the colon ixs dilated during the procedure and gets decompressed after the procedure, or a long segment of bowel is left outside the skin. Surgical treatment is necessary, i.e. the stoma is detached fully, and the stoma is reconstructed away from the original site (**Fig. 16.26B**).

Snapshots in Gastroenterology

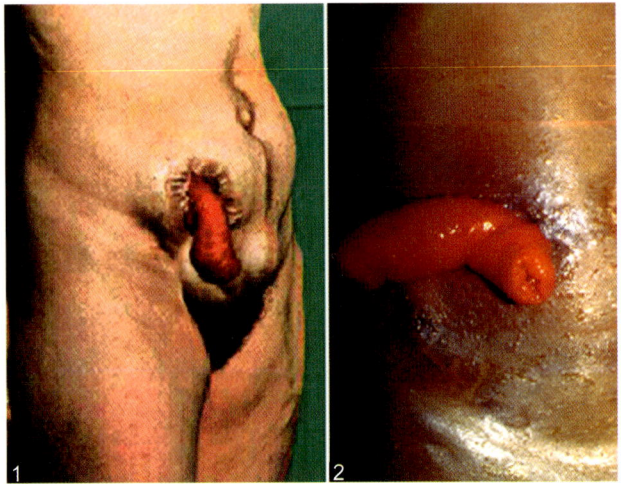

Fig. 16.26A: Prolapse of (1) End ileostomy; (2) Loop ileostomy

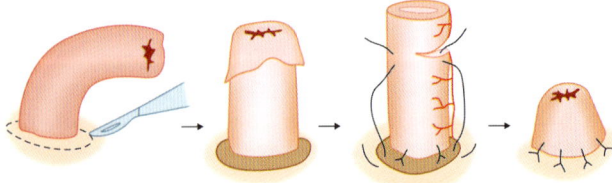

Fig. 16.26B: Operative treatment of ileostomy prolapse

Parastomal Hernia

When the stoma is not created through the rectus muscle, and left without muscular support, the paracolic part of the abdominal wall may show weakness and a hernia may result. This presents with a reducible swelling in the parastomal region (**Fig. 16.27A**). They can be managed with special corsets and girdles. The stoma needs revision, with strengthening of the muscle layers with a synthetic mesh (**Fig. 16.27B**). Mercedes repair is one of the surgical methods to treat parastomal hernia (**Fig. 16.27C**).

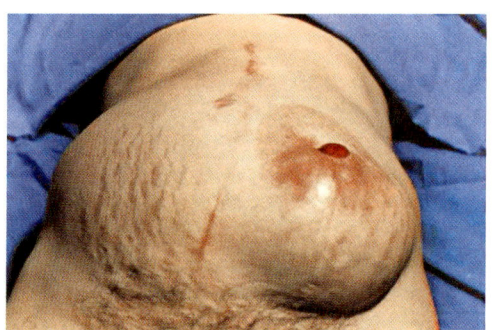

Fig. 16.27A: Paracolostomy hernia

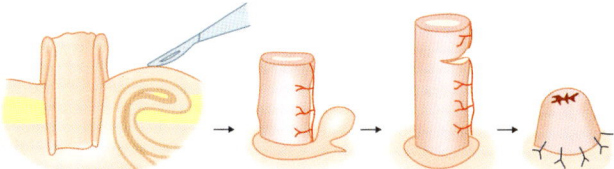

Fig. 16.27B: Operative repair of parastomal hernia

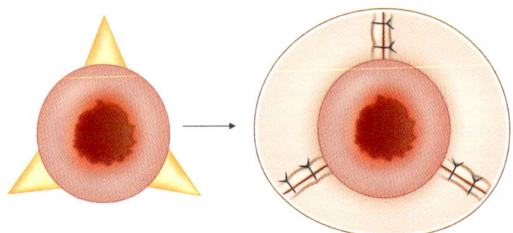

Fig. 16.27C: Mercedes repair of parastomal hernia

Fistula Formation

Deep sutures between the bowel and the rectus fascia cause infection and an abscess, when opens spontaneously or surgically results in a parastomal fistula (**Fig. 16.28**). Fistulogram may be necessary for confirmation. If the external opening of fistula is close to the stoma, no treatment may be required. If the opening is far away and interferes with the application of the bag, fistulectomy is needed, and the entire stoma may have to be revised.

Perforation

Careless irrigation technique using a rigid tube can cause perforation of the colon near the stoma. Leaking of contents may cause peritonitis. Revision of stoma is necessary.

Diversion Colitis

Inflammation of distal bypassed colon after ileostomy or colostomy occurs due to luminal nutrient deficiency, and factors like dietary constituents or bacterial products. Local pain is the presentation.

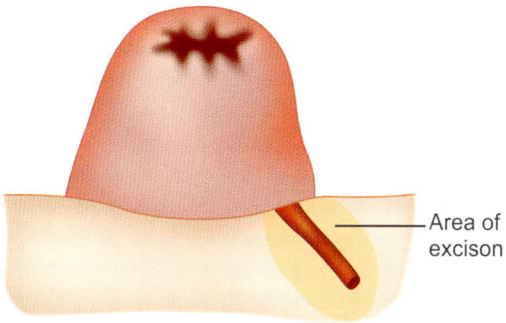

Fig. 16.28: Operative treatment of paraileostomy fistula

Endoscopy is diagnostic and differentiating from Crohn's disease may be difficult, and rectal sparing may be useful.

Clinical Pearls

- Despite similarities, each stoma presents with different problems
- Since the average person is repelled by the thought of an artificial anus, and does not even understand about the incontinent ostomy, many sittings may be required or an interaction with another ostomate (through ostomy clubs) may be necessary
- It should be highlighted that the patient can go back to his profession and activities as in the preoperative situation
- The patients with stoma, called ostomates, gain experience every day, managing their stoma, and become more knowledgeable than the doctors who treat them
- The fascial incision should be made larger, because a late hernia is preferable to early necrosis and retraction of stoma

- Loop end ileostomy may be used as a primary procedure for the definitive stoma for patients with ileal urinary conduits, and for conversion of previous loop ileostomy to end-loop ileostomy by transecting and closing the efferent limb to leave it inside the peritoneal cavity.

CONTINENT ILEOSTOMY

The continent ileostomy, which was first reported by Nils Koch in 1969 involves the construction of an internal reservoir using the terminal ileum; a reverse nipple outflow valve is made by intussuscepting the last few centimeters of ileum, and placing the stoma discretely out of sight in the suprapubic area. This procedure can be done at the time of total colectomy for ulcerative colitis and familial polyposis, or later if the patient fails to adapt to a conventional ileostomy.

Postoperative Management

The patient comes out of the operation theater with a plastic catheter in the ileostomy and connected to a urobag for continuous drainage and this needs special care.

The ileal mucosa exposed at the stoma needs to be examined periodically for the first 24–36 hours for pink color for its viability. The discharge through the tube in the first 2 or 3 days is bloodstained. The fluid assumes a fecal character and thenceforth it is satisfactory. When the fecal matter does not appear, it should be suspected for:
- Paralytic ileus
- Mechanical obstruction proximal to the reservoir
- Retention of feces due to faulty siting of tube
- Retention of feces due to slipping of tube associated with edema of the valve.

The tube may be manipulated carefully, and its position can be confirmed with a contrast study. If the ileostomy continues to be inactive beyond 5 or 6 days, the need for reoperation will arise.

The tube is kept for about 4 weeks, and a pantaloonogram obtained. Intermittent clamping is done for 10 minutes every 3 hours for 7–10 days. After 4 weeks the indwelling tube is removed and intermittent catheterization practised, at every 3 hours during the day and once at night. The night intubation may be omitted gradually and the day intubations are done rather frequently.

The convenient tube for intermittent intubation is a translucent 28F. While the patient stands or sits, the lubricated tube is introduced into the stoma, directed backwards, inwards and slightly downwards, or in any direction the patient is experienced. When the tube enters the reservoir, usually at about 10 cm, the intestinal contents gush out of the tube, and the external end of the tube is held in a mug or kidney tray to catch the discharge. Washes may also be given with the tube, till complete evacuation is achieved. The stoma may be closed with a gauze and strapped. If there is leakage, ordinary ileostomy bag may be worn for some part of 24 hours.

COMPLICATIONS

Nipple Valve Slippage

This is the most common complication after continent ileostomy, which may require surgical revision.

Leakage from Suture Lines

Breakdown of suture lines may cause leakage of intestinal contents into the peritoneal cavity causing peritonitis. Clinically, the patient may present with tachycardia, abdominal distension and signs of peritonitis. Small leaks resolve without any specific treatment. Relaparotomy may be required for peritoneal toileting and convert the pouch into a conventional ileostomy.

Necrosis of the Exit Conduit

Avascularity of the conduit may give rise to necrosis. Clinically, it presents with bloody discharge, and the mucosa may turn blue or black. Some may settle spontaneously, but severe necrosis results in converting a reservoir to a conventional ileostomy.

Fecal Incontinence

Fecal incontinence occurs due to deterioration in the efficacy of the valve because of partial or complete extrusion, and development of a perforation or a fistula. When the incontinence is minimal, intermittent intubation is sufficient. When the incontinence is gross, intubation is never easy as the exit conduit is angulated due to extruded valve, and wearing a ileostomy bag is the only option.
For gross incontinence, surgical procedures can help. They are:
- Reconstruction of the original nipple-valve
- Construction of a new nipple-valve
- Creating a new reservoir
- Use of indwelling ileostomy valve device.

Retention

Extrusion of valve and stomal stenosis can create a situation of total obstipation, not passing flatus or feces. Careful and meticulous intubation if attempted may give relief. Surgical procedures mentioned for managing fecal incontinence will help.

Profuse Diarrhea

Inflammation of the pouch, called pouchitis, with associated bacterial overgrowth can cause profuse diarrhea. Antibiotics will help.

Volvulus of Reservoir

Due to the weight, the entire reservoir can twist around its axis, and cause torsion. Plain X-rays may show a distended reservoir, with air fluid level. Treatment is to do detorsion and if the viability is lost, revision of pouch or converting it into a conventional ileostomy is the only answer.

The advantages of Koch's continent ileostomy are:
- The patient need not wear an appliance
- The patient is continent between irrigations
- No stoma complications
- Better quality of life.

The disadvantages of Koch's continent ileostomy are:
- Not all patients are continent
- Require multiple intubations during the day
- Can be difficult to intubate
- Surgery is prolonged
- If the procedure fails, the patient will lose a significant amount of small intestine.

Clinical Pearls

- A thorough search for Crohn's disease should be done in the proximal bowel before contemplating for a continent ileostomy pouch, because of the increased risk of disease in the pouch
- A detailed discussion is necessary with the patient about the potential complications of pouch, which may end up in a conventional Brooke ileostomy.

Chapter 17

Liver

SURGICAL ANATOMY

The liver is the larger organ in the body occupying the right upper quadrant of the abdominal cavity. An imaginary line (Cantlie's line) running from the medial aspect of the gallbladder fossa to the medial side of inferior vena cava, which marks the course of middle hepatic vein divides the liver into left and right lobes. The liver is divided into eight segments based on the portal triads (hepatic artery, portal vein and biliary duct) and hepatic veins. Of the eight segments,

- Segments I–IV constitute the left lobe of the liver and
- Segments V–VIII constitute the right lobe of the liver.

Right hepatic vein subdivides the right liver into anterior (segments V and VIII) and posterior (segments VI and VII) sectors. Umbilical fissure subdivides the left liver into medial sector (segment IV) and left lateral segment (segments II and III).

Segment I is named the caudate lobe and sometimes segment IV of Couinaud's classification is called in Anglo–Saxon system as a quadrate lobe.

Of the many classifications, those described by Couinaud and Bismuth are compared in **Table 17.1**.

Table 17.1: Classifications of Couinaud and Bismuth (**Figs 17.1A and B**)

	Classifications			
	C. Couinaud (1957)		**H. Bismuth (1982)**	
Part	Sector	Segment	Sector	Segment
Dorsal	Caudate lobe	I	Caudate lobe	I
Left	Lateral	II	Posterior	II
	Paramedian	III	Anterior	III
		IV		IVA, IVB
Right	Paramedian	V	Anteromedial	V
		VIII		VIII
	Lateral	VI	Posterolateral	VI
		VII		VII

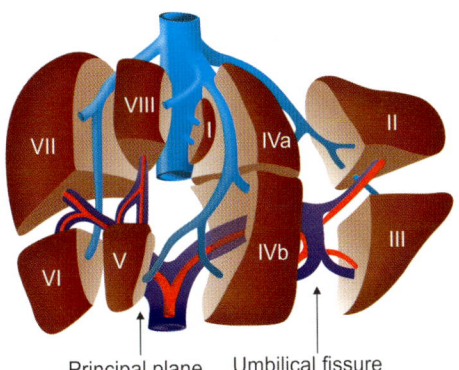

Fig. 17.1A: Bismuth classification of liver segments

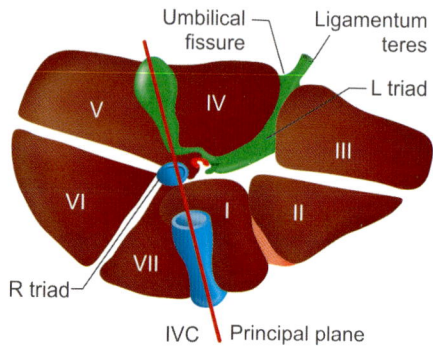

Fig. 17.1B: Bismuth classification of liver segments (ventral view)

Portal Circulation

Portal vein is formed by the confluence of splenic vein and superior mesenteric vein. This runs in the hepatoduodenal ligament posteromedial to the common bile duct. This divides into left and right branches before entering the liver substance. The right branch divides into anterior and posterior sectoral branches. The left branch divides into branches for segments II, III and IV. Inferior mesenteric vein drains into the splenic vein, just proximal to its formation of portal vein.

Venous Drainage

Hepatic veins ultimately drain the lobules of the liver. There are three hepatic veins, left, right and middle. The right hepatic vein drains into the inferior vena cava directly, while the middle and the left

hepatic veins join to form a common trunk to drain into the inferior vena cava.
- Right hepatic vein drains the posterior sectors of right liver (segments VI and VII)
- Middle hepatic vein drains segment IV and anterior sectors of right liver (segments V and VIII)
- Left hepatic vein drains segments II and III.

Small umbilical vein runs within the umbilical fissure provides accessory drainage for segments III and IV and empties into the left hepatic vein.

Arterial Supply

The common hepatic artery arises from the celiac axis, and ascends in the hepatoduodenal ligament and gives rise to right gastric, gastroduodenal and proper hepatic arteries. The proper hepatic artery divides into right and left hepatic arteries, to supply the right and left lobes of the liver, respectively.

Biliary Drainage

Biliary tree arises within the liver from the specialized segments of the hepatic membrane, as bile canaliculi. These canaliculi progressively become larger to form segmental bile ducts. Right anterior and right posterior sectoral ducts unite to form the right hepatic duct, while ducts draining the II, III and IV unite to form the left hepatic duct. Duct of segment I drains into the left hepatic duct. The right and left hepatic ducts unite to form the common hepatic duct, which descends in the free edge of the hepatoduodenal ligament, which is joined by the cystic duct at a variable distance to form the common bile duct.

Lymphatics

Lymphatics of the superficial lobules follow the subcapsular course to the diaphragm, and the suspensory ligaments of the liver and posterior mediastinum. Lymphatics of the deeper lobules travel with the hepatic veins along the inferior vena cava or along the portal veins to the porta hepatis.

Nerves

- Sympathetic nervous system from T7 to T10 segments
- Parasympathetic from right and left vagus nerves.

Clinical Pearls

- 75% of blood supply of the liver is from the portal vein and 25% is from the hepatic artery
- Hepatic artery, portal vein and bile duct which are separate before entering the liver, enter together in a sheath within a thickened layer of Glisson capsule.

PHYSIOLOGY

Formation of Bile

The hepatocytes produce bile at a rate of 500–1500 mL/day. The volume, sodium and water content are maintained by the bile salts. Apart from bile, many other constituents like bilirubin, and anions like estrogens, sulfobromophthalein are secreted by the hepatocytes.

The columnar cells of the bile ducts secrete a fluid rich in bicarbonate by a cellular pump stimulated by secretin, VIP, and cholecystokinin. The factors, which regulate bile flow, are:

- Secretion by the liver cell
- Gallbladder concentration
- Bile duct sphincter resistance.

Composition of Bile

Bile is a complex fluid containing organic and inorganic substances. This alkaline fluid contains about 10% solids and of them, 90% is formed by bile salts, lecithin and cholesterol. The remainder consists of bilirubin, fatty acids and inorganic salts.

Bile acids are derivatives of cholesterol synthesized in the liver cell. Dietary cholesterol is converted into cholic acid and chenodeoxycholic acid, which are conjugated to glycine or taurine to form water-soluble salts, cholate and chenodeoxycholate. Intestinal bacteria convert them into secondary bile salts, deoxycholate and lithocholate, by removing the hydroxyl group, of which the former is water soluble and enters the bile, but the latter which is insoluble is excreted in the feces. Bile salts take part in the digestion and absorption of fat throughout the jejunum. In the terminal ileum, they are reabsorbed through enterohepatic circulation. Finally, about 10–15% of the total pool of bile salts is lost in the stools. Bile salts along with the phospholipids, take care of digestion and absorption of lipids and lipid-soluble vitamins and to eliminate waste products (bilirubin and cholesterol) through secretion into bile and elimination in stools.

Bilirubin Metabolism (Refer Table 8.1)

Bilirubin is a byproduct of heme synthesis, which is carried to the liver bound to albumin. In the liver, it is conjugated to glucuronic acid (two molecules), catalyzed by glucuronyl transferase to form bilirubin diglucuronide, which is excreted in the bile canaliculi.

The conjugated bilirubin is excreted in the intestine though bile as waste, which is reabsorbed in the intestine and in the kidney to form the urobilinogen and excreted in the urine. The intestinal bacteria convert the conjugated bilirubin to stercobilinogen and stercobilin to be excreted in the feces. In obstructive jaundice, conjugated bilirubinemia occurs along with the absence of urobilinogen due to the absence of conjugated bilirubin in the intestine and kidney.

Vascular Physiology

The blood flow in the liver is about 1,500 mL/min (25% of cardiac output), but it is uniform. It is regulated by many factors of which the muscular sphincters at the sinusoids are the major factors. Other factors are, the autonomic nervous stimulation, circulating hormones, bile salts and metabolites. Portal and hepatic blood become pooled at the periphery of the liver sinusoid, the hepatic arterial flow adjusts to the portal venous flow, to maintain a balance and not vice versa. This mechanism is controlled by adenosine. Since the hepatic blood flow is far less when compared to portal venous flow, sudden occlusion of hepatic arterial flow has very little impact on the hepatic function, unless associated with biliary obstruction.

APPROACH TO THE PATIENT WITH LIVER DISEASE

While most patients with liver disease present with symptoms related to the system, variety of nonhepatic manifestations provide clues to otherwise normal hepatobiliary system. Hence, meticulous history taking becomes important and carries great significance. Commonly the liver diseases present with the following symptoms:
- Yellowing discoloration of conjunctivae (**Fig. 17.2**) urine and skin (Jaundice)

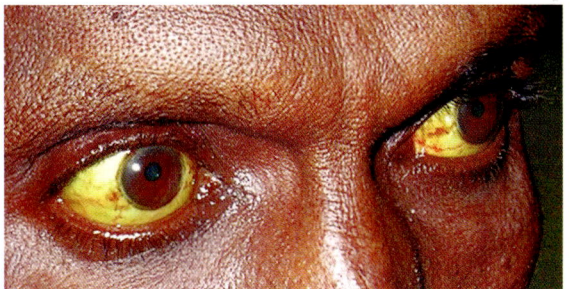

Fig. 17.2: Jaundice

- Pain in the right upper abdomen
- Appetite loss or aversion to food
- Weight loss
- Fever.

Other histories become relevant due to various reasons **(Table 17.2)**.

Symptoms

- Jaundice
  - Acute onset of jaundice, with prodromal symptoms nausea, anorexia, aversion to food—Hepatitis
  - Fluctuating jaundice may indicate choledocholithiasis or periampullary carcinoma, though the latter is painless
  - Persistent or increasing levels of jaundice may indicate obstruction of the bile ducts due to malignancy (e.g. cholangiocarcinoma, pancreatic head malignancy)
- Fever with chills indicate acute cholangitis, a severe condition
- Weight loss and appetite loss associated with jaundice may suspect a malignancy

Table 17.2: Eliciting history and its relevance

History	Symptoms	Relevance
Family history	Jaundice, anemia, splenectomy or cholecystectomy	Hemolytic anemia, congenital or familial hyperbilirubinemia, gallstones
	Tremor and neurological abnormalities	Wilson's disease
Occupational and environmental history	Contact with dogs and pets	Hydatid disease
Exposure to toxins (carbon tetracycline, beryllium and vinyl chloride)		Weil's disease, hepatitis
Consumptions of hepatotoxic drugs (chlorpromazine, contraceptives)		Drug-induced hepatitis
Travel to other countries		Endemic infections such as amebic hepatitis
Consumption of alcohol		Alcoholic hepatitis
Contact with jaundiced patients		Hepatitis B infections
Injections in the previous 6 months		
Past history	Indigestion, fat intolerance, right upper abdominal pain, jaundice	Hepatitis
Immunization against hepatic viruses		Used to eliminate hepatitis from differential diagnosis

- Pruritus is a common feature of cholestasis
- Abdominal pain
  - Acute upper abdominal pain may indicate biliary colic commonly due to obstructing calculus in the bile duct
  - Chronic upper abdominal pain may indicate a liver pathology (e.g. chronic hepatitis, liver malignancy—primary or secondary)
- Change in mental state and neurological function may indicate the level of hepatic failure.

Signs

Skin

- Ecchymosis of skin (indicates prothrombin deficiency)
- Purpura (indicates thrombocytopenia)
- Pallor (indicates anemia)
- Slate color of skin (increased melanin in hemochromatosis)
- Spider angiomas (indicate capillary fragility)
- Dilated veins around the umbilicus (caput medusae)
- Palmar erythema (indicates local vasodilation due to body androgen imbalance)
- Scratch marks (indicates severe jaundice)
- Finger clubbing
- Xanthoma of eyelids
- Flapping tremors of hands (indicates encephalopathy).

Abdomen

- Distension of abdomen (due to ascites)
- Nontender hepatomegaly
  - Smooth liver (hepatitis)
  - Nodular liver (malignancy)
- Tender hepatomegaly (hepatitis, abscess)

- Friction rub (e.g, hepatic abscess, malignancy)
- Venous hum or bruit (indicates portal hypertension).

Physical Examination

General Examination

- **General build**
    - Emaciated—Malignant causes
    - Distended abdomen—Ascites
- **Eyes**
    - Sclerae for the depth of jaundice
    - Conjunctivae for pallor and anemia
- **Skin**
    - Dry scaly skin—Malignancies
    - Scratch marks—Obstructive jaundice
    - Xanthomas
- **Examination for signs of liver failure**
    - Palmar erythema
    - Spider nevi (**Fig. 17.3A**),
    - Ascites (**Fig. 17.3B**)
    - Fetor hepaticus
    - Gynecomazia
    - Testicular atrophy
    - Clubbing of fingers
    - Pedal edema
    - Flapping tremor.

Vital Signs

- Recording of pulse and blood pressure
- Recording of temperature

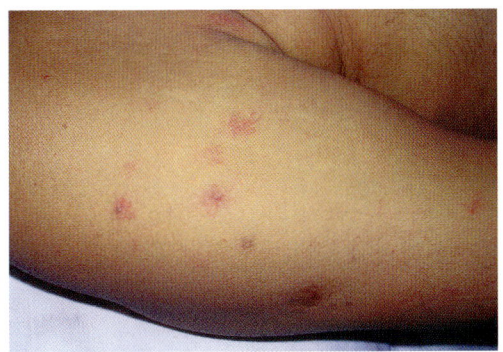

Fig. 17.3A: Spider nevi of hepatic failure

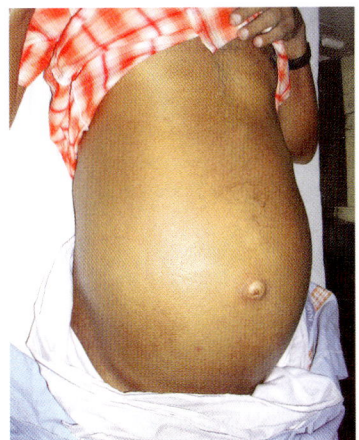

Fig. 17.3B: Ascites

– Elevated temperature (e.g. high—cholangitis, viremia, septicemia and liver abscess, mild—hepatic malignancies).

Examination of Abdomen

- Abdominal wall
  - Scars may indicate previous surgery
  - Caput medusae indicates liver failure and portal hypertension
- Abdomen: Examination should include procedures for determination of:
  - Ascites or free fluid in the abdomen (e.g. liver failure, malignancy)
  - Hepatomegaly (e.g. fine nodular liver of cirrhosis, nodular hard hepatomegaly of malignancy)
  - Splenomegaly (e.g. congenital hemolytic anemia, portal hypertension)
  - Enlargement of gallbladder (e.g. malignancy of pancreas or gallbladder)
  - Intra-abdominal lumps (e.g. malignancy, lymph node enlargement)
- Rectal examination: Rectal examination is mandatory and is useful in determining the presence of primary rectal malignancy or malignant deposits in the pouch of Douglas.

Investigations

1. **Urine examination**
   - ***Bile salts*** presence in the urine indicate bilirubinuria
   - ***Urobilinogen***—absence indicates obstructive jaundice and excess indicates hemolytic jaundice.
2. **Stool examination**
   - ***Bile pigment***—absence indicates obstructive jaundice, and excess amount indicates hemolytic jaundice

- *Positive occult blood* suggests gastrointestinal malignancy, bleeding esophageal varices.

3. **Hematology**
   - *Hemoglobin* for anemia
   - *Total and differential leukocyte count,* e.g. infections
   - *ESR* may be raised in infections and malignancies.

4. **Liver function tests**
   Tests to assess liver's capacity to transport organic anions and to metabolize drugs.
   - *Bilirubin*, a turnover product of red blood cells and its level remains constant in blood. Hyperbilirubinemia indicates several scenarios, like
     - Overproduction—*increased unconjugated bilirubin*-inherited disorders like Gilbert's syndrome.
     - Hepatocellular injury—*increased unconjugated bilirubin*—viral hepatitis
     - Obstruction to bile flow—*increased conjugated bilirubin*-obstructive lesions of bile duct.

   Tests to assess the hepatocyte injury:
   - *Transaminases (aspartate aminotransferase—AST and alanine aminotransferase—ALT)* levels are raised in hepatocellular damage (e.g. viral hepatitis). In most liver diseases ALT is greater than AST. When AST is elevated higher than ALT (ratio >2), alcoholic liver disease is suspected
   - *Alkaline phosphatase* elevation indicates injury to bile ducts, both intrahepatic and extrahepatic. It is also found in the bone, and to a lesser extent in the placenta and intestine, and its origin is not important and difficult to find. Due to its long half-life, it takes many days to normalize even after resolution of disease

- *5 nucleotidase (5NT)* is another enzyme, which parallels hepatic alkaline phosphatase, and elevation of both 5NT and alkaline phosphatase will indicate liver pathology
- *Gamma glutamyl transferase (GGT)* parallels hepatic alkaline phosphatase, and elevation of both GGT and alkaline phosphatase will indicate liver pathology. GGT is an early marker and a sensitive marker of hepatobiliary disease. It is non-specific and is elevated in alcoholic liver disease, pancreatic disease, myocardial infarction, renal failure and COPD
- *Lactate dehydrogenase (LDH)* increase is seen in hepatocellular necrosis, shock liver. ALT:LDH ratio of >1.5 may have a role in differentiating acute viral hepatitis from shock liver and acetaminophen toxicity where the ratio is <1.5.

Tests to assess liver's biosynthetic capacity:

- *Albumin* is a protein synthesized in the liver and measurement of its concentration is a reasonable test of synthetic capacity of liver. So also, loss of albumin, in renal and intestinal diseases can reduce albumin levels in the blood. This difference should be noted, while hypoalbuminemia is related to the liver. Albumin globulin ratio gets reversed in hepatocellular damage
- *Prothrombin time (PT)* measurement is a reliable marker of liver function. Excepting factor VIII, all the clotting factors are produced by the liver. Since clotting proteins require vitamin K as a cofactor, its deficiency causes prolonged PT. PT can be corrected in 12–24 hours, by administering vitamin K parenterally or as fresh frozen plasma.

5. Serological tests
    - *Hepatitis virus antigen and antibodies* (e.g. viral hepatitis)
    - *Antibodies to ANA, SMA,* etc. (e.g. autoimmune hepatitis)

- *DNA viral evaluation* for determining the viral loads
- *Alpha fetoprotein* is normally produced by the liver and fetal yolk. It is elevated in hepatoblastoma and hepatocellular carcinoma, germline tumors (testicular seminoma, teratoma, ovarian tumors), metastatic tumors of liver, active liver disease and mothers with neural tube defect children. In liver disease, its elevation is correlated with the size of HCC but not elevated in 30% of cases. Alone, its elevation is of no significance. The elevation needs to be supported by other diagnostic features like US, CT.

6. Radiology
    - *Plain X-rays of abdomen* (AP view) may show lesions like calcified hydatid
    - *US of abdomen* may be useful in assessing the liver parenchyma (e.g. fatty liver, malignant deposits, cirrhosis) and biliary system (e.g. nature and level of obstruction of biliary tree)
    - *CT or MRI scan* (e.g. fatty liver, nature and level of obstruction of biliary tree)
    - *Elastography (US/MRI)*—a method of estimating liver stiffness and measure hepatic fibrosis
    - *Contrast studies*
        ♦ *ERCP* Administration of radiopaque dye into the biliary tree by ERCP may identify the underlying cause (e.g. CBD stones, ductal malignancies)
        ♦ *MRCP* has the advantage of being noninvasive with same accuracy
        ♦ *Percutaneous transhepatic cholangiogram (PTC)* involves injection of water soluble contrast directly into the dilated intrahepatic portal radical using a fine needle is ideal for demonstrating an extrahepatic obstruction, which cannot

be reached through ERCP, and also for stenting to relieve jaundice.
7. **Radionuclide studies (HIDA):** Technetium^{99} labeled derivatives of iminodiacetic acid are excreted in high concentration in bile to produce excellent gamma camera images. Bile duct visualization is helpful in fistulas, but anatomical details are poorly displayed.
8. **Endoscopy**
    - *Upper gastrointestinal endoscopy* is important to identify the upper GI causes (e.g. esophageal varices, malignancies)
    - *Total colonoscopy* may be needed to eliminate primary colorectal cancer
    - *Proctoscopy* is an inherent part of rectal examination, and is a mandatory investigation to make a clinical diagnosis
    - *Laparoscopy* as diagnostic tool and for obtaining biopsies (e.g. cirrhosis of liver)
    - *Spyglass cholangiography* to directly visualize and treat the cause.
9. *Biopsy* image guided biopsies are now followed for accuracy, and should be done when PT is normal, and gives a definitive diagnosis (e.g. fibrosis, cirrhosis, malignant deposits).

In Summary

When liver enzymes AST and ALT are elevated, it signifies liver disease, and when serum alkaline phosphatase is elevated, it indicates biliary obstruction, and when serum alkaline phosphatase is normal, biliary obstruction is not to be considered. However, the next step is to get the ultrasound examination of the liver and look for a focal mass. The workup of a jaundiced patient with elevated enzymes and a normal alkaline phosphatase is given in **Figure 17.4**.

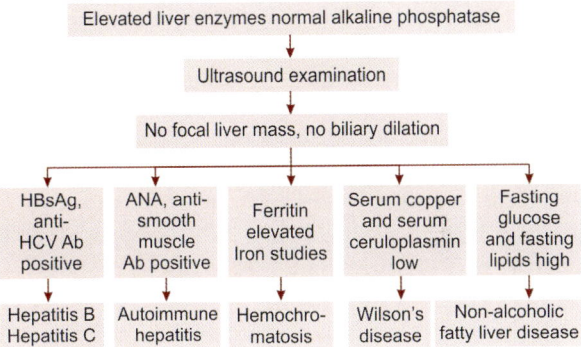

Fig. 17.4: Workup of patient with normal alkaline phosphatase

If the above tests are negative and LFT levels are deranged, undeclared alcohol excess should be considered especially when serum AST > ALT. Liver biopsy is confirmatory in all cases with a characteristic finding for each. However, the alcoholic and the non-alcoholic fatty liver disease cannot be distinguished even by histopathology. The workup of a jaundiced patient with elevated enzymes and elevated alkaline phosphatase is given in **Figure 17.5**.

HEPATOMEGALY

Introduction

The liver has limited space to expand by enlargement, as it is limited by the right dome of the diaphragm, which can be determined by percussion. The lower edge of liver is palpable, when

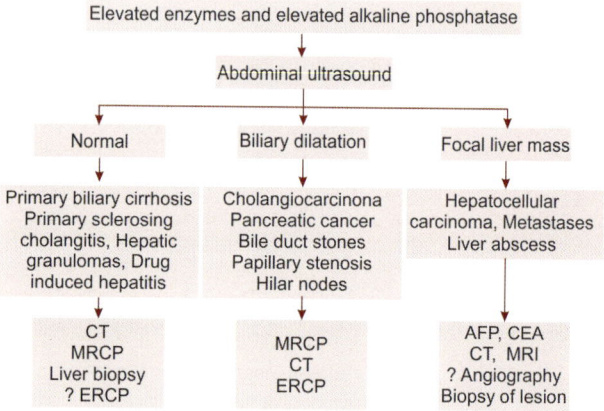

Fig. 17.5: Workup of a patient with elevated alkaline phosphatase

- It is enlarged
- It is pushed down due to:
  - Emphysema, bronchial asthma
  - Subdiaphragmatic abscess
  - Aberrant lobe of liver, e.g. Riedel's lobe
  - Visceroptosis.

Etiology

True hepatomegaly occurs due to variety of causes. They are tabulated in **Table 17.3**.

Table 17.3: Causes of hepatomegaly and their mechanisms

Etiology	Disorder	Mechanism
Cardiovascular	Congestive heart failure	Vascular congestion
	Hepatic vein thrombosis	
Obstructive	Biliary cirrhosis	Obstruction of biliary system
Infiltrative	Leukemia, lymphoma	Lymphatic infiltration of liver
	Alcoholism	Fatty infiltration of liver
	Diabetes mellitus	
	Amyloidosis	Infiltration of liver parenchyma
Inflammatory	Hepatitis	Parenchymal inflammation
	Cirrhosis	Regenerative phase
Neoplastic	Primary (hepatocellular carcinoma)	Malignant infiltration of liver parenchyma
	Secondary (metastatic)	
Miscellaneous	Simple cyst, hydatid cyst, polycystic disease	Space occupying lesion

INJURIES OF LIVER

Introduction

The liver ranks high on the list of intra-abdominal organs involved by injury.
- *Blunt injuries* are more common than the penetrating injuries, due to increase in motor traffic moving at high speeds, and are associated with fracture of lower ribs on the right side. The dome of the liver is involved with anterior-posterior tears, more on the right lobe (7:1)

- **Spontaneous rupture** of liver is seen in:
  - Primary carcinoma in adults and
  - Trauma during birth in children (postmature babies) being delivered per vaginum.

Classification

Liver injuries **(Fig. 17.6)** are classified into:
1. **Transcapsular** (blood and bile will seep into the peritoneal cavity).
2. **Subcapsular** (collection of blood between the capsule and the liver parenchyma mostly on the superior surface of liver).
3. **Central:** Bursting stellate type of laceration injury, tends to occur in the posterior and superior parts of right liver (segments VI, VII and VIII)—interruption of liver parenchyma leading to intrahepatic hematoma, abscess and hemobilia.

Grading of liver injuries is given in **Table 17.4**.

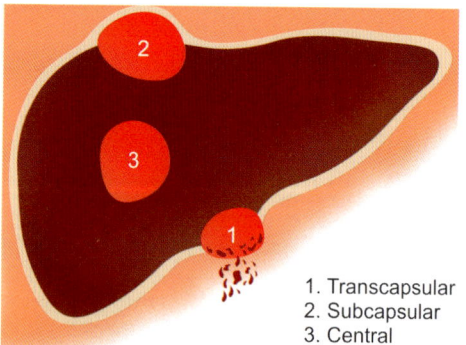

1. Transcapsular
2. Subcapsular
3. Central

Fig. 17.6: Types of liver injuries

Table 17.4: Liver injury scale

Grade	Hematoma	Laceration	Vascular
I	Subcapsular, non-expanding <10% of surface area	Capsular tear, nonbleeding <1 cm deep in parenchyma	
II	Subcapsular, non-expanding 10–50% of surface area, intraparenchymal hematoma non-expanding <2 cm diameter	Capsular tear, active bleeding; 1–3 cm deep into the parenchyma, <10 cm long	
III	Subcapsular, non-expanding >50% of surface area ruptured subcapsular hematoma with active bleeding; intraparenchymal hematoma expanding >2 cm	>3 cm deep into the parenchyma	
IV	Ruptured intraparenchymal hematoma with active bleeding	Parenchymal disruption involving <50% of hepatic lobe	
V		Parenchymal disruption involving >50% of hepatic lobe	Juxtahepatic venous injuries, i.e. prehepatic vena cava or major hepatic veins
VI			Hepatic avulsion

Diagnosis

Symptoms and Signs

1. ***Transcapsular:*** Symptoms and signs of shock and peritoneal irritation (pain right upper abdomen with reference to the right shoulder, guarding and rigidity of the right hypochondrium, absent bowel sounds, shifting dullness).
2. ***Subcapsular:*** Local tenderness and increase in area of liver dullness.

3. ***Central:*** Signs of shock may be present with hemobilia and hematemesis.

Investigations

Blood Tests

- ***Hematocrit*** may be low, but may not change when bleeding is extremely rapid, as in hepatic vein injuries
- ***Leukocytosis*** is common.

Radiology

- ***X-ray chest*** will demonstrate fracture of lower ribs on the right side
- ***Plain X-ray abdomen*** may show haziness in the area of the liver with elevation of right dome of diaphragm
- ***CT (Fig. 17.7) and MRI*** are useful in localizing the damaged areas of liver and collections of blood or bile

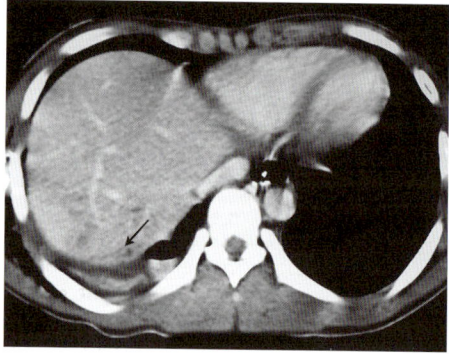

Fig. 17.7: CT—Liver injury with hemoperitoneum

- ***Peritoneal tap*** may be useful in identifying bile and blood leaks
- ***Colloidal gold Au^{198} or Technetium-sulfur colloid Tc^{99m} scans*** are useful during active bleeding.

Management

- Correction of shock
- No surgical intervention is needed for small injuries
- Early surgical intervention, sometimes amounting to hepatectomy, is needed for large injuries associated with vascular or biliary tract injuries.

Clinical Pearls

- Injury to the left liver is less common when compared to the right liver
- Serial CT scans are necessary to assess the expansion of lesion
- Sonogram does not give enough information about the extent of injury
- Angiography is not useful in the acute situation, but may be useful in the diagnosis of post-injury hemobilia.

VIRAL HEPATITIS

Introduction

Acute and Chronic Hepatitis

Acute hepatitis: It is defined as the infection of the liver and may have persistence of clinical, biochemical and serologic abnormalities for up to 6 months. However, the infections caused by A and E viruses clear from the body within 6 months and do not cause persistent infection.

Chronic hepatitis: Chronic hepatitis is defined as that infection of the liver, which lasts for more than 6 months. B, C and D viruses can lead to chronic infection, and may lead to cirrhosis ultimately.

Etiology and Pathogenesis

Currently, there are five identifiable forms of viral hepatitis; A, B, C, D and E. All these viruses primary affect the liver, and differ from those which secondarily infect the liver. Excepting the B virus, others are RNA viruses. B virus is a DNA virus.

- Hepatitis A and E viruses are transmitted via fecal oral route, and others (B, C and D) are transmitted through percutaneous, sexual, perinatal and blood routes
- Hepatitis D infection occurs only in the presence of hepatitis B infection, as a superinfection.

Hepatitis A virus (HAV) infection is typically a benign self-limited infection with the majority of patients exhibiting complete recovery within 2 months of the disease onset, and a small subset of patients will experience symptoms for more prolonged periods of time as the relapsing variant. A fulminant hepatitis A is rare and chronic hepatitis A does not exist.

Chronic hepatitis is usually defined by detectable HBsAg (Hepatitis B surface antigen) in the serum for a period of 6 months or longer. Many patients with hepatitis B virus (HBV) infection have normal liver enzymes and normal or near normal liver histology and are asymptomatic. Only a small percentage of adults become chronic carriers whereas the frequency in infants is more than 90%.

The risk factors of chronicity of hepatitis are:

- Hepatitis B, C and D virus infections (of the acute hepatitis C patients, about 40% become chronic)

- Younger age patients (neonates have a risk of 100%, healthy young adults have a risk of 1%)
- Immunologic status (immunocompromised individuals have a high risk)
- Patients on steroids have higher risk of chronic infection.

Diagnosis

Symptoms and Signs

Acute hepatitis: The classic symptoms of acute hepatitis are anorexia, nausea, vomiting, severe fatigue, abdominal pain, mild fever, jaundice, dark urine and pale stools. Some may exhibit arthralgia, arthritis and skin lesions.

Chronic hepatitis: Classically, chronic infections show fatigue as the predominant symptom. Others include the symptoms like those of acute attacks but with lesser severity.

Investigations

Blood Tests

- Serum transaminases (ALT and AST) are elevated (ALT more specific than AST), and very high levels (several thousands in B and C infection) are not uncommon
- Serum alkaline phosphatase is elevated to moderate levels
- Gamma glutamyl transpeptidase (GGT) is moderately elevated
- Bilirubin levels are raised.

Immunologic Tests

- **Hepatitis A**
  - Hepatitis A antibody (anti-HAV): Antibody directed against the viral capsid protein

- Anti-HAV IgM: Presence indicates acute infection and persists for about 3–6 months
- Anti-HAV IgG: Presence indicates post-infection or vaccination.

- **Hepatitis B**
  - Hepatitis B surface antigen (HBsAg): Protein which forms the outer coat of hepatitis B virus—presence indicates acute or chronic infection and absence indicates viral clearance or no infection
  - Hepatitis B surface antibody (HBsAb): Antibody directed towards the surface antigen—indicates past infection which has been fully cleared
  - Hepatitis B anticore antibody (HBcAb): Antibody against the core protein
    - Total HBcAb: Positivity indicates current or past hepatitis B infection
    - Anti-HBc IgM: Positivity indicates acute infection or viral reactivation
    - Anti-HBc IgG: Positivity indicates resolved past infection or with HBsAg positivity indicates chronic carrier state
  - Hepatitis B e antigen (HBeAg): Protein encoded by the precore portion of the coding domain-presence indicates wild type of infection
  - Hepatitis B e antibody (HBeAb): Antibody against HBeAg—chronic infection with HBeAg mutant
    - Branched chain DNA (bDNA): This test amplifies the signal generated by hybridization and quantifies the virus
    - Polymerase chain reaction (PCR): Most sensitive test available as it amplifies a portion of DNA itself.

- **Hepatitis C**
  - C RNA and PCR assay: C RNA assay is gold standard for hepatitis C assay. Most sensitive nucleic acid assay, can be performed by transcription mediated amplification (TMA)

- Hepatitis C assay by ELISA and RIBA: Detects the presence of antibodies to two regions of hepatitis C genome.
- **Hepatitis D**
  - Hepatitis D antibody: Antibody directed against the viral capsid protein
    - Anti-HDV IgM: Presence indicates hepatitis D viral replication
    - Anti-HDV IgG: Indicates chonic infection.
- **Hepatitis E**
  - Hepatitis E antibody (anti-HEV): Antibody directed against the viral capsid
    - Anti-HEV IgM: Presence indicates acute infection
    - Anti-HEV IgG: Presence indicates post infection or immunity.

Tissue Diagnosis

Liver biopsy is gold standard in hepatitis for evaluation of activity and fibrosis in the liver.

The clinical features of various forms of hepatitis are summarized in **Table 17.5**.

Complications

- Acute hepatitis does not cause any complication
- Chronic hepatitis causes cirrhosis and primary hepatocellular carcinoma.

Management

- Treatment of any type of acute hepatitis is mainly supportive
- Hospitalization is required only for those with complications like hepatic failure, renal failure, coagulopathy with bleeding, inability to maintain adequate nutrition and fluids
- Only chronic hepatitis requires therapy. After confirming the type of hepatitis, the treatment is targeted

Table 17.5: Clinical features of hepatitis

Feature	HAV	HBV	HCV	HDV	HEV
Transmission	Oral	Percutaneous/sexual/perinatal	Percutaneous/sexual/perinatal	Percutaneous	Oral
Incubation period (days)	15–50	60–180	14–160	21–45	15–60
Clinical illness (days)	70–80	10–15	5–10	10	70–80 adults
Fulminant	<1%	<1%	Unclear	2–8%	<1%
Acute infection	Anti-HAV IgM	HBsAg, anti-HBc IgM	HCV RNA (anti-HCV)	Anti-HDV IgM	Anti-HEV IgM
Chronic		HBsAg, anti-HBc IgG	Anti-HCV (ELISA/RIBA)	Anti-HDV IgG	
Immunity	Anti-HAV IgG	HBsAb			Anti-HEV IgG
Chronic infection	None	<5% adults >90% infants	90%		None

Hepatitis B: Patients with well compensated liver disease, with evidence of viral replication (HBV DNA or HBeAg) and ongoing hepatic necrosis as evidenced by elevated liver enzyme levels and presence of active inflammation or fibrosis in liver biopsy are to be treated **(Table 17.6)**.

There are six drugs available now for the treatment of chronic hepatitis B.

Immune Modulators

1. Interferon α 2b.
2. Pegylated Interferon α 2b (180 µg weekly SC injection for 52 weeks).

Table 17.6: Indications for antiviral therapy in chronic hepatitis B

Serology		HBV DNA	ALT level	Diagnosis	Treatment
HBsAg	Antigen/antibody				
Positive	HBcAb IgM positive			Acute hepatitis B	Observe
Positive (>6 months)	HBeAg positive HBsAb positive	Positive >20,000 IU/mL	Elevated - > twice normal	Chronic hepatitis B with wild virus	Initiate therapy
	HBeAg negative HBeAb positive	Negative or <2,000 IU/mL	Normal or less elevated	Chronic carrier	Observe
		Positive >2,000 IU/mL	Elevated - > twice normal	Chronic infection with HBeAg mutant	Initiate antiviral therapy

Oral Nucleoside Analogs

They directly inhibit viral replication without stimulating immunological response.
1. Lamivudine (100 mg/day)
2. Entecavir (0.5 mg/day)
3. Telbivudine (600 mg/day)

Oral Nucleotide Analog of Adenosine Monophosphate

It inhibits both reverse transcriptase and DNA polymerase activity and is incorporated into viral DNA, producing a chain termination.

Adefovir dipivoxil (10 mg once daily)

Pegylated interferon (polyethylene glycol added interferon) therapy for 52 weeks has the disadvantage of side effects, flu like syndrome, fever, mental depression, sleeplessness, irritability and bone marrow depression. Flu like syndrome is distressing in patients with cirrhosis.

Oral nucleoside/nucleotide analogs have varying potency and resistance profiles.

- Lamivudine has the disadvantage of intermediate potency and drug resistance (20% become resistant by the first year of therapy). It is not recommended as monotherapy and addition of adefovir may be needed
- Entecavir and telbivudine have higher potency and have better resistance profile
- Adefovir has low potency and good resistance profile.

Hepatitis C: Monitoring is done every 4 weeks for a period of 12 weeks for seroconversion or development of HCV RNA viremia. About 30% of patients clear the virus spontaneously, and require no treatment. All patients who do not clear the virus, should be started on pegylated interferon alpha (180 µg once weekly SC injection) with ribavirin (1,000 mg for 65–85 kg weight, 1,200 mg for 86–105 kg weight and 1,400 mg for >105 kg weight—divided twice daily) for 24 weeks, to prevent the development of chronic state. The pretreatment work up for hepatitis C patients should include several tests **(Table 17.7)**.

Hepatitis D: Interferon based monotherapy for 12 months, addition of lamivudine or ribavirin does not seem to change the overall outcome.

Response to Therapy

Hepatitis B: Hepatitis B infection is never totally eradicated, but it can be controlled with therapy. Undetectable viral load and e-antigen seroconversion (achieving HBeAg negativity and HBeAb positivity) indicate response to therapy. Antiviral therapy should be continued for 24–48 weeks after these parameters are achieved, and then the

Table 17.7: Pretreatment work up for hepatitis C patients

Test	To assess
• HCV RNA by PCR	• Viral load
• Serum albumin	• Liver function
• Serum bilirubin	• Liver function
• Antinuclear antibody (ANA)	• Autoimmune hepatitis
• Alpha antitrypsin phenotype	• Alpha antitrypsin deficiency
• Hepatitis B antigen (HBsAg)	• B virus coexistence
• Hepatitis C genotype	• Response to therapy
• Liver biopsy	• Severity and urgent need for therapy

therapy may be discontinued. Patients with heavy viral load and e-antigen negativity, at the time of initiation of therapy will require lifelong therapy, but the end point is appearance of HBsAb, which is rare. Interferon therapy response is long lasting with rare instances of relapse, but oral nucleoside/nucleotide therapy is for longer periods and relapses and resistances are common. E conversion is more common with interferon therapy than with oral nucleoside/nucleotide therapy.

Regardless of the therapy chosen, monitoring should be done to detect resistant strains. Levels of HBV DNA should be monitored every 3 months as long as the virus is detected, and every 6 months when viral negativity is reached. Once resistance is detected, second drug, preferably adefovir is added to lamivudine or telbivudine. If resistance is found for adefovir, lamivudine or telbivudine is added.

Hepatitis C: Normalization of enzymes indicates positive response, which should be monitored every 3 months and total response should be achieved at 12 months, which is determined by quantitative HCV-RNA assay at 4 and 12 weeks. The patients who do not achieve this at the stipulated times, are unlikely to respond well and discontinuation of therapy should be considered.

Table 17.8: Contraindications for interferon and ribavirin therapy

Interferon therapy	Ribavirin therapy
• Leukopenia and thrombocytopenia	• Pregnancy
• Psychiatric patients	• Severe myelosuppression
• Consumption of alcohol	• Ischemic heart disease
• Autoimmune diseases	• Renal insufficiency
• Comorbid conditions	
• Post-organ transplantation	

Those patients who show early response, should have continued therapy for 24 months. HCV–RNA PCR assay should be done. If no detectable virus is found, it is considered cured and treatment is discontinued. The same investigation is done 6 months after discontinuation of therapy to assess the sustained response.

Contraindications for Interferon and ribavirin therapy are listed in **Table 17.8**.

Prevention

Prevention of the disease is by avoiding incriminating agents and vaccination (immunization). The immunization can be:
- **Active immunization:** Introduction of specific antigen to provoke an antibody response which will prevent the disease
- **Passive immunization:** Introduction of antibodies produced in an animal or human by immunization or prior infection.

Related to viral hepatitis, vaccines are available commercially only to prevent hepatitis A and B.

The characteristics are given in Table 17.9.

Passive immunoprophylaxis is necessary for certain individuals and situations. They are given in **Table 17.10**.

Table 17.9: Characteristics of hepatitis vaccines

Vaccine	HAVRIX	VAQTA	ENGERIX B	TWINRIX
Type of vaccine	Inactivated A	Inactivated A	Inactivated B	Inactivated A and B
Strain	Attenuated CR326F (HAV strain)	Attenuated HM175 (HAV strain)	Purified HBsAg recombinant DNA vaccine	Attenuated HM175 (HAV strain)
Immunity	Serum anti-HAV	Serum anti-HAV	Serum anti-HBV	Serum anti-HAV and anti-HBV
Route of administration	Intramuscular	Intramuscular	Intramuscular	Intramuscular
Adult dose and time of administration	1 mL (50 U) 0 and 6 months	1 mL (1440 U) 0, 6 and 12 months	1 mL (20 mg) 0, 1 and 6 months	1 mL (720 U) 0, 1 and 6 months
Pediatric dose and time of administration	0.5 mL (25 U) 0 and 6–18 months	0.5 mL (720 U) 0, 6–12 months	0.5 mL (10 mg) 0, 1 and 6 months	Not recommended

Table 17.10: Passive immunoprophylaxis of hepatitis A and B

Hepatitis A	Hepatitis B
All children over 1 year of age	Neonates born to HBsAg positive mothers
Travelers to hepatitis A endemicity	After needlestick exposure
Chronic liver diseases	After sexual exposure
Illicit drug users	After liver transplantation in patients who were HBsAg positive before transplantation
Patients with clotting factor disorders	
Male homosexuals	

Clinical Pearls

- Viruses like CMV, HSV and EBV can cause acute hepatitis, especially in immunocompromised (congenital/acquired) individuals, and screening should be focused on this issue as well
- Acute infection by HDV and HBV is associated with higher degree of severe or fulminant liver disease
- Bilirubin levels may remain normal or mildly elevated in chronic hepatitis
- Chronic hepatitis B carriers with normal liver enzymes, negative HBeAg, positive HBeAb and non-detectable levels of HBV DNA by PCR do not require antiviral treatment
- Interferon based therapy for hepatitis B infection causes seroconversion in about 25% cases
- In pregnancy associated with chronic hepatitis B infection, interferon is contraindicated and of the oral drugs, lamivudine is the only drug recommended
- Acute hepatitis C virus infections are rare and transaminases rarely exceed 1,000 IU/L, and some patients with HCV infection may have persistently normal ALT levels, in spite of the disease being active on liver biopsy
- HCV infection once established persists in the vast majority, disease progression is largely silent and are identified during routine examination
- About 25% of patients with chronic hepatitis C progress to cirrhosis, and which patients will progress to cirrhosis are not known, all patients deserve to be treated
- Progression to cirrhosis is accelerated by alcohol consumption, coexisting B virus or HIV infection, liver disease (Fatty liver and NASH)

- Hepatitis C treatment is influenced by several factors such as age, gender, body mass index and immune status
- Hepatitis C treatment failures are common in alcoholics and obese individuals
- Ribavirin used alone as an antiviral agent is not effective against C virus, but when combined with PEG IFNα, the effectivity is greater
- Ribavirin causes dose dependent complications like hemolysis. It is also teratogenic
- Some suggest 800 mg ribavirin daily as fixed dose immaterial of body weight, weight therapy enhances good results
- Newer therapies for hepatitis C infection are protease/helicase inhibitors, RNA dependent RNA polymerase inhibitors, and immune modulators like thymosin alpha-1 and antifibrotic therapy (gamma interferon)
- Patients who are not immune for hepatitis A and B virus, should be vaccinated, before initiating therapy for hepatitis C.
- Patients coinfected with HIV should receive lesser dose of ribavirin to decrease the incidence of severe anemia
- Patients coinfected with HBV, should receive recommended doses of IFN for hepatitis B and ribavirin for hepatitis C.

AUTOIMMUNE HEPATITIS

Introduction

- Autoimmune hepatitis is defined as inflammation of liver of unknown cause in which interface hepatitis is evident on histology along with the presence of autoantibodies and hypergammaglobulinemia
- It commonly affects women before the age of 40

- There may be associated autoimmune diseases like autoimmune thyroiditis, ulcerative colitis, rheumatoid arthritis, etc.

Types of Autoimmune Hepatitis

- **Type 1:** Autoimmune hepatitis characterized by SMA or ANA. Most common type. Antibodies to actin, a subgroup of SMA supports the diagnosis
- **Type 2:** Autoimmune hepatitis characterized by antibodies to liver/kidney microsome type 1. Commonly affects the young Europeans. May have associated autoimmune diseases
- **Type 3:** Autoimmune hepatitis characterized by the presence of antibodies to soluble liver antigen (anti-SLA).

Pathogenesis

Two theories have been suggested for the development of autoimmune hepatitis. They are:
1. Antibody dependent cell mediated form of cytotoxicity
2. Cellular form of cytotoxicity.

Genetic factors: HLA DR3 and DR4 are principal risk factors

The defect is in T cell suppression of antibody-producing B cells. It is thought an environmental event, like viral hepatitis triggers B cell response to hepatic surface antigens in a genetically predisposed patient. Natural killer cells clear the antibody coated cells, exposing more autoantigens. The defective T suppressor cells fail to take the antibody response. This results in hepatic cell destruction, leading to cirrhosis. The circulating antibodies thus become the markers for diagnosis.

Diagnosis

Clinical Presentation

- There are no specific clinical features, and diagnosed only by exclusion of other conditions, especially chronic viral hepatitis, Wilson's disease, etc.
- Majority of asymptomatic patients become symptomatic sometime during the course of disease and need regular follow-up
- Fatigue and joint pains are common symptoms
- Acute fulminant hepatitis can occur.

Investigations

Blood Tests

- *Liver enzymes (AST and ALT)* are abnormally elevated.

Serological Markers

- *Smooth muscle antibodies (SMA)*
- *Antinuclear antibodies (ANA)*
- *Antibodies to soluble liver antigen (anti-SLA)*
- *Antibodies to actin (anti-actin)*
- *Antibodies to chromatin (anti-chromatin)*
- *Antibodies to liver cytosol type 1 (anti-LC1)*
- *Antibodies to asialoglycoprotein (anti-ASGPR).*

Tissue Diagnosis

Histology is characteristic: Interface hepatitis with spill over of inflammatory cells from the portal tract through the limiting plate into the liver parenchyma is the hallmark of chronic autoimmune hepatitis. Though not specific, presence of plasma cells supports the diagnosis. Histology is same in asymptomatic and symptomatic patients.

Diagnostic criteria include histologic evidence, which should rule out other granulomatous lesions.

Management

Acute autoimmune hepatitis: Corticosteroid therapy and outcome is grave if there is no response. Liver transplantation is the only option in such patients.

Chronic autoimmune hepatitis:

- Prednisolone as monotherapy or in combination with azathioprine (**Table 17.11**). Azathioprine is used as a steroid sparing strategy, which is useful in maintaining remission, even after corticosteroid withdrawal
- Liver transplantation is effective, but 40% of the patients have recurrence, which requires high dose steroids.

Response to Therapy

Response to therapy is determined by serum aminotransferases and IgG levels. However, repeat biopsy is needed.

Table 17.11: Treatment schedule for chronic autoimmune hepatitis

Dose intervals	Monotherapy	Combination therapy	
	Prednisolone	Prednisolone	Azathioprine
Week 1	80 mg daily	30 mg daily	50 mg daily
Week 2	40 mg daily	20 mg daily	50 mg daily
Week 3	30 mg daily	15 mg daily	50 mg daily
Week 4	30 mg daily	15 mg daily	50 mg daily
Maintenance dose	20 mg daily	10 mg daily	50 mg daily

Clinical Pearls

- Majority of patients with autoimmune hepatitis show positivity of SMAs and ANAs together
- Antibody titer of >1:80 has diagnostic significance, as the values seem to fluctuate in an erratic fashion
- Diagnosis of autoimmune hepatitis is only by clinical suspicion, and underdiagnosis is common
- In about 10% of cases, conventional antibodies are absent and it is called cryptogenic chronic hepatitis
- Viruses and drugs can cause autoimmune hepatitis.

ALCOHOLIC LIVER DISEASE (ALD)

Introduction

Alcohol abuse and alcohol dependence are common in developed countries, and liver being the principal site of ethanol metabolism, large quantities cause hepatocyte injury. End stage liver disease due to alcohol is the most common cause of cirrhosis in Western population.

Etiology and Pathogenesis

Ethanol gets metabolized in the liver. Ingested alcohol is absorbed from the stomach and proximal intestine and oxidized to acetaldehyde by ADH in the liver. When large quantities are ingested, it is metabolized by microsomal P450 enzymes and catalase. This reaction causes liver cell injury by causing lipid peroxidation.

$$C_2H_2OH + 2(O) \xrightarrow{ADH} CH_3COOH + H_2O$$

Types of Alcoholic Liver Disease

- *Fatty metamorphosis:* Earliest stage of alcoholic liver disease. Fat accumulation occurs within 2 days of consumption and clears within 2 weeks of cessation
- *Microvesicular steatosis:* Foamy degeneration due to mitochondrial dysfunction developing in centrilobular hepatocytes, causes jaundice, hepatic encephalopathy and death
- *Alcoholic hepatitis:* Centrilobular hepatocellular necrosis, polymorphonuclear inflammation and presence of Mallory hyaline
- *Alcoholic cirrhosis:* The end stage liver disease following alcoholic hepatitis, which may predispose to hepatocellular carcinoma.

Risk Factors

- Quantity of alcohol (more the quantity, more the damage)
- Pattern of consumption—continuous intake produces more liver damage
- Ethnicity—more common in African American population
- Genetic—Japanese AHD gene
- HCV infection
- Malnutrition.

Diagnosis

Symptoms

- Eliciting history about alcohol consumption (duration and quantity)
- Alcoholic steatosis: Nonspecific
- Alcoholic hepatitis: Malaise, nausea and fatigue
- Alcoholic cirrhosis: Variable symptoms.

Table 17.12: Interpretation of blood tests in ALD

Condition	Enzymes	Bilirubin	Prothrombin time	SGGT	Albumin	Platelet count
Alcoholic steatosis		Normal	Normal		Normal	Normal
Alcoholic hepatitis	AST > ALT	Elevated	Prolonged	Elevated	Depressed	Normal
Alcoholic cirrhosis		Elevated	Prolonged		Depressed	Depressed

Signs

- Alcoholic steatosis: Hepatomegaly
- Alcoholic hepatitis: Hepatomegaly, jaundice, ascites
- Alcoholic cirrhosis: Cutaneous stigmata of liver disease, portal hypertension.

Investigations

Blood tests (**Table 17.12**).

Tissue Diagnosis

Liver biopsy is gold standard in diagnosing alcoholic liver disease, but histology does not differ from non-alcoholic liver disease
- Alcoholic steatosis: Steatosis
- Alcoholic hepatitis: Steatosis with active inflammation
- Alcoholic cirrhosis: Fibrosis.

Management

- Abstinence from alcohol
- Nutrition

- Vitamin supplements especially Thiamine 100 mg OD (prophylaxis against Wernicke's encephalopathy)
- Glucocorticoids
- Anticytokine (tumor necrosis factor alpha) therapy
  - Pentoxifylline
  - Infliximab
  - Etanercept
- Antioxidant cocktails
- Adenosyl methionine
- Management of end stage liver disease
- Liver transplantation gives long-term success, provided patient does not return to drinking alcohol.

Prognosis

- Prognosis can be determined by using certain scores like MDF, MELD score, Glasgow alcoholic hepatitis score (GAHS) and the Lille model
  - ***Maddrey's discriminant function (MDF)*** using a modified formula. MDF = 4.6 (Prothrombin time–Control in seconds) + Serum bilirubin - µmol/L/17). A score of >32 is associated with poor prognosis of >50% at one month
  - ***Model for end-stage liver disease (MELD)*** score = (0.957 x ln [(Cr (mg%)] + 0.378 x ln [(bilirubin (mg%)] + 1.12 x ln [INR] + 0.643) x 10. A score of >18 and a change in the hospital by >2 points is associated with poor prognosis
  - ***Glasgow alcoholic hepatitis score (GAHS)*** **(Table 17.13)**.

A combined score of between 5 and 12 is obtained, and a score greater than or equal to 9 is associated with poor prognosis and accurately predicts mortality at 28/84 days when measured at days 1 and 7.

Table 17.13: Glasgow alcoholic hepatitis score

Score given	1	2	3
Age	<50	>50	–
WBC 10^9/L	<15	>15	–
Urea (mmol/L)	<5	>5	–
INR	<1.5	1.5–2.0	>2.0
Bilirubin (µmol/L)	<1 25	125–250	250

- *Lille model:* A new scoring system for predicting the prognosis. 3.19−0.101 x (age in years) + 0.147 x (albumin day 0 in g/L) + 0.0165 x (evolution in bilirubin level in) − (0.206 x renal insufficiency) − 0.0065 x (bilirubin day 0) − 0.0096 x (PT). A score of >0.45 identifies 75% of deaths. A score of >0.45 predicts a 6-month survival of 25%, versus 85% survival when the score is <0.45.

Clinical Pearls

- In alcoholics, the chances of fatty liver progressing to cirrhosis and end stage liver disease is high
- Prognosis of patients with fatty liver who stop ethanol consumption is excellent
- A biopsy is not always practical or necessary in the management of all cases of alcoholic liver disease
- Fatty liver is benign and is reversible with strict abstinence from alcohol for 4–6 weeks, but alcoholic hepatitis is potentially life-threatening with a mortality of about 50% in severe cases
- Patients with encephalopathy have very poor prognosis
- When alcohol is withdrawn, alcohol withdrawal syndrome needs to be managed.

ALCOHOL WITHDRAWAL SYNDROME

Introduction

Cessation of alcohol intake in a patient who was living an alcohol dependent life, may lead to clinical features of the severest form with a significant mortality.

Diagnosis

Symptoms

- Mental confusion
- Hallucinations (visual, auditory or olfactory)
- Agitation
- Sleeplessness
- Nausea and vomiting
- Generalized grand mal seizures.

Signs

- Tachycardia
- Systolic hypertension
- Tremor
- Dilated pupils.

Investigations

Blood Tests
- *Complete blood count*
- *Coagulation profile to assess liver function*
- *LFT to assess liver function*
- *Blood glucose to rule out hypoglycemia*
- *Blood alcohol levels*.

Radiology
- *X-ray chest* for sepsis
- *CT brain* in patients with atypical presentation or head injury.

Management

- Safe and quiet environment
- Monitoring of vital signs
- Intravenous fluids
- Thiamine 100 mg daily (oral/parenteral)
- Magnesium sulfate 1g IV/IM injections 6 hourly for 24 hours
- Benzodiazepines (Lorazepam 1 mg/diazepam 5 mg/ chlordiazepoxide 25 mg)
- Suggested schedule for chlordiazepoxide
  - Day 1–50 mg–4 hrly
  - Day 2–50 mg–6 hrly
  - Day 3–25 mg–4 hrly
  - Day 4–25 mg–6 hrly.

Clinical Pearls

- Severe form of alcohol withdrawal presenting with severe symptoms is called *Delirium tremens*
- Wernicke's encephalopathy results from vitamin B_1 deficiency, usually in alcohol dependent undernourished individuals. It is characterized by a clinical triad: Ophthalmoplegia, ataxia and cognitive impairment. Fatal, if not treated with vitamins B and C
- Death occurs due to complications like hyperthermia, electrolyte abnormalities, volume depletion, infections, hypertensive crisis or cardiac failure.

NON-ALCOHOLIC FATTY LIVER DISEASE (NAFLD)

Introduction

A generalized classification of a group of diseases marked by the presence of fat in the liver cell, mainly due to insulin resistance, without significant alcohol use. This ranges from an innocuous form of fat deposition to cirrhosis and liver failure.

It passes through three stages. They are:
1. *Simple steatosis*: Fat droplets in hepatocytes without inflammation.
2. *Non-alcoholic steatohepatitis (NASH)*: Ballooning of liver cells with inflammation. Cytoplasm may contain Mallory bodies.
3. *Cirrhosis*: Deposition of collagen in liver cells, proceeding to fibrosis.

Pathogenesis

Insulin resistance causes a complex of events in which triglycerides are not allowed to be secreted, resulting in the accumulation of fat in hepatocytes. Mechanism of conversion of simple steatosis to cirrhosis is not clearly understood. It is thought that the mitochondrial fatty acid metabolism leads to lipid peroxidation by producing reactive oxygen species. Peroxidized lipids and cytokines cause activation of collagen producing stellate cells, resulting in cirrhosis.

Diagnosis

Symptoms

- Many are asymptomatic
- Fatigue and right upper quadrant pain are common
- Jaundice.

Signs

- Hepatomegaly
- Signs of liver failure (minority).

Investigations

Blood Tests

- *Serum transaminases elevated (ALT > AST)*
- *Alkaline phosphatase is usually elevated*
- *Bilirubin and PT are usually normal unless there is cirrhosis*
- *Ferritin is elevated in 50% of patients but it is <1,000 ng/mL*
- *Negative serology for hepatitis B and C*
- *Negative ANA and SMA antibodies.*

Radiology

- *US* may show increased echogenicity
- *CT or MRI* can detect fatty changes.

Tissue Diagnosis

- *Liver biopsy*
    - Fatty change without inflammation or fibrosis (simple steatosis)
    - Fatty change with inflammation and fibrosis with stellate formation (cirrhosis).

Diagnosis of Non-alcoholic Steatohepatitis (NASH) is Made on Three Criteria

1. Liver biopsy shows macrovesicular fatty change with lobular or portal inflammation with or without fibrosis.
2. Convincing evidence that the alcohol intake is less than 40 grams/week.
3. No evidence of active infection with hepatitis B or C virus, or a secondary cause of cirrhosis.

Management

- Gradual weight reduction and exercises are useful in obese patients
- No treatment as such is now available
- Some drugs seem to play a role (statins, ursodeoxycholic acid, vitamin E, metformin).

Clinical Pearls

- About 10–15% of patients with NAFLD is said to progress to cirrhosis and require liver transplantation
- Since the donor livers also can show hepatic steatosis, about 30% steatosis is considered safe for transplantation, moderate steatosis (30–60%) is to be used with caution, and >60% steatosis is considered unsuitable for transplantation
- From the limited information available, it is seen that about 15% of transplanted livers develop de novo NASH.

DRUG-INDUCED LIVER DISEASE (DILD)

Introduction

More than 1000 drugs are implicated for the causation of liver disease. The most common drug to cause hepatotoxicity is acetaminophen, but only in doses of >10 g in non-alcoholics and lesser dose in alcoholics. The other common drugs are statins.

There are three types of liver injuries. They are:
1. Hepatocellular injury
2. Cholestatic injury
3. Mixed injury

Injury to liver occurs in about 5–90 days after initial exposure of the drug, but on withdrawal of the drug, improvement in biochemical parameters is seen in about 2 weeks for hepatocellular injury and 4 weeks for cholestatic and mixed injuries. If this recovery is not seen, it may indicate a coexistent pathology like viral, autoimmune hepatitis, primary sclerosing cholangitis, etc.

Etiology and Pathogenesis

Drug-induced liver injury is caused by two mechanisms. They are:
1. **Intrinsic:** Direct toxicity to hepatocytes (e.g., acetaminophen, carbon tetrachloride).
2. **Idiosyncratic:** Hypersensitivity reaction (usually associated with features of hypersensitivity) (e.g. halothane, isoniazid)—early or late.

In alcoholics, acetaminophen injury is possible because of alcohol induction of the cytochrome P450 2E1 system with associated malnutrition and low levels of glutathione, which is a protector of hepatocytes.

Drug-induced hepatic steatosis is of three types. They are:
1. Microvesicular steatosis (e.g. aspirin, tetracycline).
2. Macrovesicular steatosis (e.g. acetaminophen, tamoxifen).
3. Phospholipidosis (e.g. amiodarone, total parenteral nutrition).

Risk Factors

- **Age:** Young patients are more susceptible
- **Sex:** Females are more susceptible
- **Route of administration:** Parenteral route causes more instances of liver damage
- **Malnutrition:** Undernourished with low glutathione levels show more instances of liver damage

- **Drug drug interaction:** Valproic acid causes more cholestasis induced by chlorpromazine.

Diagnosis

Symptoms

- History of exposure to drug
- Nausea, vomiting and malaise are common within a few hours
- Rashes may appear if it is due to hypersensitivity.

Signs

- Right upper quadrant pain may be present
- Signs of hepatic encephalopathy may develop.

Investigations

They can be distinguished by ALT and ALP levels **(Table 17.14)**
- Aminotransferases raise, peaking above 10,000 U/L
- Bilirubin is moderately elevated.

Management

- The offending drug should be stopped
- Supportive care.
- **Specific treatment:**
    - Activated charcoal within 8 hours of ingestion

Table 17.14: Parameters of alcoholic liver injuries

Type of injury	ALT levels	ALP levels
Hepatocellular injury	>2 fold elevation	Normal
Cholestatic injury	Normal	>2 fold elevation
Mixed injury	>2 fold elevation	>2 fold elevation

- N-acetylcysteine is definitive treatment for acetaminophen overdose. (if administered within 8 hours, significant hepatotoxicity is rare)
    - Orally loading dose of 140 mg/kg body weight followed by 70 mg/kg every 4 hours for an additional 17 doses
    - Intravenous dose: 150 mg/kg (as loading dose) given for 15 minutes, followed by 50 mg/kg infusion over 4 hours and the last 100 mg/kg over the remaining 16 hours
- **Liver transplantation** is required if there is progression to liver failure and encephalopathy. The indications are, PT is greater than 100 seconds and serum creatinine greater than 3.4 mg% with grade III or IV encephalopathy or arterial pH below 7.3, irrespective of grade of encephalopathy.

Clinical Pearls

- Isoniazid-induced hepatotoxicity occurs in about 20% of patients on antitubercular therapy, but severe form is rare. The presentation is similar to acute viral hepatitis, and these infections should be excluded
- The potential for acetaminophen-induced hepatotoxicity can be calculated using the Rumack–Matthew acetaminophen nomogram (**Fig 17.8**), but it can be inaccurate if the acetaminophen is in an extended release form.

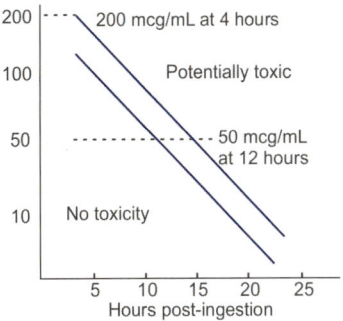

Fig. 17.8: Rumack–Mathew paracetamol nomogram

METABOLIC LIVER DISEASES

Hemochromatosis

Introduction

Hemochromatosis is an inherited disorder of overload of iron. The normal total body iron is 3–4 g. In primary or hereditary hemochromatosis it may be >20 g.

Types of Hemochromatosis

- Hereditary hemochromatosis
- Secondary iron overload
- Parenteral iron overload.

Pathogenesis

Usually, the dietary iron is absorbed when there is a deficiency and when replete, the absorption is downregulated and a balance is maintained. Normally, there is no process available to eliminate excess iron from the body. The tissue excess iron promotes the degeneration of oxygen-free radicals, to interact with lipid-rich membranes to form lipid peroxidases, resulting in membrane damage, cell death and fibrosis. The excessive fibrosis causes cirrhosis and liver failure. Hemochromatosis may manifest in various organs, such as:

- Liver—cirrhosis, hepatocellular carcinoma
- Heart—pump failure, arrhythmia
- Pancreas—diabetes
- Skin—hyperpigmentation
- Pituitary—hypogonadism
- Joints—arthritis especially of metacarpophalangeal joints.

In hereditary hemochromatosis, due to genetic disposition, (commonly cysteine to tyrosine mutation at residue 282–C282Y mutation) the second phase, the downregulation does not take place, and the iron absorption continues to take place, and blood iron values increase. When this process is occurring since birth, critical levels reach around 30 years of age, more commonly in men (women are less affected probably due to the loss of iron in menstruation).

In secondary iron overload, some cause is found to increase the intestinal absorption of iron (e.g. thalassemia, aplastic anemia).

In parenteral iron overload, iron is received commonly through large red blood transfusions especially in patients who are not iron deficient.

Triggering Factors

- Age (older age)
- Gender (men)
- Alcohol use
- Oral iron intake
- Hepatitis C infection.

Diagnosis

Symptoms

- Usually nonspecific
- Fatigue, joint pains and loss of libido are common.

Signs

- ***Hepatic:*** Signs of liver failure (hepatomegaly, skin lesions, etc.)
- Cardiovascular: Cardiomyopathy

- **Endocrine:** Diabetes mellitus, hypogonadism, panhypopituitarism, testicular atrophy
- **Dermatological:** Pigmentation (bronze diabetes), porphyria cutanea tarda
- **Skeletal:** Chondrocalcinosis, arthritis of 2nd and 3rd metacarpophalangeal joints.

Investigations

Blood Tests

- ***AST, ALT and alkaline phosphatase*** are typically normal or mildly elevated
- ***Blood glucose*** may be elevated indicating pancreatic involvement
- ***Serum iron and iron binding capacity***
- ***Transferrin saturation of >50% is suggestive (Normal 15–45)***
- ***Ferritin concentration of twice normal range (>600) is suggestive (Normal <300)***
- ***Genetic testing for C282Y mutation or compound hetero-zygotes (C282Y/H63D).***

Radiology

- ***X-rays may*** show chondrocalcinosis of joints
- ***CT and MRI*** may show the liver to be white or black, based on the amount of iron deposited in the liver.

Endoscopy

- ***Upper GI scopy***—Varices in cirrhotic patients.

Tissue Diagnosis

- ***Liver biopsy and hepatic iron*** (70 mmol/g liver) >70 (Normal < 40) and hepatic iron index >1.9 (Normal <1.5) is the gold standard of hemochromatosis.

Differential Diagnosis
- Alcoholic hepatitis.

Complications
- Hepatocellular carcinoma
- End stage liver disease.

Management
- Therapeutic phlebotomy (removal of one unit of blood—500 mL once or twice a week) until iron deficiency is achieved (Ferritin <50 ng%), and the frequency can be reduced. Once successful depletion is achieved, maintenance phlebotomy (phlebotomy every 3 weeks) should be performed
- Avoidance of alcohol
- Avoidance of iron
- Avoidance of vitamin C, as it facilitates iron absorption
- Vitamin E supplements.

Clinical Pearls

- Diagnosis is always by clinical suspicion
- Unexplained cirrhosis and heart failure should cause suspicion
- Histidine to aspartic acid mutation at residue 63 (H63D) has also been described with hemochromatosis, but less severe than the C282Y mutation
- A symptomatic hemochromatosis patient may require removal of 80 units of blood, which takes about 2 years at a rate of 1 unit of blood every week
- Once therapy is started, patients experience improvement in cardiac function, fatigue and abdominal pain, and also liver enzymes improve. Advanced cirrhosis and joint pains do not improve with phlebotomies

- Before the development of cirrhosis, hemochromatosis patients have a normal span
- When hereditary hemochromatosis is diagnosed, all first degree relatives should be screened.

Wilson's Disease

Introduction

Wilson's disease is an autosomal recessive disorder of copper metabolism, presents clinically after the age of 5, below 15, and rarely above 40.

Pathogenesis

Normally, copper is absorbed in the proximal intestine from diet and transported to liver cells. In the liver cells, it is incorporated into enzymes, including ceruloplasmin. Excess copper is bound into the complexes of metallothionine and excreted in the bile. In Wilson's disease, this process is defective. This disease occurs due to a defect in the gene located on chromosome 13 (Wilson's disease gene called ATP7B) that codes for a canalicular copper 'pump', leading to excretion of copper into bile. In the liver, the deposition of copper in the liver cells progresses to hepatitis and fibrosis. Multiple organs like liver, brain and other tissues are involved due to excessive deposition of copper, released by the dying liver cells.

Diagnosis

Symptoms and Signs
- Usually remain asymptomatic
- Younger patients present with hepatic dysfunction, and older patients with neuropsychiatric dysfunction (tremor, ataxia and personality changes)

- **Liver:** Acute/chronic hepatitis, cirrhosis
- **Brain:** Tremor, ataxia, personality changes, depression
- **Eye:** Kayser Fleischer rings (ring of 1–3 mm diameter, green/yellow/brown color) in the periphery of the cornea, best detected by slit lamp examination. Sunflower cataracts may be seen
- **Kidney:** Stones
- **Heart:** Arrhythmias
- **Joints:** Chondrocalcinosis
- **Red blood cells:** Hematologic abnormalities.

Diagnosis is usually by clinical suspicion.

Investigations

Blood Tests

- Serum ceruloplasmin concentration <20 mg% (normal 20–45% mg)
- 24 hour urinary copper concentration > 100 µg (normal <35 µg)
- Hyperuricemia shows renal involvement.

Tissue Diagnosis

- Liver biopsy and presence of excessive copper in hepatocytes is the hallmark of diagnosis. Hepatic copper concentration >250 µg/g liver (normal <50 µg/g liver)
- Kidney biopsy shows renal tubular necrosis.

Complications

- End-stage liver disease.

Management

- Chelation of copper, increasing the urinary excretion
- Penicillamine is the drug of choice and the treatment is lifelong

- Trientine is used in patients who do not tolerate penicillamine, and has lesser side effects
- Oral zinc is used as an adjunct to chelation therapy, as it interferes with copper absorption from the small intestine and increases metallothionine synthesis.

Clinical Pearls

- Young patients with abnormal liver function tests associated with neuropsychiatric disorder need to be suspected of Wilson's disease
- Since Wilson's disease is an autosomal recessive disorder, it is necessary to screen all the first degree relatives
- Prior to the use of chelating agents, the disease was invariably fatal.

Alpha1 Antitrypsin Deficiency

Introduction

An autosomal recessive condition. α1 antitrypsin is a protease inhibitor synthesized in the liver, which is responsible for inhibiting trypsin, collagenase, elastase and proteases of polymorphonuclear neutrophils.

α1 antitrypsin deficiency leads to:
- Progressive decrease in elastin in the lung which leads to premature emphysema
- Cirrhosis.

Pathogenesis

This occurs due to a genetic defect located on chromosome 14 by replacing glutamic acid by lysine at position 342. The deficiency causes liver injury related to mechanism of high levels of molecule in the endoplasmic reticulum of liver cells.

Diagnosis

Symptoms

- Usually asymptomatic
- Neonatal cholestasis and jaundice in 10% of patients.

Signs

- Icterus
- Hepatomegaly
- Signs of portal hypertension
- Signs of liver failure in late cases
- Signs of emphysema in lung involvement.

Investigations

Blood Tests

- **α1 *antitrypsin levels*** are low—<75% of lower limit of normal (80 mg%)
- ***Liver enzymes*** are elevated.

Tissue Diagnosis

- ***Liver biopsy***—PAS staining granules in hepatic cells is confirmative.

Complications

- End-stage liver disease
- Hepatocellular carcinoma.

Management

Medical

- No specific treatment is available
- Treatment is always symptomatic
- Prevention of hepatotoxic agents (alcohol)
- Adequate nutrition
- Ursodeoxycholic acid may be useful.

Surgical

- Liver transplantation.

Clinical Pearls

- Only a small percentage of patients with α1 antitrypsin deficiency develop liver disease
- Complete absence of α1 antitrypsin causes lung disease.

CIRRHOSIS

Introduction

Cirrhosis is defined as the presence of fibrous septa in the liver substance subdividing the liver parenchyma into nodules, which is the final sequel (healing process) of chronic hepatitis.

Etiology

The causes of cirrhosis are:
- Alcohol abuse
- Viral hepatitis
- Autoimmune hepatitis

- Drug-induced hepatitis
- Cholestatic diseases
- Metabolic diseases
- Hepatic vein outflow abnormalities.

Pathogenesis

Alcohol causes direct toxic injury to the liver, which is magnified by the associated protein and dietary deficiencies. It induces a specific cytochrome P450, which participates in the metabolism to acetaldehyde, having a number of deleterious effects on the liver cell, including antibody formation, decreased DNA repair, enzyme inactivation and alterations in mitochondria and plasma membrane. Acetaldehyde also produces glutathione depletion, lipid peroxidation and hepatic collagen synthesis. Increased fibroblastic activity and repair from necrosis accelerate collagen synthesis.

Hepatic necrosis stimulates the stellate cell by the production of cytokines, including IL1, IL6 and TNFα. The stellate cell activation is associated with pathologic matrix degeneration caused by overproduction of membrane-type matrix metalloproteinase 1, matrix metalloproteinase 2 and tissue inhibitors of metalloproteinases. Activated stellate cells undergo phenotypic changes and impede the portal flow, which results in increase in portal resistance by constricting the sinusoids and the cirrhotic liver. The entire process of evolution of portal hypertension is aided by endothelin 1, arginine vasopressin, eicosanoids and adrenomedullin.

The natural history of cirrhosis is unpredictable. Generally, after diagnosis, about 30% die of hepatic failure or complications of portal hypertension. The status of liver function plays a large role

Table 17.15: Differences between the types of cirrhosis

Feature	Micronodular cirrhosis	Macronodular cirrhosis	Mixed variety of cirrhosis
Septa	Thick and regular	Varying size	Mixed features
Nodules	Uniform and involves every hepatic lobule	Varying size	Mixed features

in the history of cirrhotics, which is determined by the presence of varices, and the portal pressure (Child's criteria).

Classification

- Micronodular cirrhosis
- Macronodular cirrhosis
- Mixed variety of cirrhosis.

The differences between the types of cirrhosis are tabulated in **Table 17.15**.

Diagnosis

Symptoms

- Asymptomatic (40%)
- Weight loss
- Jaundice
- Abdominal pain
- Change in sleep pattern
- Hyperirritability
- Loss of libido
- Loss of menstrual cycle
- GI bleed.

Signs

- Malnutrition
- Fetor hepaticus
- Yellow colored skin and sclera
- Signs of liver failure (spider nevi, ascites, pleural effusion, caput medusae)
- Signs of portal hypertension (bleeding varices, splenomegaly).

Investigations

Blood Tests

- **_Hematocrit:_** Normocytic normochromic anemia
- **_WBC and platelet counts_** are reduced (due to hypersplenism)
- **_Prothrombin time_** is prolonged
- **_Serum albumin_** is depressed
- **_Serum ALT and AST_** may be elevated
- **_Serum alkaline phosphatase_** may be elevated
- **_Bilirubin_** may be elevated.

Tests to evaluate the etiology
- Alcohol abuse (AST > ALT)
- Viral hepatitis (Positive hepatitis B and C serologies)
- Autoimmune hepatitis (presence of ANA and SMA)
- Cholestatic diseases (Elevated alkaline phosphatase)
- Primary biliary cirrhosis (AMA)
- Primary sclerosing cholangitis (Elevated alkaline phosphatase)
- Metabolic diseases
  - Wilson's disease (serum ceruloplasmin)
  - Hemochromatosis (Ferritin, iron studies, gene mutations test)
  - $\alpha 1$ antitrypsin deficiency (low levels of $\alpha 1$ antitrypsin levels)
- Hepatic vein outflow abnormalities (tests for hypercoagulopathy)
- NAFLD (serum lipid levels, elevated sugars).

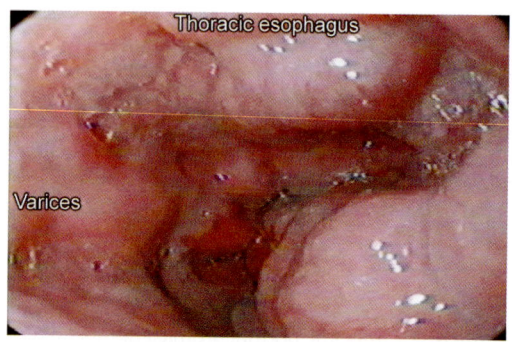

Fig. 17.9: Esophagoscopy—Varices

Endoscopy

Upper GI endoscopy may show esophagogastric varices (**Fig. 17.9**).

Tissue Diagnosis

- *Liver biopsy* is diagnostic.

Complications

- Progressive hyperbilirubinemia
- Malnutrition
- Decreased synthetic function of liver
- Portal hypertension
- Hepatic encephalopathy.

Management

- Total abstinence from alcohol
- Nutrition
- Close monitoring for complications (portal hypertension).

Clinical Pearls

- Diagnosis of cirrhosis is based on histologic findings
- A single type of cirrhosis may result from various causes, and also a single disease process can give rise to a variety of patterns
- Irrespective of etiology, cirrhosis causes right lobar atrophy, caudate lobe and left lateral segment hypertrophy, nodular surface, dilatation of portal vein, gastroesophageal varices and splenomegaly
- Normal liver function tests do not rule out the possibility of cirrhosis
- Periodic endoscopic evaluation is necessary to identify the presence of varices
- Imaging studies are useful in assessing the size and echotexture of liver, the anatomy of biliary ducts, presence of ascites and splenomegly as well as the presence of liver masses
- Cirrhosis is said to compensated when there are no manifestations of ESLD and decompensated when there are manifestations of ESLD, namely jaundice, variceal hemorrhage or uncontrolled ascites
- 30–40% of compensated cirrhotics have varices
- Compensated cirrhosis has a 10-year survival rate of about 50%
- Cirrhotics die of complications of liver dysfunction or portal hypertension.

PRIMARY BILIARY CIRRHOSIS

Introduction

Primary biliary cirrhosis is uncommon, but prevalent in women. It is a destructive disease of small, interlobular bile ducts, of autoimmune origin. Other autoimmune diseases like thyroiditis, scleroderma and rheumatoid arthritis may coexist.

Etiology and Pathogenesis

The destruction occurs due to the concentration of hydrophobic bile acids and toxins. Fibrosis is promoted by cytokines produced by inflammatory cells. Antimitochondrial antibodies (AMA) directed against bile duct epithelial cell antigens develop.

Diagnosis

Symptoms

- Majority are asymptomatic
- Fatigue is predominant in a majority
- Pruritus.

Signs

- Hepatomegaly
- Signs of liver failure in late cases
- Xanthomas around the eyes (xanthelasma).

Investigations

Blood Tests

- ***AMAs*** directed against dehydrogenase enzymes are positive
- ***LFT*** is abnormal, alkaline phosphatase is markedly elevated
- ***Serum cholesterol*** levels are elevated
- ***ANA and antithyroid antibodies*** may be present.

Radiology

- ***US or CT*** will show biliary obstruction.

Tissue Diagnosis

Liver biopsy
- Stage I: Inflammatory cells surround a bile duct with epithelial degeneration
- Stage II: Portal fibrosis
- Stage III: Fibrosis joins portal triads
- Stage IV: Cirrhotic features.

Complications

- Osteoporosis
- Steatorrhea
- Hypothyroidism
- End-stage liver disease (ESLD)
- Hepatobiliary malignancy.

Management

Medical
- UDCA is useful
- Cyclosporine has marginal benefit.

Surgical
- Liver transplantation is the most effective treatment.

PORTAL VEIN THROMBOSIS

Introduction

Thrombosis of the portal vein can occur as an isolated entity or it may be associated with splenic vein and superior mesenteric vein thrombosis. The thrombosis can be acute or chronic.

Etiology

The causes of portal vein thrombosis are:
- Cirrhosis of liver
- Portal hypertension
- Sepsis
- Malignancy
- Schistosomiasis
- Drugs
- Extrinsic compression by nodes
- Pregnancy.

Diagnosis

Symptoms and Signs

Acute portal vein thrombosis (presenting within 2 months of thrombosis)
- Acute abdominal pain
- Fever
- Signs of mesenteric infarction.

Chronic portal vein thrombosis (presents with complications of portal hypertension)
- Splenomegaly and hypersplenism
- Variceal bleeding
- Hepatic encephalopathy
- Ascites.

Investigations

Blood Tests
- ***Complete blood count*** for hypersplenism.

Radiology
- **US Doppler study** of portal vein
- **Contrast CT** of abdomen
- **EUS.**

Management

Acute portal vein thrombosis
- Anticoagulation therapy using heparin and warfarin.

Chronic portal vein thrombosis
- Surgical portosystemic shunt
- **Transjugular intrahepatic portosystemic shunt** (TIPSS) is a good alternative—this involves implantation of a metallic stent between the intrahepatic branch of portal vein and a hepatic vein radical (**Fig. 17.10**).

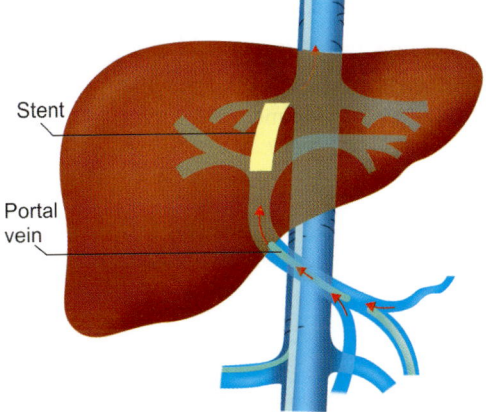

Fig. 17.10: Transjugular intrahepatic portosystemic shunt

BUDD–CHIARI SYNDROME

Introduction

Budd–Chiari syndrome is a rare disorder where obstruction of hepatic venous outflow occurs. The obstruction can occur at the small hepatic venules in the hepatic parenchyma to the main hepatic veins at its entry into the inferior vena cava even up to the right atrium.

Etiology

The causes of Budd–Chiari syndrome are:

Common causes
- Idiopathic (most common)
- Myeloproliferative disorders (polycythemia vera, thrombocytosis)
- Factor V Leiden and factor II gene mutations.

Uncommon causes
- Protein C and S deficiencies
- Antiphospholipid syndrome
- Antithrombin III deficiency
- Paroxysmal nocturnal hemoglobinuria
- Trauma
- Behçet's syndrome
- Idiopathic membranous stenosis of IVC.

Pathogenesis

Occlusion of hepatic veins results from thrombosis, as in post-sinusoidal pathology, which causes hypoxia and increase the sinusoidal pressure, which is transmitted proximally to cause hepatomegaly, varying degrees of liver failure and portal hypertension. Since there is no fibrosis in the liver parenchyma, filtration occurs to a great extent, producing marked ascites.

Diagnosis

Symptoms and Signs
- Mild and vague right upper quadrant pain
- Postprandial fullness
- Anorexia

Weeks or months later:
- Hepatomegaly
- Gross ascites is almost universal
- Hepatic failure.

Investigations

Blood Tests

- ***AST levels*** show marked elevation
- ***Bilirubin*** is slightly elevated
- ***Alkaline phosphatase*** is inconsistently abnormal.

Radiology

- ***CT and MRI*** show perfusion abnormality in the liver substance. CT shows pooling of intravenous contrast in the periphery of the liver. Caudate lobe hypertrophy may be predominantly seen
- ***Venography and Doppler studies*** demonstrate the obstructed hepatic veins
- ***CT or MRI angiography*** demonstrates the obstructed hepatic veins and also good delineation of vena cava is required to plan the portacaval shunt.

Tissue Diagnosis

Liver biopsy reveals grossly dilated central veins and sinusoids, pericentral necrosis and replacement of liver cells by RBCs.

Differential Diagnosis

- Veno-occlusive disease
- Congestive hepatopathy.

Complications

- Liver failure
- Variceal hemorrhage
- Encephalopathy.

Management

- Side to side portacaval or mesocaval shunt is useful in patients with localized hepatic vein obstruction
- In venacaval stenosis, the stenosis can be dilated by balloon angioplasty
- Obstruction of vena cava by thrombosis or compression from the liver warrants a mesoatrial shunt using a prosthetic graft
- Liver transplantation is the best treatment when there is severe hepatic decompensation either from cirrhosis or as a part of acute syndrome.

Clinical Pearls

- Since the venous drainage of caudate lobe is directly into the inferior vena cava through multiple tributaries, it is spared of the effects of hepatic venous outflow obstruction

- TIPSS cannot be done as the hepatic veins are not patent
- Patients with acute presentation may develop hepatic encephalopathy and hepatorenal syndrome, and those with chronic presentation predominantly show features of portal hypertension and cirrhosis
- When IVC is obstructed, bilateral pedal edema is the presentation.

PORTAL HYPERTENSION

Introduction

- Portal hypertension is defined as increased portal venous pressure
- Normal portal venous pressure ranges from 7–10 mm Hg. In portal hypertension, portal pressure exceeds 10 mm Hg averaging around 20 mm, sometimes rising as high as 50–60 mm Hg
- Portal venous pressure is determined by the relationship Pressure = Flow x Resistance, and portal hypertension can occur due to increased flow or increased resistance to flow
- Portal hypertension is defined as increased portal pressure of over 20 mm Hg when measured at surgery or a wedged hepatic vein pressure greater than 5 mm Hg above the inferior vena caval pressure.

Etiology

Normally, the blood flow into the liver is about 2 liters/min but from two sources: hepatic arterial and portal venous systems. Portal blood contributes about 75% of blood to the liver, which is derived from spleen, pancreas, gallbladder and the alimentary tract. The amount of portal blood averages to about 1,000–1,500 mL which reaches the liver through the portal vein, formed by the splenic and superior mesenteric veins. The portal vein does not contain valves. Portal system communicates with the systemic circulation at the gastroesophageal junction, anal canal, falciform ligament, splenic venous bed and left renal vein and retroperitoneum. When the portal pressure is normal, very little blood is shunted into the systemic circulation, but when the portal pressure increases, a large amount of blood is shunted into the systemic circulation.

The collaterals depend partly on the cause of portal hypertension.

- Extrahepatic portal vein thrombosis causes collaterals in the diaphragm and in hepatocolic, hepatoduodenal and gastrohepatic ligaments
- In cirrhotics, collaterals predominantly develop in the lower esophagus and stomach. Collaterals at other places occur later
- Isolated splenic vein thrombosis gives rise to collaterals from the spleen to gastric fundus (gastric varices without esophageal varices).

Portal hypertension is caused by a variety of causes. They are:

Increased resistance to portal blood flow

- *Hepatic (sinusoidal) causes:* Cirrhosis of liver, acute alcoholic liver disease
- *Posthepatic (post-sinusoidal) causes:* Budd–Chiari syndrome, congestive cardiac failure, constrictive pericarditis
- *Prehepatic (presinusoidal) causes:*
  - *Extrahepatic:* Portal vein and splenic vein thrombosis
  - *Intrahepatic:* Schistosomiasis, congenital hepatic fibrosis, idiopathic portal fibrosis, sarcoid

Increased portal blood flow

- Arterial portal venous fistula (traumatic/congenital)

- Increased splenic blood flow (e.g. Banti's syndrome, splenomegaly).

In general, most causes of portal hypertension cause resistance to portal flow. The commonest cause of portal hypertension is cirrhosis followed by extrahepatic portal venous thrombosis or occlusion. Posthepatic obstruction due to Budd–Chiari syndrome or constrictive pericarditis is rare.

Diagnosis

Symptoms

- Upper and lower gastrointestinal bleeds (due to rupture of collaterals)
- Jaundice and signs of hepatic failure (due to cirrhosis).

Signs

- Abdominal distension (due to ascites)
- Liver is enlarged in Budd–Chiari syndrome, not enlarged in cirrhosis and portal vein thrombosis
- Splenomegaly is a constant finding in all cases of portal hypertension.

Investigations

Blood Tests

- *Pancytopenia* indicates hypersplenism
- *Liver function tests* to establish the liver disease.

Radiology

- *Abdominal ultrasonography* demonstrates the large portal vein, which is not diagnostic of portal hypertension

- ***Doppler ultrasound*** can demonstrate the direction of portal venous flow and portal vein thrombosis
- ***Abdominal CT or MR angiography*** are capable of showing the portal vein anatomy
- ***Visceral angiography and portal venography*** are more informative
- ***Hepatic venography:*** using a balloon catheter in the hepatic vein to measure free hepatic venous pressure (FHVP) and wedged hepatic venous pressure (WHVP). Hepatic venous pressure gradient (HVPG) represents the portal venous pressure. (HVPG = WHVP–FHVP)
- ***Esophagogastroscopy*** to establish the presence of esophagogastric varices **(Refer Fig. 10.21B)**
- ***Barium swallow*** **(Refer Fig. 10.21A)** is rarely performed today.

Complications

- Ascites
- Spontaneous bacterial peritonitis
- Gastrointestinal bleeding
- Hepatorenal syndrome (portal hypertension and renal failure)
- Portopulmonary syndrome (portal hypertension and pulmonary hypertension)
- Coagulopathy
- Hepatic encephalopathy
- Hepatopulmonary syndrome
- Hepatocellular carcinoma.

Management

Acute variceal bleeding
- ICU care

- Blood transfusions
- Fresh frozen plasma and platelets for coagulopathy
- Vitamin K injections to correct prolonged prothrombin time
- Short-term antibiotics to prevent infections
- *Medical:* Vasoactive drugs to reduce portal pressure
    - Vasopressin IV 0.2–0.8 units/min
    - Terlipressin IV 2 mg every 6 hours
    - Somatostatin analogue octreotide (50 µg stat followed by 50 µg/hour) for 5 days
- *Mechanical:* Balloon tamponade with Sengstaken Blakemore tube till definitive therapy is done
- *Interventional nonsurgical*
    - Endoscopic sclerotherapy/variceal band ligation
    - Transhepatic embolization.
- *Surgical*
    - ***Emergency portacaval shunt procedures*** are needed to reverse the portosystemic flow of blood—side to side portacaval shunt is preferred for ease in the emergency situation
    - ***Esophagogastric devascularization +/- esophageal transection*** is done as an emergency procedure, when sclerotherapy or band ligation has failed. Definitive therapy for portal hypertension has to follow
    - ***Splenectomy*** is needed in cases with hypersplenism and large spleens
    - ***Liver transplantation*** provides cure for irreversible liver disorders.
- *Minimally invasive*
    - ***Transjugular intrahepatic portosystemic shunt (TIPSS)*** is a good alternative—used as a bridge procedure to liver transplantation, and not as a definitive therapy.

Snapshots in Gastroenterology

Nonbleeding Varices

Treatment aims to be prophylactic, as the risk of bleeding is about 30% with a mortality of about 25%.
- Non-selective beta blockers (Propranolol, timolol, nadolol) decrease cardiac output and cause splanchnic vasoconstriction
- Endoscopic band ligation (in patients who do not tolerate beta blockers).

Varices Bled Previously

Patients who recover from one episode of variceal bleeding, 60–70% of them bleed again, and deserve definitive therapy.
- Non-selective beta blocker therapy—Propranolol 20–160 mg daily for long period—expected to reduce variceal bleeding by 40%
- Endoscopic band ligation/sclerotherapy
- TIPSS
- Surgical procedures
  - Liver transplantation
  - Portosystemic shunts
- Devascularization procedures—Esophagogastric devascularization + esophageal transection (Sugiura–Futugawa procedure).

Clinical Pearls

- A portal pressure of >12 mm Hg is required for varices to form and subsequently bleed
- Use of beta blockers in cirrhotics without varices is debatable
- Early identification of varices and administration of beta blockers help in preventing variceal bleeds
- Variceal hemorrhage is usually intermittent
- When variceal hemorrhage is suspected/confirmed, octreotide, which decreases splanchnic pressure should be started, *and* is more effective and safer than vasopressin

- Patients with upper GI hemorrhage are prone to infections and an antibiotic effective against the enteric group of organisms, like third generation cephalosporin is to be started, which is also effective in preventing spontaneous bacterial peritonitis
- PPIs reduce gastritis but not the bleeding from portal hypertensive gastropathy
- In cirrhotics, upper GI hemorrhage is caused by variceal rupture, gastritis, peptic ulcer disease or portal hypertensive gastropathy
- TIPSS is used in patients with decompensated liver disease and shunt surgery is preferred for patients with preserved liver function
- Surgical shunt procedures are considered only in candidates not fit for liver transplantation
- Even in the absence of cirrhosis, acute alcoholic liver disease can cause portal hypertension due to centrilobular swelling and fibrosis. Liver cells engorged with fat, cause vascular channel narrowing, which results in raise in portal venous pressure
- Schistosomiasis causes portal hypertension by depositing the ova in the small portal venules, and cause obstruction to flow
- In cirrhotic patients, portal blood flow drops to about 30% of normal, ranging from 0 to 700 mL/min
- TIPSS has reduced the number of shunt procedures performed, but shunt procedures continue to be more reliable and durable

ASCITES

Introduction

Ascites is accumulation of serous fluid in the peritoneal cavity. It can result from various causes (**Table 17.16**), and is a manifestation of chronic liver disease.

Table 17.16: Causes of ascites

Causes	Mechanism
Parenchymal liver disease (cirrhosis, alcoholic liver disease)	Portal hypertension
Right heart failure	
Constrictive pericarditis	
Veno-occlusive disease	
Budd–Chiari syndrome	
Portal vein thrombosis	
Spontaneous bacterial peritonitis	Peritoneal inflammation
Malignant peritoneal deposits	
Connective tissue disorders	
Tuberculosis	
Pancreatic ascites	
Hypoalbuminic states (nephritic syndrome, malnutrition, protein losing enteropathy)	Reduced plasma oncotic pressure
Lymphatic obstruction (tuberculosis, lymphatic tear)	

Etiology and Pathogenesis

Ascites results due to sinusoidal hypertension, which can be due to:
- Increased formation of hepatic lymph (due to postsinusoidal hypertension)
- Increased formation of splanchnic lymph (due to splanchnic vasodilatation)
- Hypoalbuminemia
- Salt and water retention by kidneys

Diagnosis

Symptoms

- Full history is essential
- Symptoms related to cirrhosis, portal hypertension and cardiac disease
- Symptoms related to intra-abdominal malignancy (e.g. appetite and weight loss, abdominal pain/discomfort)
- Symptoms related to infection (e.g. tuberculosis, bacterial peritonitis).

Signs

- Signs of chronic liver disease (e.g. jaundice, flapping tremor, spider nevi, etc.)
- Signs of chronic cardiac failure (e.g. cardiomegaly, increased JVP)
- Signs of portal hypertension (e.g. caput medusae, splenomegaly).

Investigations

Blood Tests

- *Blood counts, LFT, ESR, CRP, coagulation profile.*

Radiology

- *Ultrasonography* for intra-abdominal pathology
- *Doppler study of portal venous system.*

Ascitic Fluid Analysis

- Color
  - Straw/yellow colored (e.g. portal hypertension, tuberculosis)
  - Blood suggests bloody tap or malignancy
  - White color suggests chylous ascites

- White cell count increase
  - Neutrophil increase (e.g. bacterial peritonitis)
  - Lymphocyte increase (e.g. tuberculous ascites)
- Ascitic albumin: Ratio of serum to ascites >11 g/L indicates ascites due to portal hypertension and differentiates from non-portal hypertension
- Bacterial count and culture: Bacterial peritonitis including tuberculosis
- LDH levels: Ratio of ascites to serum > 0.6 suggests malignancy or infection
- Amylase: High level suggests pancreatic disease
- Cytology: Malignant ascites.

Further tests are tailored to the results of the above tests and clinical presentation. The diagnosis of cause of ascites can be made utilizing the algorithm given in **Figure 17.11**.

Management

Medical

- Salt restriction
- Diuretics: Spironolactone (aldosterone antagonist and distally acting diuretic) 50–400 mg/day as a single dose to inhibit sodium reabsorption and to simulate weight loss. When this is not enough, furosemide (a loop diuretic) is added. The usual dose is spironolactone (100 mg) and furosemide (40 mg)
- Paracentesis to relieve tense ascites and respiratory embarrassment. Aspiration of more than 5 liters require plasma volume expander to prevent circulatory dysfunction.

Surgical

- **Portosystemic shunt:** A total shunt like side to side portacaval, H-mesocaval or central splenorenal shunt can be performed

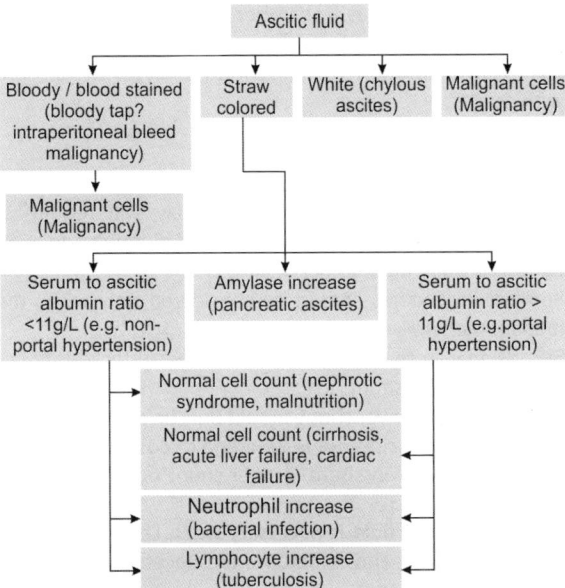

Fig. 17.11: Algorithm for the cause of ascites

mainly to reduce the sinusoidal and the splanchnic venous pressures, but not advocated exclusively to treat ascites
- *TIPSS* is a good therapeutic procedure for treating ascites, and a good alternative for repeated paracentesis but has the disadvantage of encephalopathy
- *Peritoneal jugular shunt (LeVeen shunt, Denver shunt):* A silastic catheter with a unidirectional valve—used to transport the ascitic fluid to the jugular vein (LeVeen shunt has no chamber

and Denver shunt has a chamber which can be compressed to direct the flow when blocked)
- ***Liver transplantation*** is the definitive treatment for cirrhotics with ascites.

Clinical Pearls

- Urinary sodium output of <5 mEq/day will require strong diuretics, 5–25 mEq/day will require mild diuretics and >25 mEq/day will require no diuretics at all
- Surgical procedures should be considered only when medical management fails entirely
- Surprisingly, in practice, Denver shunt gets blocked more often than the LeVeen shunt
- LeVeen shunt/Denver shunt should only be considered for those with refractory ascites not responding to doses of 400 mg/day
- Blockage of LeVeen shunt/Denver shunt occurs less when the ascitic fluid is clear
- Culture of ascitic fluid is necessary when LeVeen shunt/Denver shunt is planned and antibiotics are necessary at least during insertion
- LeVeen shunt/Denver shunt is not enough as a single procedure to decompress the ascites, and patients usually require some diuretics
- When the valve gets blocked, it needs replacement
- Malignant ascites is refractory and requires repeated therapeutic paracentesis
- The goal of therapy in portal hypertension is to reduce the weight by 0.5 kg/day and 1 kg/day if peripheral edema is prominent
- Pancreatic ascites requires planned surgical therapy depending on the site and nature of pathology.

HEPATIC ENCEPHALOPATHY

Introduction

Hepatic encephalopathy is a neuropsychiatric disorder with central nervous system abnormalities associated with chronic liver disease or liver failure. This can occur due to diversion of portal blood into the systemic circulation either due to disease process or following surgery like portacaval shunts.

Etiology and Pathogenesis

Portosystemic or hepatic encephalopathy occurs due to several factors. They are:
- *Conditions which increase the toxin levels:*
    - Portosystemic shunt
    - Decreased liver function
    - Intestinal protein load
    - Azotemia
    - Intestinal flora
    - Constipation.
- *Factors with increased CNS sensitivity:*
    - Old age
    - Hypokalemia
    - Diuretics
    - Alkalosis
    - Infection
    - Hypoxia, hypoglycemia.

Chemical agents or toxins, which are formed by colonic bacterial action are not degraded by the diseased liver, and is directly shunted into the systemic circulation though the natural portosystemic collaterals or through operative shunts. The continued exposure of these toxins to the brain causes a metabolic neuropathy, which is reversible. This syndrome is believed to be associated with four chemical mediators. They are:

- *Gamma aminobutyric acid (GABA):* This is produced in the colon by the bacteria not degraded in the liver with chronic pathology, and this inhibitory neurotransmitter, which reaches the brain through the portosystemic shunting, causes abnormalities of CNS
- *Ammonia:* Ammonia which is also produced by bacterial degradation in the colon reaches the brain by the same route as GABA
- *False neurotransmitters:* Octopamine and phenyl ethanolamine replace the normal neurotransmitters to cause inhibition of CNS function. So also, the aromatic amino acids which are the precursors of the false neurotransmitters cross the blood-brain barrier to give the similar effect
- *Synergistic neurotoxins:* Neurotoxins like the ammonia, mercaptans and fatty acids produce a synergistic effect on the brain function, but as a single agent they are not capable of producing this effect.

In essence, ammonia causes astrocyte swelling and cerebral edema, causing neurologic symptoms of hepatic encephalopathy.

Diagnosis

Symptoms and Signs

- Lethargy to coma (**Table 17.17**)
- Minor psychological disturbances to psychosis
- Asterixis to paraplegia.

Investigations

- Investigations related to liver pathology
- US or CT will show signs of portal hypertension.

Table 17.17: Grades of hepatic encephalopathy (West Haven criteria)

Grade	Features	Liver flap
1	Impaired higher functions but no effect on consciousness	Usually absent
2	Disorientation and personality change with inappropriate behavior	Usually present
3	Confusion and gross disorientation with increased somnolence	Present
4	Coma	Usually absent

Management

Acute hepatic encephalopathy
- Withdrawal of protein food in the acute stage
- High calorie carbohydrate diet
- Proper hydration (to prevent prerenal uremia)
- Lactulose (orally, rectally or through NG tube) 60–90 g/day titrated to 5 loose stools per day
- Antibiotics (neomycin, metronidazole, rifaximin)
- Vitamin K to correct the prothrombin time
- Probiotics.

Chronic hepatic encephalopathy
- Protein restricted/carbohydrate rich food
- Avoidance of constipation, by lactulose
- Intermittent courses of antibiotics.

Clinical Pearls

- Patients with alcoholic liver disease do better than those with postnecrotic liver disease, when treated for hepatic encephalopathy

- Incidence of encephalopathy is maximum with total shunts and least with selective shunts like Warren shunt
- Use of disaccharides (e.g. lactulose) is important as they have the ability to reduce intraluminal pH, facilitating the conversion of ammonia to ammonium and expel it out of the colon
- There is no correlation between serum ammonia levels and grades of encephalopathy
- Progression of encephalopathy carries a very high risk of cerebral edema, which may progress to death.

HEPATORENAL SYNDROME

Introduction

Defined as renal failure secondary to hepatic failure. This is characterized by intense renal vasoconstriction and histologically near normal kidney status in patients with liver disease.

The criteria required to diagnose hepatorenal syndrome are:
- Chronic or acute liver disease with portal hypertension
- Serum creatinine >1.5 mg% or creatinine clearance <40 cc/min
- No evidence of shock, infection, dehydration or recent use of nephrotoxic drugs
- No sustained response to 1.5 liters of saline as a challenge
- Proteinuria <500 mg/day
- No evidence of obstructive nephropathy in US.

Classification

- Type 1: Rapidly worsening renal status with doubling of initial serum creatinine (50% worsening in 2 weeks)
- Type 2: Steady deterioration over weeks or months.

Pathogenesis

Though exact mechanism is not known, dehydration, paracentesis, excessive diuresis, bleeding, NSAID use are said to be precipitate the syndrome.

Diagnosis

Symptoms and Signs
- Signs of acute renal failure
- Signs of end-stage liver disease.

Management
- No effective cure is available
- Improvement in liver function is the only hope for improving the renal function
- Liver transplantation may be useful, the renal function may deteriorate after liver transplantation.

Clinical Pearls
- Some patients of type II disease can develop type I disease at a later date
- Immaterial of the type, prognosis remains very poor, and spontaneous recovery is rare.

FOCAL LIVER MASSES

Introduction

A focal mass in the liver is a space-occupying lesion. This can be present as a single mass or multiple masses and involve one or

Table 17.18: Differential diagnosis of focal liver masses

Tissue of origin	Benign	Malignant
Epithelium	• Hepatic adenoma • Bile duct adenoma • Biliary cystadenoma	• Hepatocellular carcinoma • Cholangiocarcinoma • Biliary cystadenocarcinoma
Mesenchyme	• Hemangioma	• Angiosarcoma • Primary lymphoma of liver
Others	• Focal nodular hyperplasia • Liver abscess • Regenerative nodules of cirrhosis • Simple hepatic cyst	• Metastatic tumors

both lobes of liver. They originate from various tissues and they are tabulated in **Table 17.18**.

Diagnosis

History

- History of viral hepatitis or cirrhosis suggests malignant transformation
- Patient with a malignant disease in the past suggests metastatic disease
- Use of oral contraceptives may suggest hepatic adenoma.

Symptoms and Signs

- Many focal lesions may remain asymptomatic
- Associated with diseases like cirrhosis, can present with symptoms of liver failure.

Investigations

Blood Tests

- *Serum bilirubin* is elevated, if associated with chronic hepatitis (indirect bilirubinemia) or while causing biliary obstruction (direct bilirubinemia)
- *Liver enzymes* remain normal, unless associated with active hepatitis or cirrhosis
- *Alkaline phosphatase* is usually elevated in malignant lesions, but large benign lesions can also elevate due to biliary obstruction
- *Hepatitis virus profile* is needed to complement the diagnosis.

Serological Markers

- *Serum alpha fetoprotein (AFP)* levels above 200 ng/mL are highly suggestive of hepatocellular carcinoma, but lesser levels may indicate hepatitis. The level remains normal in a third of patients of HCC, especially when the tumor size is <2 cm
- *CA 19/9* is used in the diagnosis of cholangiocarcinoma. A level of > 100 U/mL is found in about 50% patients. Elevations can also be seen in bacterial cholangitis, pancreatic carcinoma.

Radiology

- *Ultrasound* examination is the first investigation and the lesion is found accidentally during routine workup. It can differentiate a cystic lesion from a solid lesion
- *CT* is useful to study focal liver masses in detail. Triphasic CT has the added advantage of rapidity and can be done in a single breath hold, which allows the contrast injection to be viewed in unenhanced arterial, portal and delayed phases of perfusion
- *MRI* is also helpful in studying the lesion in detail, with a sensitivity similar to CT. Similar to the triphasic CT, breath hold

T1 weighted images and fast spin echo T2 weighted images eliminate respiratory motion for finer clarity
- ***MRI angiography*** is useful for vascular lesions
- ***Endoscopic ultrasound*** is found useful in experienced hands
- ***PET scan*** is also useful for metabolically active tumors
- ***Spyglass cholangioscopy*** is useful when biliary tract is involved.

Tissue Diagnosis

- ***Biopsy of the lesion:*** FNAC is useful but controversial.

The algorithm for diagnosis of focal hepatic lesions is given in **Figure 17.12**.

Management

Management depends on the diagnosis.

Clinical Pearls

- Most liver masses are asymptomatic and are diagnosed during routine workup
- Most liver masses occur in cirrhotic livers secondary to hepatitis B and C virus infections
- Abdominal ultrasonography is the best screening method to identify liver masses
- CT, MRI and angiography only complement the diagnosis by ultrasonography
- PET scan is not the useful investigating modality in differentiating liver masses
- Biopsy of the liver lesion is indicated only when surgical treatment is contemplated.

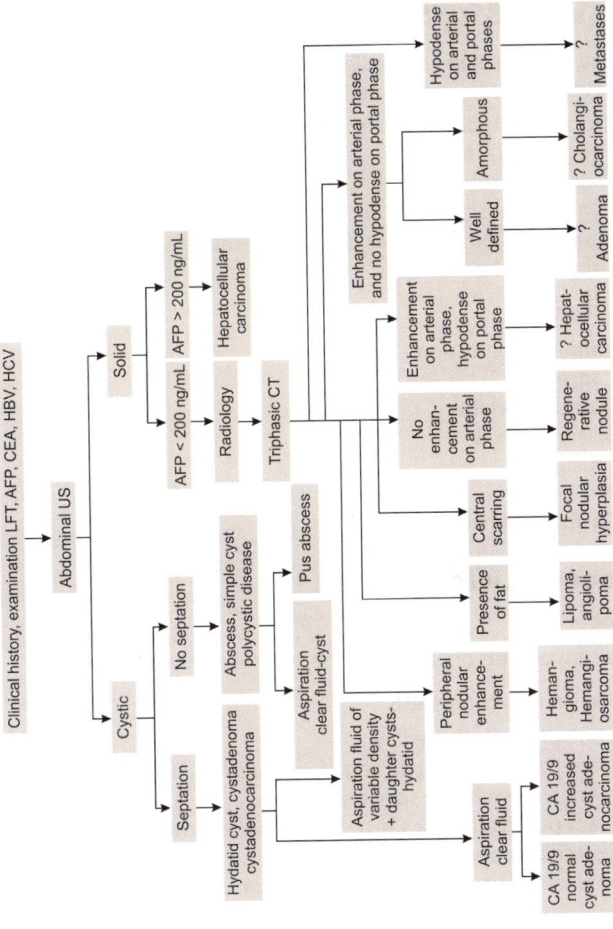

Fig. 17.12: Algorithm for diagnosing focal liver masses

LIVER ABSCESS

Due to the dual blood supply (systemic and portal), the liver is prone to develop abscesses of bacterial origin from other tissues.

The two major types of liver abscess are:
1. Pyogenic liver abscess
2. Amebic liver abscess

Pyogenic abscesses arise usually from intra-abdominal and systemic infections, whereas, amebic abscesses arise from colonic and appendicular infections.

Risk Factors
- Immunosuppression
- Cancer
- Diabetes mellitus
- Biliary diseases
- Old age
- Alcoholism
- Gastrointestinal infections.

Pyogenic Liver Abscess

Introduction

These are pockets of pus within the liver substance.

Etiology and Pathogenesis

Infection of liver is caused by:
- Gram-negative aerobes (e.g. *E. coli*, *Klebsiella* species, *Proteus* species, *Enterobacter* species)
- Gram-positive aerobes (e.g. *Streptococcus fecalis*, staphylococci, *Clostridium* species)
- Anaerobes (e.g. *Fusobacterium nucleatum*, *Bacteroides* species)

This occurs as a sequel of:
- **Direct spread**
  - Biliary tract infection (e.g. cholangitis)
  - Interventional procedures of liver or biliary tree (e.g. ERCP)
  - Obstructive biliary tract diseases (e.g. pancreatic malignancy)
  - Parasitic infections of biliary tract.
- **Portal venous blood spread**
  - Colonic diverticulitis
  - Acute appendicitis.
- **Hepatic arterial blood spread**
  - Septicemia.
- **General cause**
  - Immunosuppression
  - Diabetes mellitus.

The liver abscesses may be single or multiple, and right lobe is involved in the majority of patients, due to preferential blood flow from the mesenteric and portal venous system. Involvement of the left lobe is common with intrahepatic biliary calculi.

Diagnosis

Symptoms

- Constitutional symptoms with high-grade fever, tachycardia and sometime shock
- Right upper quadrant pain
- Less commonly, nausea, vomiting and weight loss, jaundice.

Signs

- Tender hepatomegaly may be present
- Intercostal tenderness is pathognomonic of a right lobar liver abscess
- Pleural and pericardial effusion may be present.

Investigations
- ***Leukocytosis*** indicates infection
- ***ESR*** may be raised
- ***Transaminases and bilirubin*** may be elevated, but to moderate levels
- ***Hypoalbuminemia*** may be present
- ***Blood culture*** may show the organism, in about 50% of septicemic patients
- ***Plain X-ray of abdomen or X-ray chest*** will reveal elevation of the right dome of diaphragm, Right pleural effusion is common, right lower lobe atelectasis may be present
- ***Fluoroscopy*** will show reduced mobility of the right dome of diaphragm
- ***US*** is the primary investigation as it differentiates cystic lesions from solid lesions and is diagnostic in liver abscess
- ***CT*** (Fig. 17.13A) is diagnostic

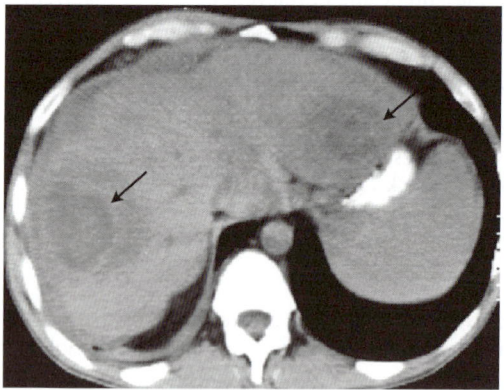

Fig. 17.13A: CT—Abscesses both lobes of liver

- *MRI* complements the CT features without any added advantage
- *Scintigraphy* (Techneitium and Gallium scans) is sensitive but may not be required
- *Aspiration* is confirmatory
- **Isolation** *of organism in culture* is required.

Differential Diagnosis

- Amebic liver abscess
- Malignant lesion with degeneration.

Complications

- Rupture into:
  - Peritoneal cavity (to cause localized peritonitis and subphrenic abscess)
  - Pleural space (to cause empyema)
  - Pericardial space (to cause pericarditis and tamponade).
- Spread by blood and cause:
  - Septic emboli in the lungs, brain and eyes.

Management

- Parenteral antibiotics
- Drainage under US guidance with broad-spectrum antibiotics
- Open drainage may be required for large and inaccessible abscesses
- Growth of pyogenic organisms in culture of pus requires appropriate treatment.

Indications for aspiration of hepatic abscess

- When pyogenic and amebic abscess cannot be differentiated
- Large abscess with impending rupture or causing severe symptoms like high-grade fever and pain.

Clinical Pearls

- Abscesses which develop due to cholangitis require definitive therapy for the primary cause
- In liver transplant patients, liver abscesses are due to hepatic artery thrombosis or severe cholangitis
- Abscesses secondary to biliary infection, tend to be small and multiple and involve both lobes of the liver, whereas abscesses secondary to portal pyemia tend to localize to the right lobe of the liver, as most of the portal blood goes to the right lobe of the liver
- Pyogenic abscesses of liver due to systemic causes are associated with splenic abscess and brain abscess
- Though rare, liver abscess caused by *Klebsiella* can have associated endogenous endophthalmitis, which may lead to visual loss
- Once a diagnosis of liver abscess is made, antibiotics should be started empirically
- Open drainage is limited to those patients who have not responded to percutaneous aspiration and antibiotics
- Hepatic resections are required for patients who have liver abscesses secondary to recurrent intrahepatic biliary lithiasis
- Prognosis depends on prompt diagnosis, treatment and general condition of patient.

Amebic Liver Abscess

Introduction

Infection of the liver parenchyma secondary to the intestinal infection caused by the parasite *Entamoeba histolytica*, common in tropical and subtropical climates.

Pathogenesis

The cystic form of the parasite is in a vegetative state, and once swallowed remains in the colon and develops into the trophozoite form, which invades the colonic mucosa, giving rise to ulcers, which are typically 'flask shaped'. The trophozoites reach the liver via the portal circulation and colonize and infect the liver parenchyma. Proteolytic enzymes destroy the parenchyma and cause abscesses. The contents remain sterile and bacterial superinfection can occur in about 20% of cases. Majority present as a solitary lesion usually in the right lobe, as majority of portal circulation reaches the right lobe of liver.

Diagnosis

Symptoms

- Constitutional symptoms like fever, toxicity
- Pain in the right upper abdomen referred to the right shoulder
- History of diarrhea or dysentery in the recent past may be present.

Signs

- Mild icterus may be present
- Liver is enlarged and acutely tender
- Marked tenderness and pitting edema are noted on application of pressure on the lower intercostal spaces on the right side (intercostal tenderness)
- Rarely, the abscess can present as a visible swelling in the abdomen.

Investigations

- *Plain X-ray of abdomen or X-ray chest* will show elevation of the right dome of diaphragm. Right pleural effusion is common

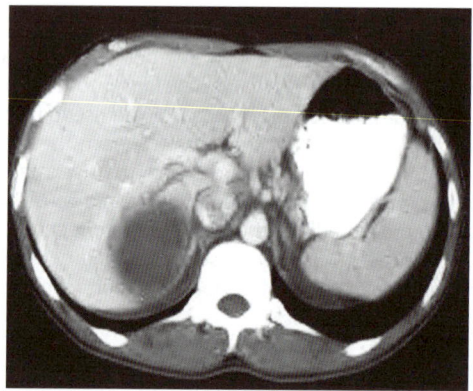

Fig. 17.13B: CT—Amebic liver abscess right lobe

- *Fluoroscopy* will show reduced mobility of the right dome
- *US and CT* (**Fig. 17.13B**) are diagnostic
- *Aspiration* is confirmatory
- *Stool examination* is routine
- *Serologic tests* are positive in majority of cases and differentiate from pyogenic abscesses, with a sensitivity of 95%
  - Hemagglutination test
  - Indirect immunofluorescence test
  - Counterimmunoelectrophoresis test
  - Immunoelectrophoresis test
  - Gel diffusion precipitin test
  - Complement fixation test
  - Latex agglutination test
  - Enzyme-linked immunosorbent assay.

Differential Diagnosis

- Pyogenic liver abscess
- Malignant lesion with degeneration.

Complications

- Rupture into:
  - Peritoneal cavity (to cause localized peritonitis and subphrenic abscess)
  - Pleural space (to cause amebic empyema)
  - Pericardial space (to cause amebic pericarditis and tamponade).
- Spread by blood and cause:
  - Septic emboli in the lungs, brain and eyes.

Management

- **Antiamebic drugs** (metronidazole or tinidazole) cure small abscess and hepatitis
- Chloroquine (600 mg/day for 2 days followed by 300 mg/day for 3 weeks) may be administered when there is no response with metronidazole
- **Drainage under US guidance**, under cover of broad-spectrum antibiotics and antiamebic drugs is curative for a large abscess
- **Growth of pyogenic organisms in culture of pus** requires appropriate treatment.

Indications for percutaneous drainage

- No improvement with medical management
- Impending rupture
- Large left lobe abscess (>5–7 cm)
- Suspicion of bacterial superinfection.

Clinical Pearls

- Compared to pyogenic liver abscess, amebic liver abscess presents with a subacute clinical presentation, and may take weeks or months to manifest
- Open surgical drainage is reserved for difficult cases with abscesses at inaccessible areas
- Only in a small percentage of patients, the pus of amebic liver abscess resemble anchovy sauce, but it is characteristically odorless
- Foul smelling pus on aspiration indicates pyogenic abscess or infected amebic abscess
- In amebic liver abscess, when aspirated only about 20% exhibit trophozoites of *E. histolytica*
- Amebae do not survive in bile, and infection of gallbladder and bile ducts do not occur, whereas pyogenic organisms survive in bile to cause cholangitis
- Serologic tests are negative in asymptomatic carriers, but positive only in invasive amebiasis like hepatic abscess and colitis.

CYSTIC LIVER DISEASES

Introduction

Cystic lesions of liver are generally picked up during routine screening and many of these patients are asymptomatic. The cysts can vary in number.

Classification

Congenital liver cysts
- Simple
- Polycystic disease
- Biliary hamartoma.

Parasitic liver cysts
- Hydatid disease.

Neoplastic liver cysts
- **Primary**
  - Cystadenoma
  - Cystadenocarcinoma
  - Cystic mesenchymal hamartoma
- **Secondary**
  - Cystic metastases
  - Large necrosed primary HCC.

Acquired liver cysts
- Post-traumatic hematoma or bileoma
- Liver abscess.

Characteristics of common cystic liver lesions are given in **Table 17.19**.

Table 17.19: Characteristics of common cystic liver lesions

Characteristic	Cystic lesion		
	Congenital cyst	Hydatid cyst	Cystadenoma
Stay in endemic areas	Not relevant	Relevant	Not relevant
Eosinophilia	Absent	Variable	Absent
Serological test	Negative	Usually positive	Positive in overt malignancy
Radiological Features			
Number of cysts	Solitary/multiple	Solitary/multiple	Solitary
Septations	Absent	Irregular	Irregular
Papillary projection	Absent	Absent	Present
Calcification	Absent	Present	Possible

Contd...

Contd...

Characteristic	Cystic lesion		
	Congenital cyst	Hydatid cyst	Cystadenoma
Split wall	Absent	Present	Absent
Communication with biliary tree	Absent	Common	Possible
Nature of cystic fluid	Serous	Variable	Mucinous
Natural History			
Malignant transformation	Rare	Not possible	Common
Recurrent after partial excision	Possible	Common	Common

CONGENITAL LIVER CYSTS

Introduction

Simple cyst: This lesion is filled with clear fluid with no communication with the intrahepatic bile ducts, and considered to develop due to the dilatation of aberrant intrahepatic bile ducts during embryogenesis. They are lined by single layer of columnar cells and surrounded by normal liver tissue. They can vary in number.

Polycystic liver disease: It is an inherited autosomal recessive disease, and is characterized by multiple cysts scattered in the liver parenchyma. They are thought to develop from cystic dilatation of biliary microhamartomas that originate from von Meyenburg complexes. It is usually associated with polycystic kidney disease (PKD) and cerebrovascular aneurysms. Prognosis depends on the renal status due to PKD.

Classification

They are divided into three types based on CT findings:
- **Type I:** Limited number (<10) of large cysts (>10 cm).
- **Type II:** Diffuse involvement of the liver parenchyma by multiple medium sized cysts with large areas of normal liver parenchyma.
- **Type III:** Massive diffuse involvement by small and medium sized cysts with few areas of preserved liver parenchyma.

Diagnosis

Symptoms and Signs

- *Simple cysts:* Most are asymptomatic, unless complicated by infection or hemorrhage
- *Polycystic liver disease:* Most are asymptomatic, unless complicated by infection or hemorrhage. Sometimes the clinical course is slowly progressive resulting in gross hepatomegaly.

Investigations

- *Simple cysts:*
  - *US* **(Fig. 17.14A)** appearance is characteristic as well defined echo-free lesion with thin wall without thickening or nodularity with septation, and spaces containing homogenous clear fluid with posterior acoustic enhancement
  - *CT* **(Fig. 17.14B)** complements the diagnosis
  - *MRI* shows low signal density on T1 weighted images with high signal density on T2 images which is characteristic
  - *FNAC* shows clear serous fluid
- *Polycystic liver disease:*
  - *US* appearance is characteristic.

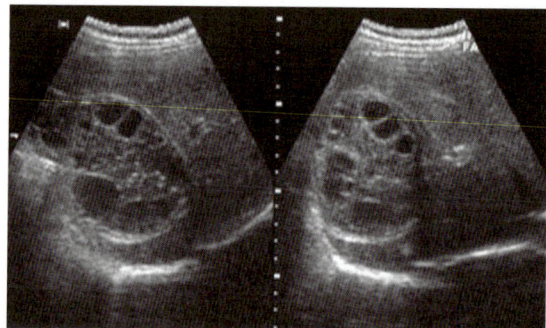

Fig. 17.14A: US—Multiloculated simple cyst of liver

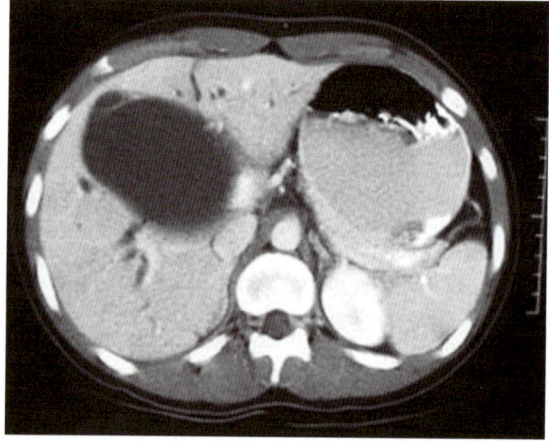

Fig. 17.14B: CT—Simple liver cyst

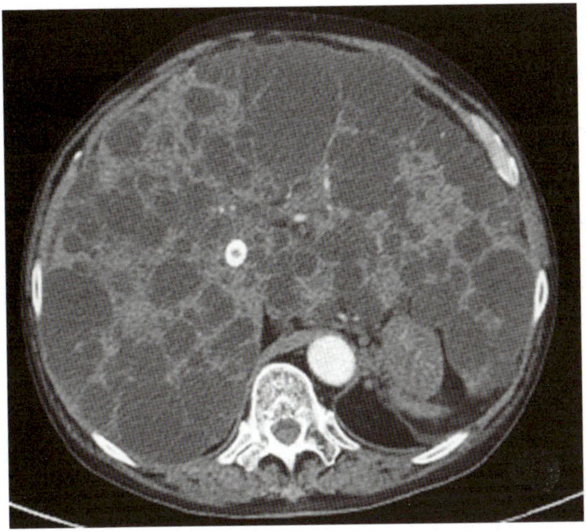

Fig. 17.14C: CT—Polycystic liver disease

- **CT (Fig. 17.14C)** complements the diagnosis, serial CT is useful to perform the liver volumetry
- **FNAC** shows clear serous fluid.

Complications

- Pressure effects on adjacent structures
- Pressure effects on intrahepatic structures (biliary obstruction, portal hypertension, IVC obstruction, Budd–Chiari syndrome)
- Intracystic hemorrhage
- Infection
- Rupture (into biliary tree, into peritoneum).

Management

- *Simple cysts:*
  - Simple aspiration will suffice, though recurrences are common
  - Alcohol sclerotherapy is effective
  - Surgical deroofing/removal is alternative therapy.
- *Polycystic liver disease:*
  - Type I disease: Simple aspiration, laparoscopic fenestration, alcohol sclerotherapy
  - Type II disease: Open fenestration ± liver resection/transplantation
  - Type III disease: Liver transplantation is the only choice, when the liver parenchyma is replaced.

Clinical Pearls

- A cystogram is necessary to rule out any biliary communication, if alcohol sclerotherapy is undertaken
- Alcohol sclerotherapy can also be undertaken using US or CT guidance or by laparoscopy
- Open surgical procedures are performed when neoplasia cannot be ruled out.

HYDATID CYST OF LIVER

Introduction

Parasitic infection caused by *Echinococcus granulosus*, with dog as the primary host.

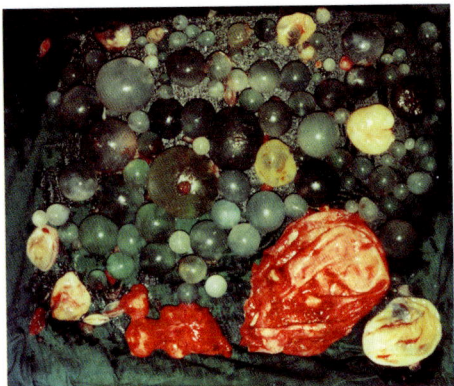

Fig. 17.15: Hydatid cysts of liver

Pathogenesis

- Close handling of dogs in a contaminated environment leads to oral ingestion of ova, which penetrate the bowel wall and through the portal circulation reach the liver and get trapped in the liver sinusoids and form cysts
- Hydatid cyst has many daughter cysts (**Fig. 17.15**) within, and the fluid is allergenic
- Usually occupies the upper pole of the right lobe and are slow growing.

Diagnosis

Symptoms and Signs

- Generally asymptomatic
- Constitutional symptoms and tenderness occur when cysts are infected

- Hepatomegaly (upward enlargement), with a localized smooth rounded swelling in the right hypochondrium
- Jaundice and cholangitis result when cyst ruptures into the biliary tree.

Investigations

- *Plain X-ray* (**Fig. 17.16A**) demonstrates the calcified cyst
- *US* gives the double line sign which reflects the pericyst and the cyst wall. The cyst contains homogeneous or heterogeneous fluid with daughter cysts. Calcification may be seen
- *CT* (**Fig. 17.16B**) is diagnostic. It shows multiple septa and loculations with daughter cysts. Calcification may be seen
- *MRI* shows markedly hypointense on T2 weighted images due to the fibrous content of the wall and differentiates other hepatic cysts
- *Casoni's* test is positive
- *FNAC* may show clear watery fluid.

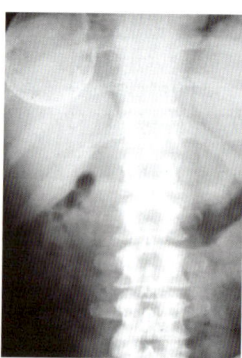

Fig. 17.16A: X-ray abdomen—Calcified hydatid cyst of liver

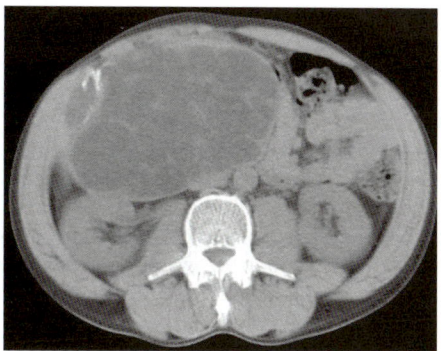

Fig. 17.16B: CT—Liver hydatid

Complications

- Rupture (into peritoneal cavity or biliary tree)
- Infection
- Calcification.

Management

- *Calcified cysts need no treatment, as they are dead*
- *Chemotherapy:* Mebendazole or albendazole are useful for small cysts, centrally located in the liver or in the peritoneal cavity and also in patients who are not fit for surgery
- *Scolicidal treatment:* 20% hypertonic saline in patients with cysts which have no communication with biliary tree or have not ruptured
- *US or CT guided percutaneous aspiration* injection reaspiration (PAIR) technique is gaining popularity
- *Excision* is curative for large symptomatic cysts.

Clinical Pearls

- The incidence of dissemination, peritoneal spillage and anaphylactic shock after hydatid cyst aspiration is extremely low and is considered theoretical
- Chemotherapy is contraindicated in large cysts, multiple septa, honeycomb like cysts, infected and inactive cysts, calcified cysts and coexistent chronic liver disease
- Laparoscopy can be used for scolicidal injections or excision
- Preoperative determination of cystobiliary communication is necessary to avoid postoperative complications
- Determination of cyst growth is the only reliable marker for assessing the recurrence
- Formalin is no longer preferred as a scolicidal agent due to the risk of biliary damage if there is a communication with biliary tree.

NEOPLASTIC LIVER CYSTS

Introduction

- Cystadenoma of liver is rare
- More common in women
- A solitary lesion, usually large and multiloculated cyst containing PAS positive fluid, with irregular septations
- Microscopically, it contains mucin secreting cuboidal epithelium with vacuolated cells with papillary projections
- Malignant transformation is known.

Diagnosis

Symptoms and Signs

- Abdominal pain
- Abdominal discomfort

- Pressure effects on adjoining structures
- Hepatomegaly.

Investigations

- **US and CT** are diagnostic and demonstrate multiloculated lesions with heterogeneous fluid and intracystic projections. Contrast enhances the septations, cyst wall and nodules in the cyst wall. Calcifications may be seen
- **FNAC** may show bloody or mucoid fluid
- **CA 19-9** estimation in aspirated fluid is diagnostic.

Management

- Complete excision.

Clinical Pearls

- Recurrence is common, when excision is partial
- If the cystic tumor is diagnosed to be a cystadenocarcinoma, aspiration should be avoided for the fear of tumor seeding.

BENIGN LIVER TUMORS

Introduction

Common benign tumors of the liver are:
- **Hemangioma:** Most common benign focal lesion, occurring in 1% of population. The commonest variety is the capillary hemangioma followed by the cavernous type
- **Focal nodular hyperplasia:** Most frequently seen in women of reproductive years, with weak association to oral contraceptives,

without any risk of malignant change. It is well circumscribed, firm, solitary and subcapsular in location, about 2–3 cm in diameter
- *Adenoma:* –Rare liver tumors. Closely linked to oral contraceptives in women and androgen therapy in men. The risk factors being galactosemia, type 1 glycogen deposits, Turner's and Klinefelter's syndromes. Have a potential to grow, bleed and rupture especially during pregnancy. Malignant transformation is a possibility.

Rare benign tumors of liver:
- Biliary hamartoma
- Solid fibrous tumor
- Benign mesothelioma
- Lipoma (angiolipoma, myolipoma)
- Mesenchymal hamartoma
- Myxoma
- Teratoma.

Diagnosis

Symptoms and Signs

- *Hemangioma:* Majority are solitary and asymptomatic. Large lesions cause hepatomegaly. The other symptoms are due to intratumoral bleeding or thrombosis resulting in rapid enlargement of liver compressing the adjacent organs. Intraperitoneal bleed is exceedingly rare
- *Focal nodular hyperplasia:* Vague abdominal pain in a small minority of patients. Hepatomegaly may be present
- *Adenoma:* Usually asymptomatic, but severe abdominal pain indicates complications (rupture, massive bleeding).

Investigations

Blood Tests
- Liver function tests and AFP levels are normal.

Radiology
- *Hemangioma:*
  - *US* shows hyperechogenicity with well-defined borders which is characteristic
  - *CT* (**Fig. 17.17A**): show homogenous hypodensity before contrast injection. Contrast fills irregularly from periphery to center and persists longer than the liver substance which is typical
  - *MRI* shows the lesion hyperintense on T2 weighted images, with peripheral filling of gadolinium contrast as in CT.
- *Focal nodular hyperplasia:*
  - *US* shows this as an echogenic lesion, and rarely the central scar is seen
  - *CT* (**Fig. 17.17B**) and MRI show this lesion as homogenous, outlining a radial central scar with a 'cartwheel' aspect.
- *Adenoma:*
  - *US* shows this as an echogenic lesion
  - *CT* (**Fig. 17.17C**) shows the lesions hyperdense prior to contrast and variable intensity after contrast injection
  - *MRI* shows the lesion hyperintense in T1 weighted image and isodense in T2 weighted image and becomes prominent on gadolinium use.

Tissue Diagnosis

- *Hemangioma:* Biopsy *is not advised* due to risk of complications
- *Focal nodular hyperplasia:* It contains a central stellate scar with radiating fibrous septa, which make the lesion into lobules.

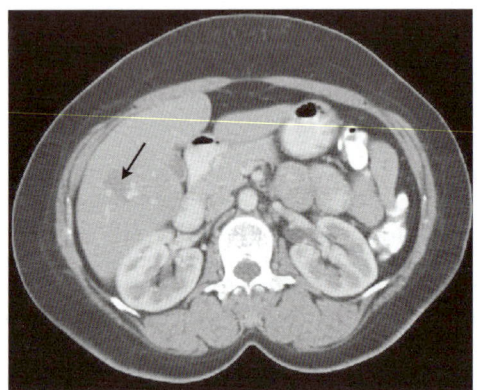

Fig. 17.17A: CT—Hemangioma of liver

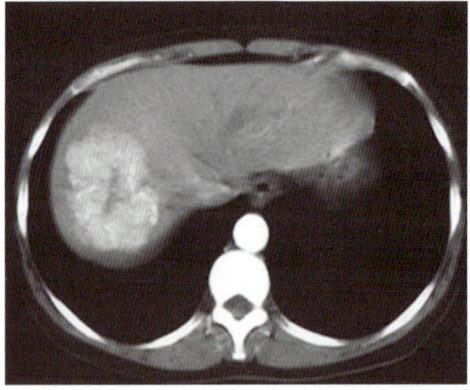

Fig. 17.17B: CT—Focal nodular hyperplasia

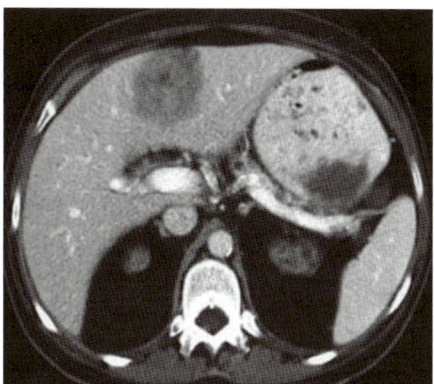

Fig. 17.17C: CT—Hepatic adenoma

Histologically, hepatocytes are normal with nodular aggregations without central veins or portal triads. The nodules contain proliferated bile ductules. Biopsy is many times inconclusive
- *Adenoma:* Typically, well-circumscribed nodule that consists of sheets of hepatocytes with a bubbly vacuolated cytoplasm. The hepatocytes are on a regular reticulin scaffold and less or equal to three cell thick. Cells resemble normal hepatocytes and are traversed by blood vessels but lack portal tracts or central veins.

Management

- *Hemangioma:* Majority need no treatment. Arteriographic embolization, hepatic artery ligation and perihepatic packing for acute bleeds and surgery (enucleation) is indicated for very large symptomatic lesions or when the diagnosis is uncertain

- ***Focal nodular hyperplasia:*** Needs no treatment, discontinuance of oral contraceptives, surgery if done it is enucleation
- ***Adenoma:*** Lesions > 10 cm in size requires surgical resection for fear of malignant transformation (enucleation/wedge resection/local ablation). Oral contraceptives should be discontinued.

Summary

In summary, the focal nodular hyperplasia and hepatic adenoma have distinct differences **(Table 17.20)**.

Clinical Pearls

- Hemangioma is the most common solid lesion found in the liver
- Hemangiomas of >10 cm diameter are called as giant hemangiomas
- Good quality ultrasonogram is sufficient to make a diagnosis of hemangioma of liver
- Resection of hemangioma is indicated only if there is pain or for diagnostic purpose

Table 17.20: Differentiating features of focal nodular hyperplasia and hepatic adenoma

Feature	Focal nodular hyperplasia	Hepatic adenoma
Mean size	<5 cm	10 cm
Kupffer cells	Yes	No
Central scar	Common	Rare
Symptoms	Nil	Present
Sulfur colloid scan	Positive uptake in 60%	Cold defect
Complications	Nil	Bleeding, malignancy
Treatment	Nil	Resection for >10 cm size

- Majority of patients with accidental diagnosis of hemangioma do well and remain stable on follow-up
- Progressive growth of asymptomatic hemangioma in a short span, especially in the young, is a relative indication for resection
- MRI is the most specific and sensitive investigation for diagnosing liver hemangioma, and is suggested when the hemangioma is of >3 cm in size with typical presentation or when <3 cm in size with atypical presentation
- Diagnosis of focal nodular hyperplasia can be easily made in a CT scan, but differentiating it from hepatic adenoma can be difficult. MRI also has similar problems
- Though modern available investigations can differentiate majority of hepatic neoplasms as benign or malignant, it is difficult to differentiate adenomas from focal nodular hyperplasia and well-differentiated hepatocellular carcinoma, by any investigation, excepting from a resected specimen
- Focal nodular hyperplasia does not require excision, but initial follow-up is recommended by radioimaging
- The risk of developing hepatic adenomas in women on oral contraceptives depends on the concentration of estrogen, duration of use (>2 years) and age (>30 years)
- Focal nodular hyperplasia is not prone to complications like malignant transformation, bleeding, necrosis or abscess, etc. whereas hepatic adenomas are prone to such complications
- When liver lesions are discovered incidentally, it should be differentiated as cystic and solid lesions. Solid lesions should be investigated to differentiate between benign and malignant lesions, by appropriate radiological and biochemical investigations.

HEPATOBLASTOMA

Introduction

- Most common primary hepatic malignancy in children
- An aggressive tumor with poor prognosis
- Cells resemble fetal or mature liver cells or bile ducts.

Etiology and Pathogenesis

They originate from immature liver precursor cells, usually unifocal and affect the right lobe of the liver more often than the left lobe, and have a potential to metastasize. Beta-catenin mutations have been shown to be common in sporadic hepatoblastomas. Its origin is suggested from a pluripotent stem cell.

Risk Factors

- Focal adenomatous polyposis (FAP)
- Low birth weight.

Diagnosis

Symptoms and Signs

Abdominal swelling, weight loss and failure to thrive.

Investigations

- **Serum AFP** is almost always elevated (>500 ng/mL)
- **US abdomen** *in informative*
- **CT abdomen** (**Fig. 17.18**) is diagnostic.

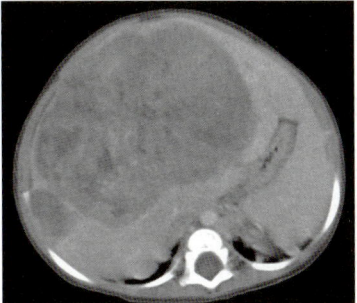

Fig. 17.18: CT—Hepatoblastoma

Management

- Resection for small encapsulated tumors
- Liver transplantation is the only option for cure.

Clinical Pearl

- When AFP is not elevated at diagnosis, the prognosis is poor.

PRIMARY LIVER MALIGNANCY

Primary liver malignancies are of many types depending on the tissue of origin. They are:
- Hepatocellular carcinoma (from hepatocytes)
- Intrahepatic cholangiocarcinoma (from biliary epithelial cells)
- Mixed HCC and cholangiocarcinoma (from hepatocytes and biliary epithelial cells)
- Primary malignancies of liver can arise from endothelial cells, stellate cells, neuroendocrine cells and lymphocytes but they are rare

- Angiosarcoma of the liver is extremely rare, and occurs in individuals exposed to vinyl chloride for prolonged periods of time.

HEPATOCELLULAR CARCINOMA

Introduction

- Hepatocellular carcinoma (HCC) is a malignancy of the hepatocytes
- Peak incidence between 40–60 years
- Male predominance of 2:1
- High incidence in hepatitis B endemic areas
- Affects men who have used androgenic anabolic steroid for body building
- HCC may form a part of paraneoplastic syndromes.

Risk Factors

- Cirrhosis of any etiology
- Chronic liver diseases caused by hepatitis B and C
- Hemochromatosis
- Aflatoxin (mycotoxin produced by fungus *Aspergillus flavus*) exposure
- Exposure to thorotrast (radiographic contrast)
- Tobacco smoking
- Alcoholism.

Types of Hepatocellular Carcinoma

- *Single:* A single predominant massive lesion demarcated from the surrounding liver, common in non-cirrhotic liver. Satellite nodules may be present

- ***Nodular:*** Multiple nodules in cirrhotic liver
- ***Diffuse:*** Infiltration of tumor throughout the liver parenchyma indistinguishable from cirrhosis
- ***Fibrolamellar:*** Multiple fibrous septa and may resemble focal nodular hyperplasia, not associated with cirrhosis.

Encapsulated tumors develop a capsule due to compression of adjacent liver tissue.

Spread of Hepatocellular Carcinoma

The tumor spreads by various routes:
- ***Direct spread:*** They grow through liver capsule, leading to invasion of adjacent structures viz., hepatic veins, portal vein, inferior vena cava, right kidney and adrenal, stomach and transverse colon, peritoneum and ascites
- ***Lymphatic spread:*** Hilar lymph nodes at the base of liver and portal nodes may be involved
- ***Hematogenous spread:*** Metastases to lungs (common), bone, skin and brain (uncommon).

Diagnosis

Symptoms and Signs

- Many are asymptomatic till the tumor grows to a large size and cause compressive symptoms
- Malaise, appetite and weight loss, abdominal discomfort, pain and jaundice
- Acute epigastric pain may indicate intratumoral bleed
- Symptoms of shock and peritonitis may be present when the tumor bleeds into the peritoneal cavity

- A hormone like substance can be produced by HCC and symptoms of a paraneoplastic syndrome may be seen (diarrhea, hypercalcemia)
- Clinical examination may reveal hepatomegaly.

TNM Classification of Hepatocellular Carcinoma

It is given in **Table 17.21.**

Table 17.21: TNM classification of hepatocellular carcinoma

Tumor status	
T_X	Primary tumor cannot be assessed
T_0	No evidence of primary tumor
T_1	Solitary tumor without vascular invasion
T_2	Solitary tumor with vascular invasion or multiple tumors not more than 5 cm
T_3	Multiple tumors more than 5 cm with invasion of portal or hepatic veins
T_{3a}	Multiple tumors more than 5 cm
T_{3b}	Single or multiple tumors of any size involving a major branch of the portal vein or hepatic vein
T_4	Tumor with invasion of adjacent structures other than gallbladder or with perforation of visceral peritoneum
Lymph node status	
N_X	Regional lymph nodes cannot be assessed
N_0	No regional node metastasis
N_1	Regional lymph node metastasis
Metastatic status	
M_0	No distant metastasis
M_1	Distant metastasis

Contd...

Contd...

Stage grouping			
Stage	T	N	M
I	T_1	N_0	M_0
II	T_2	N_0	M_0
III A	T_{3a}	N_0	M_0
III B	T_{3b}	N_0	M_0
III C	T_4	N_1	M_0
IV	Any T	Any N	M_1
IV A	Any T	N_1	M_0
IV B	Any T	Any N	M_1

Investigations

- *Raised alpha-fetoprotein levels* (Normal <20 ng/mL) >200 ng/mL is highly suggestive of HCC, and >400 ng/mL in the presence of cirrhosis is diagnostic
- Serology for virus A, B, C and D should be performed
- *Plain X-ray* may show an elevated right diaphragm in very large right lobar tumors
- *US* (**Fig. 17.19A**) has a sensitivity of 50%, and shows as a hypoechoic, isoechoic or hyperechoic lesion, but they are generally heterogenous
- *CECT* (**Fig. 17.19B**) has better sensitivity in diagnosis, and shows enhancement in the arterial phase (30 seconds) and rapid washout in portovenous phase (90 seconds)
- *MRI and PET* may each provide additional information, especially about the local spread
- *Angiography* determines the increased vascular pattern, and venous phase of superior mesenteric angiogram may show the invasion or occlusion of portal vein
- *Isotope scan* may be informative
- *Biopsy* (percutaneous or laparoscopy) is confirmatory.

Snapshots in Gastroenterology

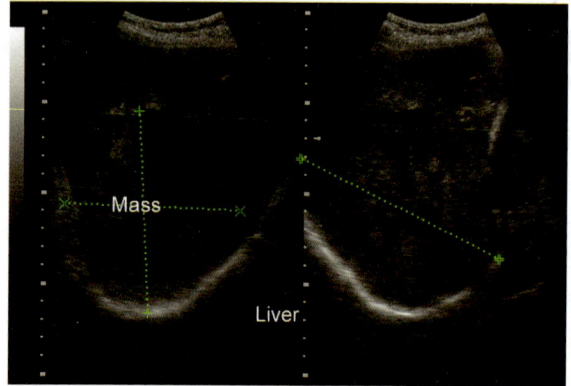

Fig. 17.19A: US—Mass in the liver (hepatocellular carcinoma)

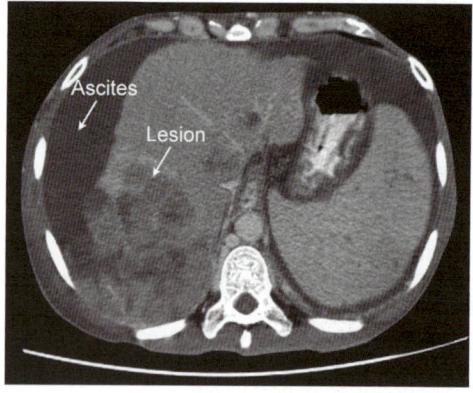

Fig. 17.19B: CT—Hepatocellular carcinoma with ascites

Paraneoplastic Syndromes Related to HCC

- Hypoglycemia
- Erythrocytosis
- Hypercalcemia
- Neuroendocrine syndromes (carcinoid)
- Cushing's syndrome.

Differential Diagnosis

- Metastatic tumors
- Benign tumors
- Abscess
- Hemangioma
- Focal nodular hyperplasia.

Management

Curative

- Surgical resection of the liver with the lesion (hepatectomy) is the primary treatment
- Liver transplantation.

Palliative (unresectable tumors)

- **Ablative procedures**
  - Percutaneous intralesional alcohol (5–20 mL of 95% alcohol) injection (US or CT guided)
  - Cryoablation
  - Radiofrequency ablation (RFA) (percutaneous, laparoscopic or laparotomy)—creates local heat to 60°C to coagulate the tumor
  - Microwave ablation (Thermal ablation).

- **Regional liver therapies**
  - Transarterial chemoembolization (TACE)—(chemotherapeutic drugs and lipiodol followed by embolization particles into the hepatic artery by percutaneous/transfemoral approach)
  - Hepatic artery chemoperfusion
  - Internal radiation therapy (Yttrium 90 microspheres infused into hepatic artery by transfemoral approach).
- **External beam radiation**
  - Stereotaxic radiosurgery
  - Intensity modulated radiotherapy (IMRT).
- **Systemic chemotherapy**
- **Multimodality therapy.**

Clinical Pearls

- Most cases of hepatocellular carcinoma occur in cirrhotic livers
- HCC is difficult to diagnose until there is widespread involvement of the liver
- The mechanisms of formation of HCC in a normal person, a chronic hepatitis patient and a cirrhotic patient may be different
- Patients with chronic viral hepatitis, hemochromatosis or alcoholic liver disease are at risk for hepatocellular carcinoma
- It takes about 30–40 years for cirrhosis and HCC to develop after the hepatitis B and C infections
- AFP levels do not correlate with tumor size and vascular invasion
- 30–40% of HCC patients have normal AFP
- Histologically, the invasion of lymphovascular tissue, liver parenchyma and bile duct and microsatellite lesions determine a poor prognosis
- PET scan using ^{11}C-acetate radio-tracer is informative compared to scans using FDG, when the tumors are well differentiated

- Multiple treatments may be required to get better benefit than one therapy, and an optimal schedule is not yet defined
- For patients with ascites, jaundice and encephalopathy, liver transplantation is the only appropriate treatment
- Child–Pugh classification of liver function is a good parameter in determining the outcome of partial hepatectomy
- Combination of RFA and chemoembolization provides better survival rate than either technique alone
- Multiple sittings may be required for RFA to be effective in large tumors
- Chemoembolization prevents a washout of the chemotherapeutic drug by the blood flow by causing ischemia
- HCC carries a very poor prognosis due to its silent growth and early spread to adjacent structures which delay treatment
- Multicentric origin of HCC interferes with effective curative treatment
- Screening for HCC in chronic hepatitis patients may reduce its incidence
- Size and number of lesions of HCC do not determine the biologic behavior
- In cirrhotics, US studies and serum AFP determinations done every yearly intervals are useful in identifying HCC when it is small.

METASTATIC LIVER DISEASE

Introduction

Primaries from which metastases of liver can develop:
- Colon
- Rectum
- Lungs

- Pancreas
- Breast
- Stomach.

Diagnosis

Symptoms and Signs

- Generally asymptomatic
- Large lesions may cause right upper quadrant pain, ascites, jaundice and anorexia
- Liver may become palpable and the hepatomegaly may be nodular and hard
- Other organs may get involved in the metastatic process.

Investigations

- **CEA** estimations may be useful in colonic adenocarcinoma
- **CA** 19/9 and CA 125 are often elevated depending on the tumor type

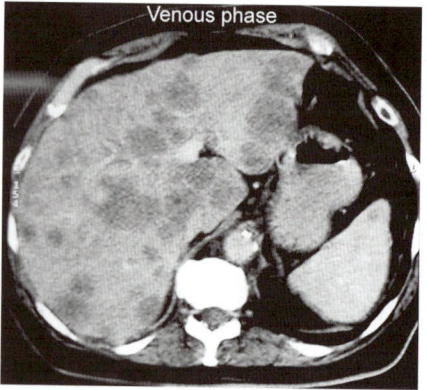

Fig. 17.20A: CT—Multiple metastases of liver

- *US and CT* (**Fig. 17.20A**) are diagnostic
- *FDG-PET* total body scan is useful in identifying extrahepatic disease (primary)
- *Intraoperative US* is useful to assess the liver for disease
- *Percutaneous guided needle biopsy* is conclusive.

Management

Curative

Surgical resection of the liver with the metastatic lesion (hepatectomy) is the primary treatment.

Palliative (unresectable tumors)

- **Ablative procedures**
  - Percutaneous intralesional alcohol (5–20 mL) injection (US or CT guided)
  - Cryoablation
  - Radiofrequency ablation (RFA) (percutaneous, laparoscopic or laparotomy)
  - Microwave ablation (Thermal ablation)
- **Regional liver therapies**
  - Chemoembolization (chemotherapeutic drugs with embolization particles into the hepatic artery by percutaneous/transfemoral approach)
  - Hepatic artery chemoperfusion
  - Internal radiation therapy (Yttrium 90 microspheres infused into hepatic artery by transfemoral approach)
- **External beam radiation**
  - Stereotaxic radiosurgery.
  - Intensity modulated radiotherapy (IMRT)

- Systemic chemotherapy is the only treatment option possible in many patients
- Multimodality therapy.

Clinical Pearls

- Untreated liver metastases carry a very poor prognosis
- While choosing the options for hepatic metastases of colorectal cancer, surgery and chemotherapy give effective and potentially curative outcome
- FDG PET is used as a routine preoperative workup of patients with colorectal metastases
- The outcome of treatment of liver metastases of colorectal cancer depends on the stage and histopathology of the primary tumor
- Liver metastases due to neuroendocrine tumors like (e.g. pancreatic endocrine tumors) have a good prognosis, and need no surgical treatment. However, patients with pain and hormonal symptoms will require excisional surgery
- Outcome depends on the micrometastases and recurrences
- For unresectable liver metastases, liver transplantation is not considered
- Peritoneal metastases and inability to achieve R0 resection are contraindications for excision of liver metastases.

SURGICAL PROCEDURES: SHUNT PROCEDURES

Introduction

The procedure involves diverting the portal blood into the systemic circulation with the aim to reduce portal pressure, and also avoid the incidence of hepatic encephalopathy.

Classification of Portosystemic Shunt Procedures

They are classified into those that shunt the entire portal system (total shunts) and those that selectively shunt blood from the gastrosplenic region while preserving the pressure flow relationships in the rest of the portal system, i.e. lower the pressure in the gastroesophageal venous plexus and preserve portal blood flow (selective shunt). They are shown in **Tables 17.22 and 17.23** and **Figure 17.20B**.

Table 17.22: Various types of total portosystemic shunts

Circulation		Shunt procedure	
Portal	Systemic	Name	Description
Portal vein	Inferior vena cava	**Portacaval shunt**	
		End to side	End of portal vein to side of IVC
		Side to side	Side of portal vein to side of IVC
Splenic vein	Left renal vein	**Central splenorenal shunt**	
		End to side	End of splenic vein to side of left renal vein (after splenectomy)
		Side to side	Side of splenic vein to side of left renal vein (spleen preserved)
Superior mesenteric vein	Inferior vena cava	**Mesocaval shunt**	
		End to side	End of IVC to side of superior mesenteric vein
		H interposition graft	Synthetic graft connecting the IVC and superior mesenteric vein

Table 17.23: Various types of selective portosystemic shunts

Circulation		Shunt procedure	
Portal	Systemic	Name	Description
Splenic vein	Inferior vena cava	**Splenocaval shunt**	
		End to side	End of splenic vein to side of IVC
Splenic vein	Left renal vein	**Distal splenorenal shunt (Warren shunt)**	
		End to side	End of splenic vein (splenic vein) to side of left renal vein + ligation of major collaterals between the portal and systemic circulation
Left gastric vein (coronary vein)	Inferior vena cava	**Coronary caval shunt (Inokuchi shunt)**	
		Interposition graft using autogenous saphenous vein	Connecting the IVC and left gastric vein

Clinical Pearls

- Total portosystemic shunts have the disadvantage of producing hepatic encephalopathy
- In patients with ascites, side to side portacaval shunt is preferred
- Warren shunt is the first choice as elective procedure but it does not improve ascites, and is not preferred for patients with ascites
- When Warren shunt and side to side portacaval shunt are not feasible, central splenorenal and H-mesocaval shunts are performed
- End-to-side H-mesocaval shunt is preferred in emergency situations
- Inokuchi shunt is technically difficult and has not become popular

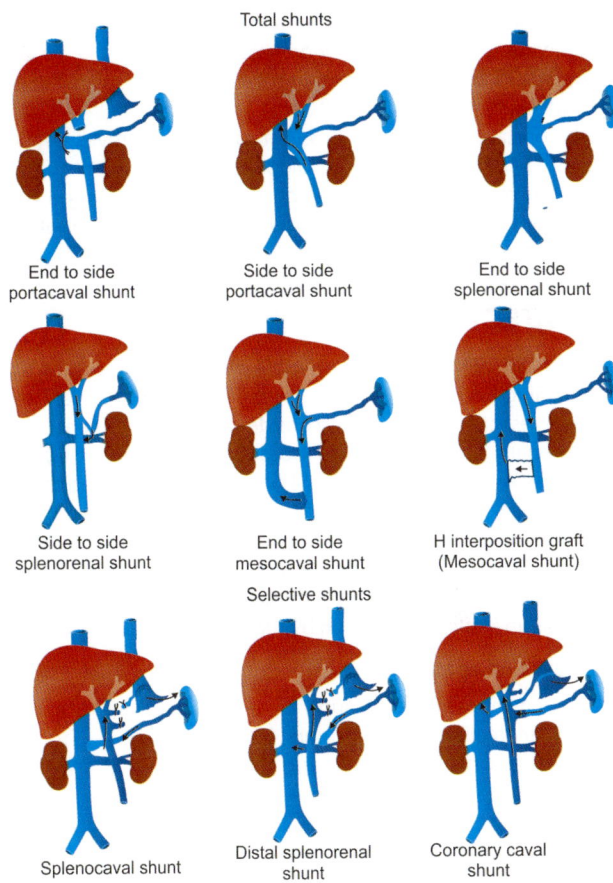

Fig. 17.20B: Portosystemic shunts

- Simple low platelet count should not be the reason for splenectomy and central splenorenal shunt
- Almost 90% of the shunts remain patent, reducing the incidence of variceal bleeding to 10%
- After portacaval shunt, the 5-year survival improves though about 15–20% develop encephalopathy
- Superior mesenteric vein—left portal vein shunt using a graft (Meso Rex shunt) is a new approach for extrahepatic portal vein thrombosis.

HEPATECTOMY

About 80–85% of the liver can be removed with the expectation that the remaining liver will regenerate for the patient to survive. These extensive resections should be considered only in patients with normal hepatic function. In other words, cirrhotics do not tolerate such extensive resections. Within 24 hours of partial hepatectomy, cell replication becomes active and continues to be active till the original volume is restored, and this process completes in about 4–6 weeks. The stimuli for such regeneration are hepatocyte growth factor, tumor growth factor α, heparin-binding growth factor, hepatopoietin B and disinhibition by tumor growth factor $\beta 1$.

Indications for hepatic resections:
- Primary malignant liver tumors
- Secondary malignant liver tumors
- Symptomatic benign liver tumors
- Liver injury
- Infection/abscess
- Metastases from colon/Wilm's tumor
- Living donor transplantation.

Table 17.24: Child–Pugh classification for hepatic functional status

Clinical finding	Points		
	1	2	3
Encephalopathy	None	Grade 1–2	Grade 3–4
Ascites	None	Mild	Moderate
Bilirubin (mg%)	<2	2–3	>3
Albumin (g/L)	>3.5	2.8–3.5	<2.8
PT (sec prolonged)	1–3	4–6	>6

Criteria for liver resection:
- Disease confined to the liver
- Disease amenable to curative resection.

Preoperative Evaluation

Though many tests are available to hepatic function, none is perfect. The Child-Pugh classification (**Table 17.24**) is the most useful parameter available and practiced to predict the mortality in cirrhotics after hepatic resection. Child–Pugh A and selected Child–Pugh B cirrhotics are good candidates for hepatic resection.
- Child's class A: 5 or 6 points—excellent survival
- Child's class B: 7, 8, or 9 points—reduced survival
- Child's class C: 10+ points—very poor prognosis.

Hepatic Resections

Classification

Nonanatomical Resections
- Wedge resection
- Enucleation.

Anatomical Resections (Couinaud) *(Figs 17.21A and B)*
- Right hepatectomy (segments V, VI, VII, VIII)
- Right lobectomy (segments IV, V, VI, VII, VIII–also called extended right hepatectomy/right trisegmentectomy)
- Left hepatectomy (segments II, III, IV)
- Left lobectomy (segments II, III)
- Extended left hepatectomy (segments II, III, IV, V, VIII–also called left trisegmentectomy).

Incisions
- Upper abdominal incision (extended right subcostal)
- Thoracoabdominal.

Procedure
- After opening the abdomen, the anterior surface of the liver is exposed by taking down the round ligament and falciform ligament
- Left coronary ligament is divided for left hepatectomy and right coronary and triangular ligaments are divided for right hepatectomy
- Gastrohepatic ligament is opened to access the replaced hepatic arteries and also take control of the vascular structures (Pringle's maneuver).

For Right Hepatectomy
- Liver is mobilized from the IVC, and short hepatic veins are divided between ligatures
- Right hilar plate dissection is done and RHA is divided between ligatures (Left hilar plate dissection is done and LHA is divided between ligatures—for left hepatectomy)
- Right portal vein is divided between vascular staplers (Left portal vein is divided between vascular staplers for left hepatectomy)

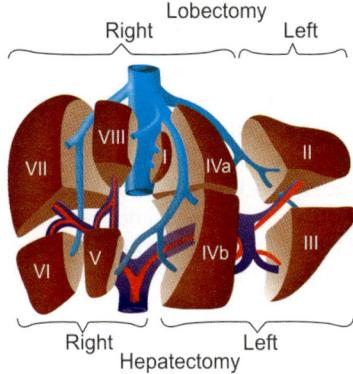

Fig. 17.21A: Hepatectomies

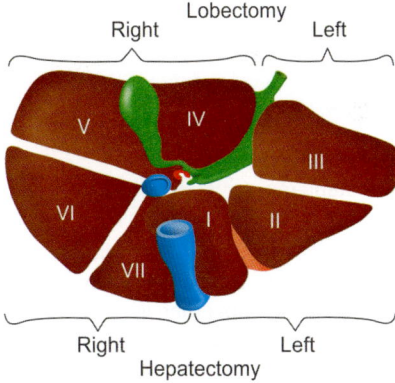

Fig. 17.21B: Hepatectomies (ventral view)

- Right hepatic duct is divided between ligatures (Left hepatic duct is divided between ligatures for left hepatectomy)
- Right hepatic vein is divided between staplers (Left hepatic vein is divided between staplers for left hepatectomy)
- Liver parenchyma is divided using crushing and vascular stapling technique, along the avascular line
- The liver surface is checked for hemostasis
- Pringle's maneuver is released and hemostasis checked and figure of eight sutures are applied for bleeding points
- A contrast cholangiogram is performed to confirm the patency of the left over hepatic duct
- A tube drain is placed in the right subphrenic space.

The liver parenchyma can be divided using various devices:
- Blunt finger fracture and hemoclips
- Crushing clamps
- Cautery (monopolar/bipolar)
- Argon beam coagulator
- CUSA ultrasonic dissector
- Hydrojet dissector
- Harmonic scalpel
- Ligasure
- Gyrus PK cutting forceps
- Endovascular staplers.

Postoperative Course

- Raising bilirubin levels should raise concern for perihepatic collection (biloma) and impending liver failure
- Prolonged INR warrants platelet administration
- Enzymes increase in the first few days and normalize thereafter
- Alkaline phosphatase may show delayed increase and stay elevated several weeks after surgery.

Laparoscopic liver resections are becoming increasing popular, but as of now, open surgical procedures remain the standard.

Complications

- Bleeding
- Bile leak and biloma
- Hepatic insufficiency
- Pulmonary complications.

Clinical Pearls

- Even if technically feasible, multiple tumors in the liver and vessel invasion are prognostically bad
- Anatomical resections have the advantage of removal of lobes with the afferent and efferent vessels without injury to the vessels and bile ducts supplying the residual liver tissue
- Unisegmentectomy is not applicable to segment I, because access to this segment requires removal of segments II and III
- Removal of segments II and III together is more easy than removing one of the segments
- Resection of segment VI alone is rarely performed
- Segment VIII alone is difficult because it is connected with infrahepatic IVC and segment I
- Segments IV and V (Bisegmentectomy) can be removed in patients with carcinoma gallbladder extending into the liver or Klatskin's tumor. Segment VI can also be added
- Anatomical resections have lower blood loss when compared to nonanatomical resections
- Anatomical resections when performed for malignancy, have a lower incidence of positive resection margins
- Centrally located lesions will require larger resections

- If gross tumor is left behind or if the resected margins are microscopically involved, progression of disease is the rule
- A small, solitary, asymptomatic tumor with well-preserved liver function are good predictors of outcome after hepatectomy, whereas large tumor (>5 cm), satellite lesions, markedly elevated AFP (>2,000 ng/mL) are associated with poor outcome
- Intraoperative ultrasound is necessary to identify small lesions and the major vasculature to guide the operation.

LIVER TRANSPLANTATION

Liver transplantation is a viable option for patients with advanced or end stage liver disease of any etiology. The common indications for liver transplantation are:
- **Chronic liver diseases**
  - Chronic viral hepatitis
  - Alcoholic liver disease
  - Autoimmune hepatitis
  - Primary biliary cirrhosis
  - Primary sclerosing cholangitis
  - Hepatocellular carcinoma
  - Drug-induced liver disease
  - Budd–Chiari syndrome
  - Nonalcoholic steatohepatitis
  - Acute fatty liver of pregnancy.
- **Metabolic liver diseases**
  - Wilson's disease
  - Hemochromatosis
  - $\alpha 1$ antitrypsin deficiency.
- **Others**
  - Hepatoblastoma
  - Hemangioendothelioma
  - Retransplantation.

Contraindications for liver transplantation are:
- **Absolute**
  - Extrahepatic malignancy
  - Active uncontrolled sepsis
  - Advanced heart or lung disease
  - Active alcohol abuse.
- **Relative**
  - Severe obesity
  - Advanced age
  - HIV infection
  - Cholangiocarcinoma.

Pretransplant evaluation of liver transplantation:

- Routine hepatic, renal, thyroid and hematological evaluations
- Serology of HIV, hepatitis B and C virus, CMV
- Cardiac evaluation
- Doppler study of hepatic vasculature
- Contrast enhanced CT of abdomen
- Substance abuse evaluation.

The primary aim of liver transplantation is that the patient should survive the procedure and benefit from the procedure with a longer lifespan.

Child's score predicts survival for patients with advanced cirrhosis of liver, and MELD (Model for End stage Liver Disease) score predicts survival using serum bilirubin and creatinine levels and the international standardized ratio (INR)

- MELD score predicts 90 days mortality, and patients with high MELD score have high priority index of liver transplantation. MELD score is used to prioritize the patients for transplantation
- Comorbid conditions add to the seriousness of liver transplantation.

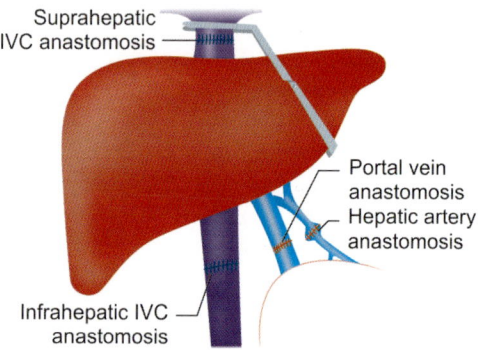

Fig. 17.22: Orthotopic liver transplantation

Operative Technique

Liver transplantation is an orthotopic procedure, meaning the recipient organ is placed at its original site, after removing the diseased organ (**Fig. 17.22**). The operation is done in three phases:

1. ***Dissection phase:*** The attachments of the liver are dissected and vascular structures are prepared for resection.
2. ***Anhepatic phase:*** From the time host liver is removed and the donor liver is vascularized.
3. ***Reperfusion phase:*** During which the blood is circulated through the new organ and the biliary tree is reconstructed.

The diseased liver is removed by dividing the attachments en bloc with the vena cava, and a venovenous bypass is maintained to overcome decreased venous return when the vena caval and portal circulations are interrupted.

- The new liver is kept in place, and the vena caval anastomosis is made end to end both above and below the new liver. An

alternate method is to dissect the liver off the vena cava and clamp and divide the main hepatic veins without occluding the vena cava. The liver is sutured by the vena cava to vena cava technique side to side, which avoids the venovenous bypass. This is called piggy back technique, as the donor cava sits directly on the recipient cava
- Biliary reconstruction is made by end to end choledochocholedochostomy if the bile duct is intact. If the bile duct is not normal, or fit for anastomosis, a Roux-en-Y choledochojejunostomy is preferred. Stenting across the biliary anastomosis is optional
- Hepatic artery and portal vein are anastomosed to the respective blood vessels in the recipient. When aberrations are found, especially in the donor, which is common with hepatic artery, proper anastomosis is planned.

Living Donor and Split Liver Transplantations

Shortage of donor livers and the necessity for smaller livers have brought in the concept of taking half the liver for transplantation. It has the flexibility of taking the left lateral lobe of liver for a child or a small adult and the right lobe for an adult. This is possible from living donors, to donate one-half of the liver. This is termed 'living donor liver transplantation'.

When the same is applied to the deceased donor, as it has the advantage of supplying livers to a child and an adult at the same time. This is termed *'split liver transplantation'*.

Post-transplant Management

- Immunosuppressants
- Tacrolimus

- Cyclosporine
- Azathioprine
- Mycophenolic acid
- Mycophenolate mofetil
- Corticosteroids
- Sirolimus
- OKT3
- Daclizumab.

The immunosuppression therapy includes tacrolimus (calcineurin inhibitor) or cyclosporine and a secondary agent such as mycophenolate mofetil, mycophenolic acid or azathioprine. Corticosteroids are also used as first line therapy as immunosuppression.

Complications

Complications following liver transplantation are common, but many of them can be effectively treated.

- Coagulopathy occurs during anhepatic phase, and continued bleeding after liver transplantation requires resurgery
- Primary nonfunction in which new liver does not recover to function is dangerous and death results, and this situation requires retransplantation
- Thrombosis of hepatic artery requires thrombectomy, and if not recognized, will lead to liver necrosis, which will require retransplantation
- Thrombosis of portal vein is documented by Doppler study which requires thrombectomy
- Biliary leaks are common, occurring in about 20%, can be handled by ERCP stenting
- Biloma requires drainage

- Biliary stricture rarely produces intrahepatic biliary dilatation in a transplanted liver, and high degree of suspicion is necessary, supported by elevated bilirubin and alkaline phosphatase levels, supported by MRCP. Strictures can be managed by ERCP biliary stenting and balloon cholangioplasty
- CMV infection is a problem, especially in those recipients who have not had CMV infection in the past. Antivirals like ganciclovir or valganciclovir are administered for months following liver transplantation for all those patients at risk
- Acute allograft rejection—indicated by elevated liver enzymes. Liver biopsy demonstrates mixed cellular infiltrate with injury to bile duct epithelium, which is diagnostic. Mild rejection requires corticosteroid pulse therapy or increased doses of immunosuppression. Antilymphocyte preparation is given for those do not respond to steroids. Retransplantation is the ultimate.
- Chronic allograft rejection—indicated by gradual increase of alkaline phosphatase and bilirubin—uncommon and usually occurs with patients noncompliant with immunosuppression
- Recurrence of disease (e.g. hepatitis C infection)
- *Metabolic complications*
  - Diabetes—due to corticosteroids
  - Hypertension—due to cyclosporine and tacrolimus
  - Renal insufficiency—due to cyclosporine
  - Hyperlipidemia—due to corticosteroids, sirolimus and cyclosporine
  - Cardiovascular and cerebrovascular disease–due to diabetes and hypertension
  - Osteopenia—due to corticosteroids
- *Malignancy*
  - Skin cancer due to ultraviolet ray (sunrays) exposure
  - Immunoproliferative disease (large B cell lymphoma).

Clinical Pearls

- Hepatitis C recurs invariably after liver transplantation, but it is not a contraindication for liver transplantation
- Regarding HCC, there are set criteria to follow for better survival rates, and they are: single tumor <6.5 cm, maximum three tumors with none > 4.5 cm, cumulative tumor size <8 cm.
- Live donor liver transplantation (LDLT) has the advantage of reducing the waiting time for availability of donor liver
- Renal insufficiency occurs more commonly in patients who are aged, hypertensives, diabetics and renal disease in the pretransplant period
- Retransplant is considered in patients with hepatitis C recurrence, but long-term survival is low
- Long-term immunosuppression has the risk of opportunistic infection, especially fungal, which can be prevented by the use of nystatin
- The liver is unique that it does not require long-term immunosuppression, as it has the capability of tolerance, in contrast to renal, cardiac, pulmonary and pancreatic grafts.

Chapter 18

Gallbladder and Bile Ducts

ANATOMY

Gallbladder

A diverticulum appears on the foregut, the cranial part of which develops into the liver and the caudal part develops into the ventral pancreas. The intermediate bud develops into the gallbladder.

The gallbladder is a pear-shaped organ about 7–10 cm long with a capacity of about 50 mL, when distended can expand up to 300 mL. It is situated at the undersurface of the liver at its fossa, which divides the liver into left and right lobes. The gallbladder is divided into fundus, body, infundibulum and neck. The fundus is the rounded blind end of the organ, which contains most of the smooth muscle and elastic tissue. The body via the infundibulum (Hartmann's pouch) tapers like a funnel to join the cystic duct. The gallbladder is lined by single, highly folded tall columnar epithelium containing cholesterol and fat globules. The tuboalveolar glands present in the mucosa of the infundibulum and neck secrete the mucus. The epithelial lining is supported by lamina propria, the circular, longitudinal and oblique muscle fibers. The subserosa contains the connective tissue, nerves, blood vessels, lymphatics and adipocytes. The outermost layer is the serosa. The gallbladder differs from the GI tract that it lacks a muscularis mucosa and submucosa.

Bile Ducts

The extrahepatic bile ducts consist of the left and right hepatic ducts, which join to form the common hepatic duct, which is joined by the cystic duct to form the common bile duct (CBD). The CBD is about 7–10 cm in length and runs in the free edge of the lesser omentum, and runs behind the first part of the duodenum to open in the medial aspect of the second part of the duodenum, through a thick coat of circular muscle, the sphincter of Oddi, at the ampulla of Vater. The CBD is joined at its terminal part by the pancreatic duct (PD) to form a common opening. In about 10%, the CBD and PD open separately into the duodenum.

Arterial Supply

The arterial supply is from the cystic artery, a branch of right hepatic artery, and the cystic artery passes behind the hepatic duct before entering the Calot's triangle and divides into anterior and posterior branches once it reaches the neck of the gallbladder.

Venous Drainage

Venous drainage of the gallbladder is directly into the liver, and there is no specific cystic vein.

Nerve Supply

The biliary tree receives both sympathetic and parasympathetic nerve supplies.
- Sympathetic nerve supply mediates the pain of biliary colic
- Parasympathetic nerve supply contains motor fibers to the gallbladder.

PHYSIOLOGY

When food is not consumed, bile is stored in the gallbladder, where it is concentrated to cause changes in concentration and composition. After a meal, the gallbladder contracts, sphincter relaxes and bile is forcibly pushed into the duodenum. This postprandial gallbladder contraction is maintained by cholecystokinin. Gallbladder bile contains about 10% solids with a bile salt cconcentration of 200 mmol/L.

ANOMALIES

Normal biliary anatomy is found in only about 25% of the population. *Gallbladder anomalies* can be that, the gallbladder be:
- Intrahepatic
- Rudimentary
- Have anomalous forms
- Duplicated (with two cystic ducts opening separately or combine to form a single cystic duct)
- Totally absent (extremely rare)
- Left-sided gallbladder opening into the left hepatic duct (extremely rare).

Cystic duct anomalies **(Fig. 18.1A)** are common. It can be:
- Long or short or absent
- Join the CBD at different levels
- Take devious route to join the CBD or CHD at different levels.

Hepatic artery and cystic artery anomalies **(Fig. 18.1B)** are common.
- Cystic artery from superior mesenteric artery
- Two cystic arteries (one from the right hepatic and other from common hepatic arteries)
- Two cystic arteries (one each from the right and left hepatic arteries)

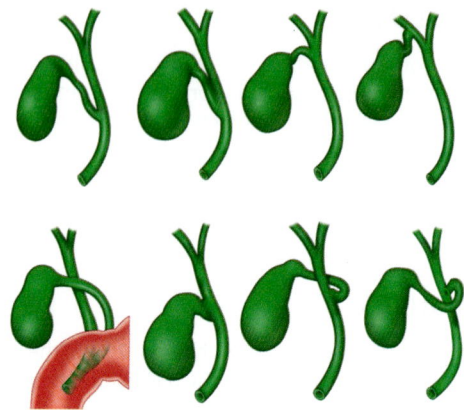

Fig. 18.1A: Cystic duct anomalies

- Cystic artery from right hepatic artery and runs anterior to the common hepatic duct
- Two cystic arteries (both arising from the right hepatic artery).

BILIARY ATRESIA

Introduction

Congenital anomaly affecting 1:15,000 live births, with fibrosis and destruction of biliary radicles at different sites:
- There are two types of biliary atresia
  i. Fetal type: present at the time of birth.
  ii. Perinatal type: develop around 2nd to 4th week of life.

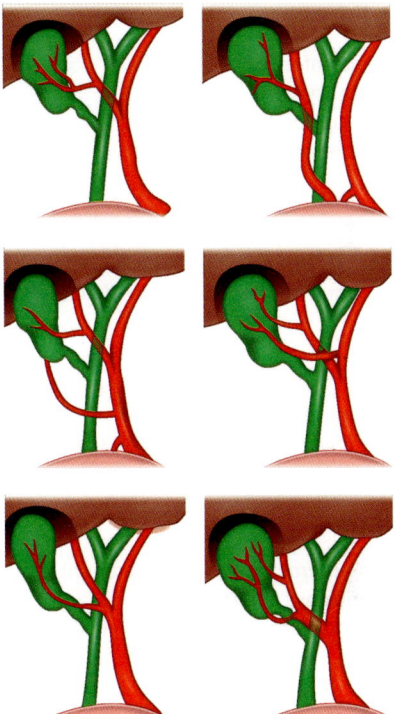

Fig. 18.1B: Cystic artery anomalies

Based on the region of involvement, it can be divided into three types:
1. Type I—common bile duct
2. Type II—common hepatic duct
3. Type III—liver hilum (85% of cases).

Triggering Factors

- Viral or bacterial infection
- Immune deficiency
- Abnormal bile component
- Error in development of biliary system.

Diagnosis

Symptoms

Persistent and progressive jaundice beyond first 2 weeks after birth.

Investigations

- ***Serum bilirubin*** (serial estimations) levels are diagnostic
- ***US and CT*** are informative
- ***Hepatobiliary iminodiacetic acid (HIDA) scan and liver biopsy*** are confirmatory.

Management

- ***Hepatic porto-enterostomy*** (Kasai operation) is the treatment of choice within 60 days of birth
- ***Liver transplantation*** is warranted for deteriorating liver functions.

CHOLEDOCHAL CYSTS

Introduction

- Uncommon cystic dilatations of the biliary system
- Can involve the extrahepatic or intrahepatic radicles or both
- Reported frequency rates range from 1 case per 100,000–150,000 to 1 case per 2 million live births

- 60% present clinically in the first decade of life
- Presentation in adulthood is uncommon, and is often due to complications
- Choledochal cysts are relatively rare in Western countries, but more prevalent in Asia
- Shows female predominance
- No definite etiology is known.

Etiology and Pathogenesis

- Pathogenesis is probably multifactorial
- Long common channel theory is the most accepted therory:
  - Anomalous junction of pancreatic duct with the bile duct, which is characterized by the entry of pancreatic duct into the CBD 1 cm or more proximal to where the CBD reaches the ampulla of Vater. Seen in 90% of patients with choledochal cysts
  - This anomalous entry of pancreatic duct leads to reflux of enzyme rich pancreatic secretion into the CBD, which is in a relatively alkaline condition. Pancreatic juice causes activation of pancreatic proenzymes, damaging and weakening the bile duct wall
- Defects in epithelialization and recanalization of the developing bile ducts and congenital weakness of the ductal wall also have been implicated in the pathogenesis of choledochal cysts.

Classifications

Alonso–Lej et al. (1959) classified choledochal cysts as:
- Type I: Choledochal cyst
- Type II: Diverticula
- Type III: Choledochocele
- Type IV: Combination of extra- and intrahepatic cyst
- Type V: Only intrahepatic cysts.

Todani et al. modified the above classification. Five major classes of choledochal cysts (**Fig. 18.2**) exist (i.e. types I-V), with subclassifications for types I and IV (i.e. types IA, IB, IC; types IVA, IVB).

- Type I cysts are the most common and represent 80–90% of choledochal cysts. They consist of saccular or fusiform dilatations of the common bile duct, which involve either a segment of the duct or the entire duct.
  - Type IA is saccular in configuration and involves either the entire extrahepatic bile duct or the majority of it
  - Type IB is saccular and involves a limited segment of the bile duct

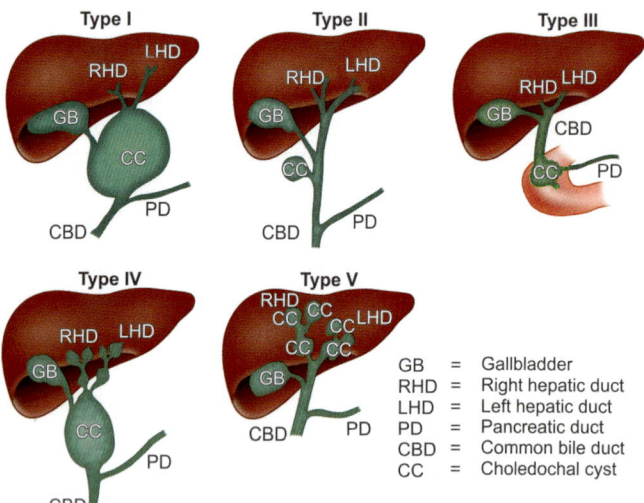

Fig. 18.2: Choledochal cysts

- Type IC is more fusiform in configuration and involves most or all of the extrahepatic bile duct.
- Type II cysts appear as an isolated diverticulum protruding from the wall of the common bile duct. The cyst may be joined to the common bile duct by a narrow stalk (incidence < 5%)
- Type III cysts arise from the intraduodenal portion of the common bile duct and are described alternately by the term 'choledochocele' (incidence <5%)
- Type IV cysts are multiple dilatations of bile ducts (incidence 5–10%)
  - Type IVA cysts consist of multiple dilatations of the intrahepatic and extrahepatic bile ducts
  - Type IVB cysts are multiple dilatations involving only the extrahepatic bile ducts
- Type V (*Caroli's disease*) consists of multiple dilatations limited to the intrahepatic bile ducts (incidence <1%).

Diagnosis

Symptoms and Signs

Can present at any age.

In Infants

- Jaundice and acholic stools. In early infancy, this may prompt a workup for biliary atresia
- Palpable mass in the right upper quadrant of the abdomen, accompanied by hepatomegaly.

In Children

- Clinical picture of intermittent biliary obstruction or recurrent bouts of pancreatitis

- A palpable right upper quadrant mass and jaundice
- Intermittent attacks of colicky abdominal pain.

In Adults

- Adults with choledochal cysts can present with one or more severe complications
- Frequently, adults with choledochal cysts complain of vague epigastric or right upper quadrant pain and can develop jaundice or cholangitis
- The most common symptom in adults is abdominal pain.

Investigations

- ***Leukocytosis*** in cholangitis
- ***Raised alkaline phosphatase*** in some cases
- ***Serum amylase*** may be increased when there is pancreatitis
- ***US abdomen*** is informative
- ***CT (Fig. 18.3) and MRI abdomen*** can delineate the biliary anatomy

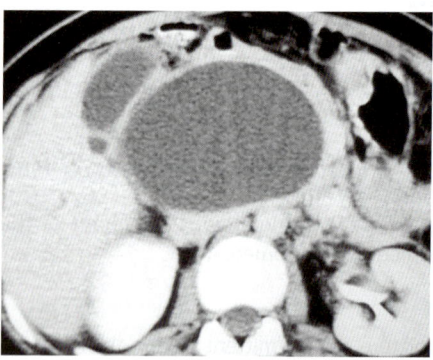

Fig. 18.3: CT—Choledochal cyst

- *MRCP* has very high sensitivity
- *ERCP* and *PTC* are useful investigations.

Complications

- Cholangitis
- Hepatic abscesses
- Recurrent pancreatitis
- Hepatocellular damage
- Cholelithiasis
- Cholangiocarcinoma
- Carcinoma of gallbladder.

Management

- Antibiotics when cholangitis or pancreatitis occur
- *Excision of cyst with biliary enteric anastomosis,* and varies according to type
  - *Type I:* Complete excision of the involved portion of the extrahepatic bile duct with Roux-en-Y hepaticojejunostomy
  - *Type II:* The dilated diverticulum comprising a type II choledochal cyst is excised in its entirety. The resultant defect in the common bile duct is closed over a T-tube
  - *Type III* (**choledochocele**): The choice of therapy depends upon the size of the cyst.
    - Choledochoceles measuring 3 cm or less can be treated effectively with endoscopic sphincterotomy
    - Lesions larger than 3 cm typically produce some degree of duodenal obstruction. These lesions are excised surgically through a transduodenal approach. If the pancreatic duct enters the choledochocele, it may have to be reimplanted into the duodenum following excision of the cyst

- *Type IV:* The dilated extrahepatic duct is completely excised and a Roux-en-Y hepaticojejunostomy is performed to restore continuity. Intrahepatic ductal disease does not require dedicated therapy unless hepatolithiasis, intrahepatic ductal strictures, and hepatic abscesses are present. In such instances, the affected segment or lobe of the liver is resected
- *Type V* (Caroli's disease): Disease limited to one hepatic lobe is amenable to treatment by hepatic lobectomy. When this occurs, the left lobe is usually affected. Hepatic functional reserve should be examined carefully in all patients before committing to such therapy. Patients with bilobar disease who begin to manifest signs of liver failure, biliary cirrhosis, or portal hypertension may be candidates for liver transplantation.

Lilly technique: Occasionally, the cyst adheres densely to the portal vein secondary to long-standing inflammatory reaction. In this situation, a complete, full-thickness excision of the cyst may not be possible. In the Lilly technique, the serosal surface of the duct is left adhering to the portal vein, while the mucosa of the cyst wall is obliterated by curettage or cautery. Theoretically, this removes the risk of malignant transformation in that segment of the duct.

Clinical Pearls

- Bile duct malignancy is reported to be enhanced by biliary cystic–enteric anastomosis performed for choledochal cysts, which allows easy regurgitation of pancreatic juice through the anomalous entry
- Excision and biliary reconstruction is recommended as the internal drainage procedure seems to increase the incidence of malignancies.

GALLSTONES (CHOLELITHIASIS)

Introduction
- Cholelithiasis is defined as presence of stones in the gallbladder
- Gallstones are congregations of cholesterol, bilirubin and bile salts
- The prevalence varies in different regions of the same country and different parts of the world.

Etiology and Pathogenesis
Bile contains three lipid species:
1. Cholesterol (5%)
2. Phospholipids as phosphatidyl choline commonly known as lecithin (25%)
3. Bile salts (70%).

Bilirubin and protein are also present in small quantities.
The formation of gallstones has many factors (**Fig. 18.4**). They are:
- Cholesterol is not water soluble (hydrophobic), whereas bile salts and lecithin are water soluble
- The biliary cholesterol is carried in a stable form as particles (micelles) made up of lecithin and bile salts
- When the capacity of lecithin and bile salts to keep the cholesterol in the soluble form is exceeded, supersaturation of bile occurs. And also there is excess of cholesterol secretion into bile
- The liquid cholesterol transforms into solid cholesterol crystals, a process called nucleation. The nucleating factor is the gallbladder mucus
- Hypotonicity and hypomotility of gallbladder produces stasis, which alters the bile composition and accelerates crystallization

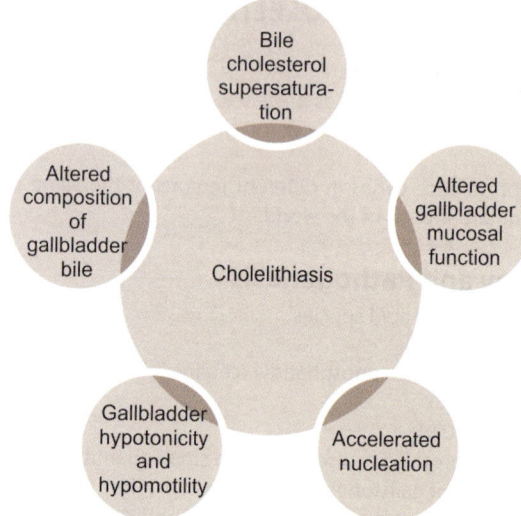

Fig. 18.4: Formation of gallstones

- The mixture of gallbladder mucus and small cholesterol or calcium bilirubinate crystals is formed in the redundant bladder called *biliary sludge*
- Macroscopic stones are conglomerations of components of biliary sludge
- 75% of patients with gallstones have cholesterol predominant stones (75–90%), which are called cholesterol stones. The remainder contains pigment stones.

The gallstones have different characteristics (**Table 18.1**).

The formation of pigment stones is shown in **Figure 18.5**.

Gallbladder and Bile Ducts

Table 18.1: Characteristics of gallstoness

Type of stones	Composition of stones	Characteristics of stones	Pathology
Cholesterol stones	Cholesterol (pure) (Uncommon)	Single, large with smooth surface Yellow (radiolucent)	Supersaturation of cholesterol in the bile
	Cholesterol (predominantly) + variable amounts of bile salts and calcium (Most common)	Multiple, variable size, may be hard and faceted or irregular, mulberry shaped and soft. Whitish yellow and green to black in color	
Pigment stones	Predominantly bile salts and calcium (cholesterol <20%)	Small, brittle, black and spiculated	Supersaturation of calcium bilirubinate, carbonate and phosphate, commonly secondary to hemolytic disorders and cirrhosis
		Less than 1 cm, brownish yellow and soft and mushy	In the gallbladder or bile ducts, secondary to infection caused by bile stasis

Note: Majority of the gallstones are of the mixed variety [cholesterol + bile pigments (calcium bilirubinate) + calcium salts]

Risk Factors

- Age >50 years
- Females
- Estrogen replacement therapy
- Obesity
- Family history

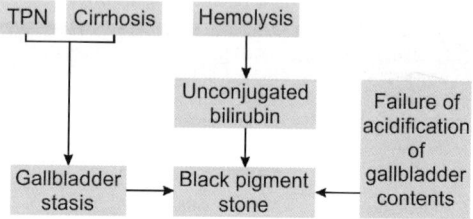

Fig. 18.5: Formation of pigment stones

- Pregnancy
- High fat and high cholesterol diet
- Crohn's disease
- Lack of exercise
- Increased triglyceride levels
- Total parenteral nutrition
- Gastric bypass surgery.

Diagnosis

Symptoms and Signs

Gallstones clinically behave in a variety of ways. They can cause:
- No symptoms
- Symptoms of non-life threatening situations
  - Biliary colic
  - Acute cholecystitis
  - Chronic cholecystitis
  - Mucocele of gallbladder
  - Obstruction of biliary duct
  - Perforation into neighboring luminal structure (e.g. duodenum)

- Symptoms of life-threatening situations:
  - Cholangitis due to obstruction of biliary duct
  - Empyema of gallbladder
  - Perforation of gallbladder and biliary peritonitis
  - Gangrenous cholecystitis
  - Mirizzi's syndrome
- Symptoms mimicking other disorders
  - Acid peptic disease
  - GERD
  - Upper abdominal dyspepsia
  - Right lung inflammations
  - Myocardial ischemia.

Investigations

Abdominal ultrasonography has about 95–98% sensitivity in diagnosing gallstones, either during or without symptoms. Apart from demonstrating stones, this investigation gives the benefit of knowing about the gallbladder thickness, pericholecystic collection during inflammations, status of the bile ducts and their dilatation, and gallbladder neoplasms, which have a close association with gallstones.

CHRONIC CHOLECYSTITIS

Introduction

- It is the chronic inflammation of gallbladder, and is the common presentation of gallstones
- Common in fat, flatulent, fertile, female of fifty (Five Fs)
- Histologically, majority will show signs of inflammation, thickening, loss of elasticity and fibrosis, but a small minority may not show any sign of inflammation.

Diagnosis

Symptoms

- Feeling of abdominal distension and flatulence, more following a fatty meal (qualitative dyspepsia), associated with belching
- Abdominal pain may be constant or colicky (biliary colic), radiating to back to the inferior angle of the right scapula. This may be associated with vomiting
- Jaundice can occur when a gallstone obstructs the common bile duct (obstructive jaundice).

Signs

- Tenderness in the right hypochondrium
- The gallbladder is usually not palpable, as it gets contracted due to recurrent inflammation (Courvoisier's law).

Investigations

- ***Transabdominal US* (Fig. 18.6A)** has a sensitivity rate of 95–98% in demonstrating gallstones
- ***EUS*** is able to detect even small stones (3 mm or less) missed by transabdominal US
- ***MRI*** has a sensitivity rate of 95%
- ***CT*** may be required rarely
- ***Plain X-rays*** may be contributory **(Fig. 18.6B)**.
- ***Isotope scan* (Fig. 18.6C)**–^{99}Tc –HIDA (technetium labeled analog of iminodiacetic acid) with gallbladder stimulation with fat, or intravenous administration of cholecystokinin (CCK) can be used to calculate the ejection fraction. Ejection fraction below 35% is considered abnormal.

Gallbladder and Bile Ducts

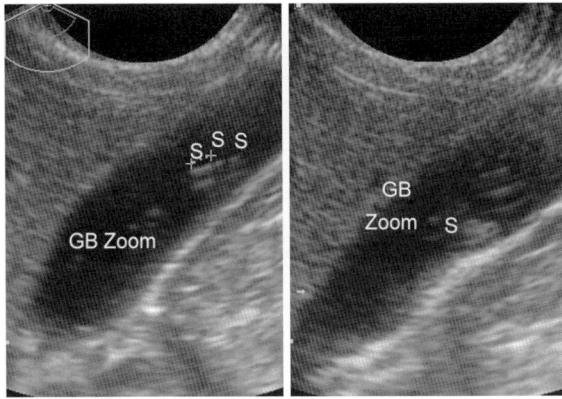

Fig. 18.6A: US—Multiple calculi in gallbladder

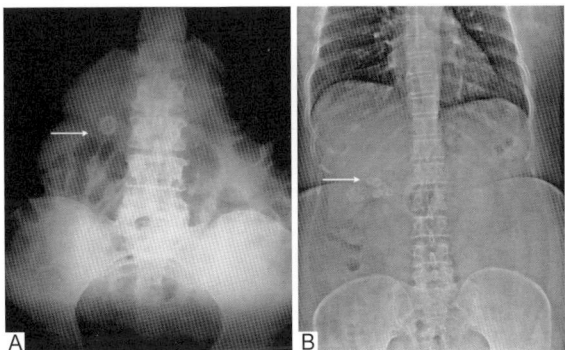

Fig. 18.6B: Plain X-ray—Radiopaque gallstones. (A) Single; (B) Multiple

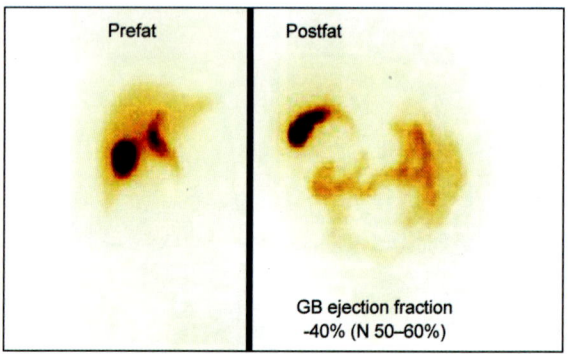

Fig. 18.6C: Isotope scan—Chronic cholecystitis

Differential Diagnosis

- Chronic duodenal ulcer
- Acid peptic disease
- Right sided radicular pain in the T6–T10 dermatomes.

Complications

- Acute cholecystitis
- Common duct stones
- Porcelain gallbladder
- Adenocarcinoma of gallbladder.

Management

Majority of the time, the treatment is surgical.

Surgical

Elective cholecystectomy (Laparoscopic or open).

Medical

Select patients who are unfit for surgery are managed by medical therapy.

Dissolution

- Cholesterol stones in the gallbladder may be dissolved by ursodeoxycholic acid, which reduces the cholesterol saturation of bile inhibiting the cholesterol secretion. The resulting undersaturated bile slowly dissolves the sole cholesterol in the gallstones. This therapy has some requisites
  - Gallstones must be small (<5 mm)
  - Should be devoid of calcium
  - Gallbladder must opacify on oral cholecystography (indicating the unobstructed flow of bile from gallbladder to CBD).

  Though some stones (50%) dissolve, it takes about 2 years to do so, but recurrences are common, and hence not preferred by many.

- ***Extracorporeal shock wave lithotripsy*** (ESWL) and dissolution—most effective in single stone of less than 2 cm in size in a normally functioning gallbladder with a nonobstructed cystic duct. Extracorporeal shock wave lithotripsy (ESWL) involves focusing shock waves, which pass through tissue and fluids, hit the gallstones and fragment by explosion of small air bubbles within interstices of the solid material of stones. The fragmented gallstones remain in the gallbladder for long time unless they are dissolved, making dissolution therapy supplementary and mandatory. The complete elimination of gallstones is attained in about 9 months in a quarter of patients.

Clinical Pearls

- The term cholecystitis is used whenever gallstones are present regardless of the histologic appearance of the gallbladder
- Many times, histological changes of inflammation are seen in asymptomatic gallstones
- If a patient has recurrent attacks of cholecystitis with the presence of sludge, cholecystectomy should be suggested
- Incidence of asymptomatic gallstones have increased probably due to the routine health checks and routine ultrasound examinations
- Majority of the asymptomatic patients remain asymptomatic for long periods of time
- Asymptomatic patients may be treated expectantly by observing them till symptoms develop
- The risk of developing gallstone related symptoms are rare (2–4%), and there is no advantage of prophylactic cholecystectomy, but once symptoms develop, cholecystectomy should be done at the earliest
- Prophylactic cholecystectomy is recommended for diabetics with silent stones, because of the higher risk of complications and increased morbidity and mortality for emergent operation
- Patients with cardiac disease especially those on anticoagulants, will require prophylactic cholecystectomy, because of the increased morbidity and mortality for emergent operation.

ACUTE CHOLECYSTITIS

Introduction

- Acute infection of gallbladder, mostly due to obstruction of cystic duct

Gallbladder and Bile Ducts

- Common in fat, flatulent, fertile, female of fifty (Five Fs)
- Infection by a variety of organisms.

Etiology and Pathogenesis

- Stones and infection work together to cause inflammation of the gallbladder. Gallstones may get colonized with bacteria, resulting in precipitation of bilirubinate salts and cause acute cholecystitis. Gallstones can be caused by infection (Bacteria are found to serve as a nidus for stone formation)
- The infected gallbladder develops subserosal edema, hemorrhage and patchy mucosal necrosis. Polymorphonuclear leukocytes appear. Resolution occurs in some cases. It is also believed that the trauma caused by gallstones causes phospholipase from the mucosal cells, which convert lecithin into lysolecithin, which is a toxic compound to cause inflammation. Bacteria seem to play a minor role as a primary cause of acute cholecystitis. Gangrene and perforation may occur.

Diagnosis

Symptoms

- Severe colicky pain (biliary colic) in the right hypochondrium, radiating to the inferior angle of the right scapula and the right shoulder
- Pain may be associated with vomiting
- Fever and jaundice are associated when there is associated cholangitis
- Symptom complex of pain, jaundice and fever with chills is called "***Charcot's triad***".

Signs

- Tenderness at the tip of the right ninth costal cartilage resulting in transient cessation of breathing due to pain during deep inspiration (**Murphy's sign**)
- There may be associated guarding and rigidity in the right hypochondrium
- The inflamed and distended gallbladder with or without the omentum may be palpable.

Investigations

- **Leukocytosis** is common during acute attacks
- **Plain X-rays abdomen**—though majority of the gallstones are not radiopaque, entities like emphysematous cholecystitis and cholecystoenteric fistula can be diagnosed by the presence of gas in the gallbladder lumen
- **Transabdominal ultrasonography (TAUS) (Fig. 18.7A)** is diagnostic. A thickened gallbladder wall of >4 mm and pericholecystic fluid is highly suggestive of acute cholecystitis. Sonographic Murphy's sign—tenderness over the gallbladder by the pressure exerted by the ultrasound probe is also diagnostic
- Rarely **CT scan (Figs 18.7B to D)** may be required, especially to localize the complications. When gas forming organisms are present, gas may seen the gallbladder lumen and wall (emphysematous cholecystitis)
- **Isotope scans** (^{99}Tc-HIDA–hydroxyiminodiacetic scan) **(Fig. 18.7E)** is contributory, when the ultrasound is inconclusive, but there is clinical suspicion. The findings are nonvisualization of gallbladder with the presence of tracer in the common bile duct and intestine, indicating cystic duct obstruction. This has a sensitivity rate about 95%.

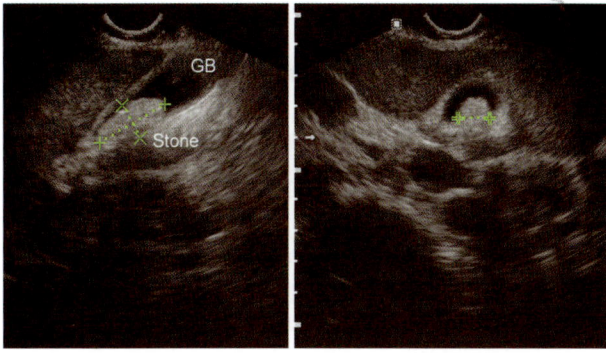

Fig. 18.7A: US—Stone in the cystic duct of gallbladder

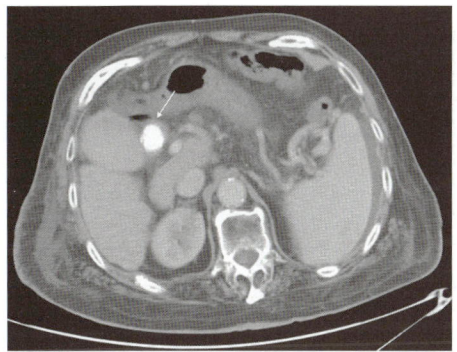

Fig. 18.7B: CT—Stone in the gallbladder

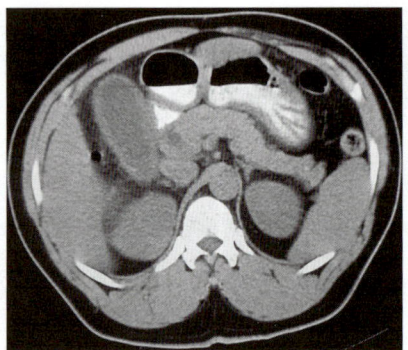

Fig. 18.7C: CT—Edematous gallbladder of acute cholecystitis

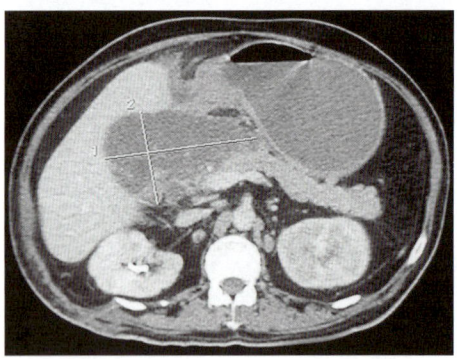

Fig. 18.7D: CT—Ruptured empyema of gallbladder

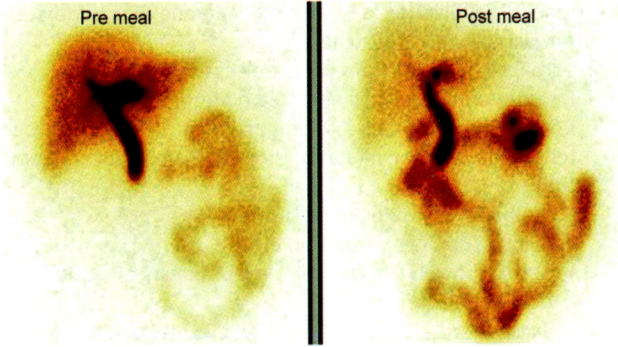

Fig. 18.7E: Isotope scan—Acute cholecystitis

Differential Diagnosis

- Acute appendicitis
- Duodenal ulcer perforation
- Acute right pyelonephritis
- Right basal pleurisy
- Myocardial infarction
- Herpes zoster of intercostal nerve
- Perihepatitis (Fitz–Hugh–Curtis syndrome).

Complications

Small stones migrate into the cystic duct: Acute obstruction of the cystic duct causes distension of gallbladder and the bile can be replaced by mucus (mucocele or hydrops) or pus (empyema).

- Distended gallbladder may lead to gangrene and perforation. Perforation can result into three forms:
  i. Localized perforation and pericholecystic abscess
  ii Free perforation with generalized peritonitis
  iii. Perforation into an adjacent organ, to cause a cholecystoenteric fistula, and the migrating stone can cause obstruction of the:
     - Stomach—vomiting of gallstones
     - Pylorus (Bouveret's syndrome)
     - Small bowel (gallstone ileus)—intestinal colic and obstruction
     - Large bowel—diarrhea provoked by entry of bile salts into the colon
- Jaundice may occur due to the extraluminal obstruction of CHD caused by an impacted stone in the cystic duct (Mirizzi's syndrome) **(Fig. 18.8A)**
- In the common bile duct—biliary colic, acute cholangitis, obstructive jaundice, acute pancreatitis.

Mirizzi's Syndrome

Multiple and large gallstones can reside chronically in the Hartmann's pouch of the gallbladder, causing inflammation, necrosis, scarring and ultimately fistula formation into the adjacent common hepatic duct (CHD). As a result, the CHD becomes obstructed by either scar or stone, resulting in jaundice.

It can be divided into four types. *Csendes classification* **(Fig. 18.8B)**:
Type I—No fistula present
- Type IA—Presence of the cystic duct
- Type IB—Obliteration of the cystic duct

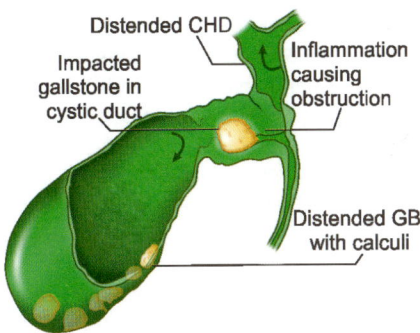

Fig. 18.8A: Mirizzi's syndrome

Pathology	Chronic cholecystitis	External compression of common hepatic duct	Cholecystocholedochal fistula		
Stages	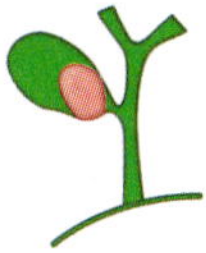	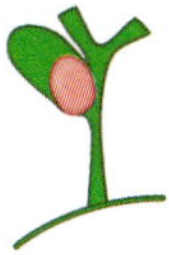	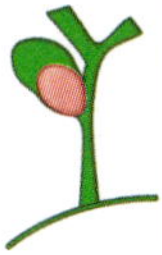	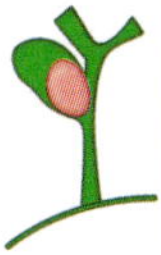	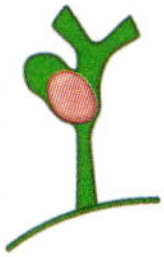
McSherry classification		Type I	Type II	Type II	Type II
Csendes classification		Type I	Type II	Type III	Type IV

Fig. 18.8B: Types of Mirizzi synrome

Types II–IV—Fistula present
- Type II—Defect smaller than 33% of the CBD diameter
- Type III—Defect 33–66% of the CBD diameter
- Type IV—Defect larger than 66% of the CBD diameter.

McSherry et al. classify only two types of Mirizzi's syndrome (**Fig. 18.8B**)
- Type I—External compression of CBD
- Type II—Cholecystocholedochal fistula

Biliary Sludge
- This is composed of microscopic precipitates of cholesterol or calcium bilirubinate, which is thought to be the earliest stage of gallstone formation. It has the potential to pass off spontaneously or also may become stones.

Management

- Acute cholecystitis is treated conservatively (nil by mouth, intravenous fluids with antibiotics and analgesics) followed by cholecystectomy (Laparoscopic or open)
- Cholecystectomy may be immediate (within 24–48 hours) or delayed (after 6 weeks), as both procedures have similar success rates, complications and conversion to open procedure
- Subtotal cholecystectomy is rarely needed when there is severe inflammation.

Management of gallstones and its complications are shown in **Figure 18.9**.

Clinical Pearls

- In diabetics, especially the elderly, the presentation of acute cholecystitis may be subtle, resulting in a delay in diagnosis

Gallbladder and Bile Ducts

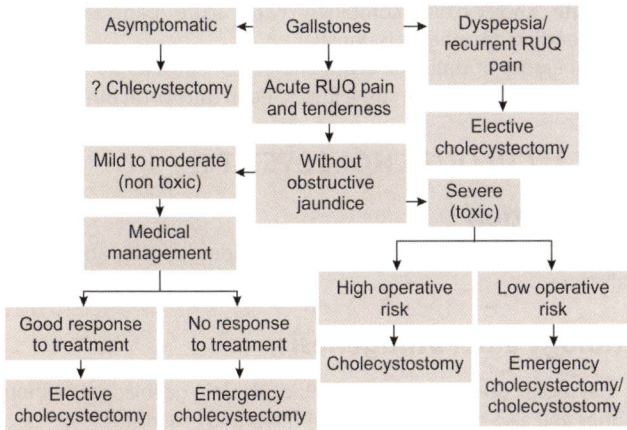

Fig. 18.9: Management of gallstones and its complications

- If US is negative for gallstones, and acute cholecystitis is suspected, isotope scan is performed. A normal HIDA scan rules out acute cholecystitis
- HIDA scan is more sensitive in the diagnosis of acalculous cholecystitis
- CT has a very limited value in the diagnosis of acute cholecystitis, but is useful in patients with a suspected neoplasm
- For patients who are not fit for surgery, the stones can be extracted by cholecystostomy, followed by elective cholecystectomy (both can be done laparoscopically)
- Symptomatic gallbladder stones and bile duct stones behave similarly
- Acute cholecystitis may produce jaundice and liver enzyme elevations in the absence of ductal pathology

- Acute cholecystitis combined with acute pancreatitis and ascending cholangitis is unusual
- In majority of patients, acute cholecystitis results due to cystic duct obstruction by a stone impacted in the Hartmann's pouch.

ACALCULOUS CHOLECYSTITIS

Introduction

Infection and inflammation of gallbladder in the absence of gallstones.

Etiology and Pathogenesis

It may occur due to dysfunctional, dyskinetic gallbladder without stones and also due to infection with typhoid organisms.

Predisposing Factors

- Abdominal surgery
- Sepsis
- Shock
- Ventilator support
- Total parenteral nutrition
- Diabetes mellitus
- Trauma.

Diagnosis

Symptoms

- Abdominal pain
- Fever.

Gallbladder and Bile Ducts

Signs

- Right upper quadrant tenderness
- Murphy's sign may be present
- Jaundice is not uncommon.

Investigations

Blood Tests

- *Leukocytosis*
- *Abnormal liver function tests*
- *Serum amylase and lipase* to rule out pancreatitis.

Radiology

- *Plain X-ray abdomen*—can identify emphysematous cholecystitis, by the presence of gas in the gallbladder and free air in the abdomen if gallbladder is perforated
- *TAUS*—reveals thickening and air in the gallbladder wall, with pericholecystic fluid collection *without gallstones in the gallbladder.* If perforated, collection of pus may be seen in the pericholecystic area. Dilated biliary ducts may indicate choledocholithiasis
- *CT scan* may show gallbladder inflammation, pericholecystic fluid or empyema of the gallbladder. Normal pancreas rules out acute pancreatitis.

Isotope Studies

HIDA scanning can be useful and may reveal nonvisualization of gallbladder.

Differential Diagnosis

- Upper abdominal dyspepsia
- Acute pancreatitis
- Biliary colic
- Choledocholithiasis.

Management

Medical

- Nil by mouth
- Intravenous fluids
- Intravenous antibiotics
- Analgesics.

Surgical

Laparoscopic or open cholecystectomy (immediate or delayed).

Clinical Pearl

Acalculous cholecystitis may occur in critically ill patients, and requires high index of clinical suspicion to diagnose, which may be difficult in that setting.

EMPHYSEMATOUS CHOLECYSTITIS

Introduction

Emphysematous cholecystitis is defined as the presence of air bubbles in the gallbladder, its wall, pericholecystic space and rarely in the bile ducts, caused by anaerobic infections (e.g. clostridia, gas forming anaerobes like *E. coli* and streptococci).

Risk Factors

- Women
- Diabetes mellitus
- Immune compromised.

Diagnosis

Symptoms and Signs

- Sudden and rapidly progressive right upper quadrant pain
- High grade fever
- High grade toxicity
- Tender mass in the right hypochondrium.

Investigations

Blood Tests

- Leukocytosis.

Radiology

- *Plain X-ray abdomen* reveals gas bubbles in and around the gallbladder, sometimes air fluid level in the gallbladder
- *CT abdomen* reveals the similar findings as plain X-rays, but is required only when X-ray findings are equivocal.

Management

Medical

- Intravenous fluids
- High dose antibiotics effective against anerobic bacteria.

Surgical

- Emergency cholecystectomy is necessary
- Cholecystostomy in critically ill patients.

Clinical Pearls

- The complications are similar to other forms of acute cholecystitis, but incidence of perforation is high
- Mortality rate is considerably high when compared to other forms of cholecystitis.

CHOLEDOCHOLITHIASIS

Epidemiology and Pathogenesis

- Stones within the common bile duct are usually formed in the gallbladder and pass on to the CBD
- Primary stones in the CBD are usually of the soft brown pigmented type and result due to stasis of bile
- About 5–10% of the patients undergoing cholecystectomy have stones in the bile ducts, the incidence increasing with age.

Choledocholithiasis is classified into:
1. Primary stones
2. Secondary stones.

Primary Stones

These stones form de novo within the bile ducts and are low in cholesterol content but have increased amounts of bilirubin. They are called **Brown stones**.

Primary intrahepatic stones, which are generally calcium bilirubinates and mixed stones, with increased amounts of cholesterol and lesser amounts of bilirubin. They form due to:
- Biliary stasis (obstructions caused by biliary stricture, papillary stenosis, tumors)
- Infection.

Risk Factors

- Low protein and low fat diet
- Malnutrition
- Parenteral hyperalimentation.

Secondary Stones

These stones resemble and have the composition of gallstones. Majority of these stones are cholesterol stones (75%) and the rest black pigment stones (25%).
- The cholesterol stones are formed due to various factors:
  - Local factors
  - Cholesterol saturation
  - Biliary stasis
  - Nucleating factors
- The black stones are formed due to:
  - Hemolytic disorders
  - Cirrhosis of liver
  - Ileal resection
  - Prolonged fasting
  - Total parenteral nutrition.

Behavioral and biologic factors play an important role in formation of these stones (**Table 18.2**).

Table 18.2: Behavioral and biologic factors for formation of secondary stones in bile duct

Behavioral factors	Biologic factors
• Nutrition • Obesity • Weight loss • Physical activity	• Increasing age • Females • Parity • Serum lipid levels • Race

Diagnosis

Symptoms and Signs

Many small stones pass into the duodenum without causing symptoms, but some enlarge in the CBD, due to stasis, and cause obstruction to bile outflow, to cause obstructive jaundice. A stone in the CBD can give rise to two varieties of obstructive jaundice:
1. Progressive jaundice due to impaction of stone.
2. Intermittent jaundice due to ball-valve action of the stone.

Gallstones obstructing the bile outflow in the bile duct can cause a variety of clinical conditions. They are given in **Table 18.3**.

Table 18.3: Clinical presentation of gallstones in the CBD

Degree of obstruction	Clinical condition	Clinical presentation
Intermittent obstruction	Biliary colic	Fluctuating jaundice
Chronic obstruction associated with infection	Ascending cholangitis	Abdominal pain, swinging pyrexia and jaundice (Charcot's triad)
Acute on chronic obstruction with severe infection	Acute suppurative cholangitis	Abdominal pain, swinging pyrexia and jaundice, toxemia
Obstruction at the duodenal papilla	Acute pancreatitis	Abdominal pain, jaundice, shock syndrome

Note:
- Presence of hypotension and mental confusion in addition to Charcot's triad is termed *"Reynald's pentad"*
- Shock with hypotension and tachycardia may be associated
- In all patients with chronic cholecystitis, the gallbladder may not be palpable as it is contracted due to repeated infections and resultant fibrosis (Courvoisier's law).

Courvoisier's Law

In a jaundiced patient, the gallbladder is not distended and palpable, when the disease is due to stones, as chronic cholecystitis leads to fibrosis and contracture and does not allow its distension. Whereas, it becomes palpably enlarged, if the obstruction is chronic and progressive as in tumors of head of pancreas (**Figs 18.10A and B**).

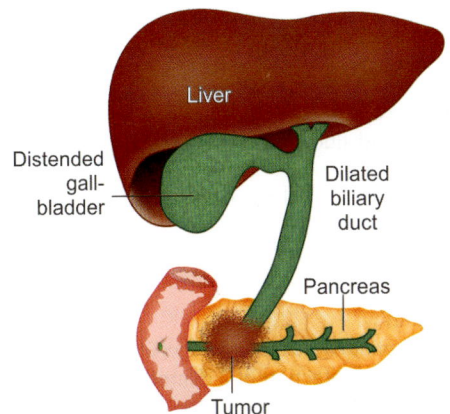

Fig. 18.10A: Distended gallbladder in obstructive tumor disease

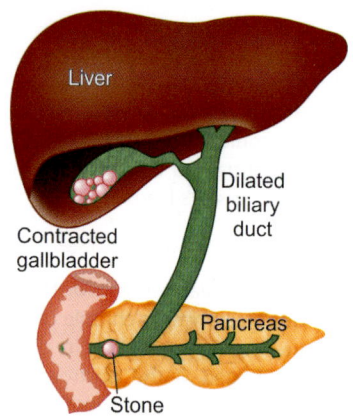

Fig. 18.10B: Contracted gallbladder in obstructive calculus disease

Investigations

Blood Tests

- Serology
  - Increased and fluctuating or persistently elevated levels of serum bilirubin
  - Raised levels of alkaline phosphatase, AST, ALT, GGT (occasionally normal).

Radiology

- Ultrasonography
  - ***Transabdominal ultrasonography (TAUS)*** has a detection rate of 70–80% for detection of a dilated bile duct, higher rate in jaundiced patients, but only 25% sensitive in detecting CBD stones

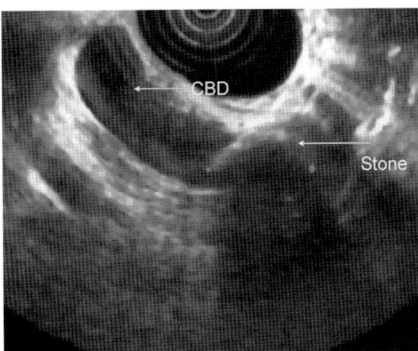

Fig. 18.11: Endoscopic US–Stone in the CBD

- ***Endoscopic ultrasound (EUS)*** **(Fig. 18.11)** has a detection rate of 98%
- ***Intraductal ultrasound*** during ERCP has a marginally better detection rate than the EUS
- ***MRCP*** has a detection rate similar to EUS, and most of the stones missed by MRCP are less than 6 mm in diameter
- ***CT cholangiography*** **(Fig. 18.12A)** has the accuracy rate less than that of either EUS or MRCP
- ***ERCP*** **(Fig. 18.12B)** detects stones in more than 90% of patients, but should be performed only as a preliminary therapeutic procedure (sphincterotomy and basketing) **(Fig. 18.12C)**, as complications like acute pancreatitis, bleeding and perforation occur
- ***PTC*** is used for establishing the upper level of obstruction caused by impacted stones, which also can be used as a drainage procedure in inoperable and very sick patients

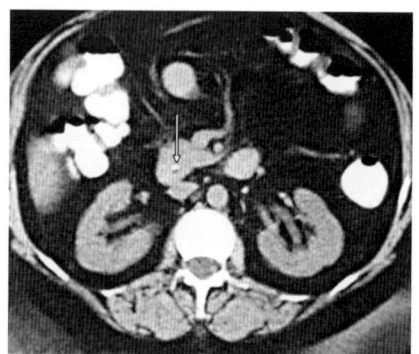

Fig. 18.12A: CT—Stone at the distal CBD

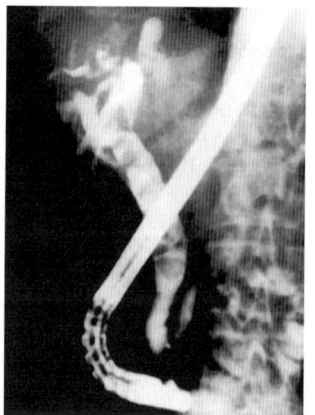

Fig. 18.12B: ERCP—Multiple stones in CBD

Gallbladder and Bile Ducts

- *Spyglass cholangiography* is almost 100% specific due to its direct visualization of stone in the bile ducts
- *Intraoperative cholangiography* performed during cholecystectomy has a very high specificity but very small stones are missed by this procedure.

Radionuclide Studies

- *Isotope studies* of biliary system will indicate the physiology.

Management

Medical
- Vitamin K injections, intravenous fluids and antibiotics
- Oral bile acids.

Endoscopic
- *ERCP sphincterotomy and basketing* is used for removal of obstructing gallstones (**Fig. 18.12C**)
- *Nasobiliary drainage/endobiliary stenting* is required to relieve jaundice caused by impacted stones, followed

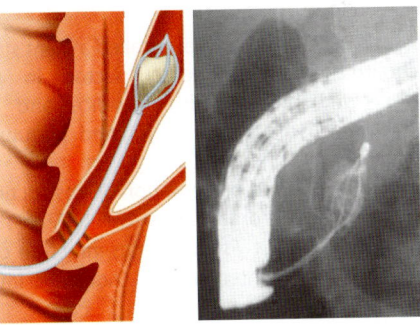

Fig. 18.12C: Basketing of common bile duct stone

by endoscopic lithotripsy during ERCP or extracorporeal lithotripsy in combination with ERCP and stone retreival
- **Urgent decompression by ERCP sphincterotomy and drainage** is required for management of suppurative cholangitis
- **PTC with stone retrieval** is an alternate method when ERCP is not possible due to previous surgery
- **Spyglass cholangioscopy** may be used for retrieval of CBD stones, and may be used for shattering the large stones.

Surgical
- **Laparoscopic transcystic CBD exploration and stone retrieval** is done by some surgeons
- **Laparoscopic choledochotomy** is a commonly done procedure for large impacted stones
- **Open CBD exploration** is rarely performed today
- **Choledochoduodenostomy** (laparoscopic/open) is performed for multiple stones and grossly dilated CBD.

An algorithm for the management of choledocholithiasis is given in **Figure 18.13**.

Clinical Pearls

- Bile duct stone of >2 cm diameter is called a giant stone
- Choledocholithiasis should be suspected in patients of cholelithiasis who present with jaundice and dark urine, extrahepatic ductal dilatation, conjugated bilirubinemia, and elevated alkaline phosphatase
- Cholangitis is the dreaded presentation of obstructing bile duct stone, and the infecting organism is usually *E. coli*, *Streptococci* species, *Klebsiella* species. *Pseudomonas* infection occurs more commonly with biliary interventions. Anerobic infections are common in the elderly

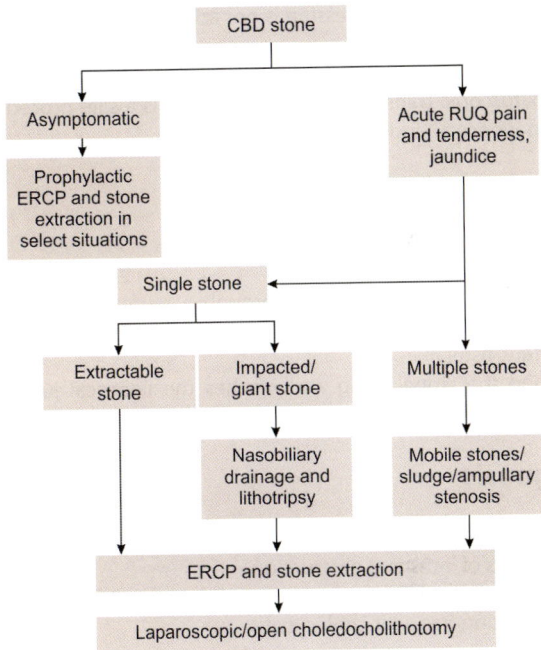

Fig. 18.13: Management of choledocholithiasis

- Drainage of the biliary tree is the mainstay of therapy for patients with acute cholangitis
- Biliary sepsis will resolve in majority of patients with conservative therapy
- Urgent decompression is needed in 10–15% of patients who fail to respond to conservative therapy

- When biliary decompression is not achieved, liver abscesses are inevitable
- When endoscopic procedure fails for retrieval of stones, laparoscopic transcystic CBD exploration is a safe procedure in experienced hands.

GALLSTONE ILEUS

Etiology and Pathogenesis

- Gallstone enters the bowel through a perforated gallbladder (post-cholecystitis) adherent to the small bowel (cholecysto-enteric fistula)
- When the stone is big and reaches the ileocecal junction, it causes small bowel obstruction.

Diagnosis

Symptoms and Signs

- Features of intestinal obstruction
- Previous history of vague attacks of right upper quadrant pain, suggesting frequent cholecystitis.

Investigations

- ***Plain X-ray abdomen*** almost always shows air in the biliary tree as bowel gas passes through the cholecystoenteric fistula. A gallstone may also be seen in the right lower quadrant, if it is radiopaque (**Fig. 18.14**)
- ***CT*** is more informative. Rarely a gallstone may also be seen in the small bowel, and also in the gallbladder if there are many.

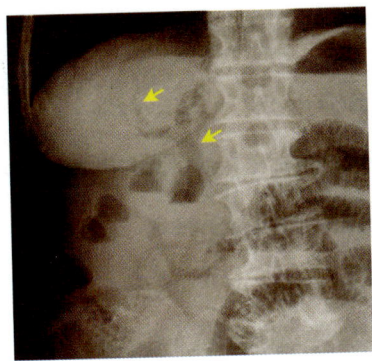

Fig. 18.14: Gallstone ileus—Air in the biliary tree

Management

During laparotomy
- Simple crushing of stone with fingers from outside the bowel may be enough if it is soft
- Simple surgical removal through an enterotomy is required if the stone is hard and big
- Cholecystectomy must be performed with closure of fistula.

INJURIES TO THE BILIARY TRACT

Introduction
- Injury can be caused to the gallbladder or extrahepatic bile ducts. Injuries to the gallbladder are extremely rare. Nevertheless, they are caused by penetrating injuries like gunshot, stabbing incidents

- Blunt injuries are extremely rare and they include laceration, rupture etc. which require cholecystectomy as therapy of choice
- Penetrating injuries of the bile ducts are rare, but when it occurs, it is associated with injury to other viscera
- Majority of bile duct injuries are iatrogenic (about 95%), and occur during cholecystectomy, more so with laparoscopic procedure.

Etiology and Pathogenesis

A number of factors are associated with such bile duct injuries during surgery, and they are:
- Associated inflammation
- Obesity
- Bleeding during surgery
- Anatomic variations of bile ducts.

The types of operative bile duct injuries are:
- Complete transection of bile duct mistaking for a cystic duct
- Partial transection by application of clamp while dividing the cystic duct too close to the CBD
- Occlusion by metal clips while applying to the cystic duct too close to the CBD.

Classifications

A number of classifications are described for bile duct injuries **(Table 18.4)**.

The *Bismuth classification system* **(Fig. 18.15A)** is based on the most distal level at which healthy biliary mucosa is available for anastomosis during repair of stricture or leak. The different types of postoperative strictures are classified based on three landmarks: 2 cm under the biliary confluence, the inferior level of the confluence, and roof of the confluence.

Gallbladder and Bile Ducts

Table 18.4: Classifications of bile duct injuries

Nature of injury	Bismuth (1982)	Strasberg et al (1995)	Stewart Way et al. (2004)	Keulemans et al. (1998)	Csendes et al. (2001)	Schmidt et al. (2004)
Bile leaks						
Cystic duct or terminal biliary radical leak		A		A		A
Bile leak from CBD/CHD without tissue loss		D	I	B1	I, II	C
Bile leak from CBD/CHD with tissue loss			II	B1	III	D
Bile leak from RHD (posterior sector)		C	IV	B2		
Transection or occlusion of CBD/CHD			III	D	III	B or D
Strictures						
CBD stricture						E

Contd....

Contd....

Nature of injury	Bismuth (1982)	Strasberg et al (1995)	Stewart Way et al. (2004)	Keulemans et al. (1998)	Csendes et al. (2001)	Schmidt et al. (2004)
CHD stricture, >2 cm CHD intact below the confluence	I	E1	III	C	III, IV	E
CHD stricture, <2 cm CHD intact below the confluence	II	E2	III	C	III, IV	E
Hilar stricture but confluence intact	III	E3	III	C	III, IV	E
Hilar stricture but confluence disruption	IV	E4	III	C	III, IV	E
Obstructed right posterior hepatic duct with or without CBD/CHD stricture	V	B/E5	IV	C		E

Note: None of the above classifications describes the injury involving the excision of extrahepatic biliary tree with separation of the right and left ducts.

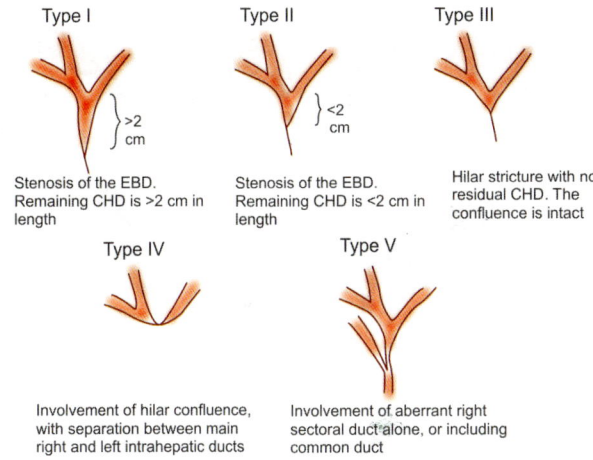

Fig. 18.15A: Bismuth classification of bile duct injuries

Strasberg and colleagues (**Fig. 18.15B**) modified the original Bismuth classification into a more comprehensive system. This classification system stratifies injuries from type A to E with type E injuries being further subdivided into E1 through E5 according to Bismuth classification.

The *Stewart-Way classification* (**Fig. 18.15C**) is based primarily on the anatomic pattern and mechanism of a particular injury. Unlike earlier classifications, both Stuart-Way and the recently proposed classification by *Lau and Lai* (2007) include the presence of associated vascular injuries, which are associated with high morbidity and common with higher bile duct injuries.

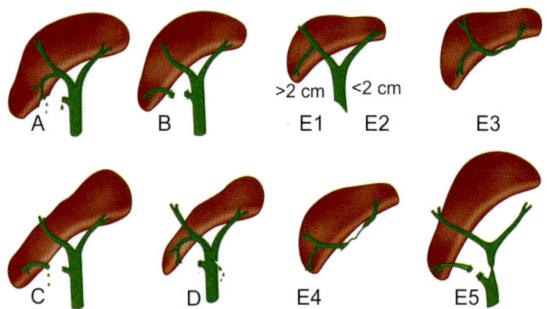

Fig. 18.15B: Strasberg classification of bile duct injuries

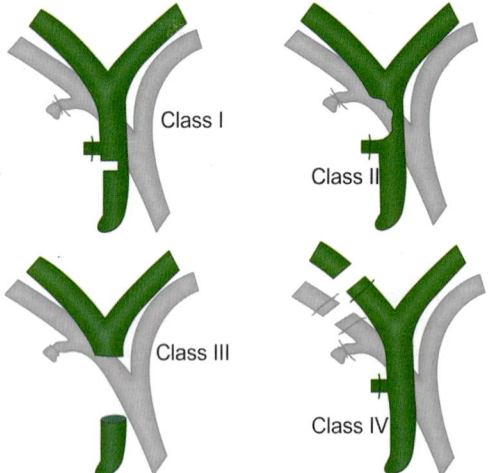

Fig. 18.15C: Stewart–Way classification of bile duct injuries

Diagnosis

Symptoms and Signs

- Only about 25% of major bile duct injuries are identified during surgery, which is recognized by the bile leak
- Some patients present with a bile leak in the immediate postoperative period
- About 60% of the patients will present within the first month after surgery
- About 15% will present months or years after surgery
- Jaundice, abdominal pain, peritonitis or sepsis.

Investigations

Blood Tests

- *Alkaline phosphatase and bilirubin* levels raise progressively.

Radiology

- *Transabdominal US (TAUS)* may show bile collection biloma
- *CT scan* may show bile collection around the area of surgery (biloma) or in the peritoneal cavity, dilatation proximal to injured site
- *MRCP* gives the site and nature of bile leak
- *ERCP* is indicated when MRCP cannot be done, or when MRCP demonstrates stones in the CBD
- *MR or CT angiography* may be needed when reparative procedures are planned to rule out associated arterial injury.

Differential Diagnosis

- Choledocholithiasis.

Complications

- Biliary peritonitis
- Biloma
- Abscess
- Anastomotic stricture
- Post-traumatic stricture
- Internal biliary fistula
- External biliary fistula.

Management

This depends on the type, extent and level of injury.

Surgical

If the damage is identified during surgery, and when the injury is:
- **Cystic duct tear**
  - A simple leak from the cystic duct stump found during laparoscopic cholecystectomy can usually be corrected with placement of an additional clip or a suture ligature loop, often without conversion to laparotomy
- **Transected bile duct**
  - Of <3 mm it can be safely ligated, as it should be an accessory duct
  - >4 mm in size, needs to be reimplanted, as it may drain more segments of entire lobe
  - With loss of duct tissue, end to side Roux-en-Y choledochojejunostomy, or Roux-en-Y hepaticojejunostomy (with stenting)

- **Lateral injury**
  - Small lateral ductal injury (Strasburg type D) can be managed by T tube drainage, introduced into the duct through the rent, as long as there is no evidence of significant ischemia or cautery damage at the site of injury. A Kocher maneuver to mobilize the duodenum can help to reduce tension on the repair
  - Large lateral injury can also managed by the above technique, but proper repair should be done by suturing to prevent stricture
  - Injury with significant tissue loss require biliary enteric anastomosis (Roux-en-Y hepaticojejunostomy) over a feeding tube to serve as a biliary stent.

Endoscopic

ERCP with stenting or sphincterotomy is useful when the bile leak is from the cystic duct or from a terminal biliary radical.

Clinical Pearls

- Bile duct injuries have to be identified early if the repair has to be successful, and high level of suspicion is required during or soon after surgery
- The extent of injury determines the operative course of action
- If the recovery of a patient who has undergone laparoscopic cholecystectomy is delayed, biliary duct injury should be suspected
- Biliary injuries have a mortality of 5%
- After biliary surgery, if systemic inflammatory respose syndrome (SIRS) develops, bile duct injury should be strongly suspected and worked up accordingly

- In about a third of cases of bile duct injuries, hepatic arterial and portal venous injuries are associated
- Localized intra-abdominal collections of bile can be drained by radiologic guidance
- Laparoscopic approach to these injuries should be undertaken only by experienced laparoscopic surgeons and not by the inexperienced attempting to minimize the event.

BILE DUCT STRICTURES

Introduction

- Of the numerous causes for bile duct strictures, operative injury of the bile ducts is the commonest
- Strictures are classified by Bismuth (**refer Fig. 18.15A**)
- Other benign causes:
    - Fibrosis of chronic pancreatitis
    - Acute cholangitis
    - Mirizzi's syndrome
    - Sclerosing cholangitis
    - Cholangiohepatitis
    - HIV cholangiopathy
- Malignant causes:
    - Cholangiocarcinoma
    - Pancreatic cancer.

Diagnosis

Symptoms

- Right upper quadrant abdominal pain, jaundice and fever.

Signs
- Jaundice
- Hepatomegaly.

Investigations

Blood Tests
- ***Alkaline phosphatase and bilirubin levels*** raise progressively.

Radiology
- ***US and CT*** may reveal the dilated intrahepatic radicals
- ***ERCP (Fig. 18.16A) and MRCP (Fig. 18.16B)*** will reveal the level and severity of stricture
- ***PTC (Fig.18.16C)*** is useful in impassable strictures
- ***MDCT with MPR technique (Fig. 18.16D)*** has sensitivity of about 90–95% in localizing the causes of biliary obstruction.

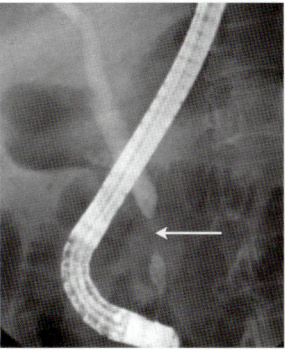

Fig. 18.16A: ERCP—Benign stricture of CBD

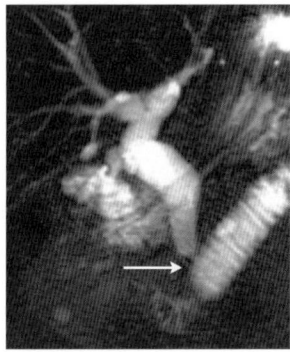

Fig. 18.16B: MRCP—Benign stricture of CBD

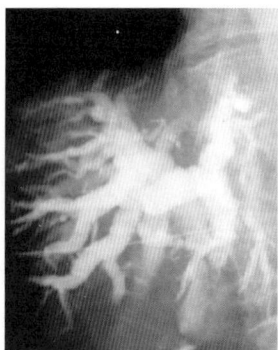

Fig. 18.16C: PTC—Grossly dilated intrahepatic bile ducts due to CBD obstruction

Gallbladder and Bile Ducts

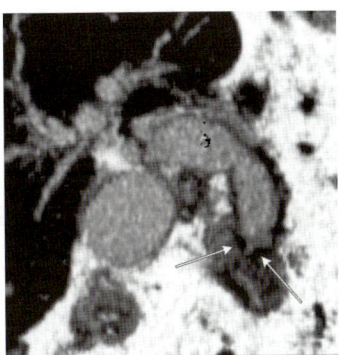

Fig. 18.16D: MDCT—Stricture due to cholangiocarcinoma

Differential Diagnosis

Choledocholithiasis.

Complications

Episodic cholangitis and secondary liver disease.

Management

- Stenting of the bile duct is the preferred treatment
- Surgical treatment is required for impassable strictures
    - Resectable strictures can be resected with primary anastomosis
    - Strictures of the retropancreatic region require, choledochoduodenostomy
    - Strictures of the common hepatic duct, require hepaticojejunostomy.

Clinical Pearls

- If the strictures are not repaired and obstruction is not relieved, cholangitis and secondary liver disease are inevitable
- If no treatment is given to a post-traumatic stricture, atrophy of liver should be anticipated or at least hepatic fibrosis.

PRIMARY SCLEROSING CHOLANGITIS (PSC)

Introduction

- Presence of bile duct strictures on cholangiography, and cholestatic abnormalities of LFT and by the absence of diseases which give a similar clinical picture
- Involvement of extrahepatic bile ducts exclusively is in about 10% of patients, intrahepatic bile ducts exclusively in about 15% and both ducts in about 75%
- Rare condition of autoimmune origin
- More common in men
- Results in progressive fibrosis of the biliary system
- Causes luminal narrowing and progressive obstructive jaundice and secondary cirrhosis
- Associated diseases
  - Inflammatory bowel disease, ulcerative colitis (75% of patients with PSC have inflammatory bowel disease and 7.5% with ulcerative colitis patients have PSC)
  - Cholangiocarcinoma
  - Ankylosing spondylitis
  - Autoimmune thyroiditis
  - Celiac disease
  - Colonic adenocarcinoma
  - Pancreatic adenocarcinoma
- Risk of malignant transformation (cholangiocarcinoma) is 15%.

Pathogenesis
- Characterized by inflammation and fibrosis of the intrahepatic and extrahepatic bile ducts, due to immune mechanisms.

Diagnosis
Symptoms and Signs
- Usually asymptomatic
- Progressive obstructive jaundice
- Low grade fever with chills, sweats.

Investigations
- *LFTs* abnormal, alkaline phosphatase is disproportionately elevated
- *ERCP* (Fig. 18.17A) is gold standard and classically shows diffuse stricturing and beading involving both intra-and extrahepatic bile ducts, but indistinguishable from cholangiocarcinoma
- *MRCP* is a good noninvasive alternative to ERCP

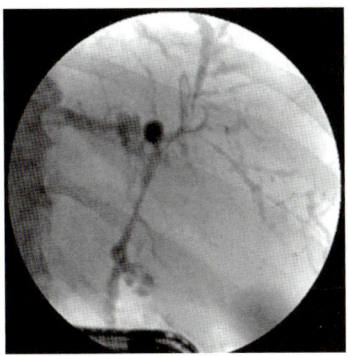

Fig. 18.17A: ERCP—Sclerosing cholangitis

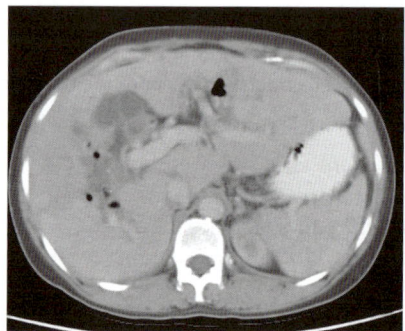

Fig. 18.17B: CT—Sclerosing cholangitis

- **PTC** though an invasive procedure is a good proximal approach which has a therapeutic advantage
- **CT (Fig. 18.17B)** gives a characteristic picture
- **Liver biopsy** may show the characteristic lesion of concentric fibrosis around small bile ducts, termed 'onion skin' fibrosis
- **Peripheral antineutrophil cytoplasmic antibody** (pANCA) is detected
- **AMA** is absent
- **Carbohydrate antigen (CA 19-9)** is useful in eliminating the diagnosis of cholangiocarcinoma.

Complications

- Cholangiocarcinoma
- End stage liver disease
- Osteoporosis.

Gallbladder and Bile Ducts

Differential Diagnosis

- HIV cholangiopathy
- Strictures from stones, surgery
- Ischemic cholangitis.

Management

- May settle spontaneously
- May respond to antibiotics, and UDCA
- Stenting of the biliary tree (**Fig. 18.18**) is very useful
- Liver transplantation is used widely for advanced disease (hepatic fibrosis).

Clinical Pearls

- Concurrent cholangiocarcinoma is seen in PSC patients in about 50%

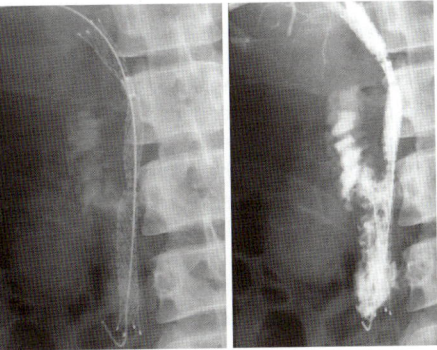

Fig. 18.18: Biliary stenting with endoprosthesis for cholangiocarcinoma

- Diagnosis of cholangiocarcinoma in the presence of PSC is extremely difficult, and high index of suspicion is required
- Excision of dominant strictures of PSC of extrahepatic ducts may prevent the formation of malignancy
- Screening colonoscopy must be advised for PSC patients as about 70% may have associated inflammatory bowel disease
- Many medical therapies have been tried and none has shown any benefit.

SPHINCTER OF ODDI DYSFUNCTION

Definition

This is a functional disorder of sphincter of Oddi, which is poorly understood.

Etiology and Pathogenesis

The sphincter of Oddi consists of muscle fibers, which surround the confluence of distal CBD and pancreatic duct and is composed of three components. They are:
1. Biliary sphincter (sphincter choledochus)
2. Pancreatic sphincter (sphincter pancreaticus)
3. Ampullary sphincter (sphincter ampullae).

These sphincters maintain the resting pressure and resist the biliary and pancreatic flow, and also prevent the reflux of duodenal contents. The sphincter is regulated by fasting and fed states. In dysfunction, there is hypertension of sphincter of Oddi causing episodic pain of pancreaticobiliary type, due to uncoordinated contractions between the gallbladder and the sphincter.

Table 18.5: Milwaukee classification of sphincter of Oddi dysfunction

Type	Biliary pain	Liver function tests	US	ERCP finding
I (Biliary stenosis)	Present	Abnormal	CBD dilated >12 mm	Delayed drainage of contrast (>45 min)
II (Biliary dyskinesia)	Present	Abnormal	CBD dilated >8 mm	Delayed drainage of contrast (>45 min)
III (Biliary dyskinesia)	Present	Normal	CBD normal	Normal drainage

Classification

The sphineter of Oddi dysfunction is classified into three types. The Milwaukee classification of the sphincter of Oddi dysfunction is listed in **Table 18.5.**

Diagnosis

Symptoms and Signs

- Epigastric and right upper quadrant pain years after cholecystectomy. The pain may radiate to the back associated with nausea and vomiting
- Pancreatitis pain may develop if the pancreatic sphincter is involved
- Localized tenderness may be present.

Investigations

- *LFT* deranged during attacks
- *US, CT and MRI*—dilated CBD
- *MRCP* may exclude structural abnormalities and stones
- *ERCP and sphincter of Oddi manometry* is gold standard. Baseline pressure is <40 mm Hg with predominantly antegrade phasic

contractions. Sustained peaks of >100 mm Hg with retrograde contractions are consistent with the diagnosis
- *HIDA scan*—delayed transit time from hilum to duodenum.

Management

- *PPIs and antispasmodics* are useful in majority of cases
- *Injections of nitroglycerin, calcium channel blockers, and botulinum toxin into the sphincter* may be tried, but long-term results are not encouraging
- *ERCP sphincterotomy* if stenosis is documented by manometry.

Clinical Pearls

- About <50% patients of type III and >50% of type II patients with dyskinesia will have manometric evidence of dyskinesia of sphincter of Oddi
- ERCP sphincterotomy is indicated only when structural alternations are detected and pain is disabling, and not relieved by PPIs and antispasmodics
- ERCP sphincterotomy is effective in about 90% of patients with type I, 60% with type II and 10% in type III dyskinesia.

GALLBLADDER POLYPS

Epidemiology

- Seen in about 5% of normal subjects undergoing abdominal sonography
- Solitary sessile polyps that are 5–10 mm are more likely to turn malignant than are small multiple, pedunculated, hyperechoic polyps.

Risk Factors which Increase the Chance of Malignancy of Gallbladder Polyps

- Size > 1 cm
- Presence of gallstones
- Age > 60 years
- Increase in size on interval imaging.

Diagnosis

Symptoms and Signs
- Most patients are asymptomatic
- Chronic upper abdominal biliary type of pain is not uncommon
- No clinical finding.

Investigations

- ***Transabdominal US* (Fig. 18.19)** is diagnostic in many cases. Cholesterol polyps may be multiple and are usually pedunculated

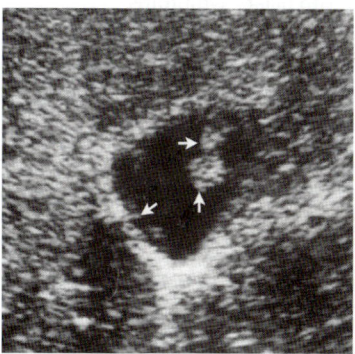

Fig. 18.19: US—Polyps of gallbladder

and hyperechoic with no acoustic shadow. Adenomas are usually solitary, sessile and isoechoic
- **EUS** is more precise and more informative in differentiating benign and neoplastic polyps
- **CT** is not useful in detecting polyps.

Differential Diagnosis

- Cholesterol polyps
- Adenomyomatosis
- Inflammatory polyps
- Adenomas
- Gallbladder carcinoma.

Management

- *Cholecystectomy* is indicated for polyps (**Fig. 18.20**) when
  - More than 1 cm in size
  - Associated with gallstones
  - In patients with biliary symptoms
  - That show increase in size on serial imaging.

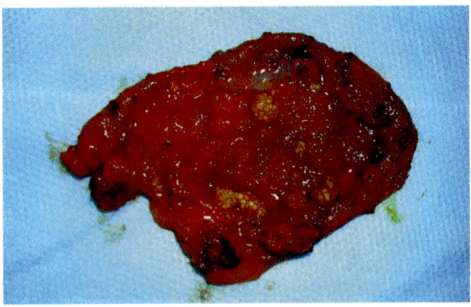

Fig. 18.20: Polyps of gallbladder

- *Observation with serial imaging* is indicated for small polyps with low risk (apparently benign) for malignancy.

Clinical Pearls
- Patients with 3 or more gallbladder polyps regardless of size should undergo cholecystectomy
- Polyps of more than 1 cm should be considered for cholecystectomy for the fear of malignancy
- Adenomyomatosis appears as a slight elevation (intraluminal convexity) in cholecystogram often with a central umbilication. When it causes abdominal pain, cholecystectomy is warranted
- Adenomas appear as pedunculated adenomatous polyps with a papillary or non-papillary etiology. May be associated with in situ malignancy of gallbladder.

CARCINOMA OF GALLBLADDER

Introduction
- Commonest biliary tract tumor
- Common between 60 and 80 years of age
- Female predominance 3:1
- 80% occur in the fundus and neck
- Morphologically, it presents as infiltrating mass
- Microscopically, they are
  - Adenocarcinomas (90%)
    - Scirrhous (60%)
    - Papillary (25%
    - Mucoid (15%)
  - Squamous cell carcinoma (10%).

Risk Factors

- Gallstones (most common)
- Gallbladder polyps (solitary, sessile, echogenic lesions >10 mm)
- Porcelain gallbladder (calcified gallbladder)
- Choledochal cysts
- Chronic *Salmonella* type infection of gallbladder.

Pathogenesis

It is thought that chronic inflammation predisposes to malignancy, but the mechanism is not known.

Spread of Gallbladder Malignancy

The tumor spreads
- Directly to adjacent liver capsule, liver parenchymal segments IV and V
- By lymphatic spread to cystic duct node, then to pericholedochal and hilar nodes and finally to peripancreatic, duodenal, periportal, celiac and superior mesenteric nodes
- By hematogenous spread to liver and lungs.

TNM Classification of Gallbladder Malignancy

It is given in **Table 18.6**.

Incidental Malignancy of Gallbladder

Incidental finding of carcinoma in the gallbladder specimen after cholecystectomy for a calculous disease is not uncommon (0.5 to 1%). T1 lesions are usually found this way, and have a 5-year survival rate of about 100%.

Table 18.6: TNM classification of gallbladder malignancy

Tumor status	
T_X	Primary tumor cannot be assessed
T_0	No evidence of primary tumor
T_{is}	Carcinoma in situ
T_1	Tumor invading lamina propria or muscle layer
T_{1a}	Tumor invading lamina propria
T_{1b}	Tumor invading muscle layer
T_2	Tumor invading perimuscular connective tissue without extension into serosa or liver
T_3	Tumor penetrates serosa (visceral peritoneum) with invasion of adjacent structures or liver
T_4	Tumor with invasion of main portal vein or hepatic artery or invades multiple extrahepatic organs
Lymph node status	
N_X	Regional lymph nodes cannot be assessed
N_0	No regional node metastasis
N_1	Regional lymph node metastasis
Metastatic status	
M_0	No distant metastasis
M_1	Distant metastasis

Stage grouping			
Stage	T	N	M
0	T_{is}	N_0	M_0
I	T_1	N_0	M_0
II	T_2	N_0	M_0
IIIA	T_3	N_0	M_0
IIIB	T_{1-3}	N_1	M_0
IVA	T_4	N_{0-1}	M_0
IVB	Any T	N_2	M_0
	Any T	Any N	M_1

Diagnosis

Symptoms

- Right hypochondrial pain
- Weight loss, appetite loss, nausea and vomiting
- Obstructive jaundice due to bile duct invasion, duodenal obstruction and lymph node metastases in the porta hepatis.

Signs

- An irregular lump may be felt in the gallbladder region
- Hepatomegaly due to liver metastases.

Investigations

Radiology

- *Transabdominal US (TAUS)* (**Fig. 18.21A**) shows thickening and irregularity of gallbladder, with loss of interface with the liver or invasion of liver, with a sensitivity of >70%
- *CT* (**Fig. 18.21B**) is useful in staging to detect liver invasion, lymphadenopathy and distant metastases
- *MRI and MRCP* are useful in mapping the tumor, vascular encasement and lymphadenopathy
- *EUS* is useful in staging and to differentiate the benign and malignant polyps.

Complications

- Abscesses in and adjacent to the tumor
- Invasion of bile duct and obstruction causes intrahepatic abscesses.

Gallbladder and Bile Ducts

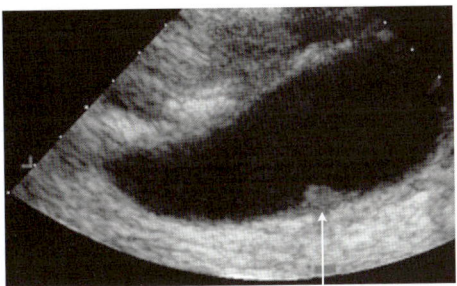

Fig. 18.21A: US—Carcinoma gallbladder

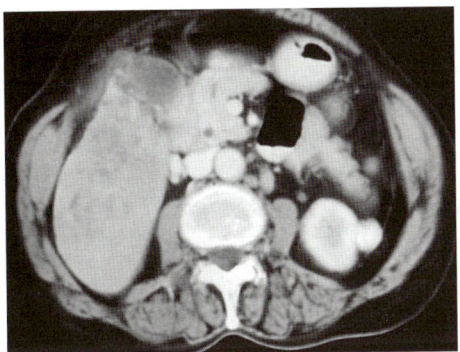

Fig. 18.21B: CT—Carcinoma gallbladder with liver secondaries

Differential Diagnosis

- Chronic cholecystitis.

Management

Curative
- ***Stage 0, I:*** Simple cholecystectomy
- ***Stage II:*** Radical cholecystectomy (lymphadenectomy of the cystic duct, pericholecochal, portal, right celiac and posterior pancreatoduodenal lymph nodes) with resection of liver (segments IV and V)
- ***Stage III, IV-T3 and T4:*** Extended radical cholecystectomy—Radical cholecystectomy, extended right hepatectomy (segments IV, V, VI, VIII and VIII).

Palliative
- Chemotherapy and radiation for unresectable tumors
- Surgical or endoscopic procedures are done to relieve jaundice and bowel obstruction.

Prognosis

Five-year survival rates depend on the stage of the disease
- T1a lesions—100%
- T1b lesions—75%
- T2 lesions—50–60%
- Stage II—30–40%
- Unresectable tumors—10–20%.

Clinical Pearls

- Heavy, thick and plate like calcification of porcelain gallbladder is not associated with gallbladder malignancy, whereas punctuate mucosal calcification of gallbladder has strong association with gallbladder malignancy and warrants cholecystectomy, even in the asymptomatic patient

- Choledochal cyst is an important risk factor for biliary tract malignancy, and gallbladder cancer incidence is highest
- At the time of diagnosis, a quarter of patients with gallbladder cancer have a localized disease, about 35% have nodal involvement and 40% have distant metastases
- Most invasive tumors have spread by the time the patient is symptomatic
- Curable lesions are small in size and they are missed by US and CT.

CHOLANGIOCARCINOMA

Introduction
- Malignancy arising from the epithelium lining the biliary ductal system
- Perihilar cholangiocarcinoma includes the intrahepatic and extrahepatic cholangiocarcinomas along with the confluence of right and left hepatic ducts
- It involves more commonly the distal extrahepatic bile ducts or at the hepatic hilum or the confluence of right and left hepatic ducts (***Klatskin tumor***)
- Common in the elderly males.

Etiology and Pathogenesis

Risk Factors

- Infestation with liver flukes (Clonorchis sinensis in Hong Kong, Opisthorchis viverrini in Thailand)
- Oriental cholangiohepatitis
- Primary sclerosing cholangitis

- Ulcerative colitis
- Hepatolithiasis
- Congenital biliary anomalies (choledochal cysts)
- Microhamartomas
- Biliary papillomatosis
- Thorotrast (historical importance only).

Pathology

- Morphologically they are divided into:
  - Nodular (most common)
  - Scirrhous
  - Diffusely infiltrating
  - Papillary
- Anatomically they are divided into:
  - Distal (lower third)
  - Proximal (middle third)
  - Perihilar (upper third)

  (Upper third tumors of extrahepatic biliary tree tend to be diffusely infiltrating, Middle third tumors tend to be nodular, Lower third tumors tend to be papillary)
- Microscopically, they are adenocarcinomas
- Spread of cholangiocarcinoma can be by various routes
  - Direct—Upper third is to the liver and lower third is to the duodenum and pancreas
  - Lymphatic—to hilar, superior mesenteric and celiac lymph nodes
  - Hematogenous—to liver, lungs and bones.

Klatskin tumor refers to hilar adenocarcinoma arising from the main hepatic duct or at the confluence of both main hepatic ducts to form the common hepatic duct.

Classification

Bismuth-Corlette classification and staging of perihilar cholangiocarcinoma (**Table 18.7**).

Diagnosis

Symptoms
- Painless progressive obstructive jaundice
- Pruritus, dark urine and pale stools
- Weight loss and weakness are common accompaniments.

Table 18.7: Bismuth-Corlette classification and staging of perihilar cholangiocarcinoma

Type	Description of tumor (Fig. 18.22)
I	Confined to common hepatic duct
II	Involving the hepatic bifurcation but not the secondary intrahepatic ducts
IIIA	Involving the hepatic bifurcation and the right secondary intrahepatic duct
IIIB	Involving the hepatic bifurcation and the left secondary intrahepatic duct
IV	Involving the hepatic bifurcation and both right and left secondary intrahepatic duct
Stage	
IA	Tumor involving only the bile duct
IB	Tumor involving periductal tissues
IIA	Locally advanced tumor that is devoid of lymph node metastases
IIB	Locally advanced tumor with adjacent lymph node metastases
III	Unresectable, locally advanced tumor
IV	Tumor with distant metastases

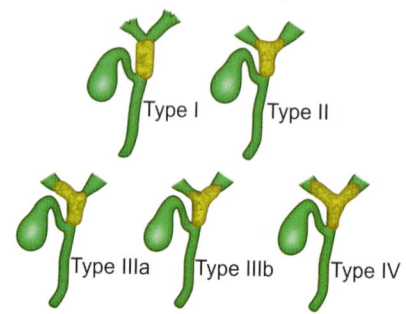

Fig. 18.22: Bismuth–Corlette classification of bile duct tumors

Signs

- Gallbladder may be palpable (positive Courvoisier's sign) (See page 907)
- Smooth hepatomegaly.

Investigations

- Serial determinations of bilirubin, alkaline phosphatase, which show marked and progressive elevation
- ***SGOT, SGPT, SGGT*** show mild elevations
- ***Tumor markers:*** Carcinoembryonic antigen (CEA) and carbohydrate antigen (CA 19/9) are usually elevated but not specific
- ***US*** shows dilated bile ducts, but lesion is not evident especially when it is distal. Gallbladder remains normal in hilar lesions, or may get dilated in distal tumors
- ***CT (Fig. 18.23A) and MRI scans*** are more sensitive and is useful in detecting the lesion and metastatic lymph nodes

- **MDCT** is useful in delineating the tumor infiltration, especially of the hepatoduodenal ligament
- **MRCP (Fig. 18.23B)** shows the level of obstruction.
- **ERCP (Fig. 18.23C)** is useful in permitting tissue diagnosis and used for temporary or permanent biliary decompression by stenting. Histopathology may be difficult due to fibrous nature of the disease, involving the duct wall
- **PTC (Fig. 18.23D)** is useful in certain situations, when ERCP is not possible
- ***Positron emission tomography (PET), endoscopic ultrasound and laparoscopic ultrasound*** are newer imaging modalities used today
- ***Spyglass cholangioscopy*** helps in visualizing the tumor and has the advantage of taking a biopsy
- ***Duodenoscopy*** to identify and confirm the lesions of the distal CBD.

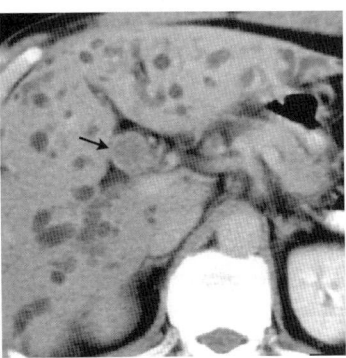

Fig. 18.23A: CT—Cholangiocarcinoma

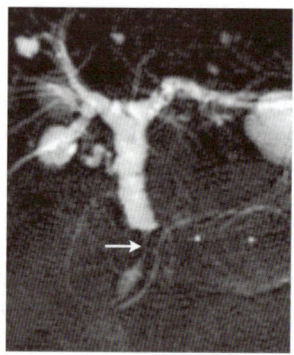

Fig. 18.23B: MRCP—Cholangiocarcinoma

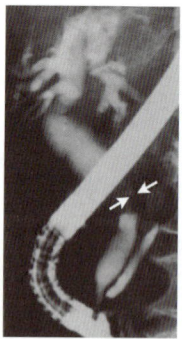

Fig. 18.23C: ERCP—Stricture due to cholangiocarcinoma

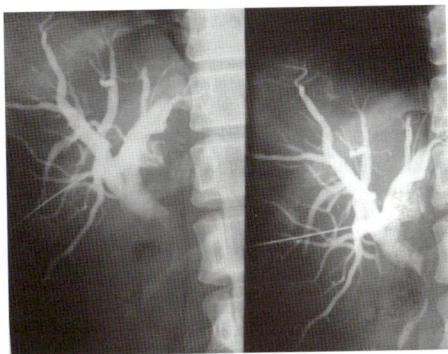

Fig. 18.23D: PTC—Cholangiocarcinoma

Differential Diagnosis

- Choledocholithiasis
- Pancreatic head malignancy
- Periampullary carcinoma
- Benign biliary strictures.

Management

It is always surgical, which may be curative or palliative.

Curative

- Local resection (with hepatic resection) and hepaticojejunostomy is done for hilar lesion
    - Bismuth–Corlette types I and II tumors with no signs of vascular involvement require local excision with portal

lymphadenectomy, cholecystectomy, CBD excision, and bilateral Roux-en-Y hepaticojejunostomies
– Bismuth-Corlette types IIIa and IIIb tumors require right or left hepatic lobectomies in addition to the resections suggested for types I and II tumors
- Pancreatoduodenectomy (Whipple's procedure) with reconstruction procedures is done for distal tumors.

Palliative

- Stenting (endoprosthesis) is useful for unresectable tumors
- PTBD is possible in most cases
- Hepaticojejunostomy (Roux-en-Y) to relieve jaundice in cases with distal tumors not amenable to endoscopic or percutaneous procedures. Gastrojejunostomy is done to prevent gastric outlet obstruction
- Choledochojejunostomy to relieve jaundice in cases not amenable to endoscopic or percutaneous procedures

Clinical Pearls

- Confluence of right and left hepatic ducts is the most common site for cholangiocarcinoma
- In most cases of cholangiocarcinoma, no risk factor is identified
- Other than cholangiocarcinoma, many rare tumors affect the bile ducts, which include biliary cystadenoma and non–Hodgkin's lymphoma
- Despite the availability of investigations, more than half the patients who undergo exploration have peritoneal implants, nodal and hepatic metastases or locally advanced disease which precludes resection

Gallbladder and Bile Ducts

- The risk factors for recurrence after resection are the positive margins and lymph node positive tumors
- Portal vein invasion is not a contraindication for surgical resection, and portal vein resection and reconstruction offers good survival benefit when compared to conservative management
- Hepatopancreaticoduodenectomy (major hepatectomy and pancreaticoduodenectomy) can be done for locally advanced tumor involving both the hepatic duct confluence and the distal intrapancreatic CBD
- Surgery is not recommended for recurrent tumors
- Metal stents have a lesser incidence of clogging and cause cholangitis when compared to plastic stents
- It is impossible to diagnose the extent of tumor during surgery, preoperative evaluation has to be precise, and the surgical resection depends entirely on this precise evaluation.

OPERATIVE PROCEDURES

- Cholecystectomy is the treatment of choice of all gallstone diseases
- When stones are found in the bile ducts, they are to be removed preferably through endoscope and when not possible by open surgical procedures
- Gallbladder malignancies require radical cholecystectomy.
- Bile duct malignancies require excision and end-to-end anastomosis, and when not possible, various bypass procedures are advocated.

Antibiotics in Gallbladder Surgery

- Wide spectrum antibiotics are necessary during the attacks of acute cholecystitis, and continued perioperatively
- Chronic cholecystitis patients require only a single dose of prophylactic antibiotic.
- When ascending cholangitis is suspected, use of antibiotics becomes essential, as the common bile duct itself behaves like an abscess, warranting immediate decompression by ERCP
- When complications like perforation, gangrene and biliary peritonitis occur, usage of antibiotics becomes mandatory and continued for at least a period of 5 days
- Combinations of extended spectrum cephalosporins and metronidazole, fluoroquinolones and metronidazole are effective in cholangitis
- Anerobic coverage is most importantly needed in the elderly and those who undergo biliary interventions.

Cholecystectomy

Cholecystectomy is the treatment of choice for any gallstone disease.

Laparoscopic cholecystectomy is the gold standard today and when cannot be done, open cholecystectomy is preferred. Operative cholangiogram is supplemented by many surgeons, and if stones are found in the bile duct, common bile duct exploration is done followed by the choledocholithotomy.

When to Operate?

The timing of the operation is scheduled at the patient's convenience in a chronic inflamed gallbladder. When acutely inflamed, it is preferred to remove the gallbladder within 48 hours of the acute episode, as the dissection of anatomic planes is relatively easier in the presence of tissue edema especially when limited to the gallbladder and cystic duct. When the inflammation becomes more severe and intense, and extends to porta hepatis, neovasculature develops, which make the cholecystectomy technically difficult.

Laparoscopic Cholecystectomy

Indications for laparoscopic cholecystectomy
- Symptomatic gallstones
  - Biliary colic
  - Acute cholecystitis
  - Chronic cholecystitis
  - Gallstone pancreatitis
- Asymptomatic gallstones
  - Gallbladder polyp >1 cm
  - Porcelain gallbladder
  - Sickle cell disease
  - Incidental cholecystectomy.

Contraindications for laparoscopic cholecystectomy
- Absolute
  - Unfit for general anesthesia
  - Refractory coagulopathy
  - Gallbladder malignancy
- Relative
  - Previous upper abdominal surgery
  - Diffuse peritonitis
  - Cirrhosis and portal hypertension
  - Chronic obstructive pulmonary disease
  - Cholecystoenteric fistula
  - Morbid obesity
  - Pregnancy.

Surgical Procedure

Procedure

- Position of the patient: Supine with left lateral tilt with head end elevated by 20° (which will help the bowel to fall down and stay away from the view)
- Anesthesia: General
- Preparation of bowel: NBM for 6 hours, mild laxatives previous night
- Technique:
  - Operating team takes positions depending on the method chosen (Surgeon and camera assistant stay on the left side of the patient in English/American set-up, surgeon stays between the abducted legs of the patient in French/European set-up) (**Figs 18.24A and B**)
  - Imaging instruments, diathermy devices, suction apparatus and instrument tables are arranged in a comfortable manner
  - CO_2 pneumoperitoneum is created, using a Verress needle at the umbilicus to distend the abdominal cavity
  - Four entry ports (**Figs 18.25A and B**) are made
    - First, a 10 mm Camera port is made at the umbilicus (for an overall view of the abdominal cavity)
    - Next, a 10mm working port is introduced at the epigastrium under vision
    - 5 mm ports are made at the right midclavicular line (A) and anterior axillary line for grasping the gallbladder (B)
    - Through the port 4, the fundus of the gallbladder is grasped and retracted cephalad (**Fig. 18.26**)
    - Through the port 3, the Hartmann's pouch of the gallbladder is grasped and retracted downwards (**Fig. 18.26**)

Gallbladder and Bile Ducts

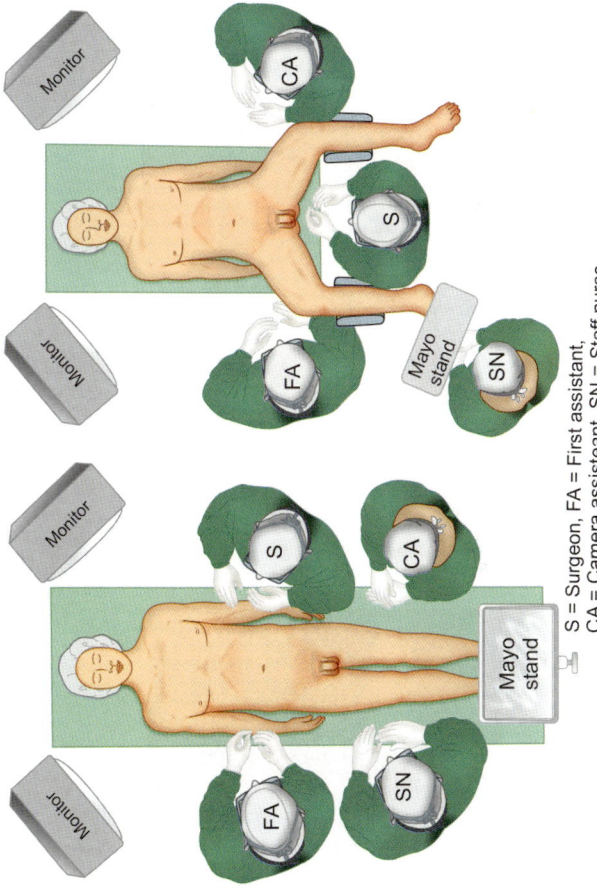

Figs 18.24A and B: Positions of operating team. (A) American; (B) French

S = Surgeon, FA = First assistant,
CA = Camera assistant, SN = Staff nurse

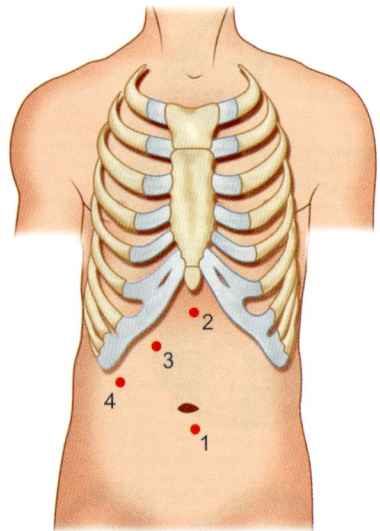

Fig. 18.25A: Port positions for laparoscopic cholecystectomy

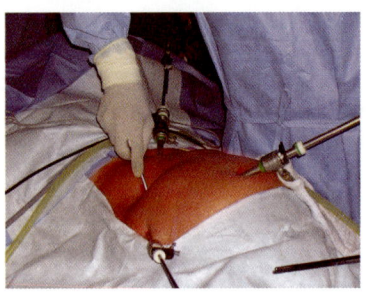

Fig. 18.25B: Ports for laparoscopic cholecystectomy

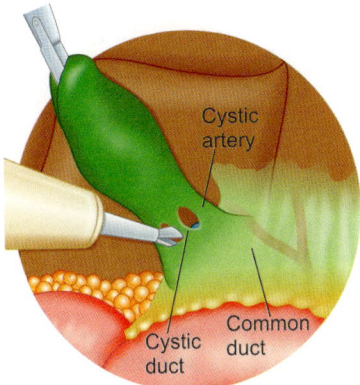

Fig. 18.26: Retraction of gallbladder cephalad

- The junction of cystic duct and CBD is at right angle, by this traction
- Calot's triangle and its structures are identified well
- Dissection should start at the infundibulum and worked towards the common bile duct
- After isolation, the cystic artery and cystic duct are divided between clips, preferably in that order (**Fig. 18.27**)
- Gallbladder is removed from its bed using a hook or spatula, using coagulation diathermy (**Fig. 18.28**)
- Hemostasis over the gallbladder bed is established
- Gallbladder is removed from the abdominal cavity through the epigastric port, if necessary by the dilatation of port site
- Saline wash and suction may be needed if there is spill of gallbladder contents

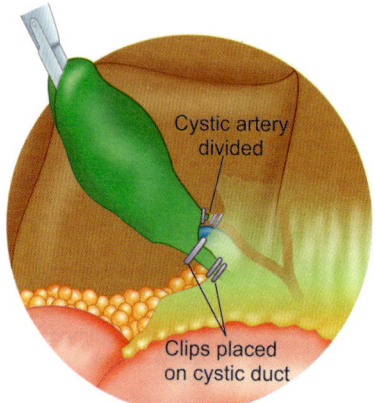

Fig. 18.27: Cystic artery and duct division

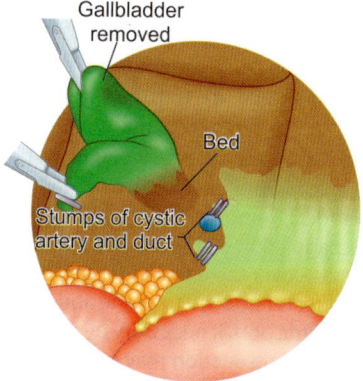

Fig. 18.28: Removal of gallbladder from its bed

- Port sites are closed with sutures, taking care of 10 mm ports by approximating the fascial defects to prevent herniation.

Complications of Laparoscopic Cholecystectomy

Surgery Related

- **Operative**
  - Gallbladder injury
  - CBD injury
  - Hepatic artery injury
- **Postoperative**
  - Hemorrhage from
    - Gallbladder bed
    - Slippage of cystic artery clip
  - Bile duct injury causing
    - Bile leak
    - Biloma
    - Biliary peritonitis
    - Subphrenic abscess
    - Postoperative stricture
    - External biliary fistula
    - Biliary enteric fistula
  - Retained CBD stones causing
    - Obstructive jaundice
    - Cholangitis
    - Pancreatitis
  - Wound infection
  - Trocar site hernia

- **Pneumoperitoneum related**
  - CO_2 embolism
  - Vasovagal reflex
  - Cardiac arrhythmias
  - Hypercarbic acidosis
- **Trocar related**
  - Abdominal wall bleeding
  - Vascular injury
  - Visceral injury
  - Trocar site hernia.

During laparoscopic cholecystectomy for acute cholecystitis, decompression of the gallbladder and aspiration of contents will be required for a perfect grasp of the fundus. During this procedure, the contents and the stones may spill into the peritoneal cavity in about one-third of patients. However, this has no impact on the incidence of postoperative infection, hospital stay or adverse long-term complications, excepting an increase in operating time of about 10 minutes required to clean the spillage by wash and aspiration. The stones need to be picked up as far as possible, but cholesterol stones pose little threat to infection, whereas pigment stones can harbor bacteria.

Conversion to Open Cholecystectomy

About 2–5% of laparoscopic cholecystectomies get converted to open procedure, more so in the elderly and in the setting of acute cholecystitis. Decision to convert to open procedure is a matter of judgment based on:

- Existing anatomy
- Local conditions
- Surgeon's experience and confidence to complete the procedure.

Gallbladder and Bile Ducts

Clinical Pearls

- Classic anatomy of biliary tree is present in only 30% of individuals, so it may be said that anomalies are the rule, not the exception
- It is always important to identify the borders of Calot's triangle and the structures that lie within it for understanding the biliary anatomy
- Right hepatic artery anomalies are the commonest
- The most dangerous variant is where cystic duct joins a low lying aberrant right sectoral duct.

How to Avoid Bile Duct Injury during Laparoscopic Cholecystectomy

- Use a 30° scope and high resolution video equipment
- Apply cephalic traction to the fundus and lateral traction to the infundibulum so the cystic duct lies perpendicular to the common bile duct
- Dissect the cystic duct well from the gallbladder
- Orient the anatomy before dividing the cystic duct
- Convert to open procedure if required.

Open Cholecystectomy

- Preparation of bowel: NBM for 6 hours, mild laxatives previous night
- Position of the patient: Supine
- Anesthesia: General
- Procedure:
  - Incision: Upper midline/right upper paramedian/right subcostal (Kocher's)

- Retraction:
    - A deep retractor is used by an assistant No. 2 to retract the liver upwards
    - Assistant No. 1 who stands at the left of the patient and opposite to the surgeon, uses his left hand to retract the duodenum downwards to stretch the hepatoduodenal ligament, and uses his right hand to retract the stomach towards him to stretch the ligament **(Fig. 18.29A)**
- After identifying the Calot's triangle and the structures within it, the gallbladder fundus is held with a sponge holder and is retracted laterally by Assistant 2
- A clamp is applied at the Hartmann's pouch to retract it downwards to make the angle between the cystic duct and CBD at right angle
- The peritoneal reflection at this angle is snipped, and dissected anteriorly exposing the contents of the Calot's triangle, the cystic artery and the lymph node
- The cystic artery is divided between ligatures or clips **(Fig. 18.29B)**
- The cystic duct is isolated well with a right angled forceps, and is divided between ligatures or clips **(Fig. 18.29C)**
- Gallbladder is dissected from its bed by blunt finger dissection and removed
- Hemostasis is established by coagulation diathermy
- Closure of the abdomen is done in layers with or without a tube drain in the subhepatic area.

Clinical Pearl

- While ligating and dividing the cystic artery and cystic duct, double ligating or double clipping is necessary to prevent complications of slippage.

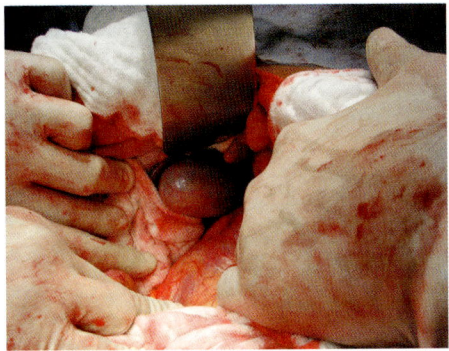
Fig. 18.29A: Isolation of gallbladder

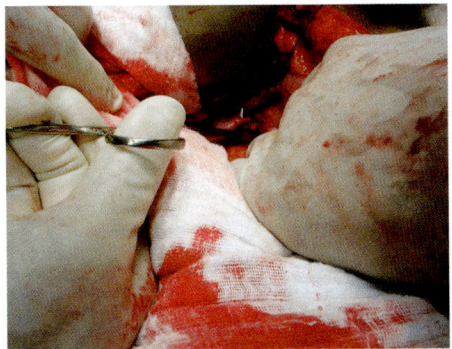
Fig. 18.29B: Isolation of cystic artery for division

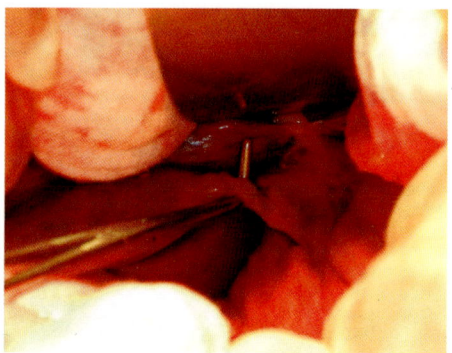

Fig. 18.29C: Isolation of cystic duct for division

Complications of Open Cholecystectomy

- Hemorrhage from
  - Gallbladder bed
  - Slippage of cystic artery ligature or clip
- Bile duct injury causing
  - Bile leak
  - Biloma
  - Biliary peritonitis
  - External biliary fistula
  - Postoperative stricture
- Retained CBD stones causing
  - Obstructive jaundice
  - Cholangitis
  - Pancreatitis
- Wound infection
- Incisional hernia.

Complications of Cholecystectomy: Hemorrhage

Introduction

Hemorrhage occurs during surgery or around the 2nd postoperative day due to:
- Slipped ligature of cystic artery or
- Ooze from gallbladder bed.

Diagnosis

Symptoms

Low grade fever, pain in the right upper abdomen.

Management

Though small collections resolve, large collections obstructing the CBD, need aspiration under US or CT guidance or open drainage.

Clinical Pearl

Application of double ligatures or double clips to the cystic artery proximally prevents hemorrhage.

Bile Leak, Biloma and Biliary Peritonitis

Introduction

Bile leak into the peritoneal cavity is called biloma, which may spill into the general peritoneal cavity to cause biliary peritonitis.

Bile leak occurs due to:
- Slipped ligature of cystic duct or ooze from gallbladder bed (during or 2–5 days after surgery)

- Sloughing of ligature of cystic duct (during or 2–5 days after surgery)
- Surgical error
- Anomalies of ductal system
- Surgery on gangrenous gallbladder.

Diagnosis

Symptoms

- Low grade fever, severe pain right upper abdomen.

Investigations

- US may identify the collection
- CT is done when US is equivocal.

Management

- Though small collections resolve, large collections obstructing the CBD, need aspiration under US or CT guidance or open drainage
- Generalized biliary peritonitis is a morbid condition and may require laparotomy.

Clinical Pearls

- Double ligature or clipping of cystic duct, proper irrigation and suction, understanding the anatomy will prevent this complication
- Biloma may leak into the general peritoneal cavity and cause generalized biliary peritonitis.

Subphrenic or Intra-abdominal Abscess

Introduction

Collection of pus in the peritoneal cavity occurs around the 5th to 7th postoperative day due to:
- Infection of collected bile or blood or both
- Collection of infected bile.

Diagnosis

Symptoms and Signs

Varying grades of fever, severe pain and tenderness right upper abdomen.

Investigations
- Ultrasonography or CT may be useful.

Management
- Though small collections resolve, large collections obstructing the CBD, need aspiration under US or CT guidance or open drainage
- Higher grade broader spectrum antibiotics, to cover gram-positive organisms (3rd and 4th generation cephalosporins), gram-negative organisms (aminoglycosides) and anaerobes (metronidazole).

Clinical Pearl

Prophylactic antibiotics and good hemostasis and measures to prevent a bile leak will prevent this complication.

External Biliary Fistula

Introduction

Leakage of bile through a fistulous tract between the gallbladder and exterior, occurs around 7th–10th postoperative day due to:
- Spontaneous leakage of bile or biloma to the exterior
- Surgical drainage of biloma
- Distal obstruction of CBD (stone or malignancy).

Diagnosis

Symptoms

High grade fever, discharge of bile from wound or drain site with or without signs of electrolyte imbalance.

Investigations

- US will demonstrate dilated biliary radicles
- CT and MRI may demonstrate the pathology at the distal CBD
- Fistulography or MR fistulography may demonstrate the pathology at the distal CBD
- MRCP is useful
- PTC is useful when the ductal system is dilated
- Isotope studies apart from the origin of fistulous tract gives the index of liver function and biliary secretion.

Management

Medical

- Correction of electrolyte and fluid imbalance
- Correction of malnutrition
- Control of skin excoriation
- Control of intra-abdominal infection.

Surgical

- Relief of obstruction of CBD (ERCP sphincterotomy and basketing of stone)
- Total disruption of CBD warrants fistulojejunostomy or choledochojejunostomy
- Malignancy requires pancreatoduodenectomy.

Biliary Enteric Fistula

Introduction

Communication between the biliary system and intestines occur due to the rupture of pericholedochal abscess into the adjoining bowel, months or years after surgery.

Diagnosis

Clinical Presentation

Clinically, they remain asymptomatic or present with symptoms of ascending cholangitis (e.g. fever, jaundice).

Investigations

- CT and MRCP are useful
- Barium studies may show the fistula
- Isotope studies are diagnostic.

Management

- Asymptomatic patients require no treatment
- Excision of fistula is required in symptomatic patients.

Stricture of Common Bile Duct

Introduction

Postoperative narrowing of common bile duct occurs due to:
- Primary closure of CBD after stone removal (in the immediate postoperative period)
- Injury to the common bile duct resulting in fibrosis and stricture (in the late postoperative period).

Diagnosis

Clinical Presentation
- Upper abdominal pain
- Obstructive jaundice
- Fever.

Investigations
- US and CT shows proximal dilatation of bile ducts
- MRCP or ERCP shows the stricture
- PTC is used when ERCP is non-contributory, especially in dilated ductal system
- Spyglass cholangioscopy is contributory
- Isotope studies are useful.

Management
- Excision of stricture and end-to-end anastomosis over a T tube
- Choledochoenterostomy is a good alternative
- Hepaticodochoenterostomy is required for strictures of common hepatic duct.

Retained CBD Stones

Introduction

Stones may remain in the common bile duct unidentified after primary gallbladder or bile duct surgery, for two reasons.
1. Overlooked stones in the common bile duct.
2. Retained stones descending from hepatic ducts.

Diagnosis

Clinical Presentation

- Upper abdominal pain
- High grade fever with rigor
- Obstructive jaundice
- Symptoms and signs of pancreatitis.

Investigations

- US shows proximal dilatation of bile ducts
- CT may show the obstructing calculus
- ERCP shows the obstructing calculus
- PTC is used when ERCP is non-contributory, especially in dilated ductal system
- Per-oral mother baby choledochoscopy is contributory.

Management

Removal of stone is necessary.
- Sphincterotomy and basketing is curative.

When the stone is impacted,
- ESWL may be used to break the stone, followed by basketing
- Extraction using per oral mother baby choledochoscope
- Dissolution of stones may be attempted

- Choledochotomy is required if endoscopic procedure fails
- Choledochoenterostomy is done for stones impacted in the lower CBD.

Trocar Site or Incisional Hernia

Introduction

Herniation occurs at the trocar site or at the incision occurs due to:
- Infection of wound in the postoperative period
- Patients with chronic cough
- In elderly and immunocompromised individuals.

Diagnosis

Clinical Presentation

Clinically it presents as a swelling in the trocar site (commonly at 10 mm port entries, especially at the umbilicus) or at the incision.

Management

Always surgical, a repair with or without a mesh.

Clinical Pearl

Closure of the fascial defect especially the 10 mm port entries with a non-absorbable sutures prevents the trocar site hernia.

Advantages and Disadvantages of Laparoscopic Cholecystectomy over Open Procedure

- *Advantages*
    - Less postoperative pain
    - Earlier return of bowel function

- Shorter hospital stay
- Earlier return to full activity
- Reduced overall cost.
- *Disadvantages*
  - Lack of depth of perception
  - View controlled by camera operator
  - More difficult to control bleeding
  - Decreased tactile discrimination
  - Potential CO_2 insufflation complications
  - Adhesions limit use
  - Increase in bile duct injuries
  - Trocar site/incisional hernia.

MANAGEMENT OF CHOLEDOCHOLITHIASIS

The obstructing stone of the common bile duct needs removal to cure cholangitis or prevent obstructive jaundice or gallstone pancreatitis. The modalities available are:
1. Endoscopic retrograde cholangiopancreatography (ERCP) and stone extraction
2. Percutaneous transhepatic drainage and stone extraction
3. Open surgical methods of stone extraction.

Endoscopic Procedures

ERCP Stone Extraction

Stones in the common bile duct are extracted using a gastroduodenoscope. By performing the ERCP, the presence of stone is confirmed. The details regarding the location, size and number are noted and appropriate procedure is performed. The stone can be extracted using a Dormia basket or a balloon catheter.

Complications of ERCP

- Cardiopulmonary complications
- Arrhythmias
- Hyperventilation
- Perforation
- Bleeding
- Cholecystitis
- Gallstone pancreatitis.

Clinical Pearls

- ERCP is a relatively safe endoscopic, diagnostic or therapeutic tool, but it is not without complication, which vary from center to center
- Dormia basket exerts better traction than the balloon catheter
- Balloon catheter occludes the bile duct lumen after inflation and prone for bile duct injury during traction
- Dormia basket is used for stones above 1 cm size and Balloon catheter is used for small stones and gravel
- Both procedures cannot be utilized for extracting stone proximal to a stricture
- Both procedures are not possible when the stones are multiple in number and impacted

Endoscopic Sphincterotomy and Stone Extraction

This involves the division of papilla and sphincter muscles to widen the distal end of common bile duct with the use of sphincterotome, a device consisting of a Teflon catheter with exposed cautery wire at the tip. The length of the intraduodenal part of common bile duct limits the extent of the cut.

Balloon Sphincteroplasty

This procedure involved the stretching of the sphincter muscles and dilatation of papilla with a hydrostatic balloon of either 6 or 8 mm diameter, which uses a high pressure to do this procedure.

Endoscopic sphincterotomy and stone extraction by the above procedures give successful results in about 80–90% patients.

Clinical Pearl

Balloon sphincteroplasty creates a limitation in size of opening as compared to sphincterotomy.

Lithotripsy

When stones are large and not extractable, mechanical, hydrophilic, laser or extracorporeal shock wave lithotripsies are performed to break the stones so that extraction is possible and easy. These procedures increase the success rate to over 95%.

Mechanical Lithotripsy

This is used to fragment the stone by using the dormia basket. This spiral device is used to trap the stone within the wires, crush it using a metal sheath by applying tension to the wires by the use of crank handle.

Intraductal Short Wave Lithotripsy (ISWL)

- First the duodenoscope is passed to identify the papilla

- A choledochoscope is passed through the main channel of duodenoscope (Spyglass cholangioscope)
- A flexible lithotripsy probe is then passed into the CBD through the working channel of choledochoscope
- Stones are grasped at the tip of lithotomy probe by electrical (electrohydrophilic lithotripsy) or light energy (laser lithotripsy)
- Impulses are fixed on the surface of the stones, which will break the stones.

Complication

Bile duct injury.

Results

About 80–95% in good hands.

When the presence of stone is questionable, but the patients are symptomatic supported by laboratory parameters, the bile is tested for microlithiasis.

Percutaneous Transhepatic Biliary Drainage (PTBD) with Stone Extraction

This procedure is limited to hilar cholangitis with hepatolithiasis, where ERCP is not possible.

Open Surgical Procedures

Open surgical procedures to remove calculi are rarely done today. Endoscopic procedures have become common in most centers and have yielded good results in best hands. This has reduced the morbidity and mortality of the open procedures. However, when stones are big and are not able to be removed or crushed by endoscopic procedures, open procedures are planned. Nevertheless, laparoscopic procedures have also gained momentum, and most procedures, which were done by open technique, are being done laparoscopically now.

Choledocholithotomy

Principle

To remove the obstructing stones in the common bile duct, to prevent or relieve obstructive jaundice and its effects, by directly opening the CBD.

Opening the common bile duct is required when:
- Impacted stone at the ampulla
- Papillary stenosis
- Multiple stones
- Stones detected during intraoperative cholangiography.

Procedure

- Position of the patient: Supine with left lateral tilt with head end elevated by 20°
- Anesthesia: General
- Preparation of bowel: NBM for 6 hours, mild laxatives previous night
- Technique:
  - The structures in the free edge of lesser omentum are identified and isolated
  - The CBD is isolated well and confirmed if necessary by aspirating bile
  - The stone is palpated well and its presence confirmed
  - A vertical incision is made on CBD between stay sutures (3/0 silk) at the level of the stone or slightly above the stone
  - The stone is milked and is extracted

- If the stone is not mobile, a Desjardin's stone holding forceps is used to extract the stone or stones
- A T tube is introduced into the CBD through the choledochotomy, and the CBD is sutured in interrupted fashion, so that all sutures lie on one side of the tube
- The vertical limb of the T tube is brought out through the skin through a separate stab incision.

Note: The same procedure can be done laparoscopically.

Cholecystectomy after CBD Clearance

Cholecystectomy is recommended after ERCP sphincterotomy and bile duct clearance, to prevent recurrence of symptoms, as the studies show that

- Risk of developing biliary problems ranges from 4–12% with patients with CBD stones
- About 40% of patients who were on wait and watch regimen will ultimately need cholecystectomy.

Surgical Biliary Drainage Procedures

These procedures are required when the obstructing stone is not easily extractable or there is distal obstructive pathology.

Transduodenal Sphincterotomy

Principle

To remove the obstructing stones affected in the distal common bile duct or in the ampulla of Vater, to prevent or relieve obstructive jaundice and its effects.

This procedure is indicated in:

- Impacted stone at the ampulla
- Papillary stenosis
- Multiple stones
- Non-dilated CBD.

Procedure

- Position of the patient: Supine with left lateral tilt with head end elevated by 20°
- Anesthesia: General
- Preparation of bowel: NBM for 6 hours, mild laxatives previous night
- Technique:
  - The duodenum is identified well and Kocherized completely
  - A vertical incision of about 2 inches is made on the anterior wall of the duodenum
  - The ampulla is located by passing a biliary Fogarty catheter through CBD into the duodenum
  - The papilla identified by its characteristic appearance on the inner wall at 4 o'clock position
  - A probe is introduced into the papilla without any pressure
  - Absorbable sutures are placed on the lateral wall of ampulla
  - A diathermy cut is made at 11 o'clock position, and extended with sequential placement of sutures along the incision
  - A free flow of bile and the contents of the CBD indicates adequate drainage
  - Duodenotomy is closed transversely to prevent stenosis
  - A drain is left near the duodenotomy closure to take care of a leak if it happens.

Choledochoduodenostomy (CDD)

Principle

To remove the obstructing stones in the common bile duct, and create a side to side anastomosis between the dilated CBD and the duodenum to prevent or relieve obstructive jaundice and its effects. This procedure is indicated in:

- Impacted or giant stone

- Recurrent stones requiring repeated interventions
- Biliary sludge
- Ampullary stenosis
- Funnel syndrome.

Clinical pearl: Since stones in Funnel syndrome occur due to biliary stasis and primary in nature any procedure to remove the stones alone has a temporary effect and a biliary drainage procedure is mandatory.

Procedure

- Position of the patient: Supine with left lateral tilt with head end elevated by 20°
- Anesthesia: General
- Preparation of bowel: NBM for 6 hours, mild laxatives previous night
- Technique:
    - The structures in the free edge of lesser omentum are identified and isolated
    - Duodenum is Kocherized well
    - The dilated CBD is isolated well and confirmed if necessary by aspirating bile
    - The stone is palpated well and its presence confirmed
    - A vertical incision is made on anterior wall of distal most part of supraduodenal CBD between stay sutures (3/0 silk) at the level of the stone or above the stone (when stone is totally impacted or presence of sludge)
    - The stone is milked out of the incision and CBD exploration is done
    - A longitudinal incision of about 2 cm is made on the superior aspect of the 1st part of duodenum between stay sutures

- The side to side single layered anastomosis is completed so it ends up in the shape of a diamond
- A tube drain is better left near the anastomosis.

Clinical pearl: Both the transduodenal sphincterotomy and choledochoduodenostomy can be performed as elective or emergency procedures.

Complications

- Cholangitis due to:
  - Ascending reflux of duodenal contents into biliary tree
  - Stenosis of anastomotic stoma
- Sump syndrome
  - Caused by food and debris accumulating between the stoma and the ampulla of Vater, leading to contamination of bile ducts with recurrent cholangitis.

Clinical pearl:
- Stomal patency is the most important factor for preventing both cholangitis and sump syndrome
- A CBD diameter of at least 1.2 cm is necessary for an effective biliary drainage by choledochoduodenostomy and a stoma of about 14 mm is necessary in preventing both cholangitis and sump syndrome.

Choledochojejunostomy (CDJ)

CDJ is a good alternative to CDD which can be done with either a loop of jejunum or using a Roux-en-Y configuration, but for loop jejunostomy, a side to side jejunojejunostomy is done to prevent intestinal reflux and secondary cholangitis. When Roux-en-Y configuration is followed, it is done in the retrocolic fashion using a 60 cm afferent limb to prevent intestinal reflux and secondary cholangitis.

T tube splinting can be utlized for the CDJ, but a drain is placed near the anastomosis to care of the leak if any.

Complications

Cholangitis due to stricture of anastomotic stoma or residual stones.

Clinical pearl:
- CDD is preferable to CDJ for it is easier and faster to perform and also allows easy endoscopic intervention if needed in future
- Choice between CDD and CDJ is dictated by anatomy and feasibility of creating a tension free anastomosis
- Roux-en-Y CDJ and CDD are possible using laparoscopy and have been done successfully.

Chapter 19

Pancreas

ANATOMY AND PHYSIOLOGY

Pancreas is a retroperitoneal organ, which lies in an oblique position, sloping upwards from the C loop of the duodenum to the splenic hilum. It is divided into head, neck, body and tail. The head of the pancreas is related posteriorly to the inferior vena cava, right renal artery and both renal veins. The neck of the pancreas lies over the portal vein. The splenic vein travels along the inferior border of the pancreas and joins the superior mesenteric vein to form the portal vein. Inferior mesenteric vein joins the splenic vein near the confluence of splenic vein and superior mesenteric vein. Superior mesenteric artery is just parallel to the superior mesenteric vein. Uncinate process of pancreas wraps around the right side of the portal vein.

Common bile duct runs in a deep groove in the posterior aspect of the head and joins the main pancreatic duct at the ampulla of Vater.

The anterior surface of the pancreas is covered by the peritoneum.

Pancreatic Duct Anatomy

Pancreas is formed by the fusion of smaller ventral bud (arises from the hepatic diverticulum) and the larger dorsal bud (arises from the duodenum). The duct from the dorsal bud (duct of Santorini) drains directly into the duodenum (as accessory papilla), and the duct of ventral bud (duct of Wirsung) directly joins the CBD and opens into the duodenum (as greater papilla—ampulla of Vater). By the rotation of gut, the two buds fuse and the ventral anlage becomes the head and uncinate process whereas the dorsal bud becomes the body and tail of pancreas. The ducts fuse usually and most of the pancreas drains through the ventral duct, or main pancreatic duct, into the common channel formed with the CBD. The dorsal duct, the duct of Santorini persists as the lesser pancreatic duct and drains through the accessory papilla. Normally, the opening of the minor papilla is 2 cm proximal to the major papilla, in the medial part of second part of duodenum.

When the ducts fail to fuse, resulting in the drainage of majority of pancreas through the duct of Santorini at the minor papilla and the head and uncinate process draining through the duct of Wirsung at the major papilla separately, result in a condition called *Pancreas divisum*. In some patients, this minor papilla can be inadequate to handle the outflow of pancreatic secretions and cause pancreatitis. Sphincterotomy of the minor papilla can give a curative effect.

Normally, the intrapancreatic duct pressure is twice that of the intrabile duct pressure, thereby preventing a reflux of bile into the pancreatic duct. The bile flow is unidirectional into the duodenum and the reflux of duodenal contents into the bile duct is prevented by muscle fibers around the ampulla of Vater, which form the sphincter of Oddi.

Vascular and Lymphatic Anatomy

The blood supply to the pancreas is from multiple branches of celiac (superior pancreaticoduodenal—a branch of gastroduodenal) and superior mesenteric arteries (inferior pancreaticoduodenal—a branch of superior mesenteric artery). The superior and inferior pancreaticoduodenal arteries form two arches (anterior and posterior—in relation to head of pancreas) along the inner border of C loop of duodenum and supply the head of pancreas and uncinate process. The body and tail are supplied by the splenic artery branches, dorsal pancreatic, pancreatica magna and caudal pancreatic arteries. The venous drainage follows the pattern of the arterial supply. The lymphatic drainage is diffuse and widespread, along the blood vessels.

Neuroanatomy

Pancreas is innervated by sympathetic and parasympathetic nervous systems. The parasympathetic nervous system stimulates endocrine and exocrine secretions and the sympathetic system inhibits secretions. Pancreas has a rich afferent sensory fibers, which are responsible for pain with pancreatic diseases (e.g. acute and chronic pancreatitis, pancreatic cancer).

Histology and Physiology

Pancreatic cells secrete enzymes (exocrine pancreas) and hormones (endocrine pancreas). These functions seem to be interrelated.

Exocrine Pancreas

This secretes about 750 mL of colorless, odorless, alkaline, iso-osmotic pancreatic juice, containing amylase (digest carbohydrates), protease (digest proteins) and lipase (digest fats).

Amylase is secreted in its active form and hydrolyzes starch and glycogen to glucose, maltose, maltotriose and dextrins. These simple sugars are transported across intestinal brush border.

Proteases are secreted in inactive forms. Trypsinogen is converted into its active form, trypsin, by enterokinase. Chymotrypsinogen is converted into chymotrypsin. Trypsin helps in the activation of elastase, carboxypeptidase A and B and phospholipase. The individual amino acids and small dipeptides are actively transported into the intestinal epithelial cells.

Lipase is secreted in its active form and hydrolyzes triglycerides to 2-monoglyceride and fatty acid. The activity of lipase is increased by another enzyme colipase. The hydrolyzed fat is transported into the intestinal epithelial cell as micelles.

The pancreatic juice rich in enzymes, water and electrolytes especially bicarbonate, secreted by the pancreatic acini is transported in the pancreatic ductal system into the duodenum. Diseases affecting the ductal system (e.g. fibrosis of chronic pancreatitis, obstruction by pancreatic calculi) may ultimately destroy the exocrine pancreas and cause exocrine pancreatic insufficiency.

Endocrine Pancreas

There are a large number of islets of Langerhans in the pancreas and larger islets are situated near the major ducts and smaller islets near the minor ducts. Most islets contain five major types:
1. *Alpha cells*—secrete *glucagon*—increase gluconeogenesis, glycogenolysis (opposite effect of insulin).
2. *Beta cells*—secrete *insulin*—decrease gluconeogenesis, glycogenolysis, fatty acid breakdown and ketogenesis.
3. *Delta cells*—secrete *somatostatin*—inhibits GI secretion a nd all peptides.
4. *Epsilon cells*—secrete *ghrelin*—decrease insulin release and action.
5. *PP cells*—secrete *polypeptide*—inhibits pancreatic exocrine secretion and secretion of insulin.

Beta cells are located in the central part of each islet cells and make the majority of the cell mass (75%), and the others (alpha cells–15%, PP cells 4%, and delta cells 5% and epsilon cells <1%) at the periphery.

Clinical Pearls

Beta cells and delta cells are evenly distributed in the pancreas, and islets in the head and uncinate process have a higher percentage of PP cells and lesser alpha cells, whereas islets in the body and tail have lower percentage of PP cells and high alpha cells. This explains the higher glucose intolerance after pancreatoduodenectomy.

APPROACH TO A PATIENT WITH PANCREATIC DISEASE

Pancreas is relatively inaccessible for direct examination, and the gland is not palpable even when it is diseased. However, abdominal pain is the presenting symptom in inflamed situations, the presentation may be classical. The clinical manifestation of acute and chronic pancreatitis and pancreatic insufficiency are protean. Furthermore, there is very large reservoir or pancreatic exocrine function, and the symptoms related to exocrine dysfunction are late manifestations. To demonstrate protein and fat maldigestion, more than 90% of pancreas should be damaged, and hence the difficulty in getting the objective evidence for disease.

Commonly the pancreatic diseases present with the following symptoms:
1. Pain in the upper abdomen radiating to the back and relieved by stooping forwards.
2. Yellowish discoloration of conjunctivae, urine and skin (Jaundice), when bile duct is obstructed.
3. Appetite loss or aversion to food.

4. Weight loss.
5. Fever.

Signs

Abdomen

- Distension of abdomen (in acute pancreatitis)
- Hepatomegaly
  - Smooth liver (chronic hepatomegaly in chronic pancreatitis)
  - Nodular liver (metastatic liver due to pancreatic primary)
- Enlarged gallbladder (pancreatic head malignancy—Courvoisier's law)

Physical Examination

General Examination

- General build
  - Emaciated—Malignant pancreas
  - Distended abdomen—Ascites
- Eyes
  - Sclerae for the depth of jaundice
  - Conjunctivae for pallor and anemia
- Skin
  - Dry scaly skin—Malignancies
  - Scratch marks—Obstructive jaundice
  - Xanthomas.

Vital Signs

- Recording of pulse and blood pressure
  - Tachycardia (e.g. acute pancreatitis)
  - Hypotension (e.g. shock in acute pancreatitis)

- Recording of temperature
  - Elevated temperature (e.g. acute pancreatitis, pancreatic abscess).

Examination of Abdomen

- Examination of abdominal wall
  - Scars may indicate previous surgery
  - Cullen's sign in acute pancreatitis
  - Umbilical nodule in pancreatic carcinoma (e.g. Sister Mary Joseph nodule).
- Examination of abdomen: Examination should include procedures for determination of
  - Ascites or free fluid in the abdomen (e.g. malignancy)
  - Hepatomegaly (e.g. fine nodular liver of cirrhosis, nodular hard hepatomegaly of malignancy)
  - Enlargement of gallbladder (e.g. malignancy of pancreas)
  - Intra-abdominal lumps (e.g. malignancy, lymph node enlargement).

Investigations

1. **Urine examination**
   - Bile salts: Its presence in the urine indicate bilirubinuria
   - Urobilinogen: Its absence indicates obstructive jaundice.
2. **Stool examination**
   - Bile pigment: Its absence indicates obstructive jaundice.
3. **Hematology**
   - Hemoglobin for anemia
   - Total and differential leukocyte count, e.g. acute pancreatitis
   - ESR may be raised in infections and malignancies.
4. Pancreatic function tests.

Pancreatic Enzymes in Body Fluids

Amylase: Pancreas produces 40% of serum amylase and the rest by salivary glands. The increase occurs 6–12 hours after onset of acute pancreatitis, and levels of >1,000 Somogyi units is indicative of acute pancreatitis. Elevated levels but <1,000 Somogyi units occur in many intra-abdominal conditions like acute cholecystitis, perforation of viscus and salpingitis. Chronic increase of serum amylase occurs in macroamylasemia. Diagnosis of acute pancreatitis should not be done solely on the amylase level, which may not be elevated in the presence of pancreatic insufficiency. Levels of amylase may be elevated in various tissue fluids, such as:
- Serum: Pancreatic inflammations
- Urine: Pancreatic inflammations with increased renal clearance
- Ascitic fluid: Disruption of gland or main pancreatic duct
- Pleural fluid: Exudative effusion in pancreatitis.

Lipase

- Serum: Elevated in pancreatic inflammation.

Tests Pertaining to Pancreatic Structure

Radiology

- ***Plain X-rays of abdomen:*** Presence of calculi or calcification in pancreas in chronic inflammation
- ***Contrast X-rays of upper GIT:*** Widening or displacement of duodenum in pancreatic head malignancy
- ***Abdominal ultrasonography:*** Information like edema, inflammation, calcification, pseudocysts and mass
- ***Endoscopic ultrasonography:*** Information obtained in abdominal ultrasonography with advantage of obtaining biopsies, with more sensitivity

- *Computed tomography:* Visualizing pancreas and surrounding structures
- *Magnetic resonance imaging:* Visualizing pancreas and surrounding structures
- *MRCP:* Visualizing the ductal system of pancreas and biliary system
- *Selective angiography:* Vascularity of pancreatic mass
- *PET scan:* It is needed in selected cases to assess the extent of the disease.

Endoscopy

- *Upper GI endoscopy:* Infiltration of pancreatic malignancy, periampullary carcinoma
- *ERCP:* Visualizing the ductal system of pancreas and biliary system with the advantage of performing the sphincterotomy and therapeutic procedures (basketing of pancreatic stones).

Tests of Exocrine Pancreatic Function

- Direct tests
  - Secretin pancreozymin test
  - Endoscopic pancreatic function test (ePFT).
- Indirect tests (measurement of pancreatic enzymes or their metabolites in the serum, urine or stool or breath after oral administration of a compound). More advanced is the disease more is the specificity.
  - Serum
    - Serum trypsinogen (very low 20 ng/mL in patients with CP)
    - NBT-PABA test
  - Urine
    - Pancreatolauryl test
    - Bentiromide test

- Fecal tests
    - Fecal fat quantification (van de Kamer test)
    - Fecal levels of pancreatic enzymes
- Breath tests.

Liver Function Tests

- Bilirubin—increased conjugated bilirubin—obstructive lesions of bile duct by pancreatic mass
- Alkaline phosphatase elevation indicates bile duct obstruction.

Serological Tests

CA 19 /9 may be elevated in pancreatic malignancy

Laparoscopy

Laparoscopy is useful in diagnosing metastases in liver and peritoneum.

Biopsy

Histopathology is possible with ERCP brushing, or fine needle aspiration guided by EUS, CT.

ACUTE PANCREATITIS (AP)

Introduction

Acute pancreatitis is an inflammatory disease of pancreas with no or little fibrosis of the gland, which has a mild, sefl-limited course to a rapidly progressive, severe illness.

Etiology

Common causes of acute hemorrhagic pancreatitis:
- Common causes are (mnemonic: *I get smashed*)
  - **I**-Idiopathic
  - **G**-Gallstone (in the ampulla of Vater)
  - **E**-Ethanol
  - **T**-Trauma
  - **S**-Steroids
  - **M**-Mumps (paramyxovirus, Epstein Barr virus, cytomegalovirus)
  - **A**-Autoimmune (Polyarteritis nodosa, systemic lupus erythematosus)
  - **S**-Scorpion sting (Tityus trinitatis), snake bite
  - **H**-(Hypercalcemia, hyperlipidemia, hypertriglyceridemia, hypothermia)
  - **E**-ERCP
  - **D**-Drugs (**SAND**-steroids and sulfonamides, azathioprine, NSAID, diuretics).
- Less common causes are:
  - Pancreas divisum
  - Long common duct
  - Carcinoma of the head of pancreas
  - Ascaris blocking pancreatic outflow
  - Chinese liver fluke
  - Ischemia from bypass surgery
  - Fatty necrosis
  - Pregnancy
  - Infections other than mumps, including varicella zoster
  - Repeated marathon running
  - Cystic fibrosis.

- Most common causes of pancreatitis, by demography are as follows:
  - Western countries—Chronic alcoholism and gallstones
  - Eastern countries—Gallstones.

Pathogenesis

Phase I

Acute necrotizing pancreatitis: The initial damage which occurs in the acini of pancreas is presumed to be due to inappropriate activation of trypsinogen, trypsin and other proteases, but trypsin does not affect living cells. The causative agents are phospholipase A, lipase A and elastase. Phospholipase A with small amounts of bile salts attack the phospholipids (e.g. lecithin) and produce extremely potent lysocompounds (e.g. lysolecithin) which is the cause for severe necrotizing pancreatitis.

Acute hemorrhagic pancreatitis: At the same time, elastase which is elastolytic and proteolytic, is secreted in inactive form and digest the walls of blood vessels and cause hemorrhagic pancreatitis.

Whatever the mechanism, the final cause is autodigestion causing edema, hemorrhage and sterile pancreatic and peripancreatic necrosis.

Septic syndrome: This is mediated by the release of multiple inflammatory mediators from activated leukocytes and macrophages, including the proinflammatory cytokines IL1, IL6, IL8 and TNF soluble receptors and IL1 receptor antagonist.

The disease resolves quickly in majority of patients, and only a quarter progresses to severe disease. The inflamed pancreas may return to normal, but may recur, under two circumstances:

1. The initiating cause has not been removed (e.g. gallstones, alcohol consumption).
2. Major pancreatic necrosis, resulting in chronic pancreatitis or stricture of main pancreatic duct.

Phase II

Infection of necrosis: The necrosis is sterile to start with. The infection is caused by the enteric microorganism increasing the seriousness of the situation.

Phase III

The necrosis can liquefy and can take one of three following forms:
1. Resolution of symptoms over a period of 1–3 months.
2. Wall off and organize into sterile liquefied necrosis, which may require some surgical intervention.
3. Infection of sterile liquefied necrosis forming an abscess, which will require some surgical intervention.

Classification

The disease is divided into two types:
1. Mild disease (without local or systemic complications and has a self limited course).
2. Severe disease (with local or systemic complications).

Diagnosis

Symptoms

- Very severe, unbearable constant epigastric pain radiating to the back, relieved by sitting and bending forwards
- Nausea and vomiting are marked, frequent and persistent.

Signs

- Shock and cyanosis are marked
- Elevated temperature, tachycardia, tachypnea
- Epigastric tenderness but guarding and rigidity are not marked
- Retroperitoneal hemorrhage may lead to characteristic discoloration
  - Around the umbilicus (*Cullen's sign*) **(Fig. 19.1A)**
  - Of the flanks (*Grey Turner's sign*) **(Fig. 19.1B)**

(These signs are not pathognomonic of pancreatitis, as they can be seen with ruptured ectopic pregnancy as well).

Investigations

- **Elevation of serum amylase** over 400 Somogyi units is indicative and more than 1,000 Somogyi units is diagnostic— three times the upper limit of normal (It usually rises 2–12 hours from the

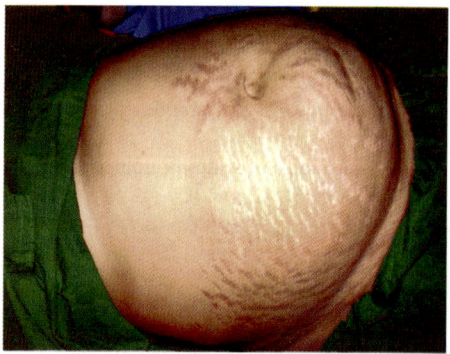

Fig. 19.1A: Cullen's sign

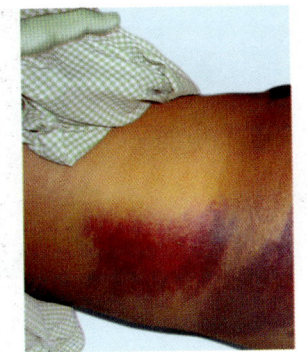

Fig. 19.1B: Grey Turner's sign

onset of symptoms, peaks at about 24 hours and normalizes within 48–72 hours)
- **Serum lipase levels** are elevated (It rises 4 to 8 hours from the onset of symptoms and normalizes within 7–14 days)
- **Serum CRP** levels above 150 mg/L indicate a severe attack, but the peak is reached at about 72 hours.

Note: Serum amylase may be normal (in 10% of cases) in cases of acute on chronic pancreatitis (depleted acinar cell mass) and hypertriglyceridemia. Reasons for false positive elevation of serum amylase include salivary gland disease (elevated salivary amylase) and macroamylasemia. If the lipase level is about 2.5–3 times that of amylase, it is an indication of pancreatitis due to alcohol.

Radiology

- **Plain X-rays of abdomen** show characteristic features:
    - *'Sentinel loop sign'*—duodenum—which represents a focal dilated jejunal loop in the left upper quadrant

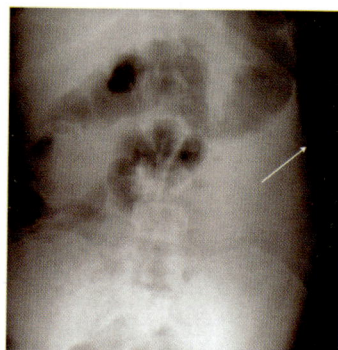

Fig. 19.2: X-ray—Colon cutoff sign

- *'Cutoff sign'—Transverse colon* (**Fig. 19.2**)—Inflammatory exudate of acute pancreatitis extends into the phrenicocolic ligament directly spreading through the lateral attachment of the transverse mesocolon causing functional spasm and/or mechanical narrowing of the splenic flexure at the level where the colon returns to the retroperitoneum

    (Absence of gas under the diaphragm eliminates the diagnosis of perforated duodenal ulcer.)
- *TAUS* may not be very useful at all times, due to the overlying abdominal gas, but can demonstrate the biliary sludge or stones, indicating biliary pancreatitis. It can also demonstrate the peripancreatic collections, but pancreatic necrosis is difficult to establish as it cannot determine the organ perfusion (**Fig. 19.3**)
- *CECT* is very useful in assessing (95% specific) the size of the pancreas (**Fig. 19.4A**), and also in determining the causes like the biliary or pancreatic duct calculi (**Fig. 19.4B**). Can accurately determine the extent of complications like necrosis (**Table 19.1**) and abscess

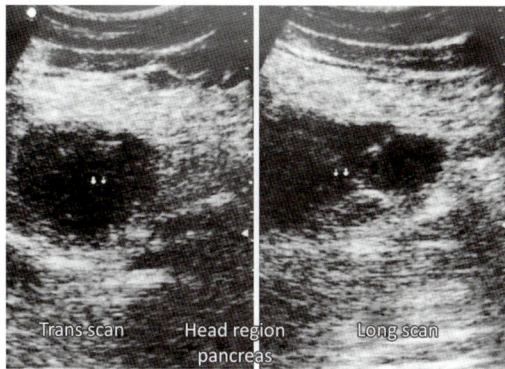

Fig. 19.3: US—Acute pancreatitis

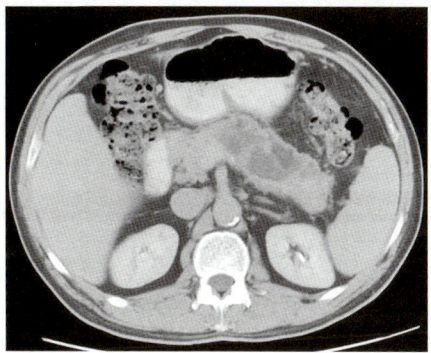

Fig. 19.4A: CT—Enlarged and edematous pancreas—Acute pancreatitis

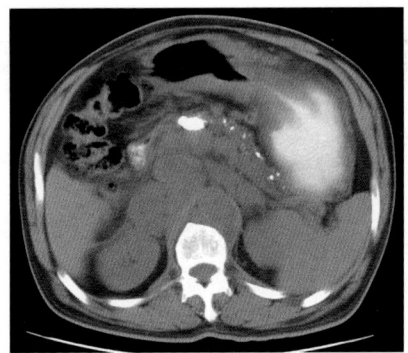

Fig. 19.4B: CT—Pancreatic calculi

Table 19.1: Balthazar computed tomography severity index

Grade of acute pancreatitis	Points
A—Normal pancreas	0
B—Enlargement of pancreas	1
C to B+—Pancreatic inflammation	2
D to C+—Single fluid collection	3
E to C+—Multiple fluid collection and/or presence of gas	4
Percentage of necrosis	**Points**
No necrosis (0%)	0
<30% of pancreas	2
30–50% of pancreas	4
>50% of pancreas	6

Grade of AP (0–4) + percentage (0–6) = Computed severity index (0–10)

Index <2 is associated with low morbidity and mortality. Score >5 is more likely to predict prolonged hospitalization and 10 times more likely to predict surgical debridement of necrosis and patient is 8 times more likely to die.

- **MRI** is comparable to CT and superior in demonstrating necrosis and peripancreatic collections
- **EUS and MRCP** are useful in determining the intraluminal causes of acute pancreatitis
- **ERCP** is considered in acute and recurrent pancreatitis, especially when the intraductal pathology is suspected and therapeutic measure is planned, but has the disadvantage of exacerbation of pancreatitis.

Criteria to Assess the Severity of Acute Pancreatitis

Ranson criteria is a clinical prediction rule introduced in 1974 for predicting the severity of acute pancreatitis by evaluating 11 clinical and laboratory parameters accumulated during the first 48 hours after the onset of acute pancreatitis (**Table 19.2**).

Interpretation
- If the score ≥ 3, severe pancreatitis likely
- If the score < 3, severe pancreatitis is unlikely
  Or
- Score 0–2: 2% mortality
- Score 3–4: 15% mortality
- Score 5–6: 40% mortality
- Score 7–8: 100% mortality.

Note: Ranson criteria is useful for patients who are at high risk of life-threatening complications, but it requires 48 hours to complete the assessment.

Glasgow (Simplified Ranson) Criteria

Predicting the severity of an attack of acute pancreatitis can be made using Glasgow or Imrie criteria (simplified Ranson criteria),

Table 19.2: Ranson criteria

Non-gallstone pancreatitis	
At admission	**At 48 hours**
• Age in years >55 years	• Calcium (serum calcium <2.0 mmol/L (<8.0 mg/dL)
• White blood cell count >16,000 cells/mm^3	• Hematocrit fall >10%
• Blood glucose >10 mmol/L (>200 mg/dL)	• Oxygen (hypoxemia pO$_2$ <60 mm Hg)
• Serum AST >250 IU/L	• BUN increased by 1.8 or more mmol/L (5 or more mg/dL) after IV fluid hydration
• Serum LDH >350 IU/L	• Base deficit (negative base excess) >4 mEq/L
	• Sequestration of fluids >6 L
Gallstone pancreatitis	
At admission	**At 48 hours**
• Age in years >70 years	• Calcium (serum calcium <2.0 mmol/L (<8.0 mg/dL)
• White blood cell count >18,000 cells/mm^3	• Hematocrit fall >10%
• Blood glucose >12.2 mmol/L (>220 mg/dL)	• Oxygen (hypoxemia pO$_2$ <60 mm Hg)
• Serum AST >250 IU/L	• BUN increased by 1.8 or more mmol/L (5 or more mg/dL) after IV fluid hydration
• Serum LDH >400 IU/L	• Base deficit (negative base excess) >5 mEq/L
	• Sequestration of fluids >4 L

which is much simpler, and requires only 8 criteria at 48 hours and as accurate as the classical Ranson criteria **Table 19.3**.

APACHE II score (**A**cute **P**hysiology **A**nd **C**hronic **H**ealth **E**valuation) can be applied at any time but it is cumbersome as it requires 15 different or biochemical criteria. A score of >6 at admission is useful

Table 19.3: Glasgow criteria

P	Arterial **P**aO$_2$ <9 kPa
A	**A**lbumin <32 g/L
N	Urea **N**itrogen >10 mmol/L
C	**C**alcium <2 mmol/L
R	**R**aised white cell count >16 mmol/L
E	**E**nzyme–lactate dehydrogenase >600 mmol/L
A	**A**ge >55 years
S	**S**ugar glucose >10 mmol/L

Presence of three or more criteria reached before or at 48 hours of an attack predicts a severe attack and two or less predicts a mild attack

in identifying the patients with severe acute pancreatitis, and can be employed at any time of the course of the disease.

Complications

- **Systemic complications**
  - Respiratory failure (due to ARDS, pleural effusion containing high amylase)
  - Renal failure (due to renal hypoperfusion progressing to acute tubular necrosis)
  - Metabolic abnormalities (hyperglycemia caused by insulin deficiency due to islet cell necrosis and/or hyperglucagonemia)
  - Coagulation disorders (diffuse intravascular coagulation)
  - Multiple organ failure
  - Shock (due to third space fluids, peripheral vasodilation and reduced ventricular perfusion)

- Retinopathy (Purtscher's) (due to occlusion of posterior retinal artery with aggregated granulocytes)
- Encephalopathy.
- **Local complications**
  - Pancreatic necrosis
  - Infection of pancreatic necrosis
  - Fungal infections
  - Hemorrhage
  - Pancreatic pseudocyst, pancreatic fistula, pancreatic abscess.

Differential Diagnosis

There are a number of clinical conditions which mimic acute pancreatitis (**Table 19.4**).

Management

Initial management is conservative.
- **Mild disease**
  - Fluid resuscitation
  - Nasogastric decompression
  - Analgesics

Table 19.4: Diseases which mimic acute pancreatitis

Acute conditions above the diaphragm	Acute conditions below the diaphragm
Myocardial infarction	Perforated peptic ulcer
Pneumonia	Leaking aortic aneurysm
Perforated esophagus	Acute cholecystitis
	Acute hyperacidity
	Mesenteric infarction

- ?Antibiotics
- Octreotide.
- **Severe disease**
  - Management in intensive care unit
  - Continuous arterial and CVP monitoring
  - Assisted ventilation if required
  - Inotropic support
  - Enteral feeding (as early as possible)
  - Parenteral feeding (when enteral feeding is withheld for more than a week)
  - Hemodialysis for renal failure if warranted.
- **Endoscopic treatment**
  - ERCP sphincterotomy and extraction of stones followed by laparoscopic cholecystectomy in patients with severe attack with jaundice and/or cholangitis.
- **Surgical procedures**
  - Pancreatic necrosectomy is the treatment of choice with questionable outcome in a grave situation (postpone to 30 days if patient is stable)
  - Lavage
  - Pseudocyst drainage.

The approach to management of acute pancreatitis is shown in **Figure 19.5**.

Clinical Pearls

- The clinical diagnosis of acute pancreatitis is almost by exclusion
- The three characteristic features of acute pancreatitis are: characteristic abdominal pain, hyperamylasemia and findings of acute pancreatitis in CT
- Most patients with acute pancreatitis have a mild disease and recover without specific therapy

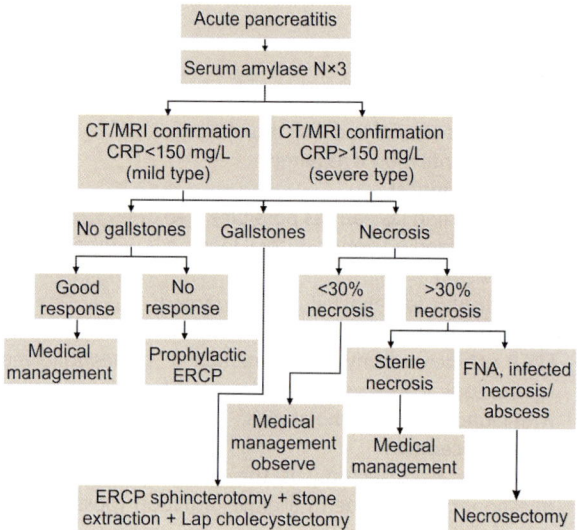

Fig. 19.5: Management of acute pancreatitis

- In traumatic pancreatitis, blunt injury is a more common cause than the penetrating trauma
- After an attack of acute pancreatitis, there is complete resolution of symptoms and the anatomy and physiology of the pancreas return to normal
- Pancreatitis recurs when the initiating cause is not removed (gallstones, alcohol)
- Patients with major pancreatic necrosis suffer from recurrent attacks probably due to stricture of the pancreatic duct
- Serum triglyceride levels of >800 mg% are needed to cause acute pancreatitis

- SIRS is considered not as a complication of acute pancreatitis but as a manifestation of disease, but a severe SIRS response will lead to multiorgan dysfunction syndrome (MODS) which determines the prognosis
- Hemorrhage in acute pancreatitis is due to erosion of intrapancreatic and peripancreatic major blood vessels
- Pancreatic necrosis of less than 30% is classified as mild variety
- Serum amylase and lipase levels have no predictive value of severity of acute pancreatitis, but CRP is a good reliable marker (>150 mg/L) in predicting severe pancreatitis at 48 hours of admission but not at admission
- Infected pancreatic necrosis is due to secondary bacterial contamination of sterile necrosis, which is the focus from which complications like SIRS and MODS develop. This condition has a mortality of 25–40%
- Infection of sterile necrosis occurs more commonly around the 2nd and 3rd weeks, and the incidence declines after the fourth week
- Pancreatic abscess is the localization of infected pancreatic necrosis and has a significantly lesser mortality rate when compared to infected necrosis itself
- Secondary fungal infections are not uncommon, but they raise the mortality rate
- While managing biliary pancreatitis, in patients who are not fit for laparoscopic cholecystectomy, ERCP can be used to prevent further attacks
- If the gallbladder is not removed, about 70% of patients will have recurrent pancreatitis
- If the etiology is uncertain, endoscopic ultrasound is suggested at resolution to look for unusual causes like small tumor or microlithiasis

- In patients with severe attack, weekly CECT is recommended to evaluate pancreatic necrosis
- When pancreatic necrosis is documented by CECT, guided FNAs for bacteria and fungi are required. If positive, necrosectomy becomes mandatory
- Routine ERCP is not recommended in mild, acute biliary pancreatitis
- Since there is a 20% risk of biliary complications within 8 weeks of acute pancreatitis, cholecystectomy is necessary, preferably within a week
- Sterile pancreatic necrosis can be treated conservatively, but progressive deterioration from SIRS with sterile pancreatic necrosis can be preferred to be treated by necrosectomy
- Necrosectomy can be performed as open technique/zipper laparostomies/minimally invasive procedures
- Surgical intervention is reserved when the collections or necrosis are infected, or to relieve pancreatic duct obstruction
- When the necrosis is walled off, surgical intervention may not be necessary, and can be delayed for up to 12 weeks
- Bleeding complicating acute necrotizing pancreatitis is best managed by angiography and transvascular embolization.

CHRONIC PANCREATITIS (CP)

Introduction

An inflammatory process leading to slow progressive destruction and fibrosis of the functional acini.
- Sometimes calcification occurs
- Both exocrine and endocrine parts of the pancreas are affected
- More common in females between 32 and 40 years of age.

Classification and Risk Factors

The classification and risk factors for chronic pancreatitis are tabulated in **Table 19.5**.

Pathogenesis

Chronic pancreatitis results due to inflammation of the pancreas leading to progressive irreversible damage to the gland.

Table 19.5: Classification and risk factors of chronic pancreatitis

Classification	Risk factors
Toxic-metabolic pancreatitis	• Alcohol consumption • Tobacco smoking • Hypocalcemia • Chronic renal failure • Toxins and drugs
Idiopathic pancreatitis	• Tropical pancreatitis • Tropical calcific pancreatitis
Genetic pancreatitis	• Autosomal dominant (mutation in *PRSS1* gene) • Autosomal recessive (*CFTR* mutation/*SPINK* 1 mutation)
Autoimmune pancreatitis	• Isolated variety • Associated with Sjögren's syndrome, IBS, primary biliary cirrhosis
Recurrent pancreatitis	• Post-necrotic • Ischemic • Post-radiation
Obstructive pancreatitis	• Pancreas divisum • Sphincter of Oddi dysfunction • Post-traumatic

Diagnosis

Symptoms

- Abdominal pain, in the epigastrium or on either side of the midline, radiating to the back. The pain may be continuous or intermittent. Recurrent attacks are common
- Anorexia, weight loss and insulin dependent diabetes mellitus (features of endocrine deficiency) are commonly seen
- 25% have steatorrhea, weight loss, peptic ulcer due to loss of bicarbonate secretion (features of exocrine deficiency).

Signs

- Tenderness in the epigastrium
- Jaundice due to biliary obstruction
- Vomiting due to duodenal obstruction
- Abdominal distension due to pancreatic ascites
- Upper GI hemorrhage due to gastric varices
- Cachexia due to ductal adenocarcinoma.

Investigations

Pancreatic Function Tests

Direct tests based on the measurement of pancreatic enzymes and bicarbonate output in samples of duodenal juice obtained after stimulation of the gland by intravenous administration of secretin and CCK or cerulein.

- ***Secretin pancreozymin test***
    - Double lumen nasoduodenal tube is placed
    - Administration of secretin and CCK or cerulein
    - Bicarbonate and enzyme output is quantified
    - (<50 mEq/L–consistent with CP, >75 mEq/L is normal, intermediate values are indeterminate).

Disadvantage: Collection may be incomplete, amount of juice lost towards the jejunum is calculated using marker (PEG), which may require a triple lumen tube.

- *Endoscopic pancreatic function test (ePFT)*
  - Intravenous secretin, upper GI scopy at 15-minute intervals and duodenal juice samples obtained for bicarbonate concentration. Concentration of <8 mM is considered abnormal.

Indirect tests (measurement of pancratic enzymes or their metabolites in the serum, urine, stool or breath after oral administration of a compound). More advanced is the disease more is the specificity.

- *Serum*
  - Serum trypsinogen (very low 20 ng/mL in patietns with CP)
  - NBT-PABA test.
- *Urine*
  - ***Pancreatolauryl test:*** Fluorescein dilaurate is split by pancreatic enzymes into lauric acid and fluorescein. The fluorescein which is absorbed by the intestine, partly conjugated in the liver and excreted in the urine. On day one, fluorescein dilaureate tablets are given and on the second day, free fluroscein tablets are given. The urine samples collected on both days and a ratio is calculated. The ratio of < 20% is considered abnormal
  - ***Bentiromide test.***
- *Fecal tests*
  - ***Fecal fat quantification*** (van de Kamer test): Gold standard for diagnosis of fat maldigestion and steatorrhea, when administered 100 g fat diet daily for 5 days, entire stool produced over the last 3 days of diet for fat estimation. Fecal fat excretion below 7.5 g/day is normal, and more than 7.5 g/day indicates pancreatic insufficiency

- **Fecal levels of pancreatic enzymes:** Quantification of fecal chymotrypsin and elastase. A concentration of higher than 200 µg/g is considered normal. Lower concentration of 100 is related to pancreatic insufficiency.
- *Breath tests*
  - Labeled substrate, mainly ^{13}C-triglycerides is given orally with a test meal
  - 13C metabolites are released by pancreatic enzymes, which are metabolized in the liver to release $13CO_2$. This is measured in the expired air by mass spectrometry or infrared analysis
  - Breath samples are collected in 10 mL tubes before (basal sample) and at 30-minute intervals for 6 hours after ingestion of the meal
  - Result is expressed as the total amount of recovered CO_2 over the 6 hours.

Radiology

Ultrasonography

- *Abdominal US* is useful in localizing enlarged pancreas and also local collections, ductal dilatations
- *Endoscopic US* is highly sensitive for chronic pancreatitis (**Table 19.6**)
- *Plain X-ray* will demonstrate calcification or calculi (**Fig. 19.6**)

Table 19.6: EUS findings of chronic pancreatitis

Ductal findings	Parenchymal findings
• Dilated main pancreatic duct	• Hyperechoic foci
• Dilated branches	• Hyperechoic strands
• Duct irregularities	• Gland nodularity
• Stones/calcifications	• Cystic lesion

- **CECT and MRI** demonstrate the ductal calculi (**Refer Fig. 19.4B**) and calcifications (**Fig. 19.7**) and enlargement of pancreas and pseudocysts

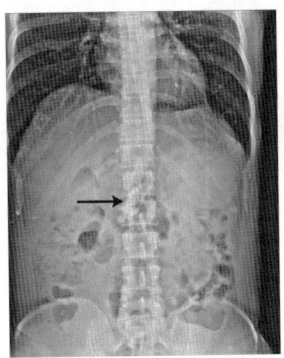

Fig. 19.6: Plain X-ray—Pancreatic calculi

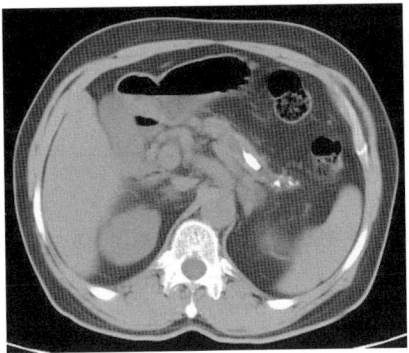

Fig. 19.7: CT—Calcific pancreatitis

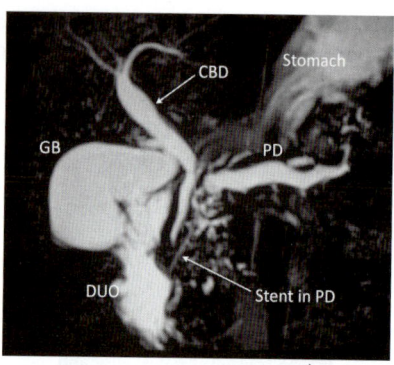

Fig. 19.8: MRCP—Dilated pancreatic duct with calcific pancreatitis

- *MRCP (Fig. 19.8) and ERCP* demonstrate the ductal dilatations, filling defects (calculi). Finding of chain of Lakes (due to stenoses and dilatations) beading of the main pancreatic duct, ecstatic side branches and intraductal filling defects are characteristic of CP. CP is graded on ERCP findings by Cambridge grading system **(Table 19.7)**.

Tissue Diagnosis

EUS-guided fine needle aspiration or Trucut biopsy are useful for making tissue diagnosis.

Diagnostic Features of Chronic Pancreatitis

The classical triad is:
1. Pancreatic atrophy
2. Enlargement of the pancreatic duct
3. Calcification.

Table 19.7: Cambridge grading system of ERCP findings of chronic pancreatitis

Grade	Main pancreatic duct	Branches
Normal	Normal	Normal
Equivocal	Normal	<3 abnormal
Mild	Normal	≥3 normal
Moderate	Abnormal	≥3 normal
Marked	Abnormal + one or more of the following • Large cavity (>10 mm) • Ductal obstruction • Severe duct dilatation • Intraductal filling defects or calculi	≥3 normal

Complications

- Exocrine and endocrine deficiencies
- Pseudocyst
- Pancreatic ascites
- Pancreatic fistula
- Ductal adenocarcinoma
- Biliary obstruction
- Macronutrient deficiencies
  - Fat malabsorption—steatorrhea
  - Protein malabsorption—azotorrhea
  - Carbohydrate malabsorption
- Micronutrient deficiencies
  - Fat-soluble vitamins deficiency
  - Vitamin B_{12} deficiency
  - Zinc deficiency
  - Copper and selenium deficiency.

Management

Medical

- Elimination of alcohol consumption and tobacco smoking
- Pancreatic enzyme supplementation (especially lipase up to 8 lakh units)
- Proton pump inhibitors
- Treatment of diabetes, analgesics and psychological support.

Endoscopic

- Stenting of biliary tree
- Drainage of pancreatic pseudocysts
- Celiac plexus block under EUS guidance.

Surgical

- Bilateral thoracoscopic splanchnicectomy.
- Surgical therapy for chronic pancreatitis should be based on:
    - Small/large duct disease
    - Inflammatory pancreatic head mass
    - Suspicion of malignancy
    - Predominantly left sided/right sided disease
    - Associated complications
    - Portal hypertension.

Drainage Procedures

Partial: Draining the Duct Partially

- ***Duval procedure*** (distal pancreatectomy, splenectomy + end to end PJ) **(Fig. 19.9A)**
- ***Leger procedure*** (distal pancreatectomy, splenectomy + side to side PJ) **(Fig. 19.9B)**

- ***Puestow–Gilesby procedure*** (distal pancreatectomy, splenectomy + invagination of tail of pancreas into the jejunum (**Fig. 19.9C**)
- ***Mercadier procedure:*** For drainage of body of pancreas in Roux-en-Y Loop of jejunum by a side-to-side anastomosis (**Fig. 19.9D**).

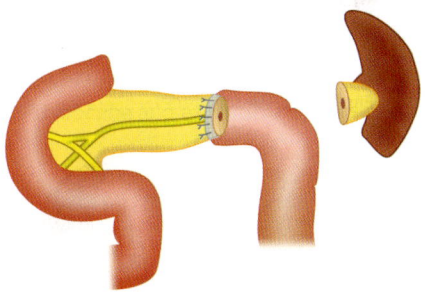

Fig. 19.9A: Duval's procedure

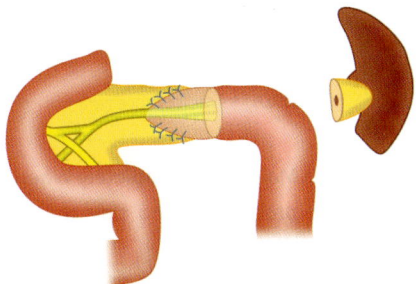

Fig. 19.9B: Leger's procedure

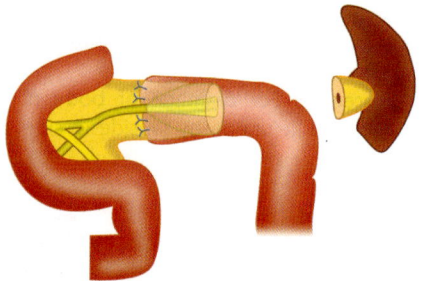

Fig. 19.9C: Puestow–Gilesby operation

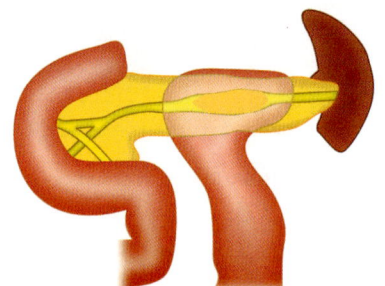

Fig. 19.9D: Mercadier procedure

Complete: Draining the Main Duct Completely When it is Dilated

- *Partington–Rochelle procedure* (long side to side PJ without resection of pancreas) **(Fig. 19.10A)**
- *Bapat's procedure* (long end to side PJ without resection of pancreas) **(Fig. 19.10B)**.

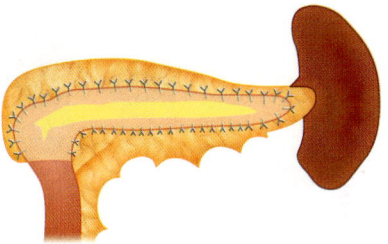

Fig. 19.10A: Partington–Rochelle operation

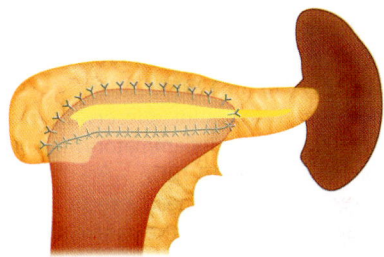

Fig. 19.10B: Bapat's procedure

Extended Drainage Procedure

Adding a pancreatic sphincterotomy to the drainage procedure

Rumpf's procedure: It is a combination of Partington's with a transduodenal pancreaticoplasty (**Fig. 19.11**).

Resectional Procedures

Resecting a part of pancreas with or without removal of adjoining organs:

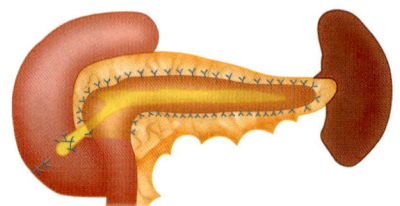

Fig. 19.11: Rumpf's operation

- ***Whipple procedure:*** Pancreaticoduodenectomy with reconstruction by a pancreaticojejunostomy/gastrostomy + gastrojejunostomy + hepaticojejunostomy **(Fig. 19.12A)**
- ***Transverse Longmire operation:*** Pylorus preserving pancreaticoduodenectomy **(Fig. 19.12B)**
- ***Beger's procedure:*** Duodenum preserving pancreatic head resection (DPPHR) for a large inflammatory mass in the pancreatic head and normal duct **(Fig. 19.12C)**
- ***Berne procedure:*** Limited local head resection (modified DPPHR) for a large inflammatory mass in the pancreatic head and normal duct
- ***Pancreatic left resection:*** Removal of tail for isolated CP in the tail
- ***Segmental resection:*** For isolated ductal stenosis in the body
- ***Total pancreatectomy:*** For disease involving the entire pancreas
- ***Total pancreatectomy with islet cell transplantation:*** For widespread small duct disease with severe pain.

Resection with Drainage

(Resection of inflammatory mass/malignant lesion + drainage for dilated pancreatic duct)

- ***Frey's procedure:*** Limited local head resection (modified DPPHR) + drainage of main pancreatic duct for an inflammatory mass

Pancreas

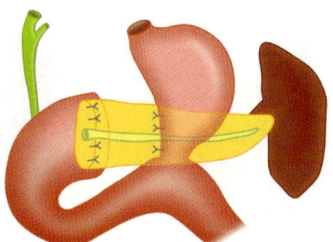

Fig. 19.12A: Whipple operation

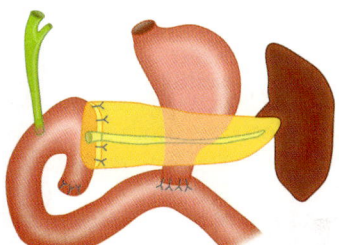

Fig. 19.12B: Transverse Longmire operation

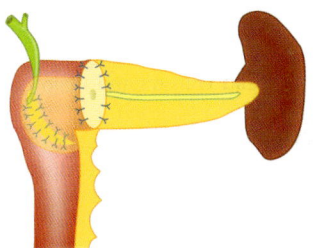

Fig. 19.12C: Hans Beger procedure

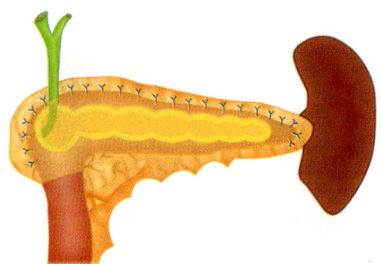

Fig. 19.13A: Frey's procedure

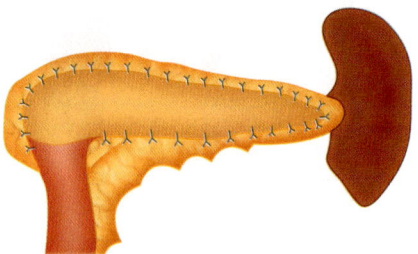

Fig. 19.13B: Izbicki's procedure

in the pancreatic head with dilated main pancreatic duct (**Fig. 19.13A**)
- *Izbicki's* "V" shaped ventral pancreatic excision with lateral pancreaticojejunostomy for small duct disease (**Fig. 19.13B**).

Denervation Procedures
- *Bilateral thoracoscopic splanchnicectomy.*

Clinical Pearls

- The rationale for various surgical procedures are:
  - Drainage procedures were developed on the basis that pain in chronic pancreatitis is due to ductal hypertension and drainage of the duct will decompress it
  - Excisional procedures and drainage procedures were expected to reduce the pain due to fibrotic pancreas causing neural inflammation
  - Combinations of these would have an additive benefit
- Pancreatic enzyme replacement is required to correct weight loss, steatorrhea related symptoms
- Treatment of pancreatic insufficiency should correct nutritional status, vitamin deficiencies and associated maldigestion
- Fecal elastase quantification is more reliable as it is highly stable during GI transit
- Calcifications are not usually seen in plain radiographs in early disease but they are specific for chronic pancreatitis
- Partial drainage procedures have been abandoned because of the small anastomosis, which soon tends to occlude. Also the concept of preservation of spleen with pancreatic tail is important, as it prevents post-splenectomy sepsis and also delays the onset of diabetes mellitus.

PANCREATIC PSEUDOCYST

Introduction

- Active collections of pancreatic fluid, rich in pancreatic enzyme content, usually associated with disruption of pancreatic duct or initial communication with the pancreatic duct

- They develop usually between 4 and 6 weeks from the attack of pancreatitis
- They can occur in any part of the pancreas, but commonly are seen near the body and tail of pancreas
- They start either as sympathetic inflammatory collections (usually in the lesser sac) or as a result of rupture of pancreatic duct or one of its tributaries
- Typically, the wall of the pseudocyst lacks an epithelial lining, and it contains pancreatic secretions rich in amylase.

Types of Pseudocyst

- *Acute pseudocyst:* Collection of fluid in the peripancreatic area surrounded by early granulation tissue without much fibrosis, following acute pancreatitis, which has occurred in about 3–4 weeks after the attack of pancreatitis
- *Chronic pseudocyst:* Collection of pancreatic fluid surrounded by normal granulation and fibrosis and persists for more than 6 weeks, arising as a consequence of chronic pancreatitis without an attack of acute pancreatitis.

Diagnosis

Symptoms and Signs

- A smooth rounded soft lump in the epigastrium
- Cyst behind the stomach push the stomach and are impalpable.

Investigations

***Barium meal series, US and CT abdomen* (Fig. 19.14)** are diagnostic.

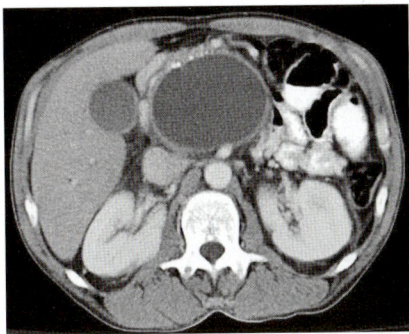

Fig. 19.14: CT—Pancreatic pseudocyst

Complications

- Infection and abscess
- Compression and obstruction of surrounding structures (causing splenic vein thrombosis, portal vein thrombosis)
- Erosion into adjacent blood vessels and cause pseudoaneurysm.

Management

- Small cysts which are asymptomatic and those which result as sympathetic reaction resolve spontaneously
- *Internal drainage procedures (cystogastrostomy, cystojejunostomy)—endoscopic or surgical (open or laparoscopic)* are required for:
  - Cysts in communication with pancreatic ductal system and large cysts, especially those which persist for more than 6 weeks
  - Cysts which are symptomatic
  - Cyst which shows progressive enlargement

- Complicated cysts (infected, hemorrhagic, causing pressure effects)
- Cysts with suspected malignancy
- ***Percutaneous drainage procedures*** for pseudocysts are rarely done
- ***Transpapillary stent insertion*** (during ERCP) can be used to drain the cysts through the communicating ductal system.

Clinical Pearls

- Usually acute pancreatic pseudocysts resolve spontaneously
- Acute pseudocysts result when the fluid collections are rich in pancreatic enzymes
- From the initial attack of acute pancreatitis, for the pseudocyst to form and mature it takes about 4 weeks
- Large pseudocysts are usually seen with acute pancreatitis and chronic pseudocysts are usually small, multiple and of variable size
- Pseudocysts can be multiple in about 15% of cases and they can be multiloculated
- Pseudocysts immaterial of the size should be decompressed if they are compressing the contiguous organs
- Cysts larger than 6 cm diameter that persist for more than 6 weeks are more often in communication with a duct.

AMPULLARY AND PERIAMPULLARY CARCINOMA

Introduction

- ***Ampullary carcinoma:*** Malignancy arising from the ampulla of Vater

- ***Periampullary carcinoma*** includes malignancies arising from distal bile duct, duodenal mucosa and the pancreas adjacent to the ampulla
- Morphologically, presents as a polypoid lesion projecting into the duodenal lumen
- Histologically, it is an adenocarcinoma.

Risk Factors

- Ampullary adenoma
- Familial adenomatous polyposis (FAP).

Diagnosis

Symptoms and Signs

Fluctuating jaundice, as the tumor is friable and tends to bleed insidiously.

Investigations

Stool Test

- Fecal occult blood test is positive in many cases.

Blood Tests

- LFT: Conjugated bilirubin and alkaline phosphatase levels are raised (may show fluctuation in serial determinations).

Radiology

- *US* may show dilated biliary system
- *EUS* helps in obtaining biopsy and determining the local invasion
- *CT* (Figs 19.15A and B) localizes the tumor and also about the lymph nodal involvement, liver metastases
- *MRCP* (Fig. 19.15C) helps in localizing the tumor.

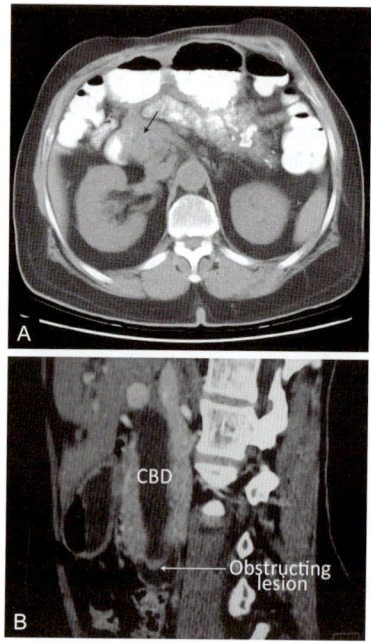

Figs 19.15A and B: CT—Periampullary carcinoma

Endoscopy
- *Duodenoscopy* (**Fig. 19.15D**) and biopsy are diagnostic.

Differential Diagnosis
- Periampullary adenoma.

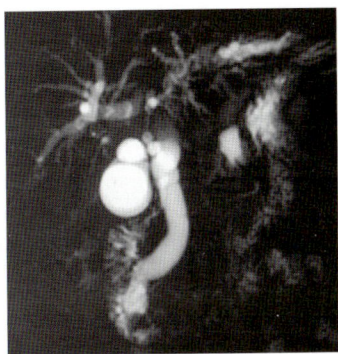

Fig. 19.15C: MRCP—Polypoid periampullary carcinoma

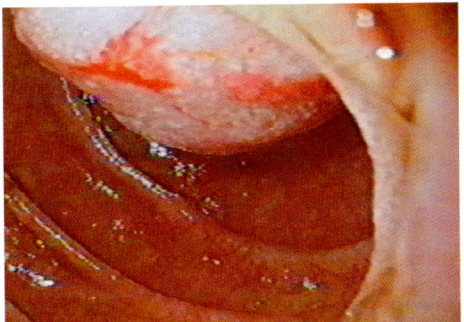

Fig. 19.15D: Duodenoscopy—Periampullary carcinoma

Management

Pancreatoduodenectomy (Whipple's operation) is the treatment of choice.

PANCREATIC MALIGNANCY

Introduction

Commonly refers to ductal adenocarcinoma:
- Occurs in the elderly
- Equal in both sexes
- More common in the head (80%), body (15%) and tail (5%)
- 90% arises from the ducts and 10% from the glandular elements.

Etiology and Pathogenesis

Risk Factors

- Tobacco smoking
- High dietary fat and meat consumption
- High coffee and/or alcohol consumption
- Familial varieties
  - BRCA2 gene mutation
  - K-RAS 2 and CDKN2 mutations
  - Peutz Jeghers syndrome
  - Familial breast and ovarian cancer
  - Ataxia telangiectasia
  - Li Fraumeni syndrome
  - Familial adenomatous polyposis.

Pathologic Features

- Morphologically, it may be well circumscribed or diffusely infiltrating the pancreas
- Microscopically, they are:
  - Mucinous adenocarcinoma (majority)
  - Signet ring cell carcinoma
  - Adenosquamous carcinoma

- Anaplastic carcinoma
- Acinar cell carcinoma
- Pancreatoblastoma
- Lymphoma.

Spread of Pancreatic Malignancy

The tumor spreads in many ways. They are:
- Tumor infiltrates diffusely through the gland
- May grow along the pancreatic duct system, eventually reaching the CBD
- May breach the capsule and invade stomach, duodenum and spleen
- Transcelomic spread leads to peritoneal deposits and ascites
- Lymphatic spread involves the pancreaticoduodenal, gastroduodenal, hepatic, superior mesenteric and celiac groups
- Distant metastases to liver, lungs, skin and brain are common.

TNM Classification of Pancreatic Malignancy

It is given in **Table 19.8**.

Diagnosis

Symptoms

- Painless jaundice (progressive or deep jaundice), as the CBD is obstructed in pancreatic head malignancy. This may be the first presenting symptom in an otherwise asymptomatic patient
- Weight loss, anorexia, fatigue, constipation, vomiting due to duodenal obstruction
- Steatorrhea is common
- Abdominal pain is common, which is 'boring' in nature forcing the patient to sit up most of the day and night

Table 19.8: TNM classification of pancreatic malignancy

Tumor status	
T_X	Primary tumor cannot be assessed
T_0	No evidence of primary tumor
T_{is}	Carcinoma *in situ*
T_1	Tumor limited to pancreas not more than 2 cm
T_2	Tumor limited to pancreas more than 2 cm
T_3	Tumor extends beyond the pancreas without involvement of celiac axis or superior mesenteric artery
T_4	Tumor extends beyond the pancreas with involvement of celiac axis or superior mesenteric artery
Lymph node status	
N_X	Regional lymph nodes cannot be assessed
N_0	No regional node metastasis
N_1	Regional lymph node metastasis
Metastatic status	
M_0	No distant metastasis
M_1	Distant metastasis

Stage grouping			
Stage	T	N	M
0	T_{is}	N_0	M_0
I A	T_1	N_0	M_0
I B	T_2	N_0	M_0
II A	T_3	N_0	M_0
II B	$T_1/T_2/T_3$	N_1	M_0
III	T_4	Any N	M_0
IV	Any T	Any N	M_1

- Foul smelling clay colored stools (due to obstruction of CBD) is common.

Signs

- Jaundice, scratch marks of obstructive jaundice, multiple bruises due to impaired coagulation
- Gallbladder may be palpably enlarged (Courvoisier's law)
- Migratory thrombophlebitis can occur (Trousseau's sign)
- Hepatomegaly may be present when liver is metastasized
- Metastasis to umbilicus (Sister Mary Joseph's sign)
- Metastasis to left supraclavicular (Virchow's node) lymph node (Troisier's sign).

Note: Carcinoma of body and tail of pancreas do not present with obstructive jaundice, unless it is metastasized to the liver.

Investigations

Blood Tests

- Increased direct bilirubin and serum alkaline phosphatase levels are in favor of obstructive jaundice
- Serum cancer antigen (CA 19/9) is elevated but not specific.

Ultrasonography

- *US* identifies the dilated biliary radicles and pancreatic duct, and also liver metastases
- *EUS* is highly sensitive in detecting small tumors and for obtaining biopsy.

Radiology

- *Barium meal series* may show widening of the duodenal 'C' loop.
- *CECT* (**Figs 19.16A and B**) is gold standard for diagnosis and staging for resectability

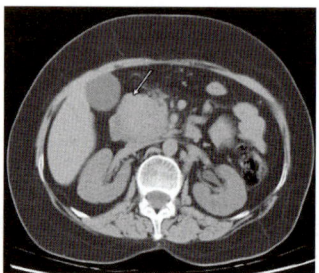

Fig. 19.16A: CT—Pancreatic head malignancy

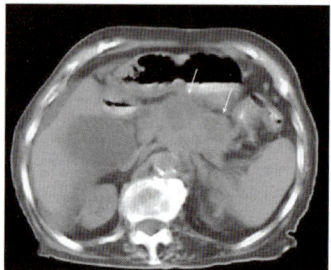

Fig. 19.16B: CT—Malignancy of body and tail of pancreas

- *MRI* gives the same information as the CT
- *MRCP* **(Fig. 19.16C)** enhances the diagnosis by revealing the double duct sign
- *ERCP* is useful for diagnosis as tissue for biopsy may be taken, if possible and also useful for stenting the biliary tree
- *PTC* is useful for determining the upper limit of the tumor obstructing the CBD
- *PET scan* is needed in selected cases to assess the extent of the disease.

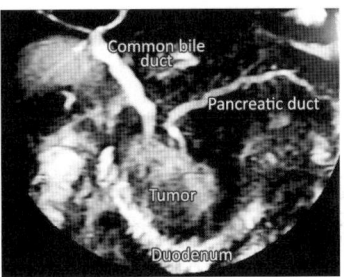

Fig. 19.16C: MRCP—Carcinoma of head of pancreas

Laparoscopy

Laparoscopy is useful in diagnosing metastases in liver and peritoneum.

Biopsy

Histopathology is possible with ERCP brushing, or fine needle aspiration guided by EUS, CT

Differential Diagnosis

- Solid tumors
  - Chronic pancreatitis
  - Distal cholangiocarcinoma
  - Periampullary tumors
- Cystic tumors
  - Pancreatic pseudocyst
  - Pheochromocytoma.

Management

Curative

- Pancreatoduodenectomy (Whipple's operation) for head and neck region tumors
- Partial or subtotal pancreatectomy for body and tail region cancers
- Left (distal) partial pancreatectomy + splenectomy for tumors in the tail
- Total pancreatectomy is reserved for large tumors
- Adjuvant chemotherapy is useful in improving survival and tumor free periods
- Modern radiotherapy use is controversial.

Palliative

- Bypass procedures (choledochojejunostomy or stenting to relieve jaundice and gastrojejunostomy to relieve duodenal obstruction) are used for inoperable cancers
- Pain management
- Palliative chemoradiation in locally advanced cases.

Clinical Pearls

- Pancreatic cancer should be suspected when the jaundice is painless and progressive, especially in the elderly
- Pancreatic cancers presenting with jaundice have a better prognosis when compared to those cancers which are in a position of pancreas, which cannot cause jaundice, as diagnosis becomes late
- Pancreatic cancer of body and tail are diagnosed late and the tumors are large, and less commonly resectable

- Majority of the pancreatic cancers are diagnosed after it has already metastasized
- Though pancreatic cancer is said to present with painless jaundice, actually many patients perceive epigastric pain which is mild and vague
- Vague abdominal pain and recent onset diabetes in a very elderly person should be suspected for a pancreatic malignancy.

CYSTIC NEOPLASMS OF PANCREAS

Introduction

- Cystic neoplasms are true cystic lesions meaning that these have an epithelial lining, and differ from the pseudocyst which is lined by inflammatory tissue and no epithelium
- True cystic lesions account for only about 10% of cystic lesions of pancreas
- The major point of differentiation in cystic neoplasms of pancreas is whether the lining epithelium is serous of mucous
    - Serous tumors:
        - Serous cystadenoma (SCA)
    - Mucinous tumors:
        - Mucinous cystic neoplasms (MCN)
        - Intraductal papillary mucinous neoplasm (IPMN)
- Serous tumors are benign and mucinous tumors are potentially or overtly malignant.

Diagnosis

Symptoms and Signs

- The clinical features and diagnostic features are tabulated in **Table 19.9**.

Table 19.9: Clinical features of pancreatic cystic tumors

Feature	Serous cystadenoma (SCA)	Mucinous cystic neoplasm (MCN)	Intraductal papillary mucinous neoplasm (IPMN)
Incidence	40%	40%	20%
Sex	Females >75%	Females >95%	Males >50%
Age	60–70 years	40–50 years	60–70 years
Presentation	Usually asymptomatic, Mass/abdominal pain. Weight loss, jaundice and gastric outlet obstruction are very rare	Many are asymptomatic, mass/abdominal pain. Weight loss, anorexia should raise suspicion of malignancy–mucinous cystadenocarcinoma	Recurrent pancreatitis.
Site	Anywhere in pancreas	Body and tail	Head
Morphology	Multiple small cysts (<2 cm) in the periphery, cut section shows honeycomb like appearance, filled with a glycogen rich, low viscosity serous fluid	Large cysts (>2 cm) with septa and peripheral calcification, with a solid component. Mucinous fluid is rich in tumor markers and low in amylase	Originates in the ductal system and may appear multicystic due to ductal dilatations. Depending on its involvement and location, they are classified into main duct type (80%) or branch type (20%)
TAUS, EUS, CT and MRI findings	Honeycomb or small cysts with a subburst calcification in a central scar	Well defined, rounded cysts composed of multiple cysts with a septum or papillary processes	Multicystic lesions (bunch of grapes appearance) with dilated pancreatic duct with atrophic pancreas

Contd....

Contd....

Feature	Serous cystadenoma (SCA)	Mucinous cystic neoplasm (MCN)	Intraductal papillary mucinous neoplasm (IPMN)
ERCP findings	Not indicated, but show no communication between the cystic mass and ductal system	Not indicated, but show no communication between the cystic mass and ductal system	Ductal dilatation and communications and mucin extruding from the ampulla of Vater, a specific finding
Cyst fluid analysis	Serous, normal amylase levels, normal CEA levels	Mucinous, increased amylase levels, elevated CEA levels	Mucinous, increased amylase levels, elevated CEA levels
Histology	Cystic areas lined by single layer of flat or cuboidal epithelium	Cystic areas lined by mucinous epithelium, which is discontinuous, proliferative with atypical cells. Only microscopy differentiates benign and malignant lesions	Pancreatic ducts lined by mucinous papillary epithelium with proliferative features with dysplastic to *in situ* to invasive carcinoma
Malignant potential	Benign	Potentially/overtly malignant	Potentially malignant

Differential Diagnosis

Solid neoplasms with cystic degeneration
- Pancreatic adenocarcinoma
- Metastatic pancreatic lesion (from ovarian carcinoma)
- Islet cell neoplasms
- Lymphangioma.

Management

- Serous cystadenomas (SCA)—no treatment
- Mucinous cystic neoplasm (MCN)—Excision
- Intraductal papillary mucinous neoplasm (IPMN)—Excision.

Clinical Pearls

- A cystic lesion in the pancreas without a previous history of pancreatic pathology should be considered to be a cystic neoplasm until proven otherwise
- Lack of previous symptoms related to pancreatic pathology strongly suggests a neoplasm
- Cystic neoplasms especially IPMN can cause pancreatitis
- A single mucinous cystadenoma can contain both benign and malignant components
- EUS guided biopsy should be done only when conservative management is comtemplated
- Cystic neoplasms of pancreas do not exhibit inflammatory changes in the surrounding parenchyma, and remain normal
- EUS-FNA carries the risk of complications like intraperitoneal tumor seeding, infection and pancreatitis
- Since IPMN communicates with the ductal system, the fluid may show increased amounts of amylase, even when it is not frankly malignant
- All mucinous tumors of pancreas should be resected
- IPMN resection warrants frozen section biopsy, and if the margins are positive, creeping resection is indicated
- After resecting serous tumors, surveillance imaging is not necessary, whereas, after resecting mucinous tumors, surveillance imaging is necessary with CT/EUS.

ISLET CELL TUMORS OF PANCREAS

Introduction

- Islet cell tumors of pancreas (also called neuroendocrine or pancreatic endocrine tumors) are uncommon
- About half the number of islet cell tumors are non-functioning
- Islet cell tumors are said to be functioning when they are associated with a clinical syndrome due to hormone release
- Many of the islet cell tumors of pancreas are malignant
- Islet cell tumors of pancreas arise from the cells which secrete the corresponding hormone
    - Insulinomas
    - Gastrinomas
    - Vasoactive intestinal polypeptidomas (VIPomas)
    - Glucagonomas
    - Somatostatinomas
    - Polypeptidomas (PPomas)
- Functioning and non-functioning islet cell tumors are associated with multiple endocrine neoplasia type 1 (MEN 1) and von Hippel Lindau
- Majority of non-functioning tumors occur in the pancreatic head.

Diagnosis

Symptoms and Signs

Incidence and symptomatology of islet cell tumors of pancreas are tabulated in **Table 19.10**.

- Presentation of malignant tumors is similar to that of pancreatic adenocarcinoma (weight loss, anorexia, abdominal pain and jaundice).

Table 19.10: Incidence and symptomatology of islet cell tumors of pancreas

Tumor	Incidence	Symptoms	Morphology and histology	Malignancy rate
Insulinomas	50%	Hunger, irritability, weakness, diaphoresis, fasting hypoglycemia	Usually single, may be multiple, malignant	< 10%
Gastrinomas		Epigastric pain, peptic ulcer symptoms, chronic diarrhea	Usually multiple present in gastrinoma triangle, majority are malignant	>70%
VIPomas	10–15%	Large volume watery diarrhea, hypokalemia, hypochlorhydria and acidosis	Small tumors	>60%
Glucagonomas	1%	Diabetes, dermatitis, depression and DVT (4D syndrome)	Small tumors	60%
Somatostatinomas		Diabetes, diarrhea, steatorrhea, gallbladder disease	Large malignant tumors	>75%
PPomas	Rare	No symptoms	Can be associated with MEN I syndrome	

Investigations

- **Serum hormone levels** may be high
- **CECT** shows an islet cell tumor as a hypervascular and hyperdense lesion, with calcifications
- **MRI** has similar sensitivity as CT.

Management

- Excision of primary tumor and low volume hepatic metastases
- Chemotherapy (streptozotocin and 5 FU) shows good response in metastatic disease.

Clinical Pearls

- Zollinger–Ellison syndrome refers to the triad of severe peptic ulcer disease, gastric hypersecretion and gastrinoma
- Non-functioning islet cell tumors are usually larger than a typical adenocarcinoma.

SURGERY OF PANCREAS: PANCREATIC RESECTIONS

- Distal pancreatectomy (removal of tail with splenectomy)
- Left pancreatectomy (removal of body and tail)
- Pancreatoduodenectomy—Whipple's operation (removal of pancreatic head including duodenum, proximal part of jejunum and distal biliary tree)
- Subtotal pancreatectomy (removal of part of head, entire body and tail of pancreas)
- Total pancreatectomy (removal of entire pancreas).

Indications

- Inflammations
- Acute inflammation with gross necrosis/sepsis
- Chronic pancreatitis with pain
- Trauma
- Neoplasms (benign/malignant).

Incisions

- Bilateral subcostal (Roof top)
- Long midline.

Surgical Technique of Pancreatoduodenectomy

- Mobilization of duodenum and head of pancreas medially with identification of superior mesenteric vein (Kocherization)
- Mobilization of gallbladder and cystic duct as in cholecystectomy (but not removed)
- Elevation of neck of pancreas from superior mesenteric and portal veins
- Division of stomach (if pylorus is to be preserved) or duodenum
- Division of common hepatic duct
- Division of pancreas at its neck
- Dissection of divided pancreas from mesenteric vessels
- Mobilization and division of proximal jejunum to create a Roux loop
- Division of mesoduodenum and attachments of uncinate process to the superior mesenteric artery, and removal of specimen
- The excised specimen contains part of common hepatic duct, gallbladder and cystic duct, entire common bile duct, entire duodenum and proximal jejunum, head and uncinate process of pancreas
- Reconstruction to restore continuity using Roux-en-Y jejunal loop (create end to side hepaticojejunostomy, end to side gastrojejunostomy, end to side pancreaticojejunostomy, end to side jejunojejunostomy).

COMPLICATIONS OF PANCREATIC SURGERY

Gastrointestinal Hemorrhage

Bleeding in the stomach occurs between 1st and 5th postoperative days due to bleeding from:
- Anastomotic area
- Small bleeding ulcer in the gastric pouch
- Erosion of ligated artery following pancreatic leak.

Diagnosis

Sign

Bloody nasogastric aspirate.

Investigations
- Hematocrit values may fall low
- Endoscopy.

Management

Medical
- Ice cold saline
- Endoscopic injection of 1:10000 adrenaline
- Blood transfusions.

Surgical

Opening of gastric pouch above the anastomosis and control of bleeding site if endoscopic injection is ineffective.

Extragastric Hemorrhage

Bleeding from sources outside stomach occurs around the 1st to 5th postoperative day due to:

- Laceration of spleen
- Injury to liver by retractors
- Injury to vasa brevia
- Hemorrhage from pancreatic bed
- Improperly secured vessel in the greater and lesser omentum.

Diagnosis

Symtoms and Signs

- Bloody discharge from the drain in the abdominal cavity
- Clear nasogastric aspirate.

Investigations

- Hematocrit values may fall low
- CT abdomen may be contributory.

Management

Medical

- Blood transfusion.

Surgical

- Exploratory laparotomy and correction of cause.

Delayed Gastric Emptying

Delay in emptying of stomach occurs around the 3rd to 5th postoperative day, due to:

- Gastric atony due to disruption of gastoduodenal neural connection
- Ischemic injury to antropyloric muscle mechanism
- Gastric dysrhythmias due to intra-abdominal leaks
- Gastric atony due to reduced levels of motilin.

Diagnosis

Clinical Presentation

Increasing nasogastric aspirate lasting for more than 2–3 weeks.

Investigations

Upper GI endoscopy after two weeks to rule out mechanical obstruction.

Management

Medical

- Prolonged gastric decompression
- Intravenous water and electrolyte substitution
- Prokinetic drugs like bethanechol, metoclopramide, erythromycin derivatives.

Biliary Leak

Leakage of bile occurs around the 3rd to 7th postoperative day due to disruption of biliary enteric anastomosis.

Diagnosis

Clinical Presentation

- Discharge of bile of bile-stained fluid through the intraabdominal drain
- Skin excoriation around the drain.

Investigations

- Diagnosis is obvious, but isotope scan can demonstrate the leak
- CT is useful in locating localized collections of bile.

Management

Medical

Most leaks heal spontaneously if there is no distal obstruction.

Surgical

- Localized collections of bile should be drained by US or CT guidance
- Open drainage of collection of bile is rarely necessary.

Pancreatic Leak

Leakage of pancreatic secretions occurs around the 3rd–7th postoperative day due to disruption of pancreaticoenteric anastomosis.

Diagnosis

Clinical Presentation

- Discharge of clear fluid through the intra-abdominal drain
- Tachycardia, hyperpyrexia, tachypnea
- Excoriation of skin around the drain
- Abdominal tenderness.

Investigations

- Leukocytosis
- Serum lactate and amylase levels may be elevated.

Management

Medical

- Replacement of fluids and electrolytes
- When the loss is less than 50 mL/day, it heals spontaneously
- Antibiotics are needed for large leaks with peritonitis

- Total parenteral nutrition is useful in large leaks
- May result in a pancreatic fistula.

Surgical
- Percutaneous drainage of localized collections
- Laparotomy and peritoneal toileting in peritonitis
- Completion pancreatectomy is rarely needed.

Chylous Ascites

Leakage of lymph in the peritoneal cavity occurs around the 10th to 15th postoperative day due to extensive retroperitoneal lymph node dissection and injury to main lymphatic channels.

Clinical Presentation
- Yellowish serous or milky discharge (chyle) through the intra-abdominal drain
- Amounts to several liters of fluid daily.

Investigations
- CT is useful in diagnosing localized collections.

Management
- Ligation of main lymphatic channel may be required if it does not resolve in a few weeks
- TPN may be required to maintain good nutritional status.

Marginal Ulcerations

Ulceration on the anastomotic margin occurs after 2 weeks due to:
- Non-performance of vagotomy
- Ulcerogenic potential of pancreatectomy.

Diagnosis

Clinical Presentation

- Upper abdominal discomfort
- Pain abdomen
- Hematemesis and melena.

Investigations

Upper GI endoscopy is diagnostic.

Management

Proton pump inhibitors.

Obstructive Jaundice

Jaundice due to obstruction in the biliary drainage occurs after 12 weeks of surgery due to following causes:
- Benign
  - Stricture of biliary enteric anastomosis
  - Common duct stones.
- Malignant
  - Local recurrence at mesenteric root
  - Recurrence of malignancy at hilum of liver.

Clinical Presentation

Yellowish discoloration of urine, sclera and skin.

Investigations

- Serum bilirubin levels are high
- MRCP will localize the level of obstruction
- CT will localize the cause of obstruction.

Management

Surgical

- Percutaneous transhepatic drainage and stenting of tumors at hilum of liver
- Second Roux-en-Y reconstruction may relieve jaundice.

Endocrine and Exocrine Insufficiency

Deficiency of endocrine and exocrine components of pancreatic secretions months after surgery due to:
- Removal of endocrine and exocrine tissues as part of pancreatic resection
- Fibrosis of pancreatic remnant leading to loss of islet cell tissue
- Stenosis at pancreatojejeunostomy site.

Diagnosis

Clinical Presentation

Severe wasting.

Investigations

- Determination of blood sugar levels (endocrine deficiency)
- Determination of enzyme levels in blood and feces (exocrine deficiency).

Management

Medical

- Replacement of insulin
- Administration of enzymes rich in lipase, fat-soluble vitamins, calcium and trace elements.

Index

Page numbers followed by *f* refer to figure and *t* refer to table.

A

Abdomen 6, 29, 732
  examination of 732
  opening 690*f*
  regions of 2*f*
Abdominal pain, acute 1
  lower 9, 10*t*, 13
    blood tests 13
    diagnosis 10
    management 14
    signs 11
    symptoms 10
  upper 3
    diagnosis 3
    management 9
    signs 6
    symptoms 3
Abdominal pain, chronic 19, 20*t*, 27*t*, 28*t*
Abdominal pain, stimuli
  chemical 1
  mechanical 1
Abdominal rectopexy 657*f*
Abdominal sigmoidectomy 657*f*
Abdominal tuberculosis 365
  classification 365
  management 369
Abdominal wall 732
Abdominoperineal resection 640, 641*f*
Abscess
  Pelvirectal, drainage of 621*f*
  paracolic 473*f*
  subphrenic or intra-abdominal 967
Acalculous cholecystitis 900
Achalasia 124*f*, 125*f*
Achalasia cardia 122, 123
  complications of 125
  management of 126
  symptoms of 123
Acid peptic disease 214, 218*t*
  complications of 220
  management of 223
  signs of 215
  symptoms of 215
Acid secretion 217*t*
Adefovir dipivoxil 749
Adenocarcinoma 184, 236, 402, 406
Adenomas 524, 834
Adhesions 423, 566
  management 424
Aerophagia 66
Albumin 734
Alcohol withdrawal syndrome 764
  management 765, 768

Alcoholic cirrhosis 760
Alcoholic hepatitis 760
Alcoholic liver disease 759
   management 761
Alkaline phosphatase 733, 811
Alkaline reflux gastritis 307
   management 309
Allergy 707
   management 707
Altemeier operation 658f
Amebic dysentery, complications of 41
Amebic liver abscess 818
   right lobe 820f
   signs 819
   symptoms 819
Amebic proctitis and ulcers 634
   management 635
Amebic ulcers of rectum 634f
Ammonia 806
Ampullary carcinoma 1026
   management 1029, 1036
   signs of 1027
   symptoms of 1027
Anal stenosis, island flap repair for 607f
Anal canal malignancy 651, 652f
Anal fissures 612
   management 614
   classification 612
   management 614
   signs of 613
   symptoms of 613
Anal fistulae 622f, 627f,
   multiple 624f
   treatment of 627
Anal fistulogram 625f
Anal malignancy 649
   management 652
   signs 651
   symptoms 651
Anal sphincter
   external 50
   internal 50
Anal sphincterotomy
   internal 615
      lateral 615
Anal stenosis
   repair for 608f
   S-anoplasty for 609f
Anastomosis
   completion of 275f
   end-to-side 418f
   second layer 557f
   third layer 557f
   stabler anastomosis
      anastomosis-1 647f
      anastomosis-2 648f
      anastomosis-3 648f
      anastomosis-4 649f
Anastomotic leakage 195, 420f, 563
Anemia 323
   management 325
   pathogenesis 324f
Angiodysplasia 400
   management 400

Anomalies 871
  congenital 437, 437f
  with vitellointestinal duct 397f
    obliteration of 397t
Anorectal abscesses 617, 617f
  management 620
  pathogenesis 618
  signs and symptoms 619
Anorectal advancement flap 627f, 630
Anorectal disease 571
  signs and symptoms of 571
Anorectal malformations 575
Anorectal manometry 57
Anorectoplasty, posterior sagittal 578
Anorectum, anatomy of 50
Antiamebic drugs 821
Antibiotics, use of 378
Antireflux surgery, preoperative assessment for 146t
Antitrypsin deficiency, alpha1 778
Appendicectomy 460, 471f
  complications of 469
  for mucocele 459f
  incisions for 461f
  laparoscopic 465
  surgery 462f
  surgical technique 460
Appendicitis,
  acute 438, 440, 446, 450, 450t, 451
    Baldwing's sign 442
    Blumberg's sign 441
    complications 451
    Cope's psoas test 442
    management 451
    Obturator sign 442
    Rovsing's sign 441
    suppurative 438f
    symptoms 439
  pre- and postileal 444t
  recurrent 452
  retrocecal 443
    and paracecal 444t
  types of 438
Appendicocutaneous fistula 474f
Appendicolith 447f, 448f
Appendicular carcinoids, TNM staging of 455t
Appendix
  crushing 464f
  division of 468f
  exposure 462f
  extraction of 469f
  in pregnant woman 445f
  ligation 464f
  neoplasms of 453
  positions of 435f
  surgery of 460
  with fecoliths 439f
Arms 576
  wingspread classification of 576t
Arterial supply 478, 723, 870
Ascites 731f, 799
  cause of 800t, 803f
Ascitic fluid analysis 801
Autoimmune gastritis 213

Autoimmune hepatitis 755
  management 758
  types of 756

B

Bacteroides species 814
Bag to flange, application of 704f
Bag
  detachment of 705
  drainable 698
  non-drainable 698
Baldwing test 443f
Balloon expulsion study 57
Balloon sphincteroplasty 975
Bapat's procedure 1018, 1019f
Bariatric surgery 261, 263
  procedures 262f
    types of 261
Barium enema 372f
Barium meal series 1024
Barium swallow 796
Barrett's esophagus 140f, 165, 168
  management 167
  pathogenesis 166
  signs 167
  symptoms 167
  therapy in 167
  types of 166
Barron ligator 593f
Barron rubber banding 595f
Basketing of bile duct stone 911f
Beger's procedure 1020
Belching 65
  management 66

Bentiromide test 1011
Beta cells 986
Bezoars 256
  management 257
  signs 256
  symptoms 256
Bianchi procedure 432f
Bile duct 870, 906t
  injuries 917t, 920f
    bismuth classification of 919f
    types of operative 916
  strictures 924
    complications 927
    management 927
    signs 925
    symptoms 924
  tumors, classification of 946f
Bile reflux gastritis 213
Bile, formation of 724
Biliary atresia 872
  classifications 875
  complications 879
  management 874, 879
Biliary cirrhosis, primary 785
  complications 787
  management 787
  signs 786
  symptoms 786
Biliary drainage 723
Biliary enteric fistula 969
Biliary fistula, external 968
Biliary leak 1047
  management 1048
Biliary peritonitis 965

Biliary sludge 882
Biliary stenting with endoprosthesis 931f
Biliary system, anatomy of 69, 73f
Biliary tract, injuries to 915
Biliopancreatic diversion 262
   advantages of 264
   complications of 264
Bilirubin metabolism 69, 70f, 725
   defects 71t
   diseases 71t
   disorders of 72
Biopsy 736
Bismuth 721t
   classification of 721f, 722f
Bismuth-Corlette classification 945t
Bleeding angiodysplasia of large bowel 106f
Bleeding colonic polyp 107f, 526f
Bleeding esophageal varices 94f, 180f
Bleeding esophagitis 94f
Bleeding
   from carcinoma of cecum 108f
   from colonic diverticulitis 104f
   from Crohn's disease of colon 105f
   from Mallory-Weiss tear 95f, 181f
Bleeding hemorrhoids 108f
Bleeding peptic ulcer, forrest classification for 93t
Bleeding ulcerative colitis 107f
Bloating 66
   etiology 66
Bloch-Paul-Mikulicz operation 685
Blood flow, increased portal 794
Blood tests 908
   in ALD, interpretation of 761t
Blunt injuries 739
Body and tail of pancreas, malignancy of 1034f
Body mass index 261t
Borrmann's classification 239f
Bowel anastomoses 411f
Bowel atresia 352
Bowel disease 350
Bowel resections, types of 551
Bowel, surgery of small 410
Brain 777
Breath tests 1012
Brooke's ileostomy 683
Brown stones 904
Budd–Chiari syndrome 790
   causes 790
   complications 792
   management 792
   signs 791
   symptoms 791

C

Calcium 350
Capsule endoscopy 29
Carbohydrates 349
Carcinoid tumor 408
   diagnosis 409
Cardiospasm 122
Catheter duodenostomy 287f
Catheter stab incision 665f

1058 Snapshots in Gastroenterology

CBD, benign stricture of 925, 926f
Cecal bascule 484f
Cecal diverticulitis 520
  management 521
Cecal volvulus 483, 484f
  management 485
  pathogenesis 483
Cecum, carcinoma 546f
Celiac disease 379
Cerebrovascular disease 663
Cervical esophagostomy 295f
Cervical esophagus 116, 171f
Charcot's triad 891
Child-Pugh classification 857t
Cholangiocarcinoma 943, 947f, 948f
Cholecystectomy 952
  after CBD clearance 978
  laparoscopic 953, 956f
  open 961
    complications of 964
  ports for laparoscopic 956f
Cholecystitis
  acute 890, 894f, 895f
  chronic 885, 888f
    complications 888
Cholecystoenteric fistula 914
Choledochal cysts 874f, 876f, 878
Choledochocele 879
Choledochoduodenostomy 979
Choledochojejunostomy 981
Choledocholithiasis 904
  management of 913f, 973
Choledocholithotomy 977

Cholelithiasis 881
Cholestasis 76
Cholesterol stones 883
Christeas operation 317f
Chylous ascites 1049
Ciprofloxacin 42
Cirrhosis 780
Colic 14
Colitis
  radiation 105f
  ulcerative 492f
Collis gastroplasty 158, 159f
Colocolic intussusception 544f
Colon, ascending 555f
Colon Cutoff sign 998f
Colon
  malignancy of 544f
  malignant growth 545f
  opening loop of 691f
  resection of 548f, 553f
  surgeries of 551
  transverse 197
Colon polyp, sigmoid 526f
Colon volvulus, transverse 486
Colonic anastomosis 564
Colonic diverticulitis 517f
Colonic fistula, external 567, 567f
Colonic malignancies 537, 538f, 540, 543t
  TNM classification of 540, 541t
Colonic pseudo-obstruction 509f
Colonic resections 553
Colonoscopic polypectomy 531f
Colonoscopy 736

Colorectal polyps 522
Colostomy 685
 created terminal 645f
 end 689f
 management of 693
 types of 686f
Constipating drugs, avoidance of 56
Constipation 50, 51
 causes of 52f, 54t
 chronic 52t
 criteria for 52t
 medical therapy of chronic 57t
 primary 53
 refractory 56
 secondary 53
Cope's psoas test 442f
Couinaud 721t
Crigler–Najjar syndrome 72, 76
 type I 77
 type II 78
Crohn's disease 369, 371, 375t
 classification of 373t
 from ulcerative colitis 375t
Cryptosporidium 42
Csendes' procedure 227f
Cullen's sign 996f
Cyclospora 42
Cystic artery
 and duct division 958f
 anomalies 871, 873f
Cystic duct anomalies 871, 872f
Cystic duct for division, isolation of 964f

Cystic duct of gallbladder, stone in 893f
Cystic liver diseases 822
Cystic liver lesions 823t
Cystic neoplasms 1037
 of pancreas 1037
Cystojejunostomy 1025
Cytomegalovirus 173

D

Defecation disorders, functional 52t
Defecation, physiology of 50
Delorme's operation 659f
Delta cells 986
Denture in thoracic esophagus 177f
Dermatome 2t
Diarrhea 38
 acute 38
  management 39
 and local tenderness 8
 causes of chronic 44t
 chronic 38, 43
 inflammatory 44t
 profuse 719
 treatment of chronic 49t
 types of 38
Dieulafoy's ulcer 258
Disposable bags 696
Disposable or non-disposable appliances 696
Diversion colitis 714
Diverticula, types of 511f
Diverticulitis 517f
 symptoms of 518t

DNA viral evaluation 735
Dubin–Johnson syndrome 72, 81*t*
Duke's classification 540*f*
Dumping syndrome 311
Duodenal diverticulum 395*f*
Duodenal stump leakage 287*f*, 289
Duodenal switch 262, 310*f*
Duodenal ulcer perforation 221*f*
Duodenal ulcer, chronic 220*f*
Duodenojejunostomy 298*f*
Duodenum
  injuries of 255
  surgeries of 265
Duval's procedure 1017*f*
Dysentery 39
  causes of 40
Dysphagia 31, 32
  causes of 33, 34*t*
  drug-induced, causes of 33

E

E. coli species 814
Edematous gallbladder 894*f*
Emphysematous cholecystitis 902
Empyema 895
Endocinch suturing system 162, 164*f*
Endocrine diseases 45
Endocrine tumors (carcinoids) 401
Endoloops, application of 468*f*
Endoscopic appearance 234*t*
Endoscopic pancreatic function test 1011
Endoscopic procedures 973
Endoscopic sphincterotomy 974
Endoscopy 736
Entamoeba histolytica 818
Enterobacter species 814
Enteroenterostomy, simple 298*f*
Eosinophilic gastritis 214
Epigastric pain 3*t*
Epigastrium 20*t*
Epiphrenic diverticulum 132*f*
Epsilon cells 986
Epstein Barr virus 173
Esophageal atresia 120*f*, 122*f*
  varieties of 121*f*
Esophageal disease 119
Esophageal diverticula 132*f*, 133*f*
Esophageal dysphagia 36
Esophageal injury 172
Esophageal malignancy 184, 185
  lower third 188*f*
  mid-third 188*f*
  TNM classification of 186*t*
  upper-third 188*f*
Esophageal pain 32
Esophageal pathology 118
Esophageal perforation, leaking dye in 172*f*
Esophageal resections 191, 192*f*
Esophageal spasm, diffuse 175
Esophageal varices 179, 179*f*
Esophageal web 127, 128*f*
Esophagojejunal anastomosis
  edema of 195*f*
  inflammation of 195*f*

Esophagojejunostomy (Roux-en-Y gastric) 272f, 294f
Esophagus 116
    abdominal part of 116
    anatomy of 31, 116
    arterial supply 117
    atresia of 119
    candidiasis of 174f
    corkscrew 175f
    corrosive strictures 170f
    diverticula of 131
    foreign bodies of 176
    infections of 173
    leiomyoma of 183f
    lipoma of 183f
    physiology 116, 118
    stricture 170f
    transection of 194
    with ulcer, lower 171f
Exocrine insufficiency 1051
Exocrine pancreatic function 991
Extragastric hemorrhage 288, 1045
Eye 777

F

Familial adenomatous polyposis 538
Fat-soluble vitamins 350
Fatty diarrhea 44t
Fatty liver disease, non-alcoholic 766
Fatty metamorphosis 760
Fecal fat quantification 1011
Fecal incontinence 50, 58
Fecal peritonitis 563f
Fecal tests 1011
Feeding gastrostomy 663
Feeding jejunostomy 663
Ferritin concentration 774
Fever, association of 4
Finney's pyloroplasty 225f
Fissure in ano, acute 613f
Fissures, operative procedures for 615
Fistula in ano 621, 624f
Fistula
    external 426
    internal 425, 425f
    multiple 426f
Fistulectomy 630
Fistulogram-ileocutaneous fistula 427f
Flatulence 67
Focal liver masses 810t
Foreign body esophagus 176f
Frey's procedure 1020, 1022f
Fusobacterium nucleatum species 814

G

Gallbladder 869
    and bile ducts 869
    anomalies 871
    carcinoma of 937, 941f
        with liver secondaries 941f
    cephalad, retraction of 957f
    complications, carcinoma of 940
    in obstructive tumor disease 907f

isolation of 963f
malignancy 938
   TNM classification of 938, 939t
management, carcinoma of 942
multiple calculi in 887f
polyps of 934, 935f, 936f
removal of 958f
stone in 893f
surgery, antibiotics in 952
Gallstone ileus 914, 915f
Gallstone pancreatitis 1002
Gallstones 881
  characteristics of 883t
  formation of 882f
  in CBD 906t
  management of 899f
Gamma aminobutyric acid 806
Gamma glutamyl transferase 80, 734
Gaseousness 65
Gastrectomy 267f
  complications of 283f
  late complications of 308f
  partial/subtotal 268
  ports for 276f
  reconstructions after 271, 271f
  steps of 270f
Gastric atony
  pathogenesis 326f
  chronic 325
Gastric banding, laparoscopic adjustable 261
Gastric cancer 239
  advanced 239f
  Japanese classification of 238f
Gastric emptying
  delayed 1046
  management 1047
Gastric inhibitory polypeptide 311
Gastric lymphoma 246
  Ann Arbor staging of 248
Gastric malignancy 236, 237
  signs of 242t
  symptoms of 242t
  TNM classification of 240, 240t
  variety of 237
Gastric polyps 232, 234
Gastric remnant carcinoma 333, 334f
Gastric remnant necrosis 292
Gastric remnant syndrome 327
Gastric surgery 266t
  complications of 281, 306, 307
  management 281
  Visick's classification of 308t
Gastric ulcer 217f, 219f
  chronic 219f
  classification of 215
  Johnson's classification of 215, 217t
  types of 216f
Gastric volvulus 205
  mesenteroaxial 207f
  organoaxial 207f
Gastritis 209
  causes of 209t
  classification of 209t

Gastroepiploic vessel, division of left 277f
Gastroesophageal reflux disease 32, 137
  therapy for 145
Gastrograffin swallow 172f
Gastrointestinal bleeding/hemorrhage 88, 103t, 1045
  causes of 90f, 100t
  lower 88, 99
    management 103
  upper 88
Gastrointestinal endoscopy
  lower 29
  upper 29, 736, 991
Gastrointestinal lymphomas, Ann Arbor staging of 404t
Gastrointestinal pathology, upper 204
Gastrointestinal stromal tumor 235
Gastrointestinal tract, upper 90t
Gastrojejunocolic fistula 338, 338f, 339f
Gastrojejunostomy 266t, 268f, 272, 663
  removal of distal stomach
    after 278f
    before 278f
  surgery steps 272
Gastroparesis 230
Gastroscopy
  bleeding from
    gastric malignancy 97f
    polyp of stomach 96f, 233f
    bleeding gastric lymphoma 96f, 249f
    bleeding gastric ulcer 95f
    Dieulafoy lesion 259f
    gastric polyps 233f
    jejunogastric intussusception 345f
    phytobezoar 257f
Gastrostomy 265f, 266t, 664
  surgery 664f
  open surgical (Witzel's type) 664, 673
Giardia 42
Gilbert's syndrome 72, 73, 76
Glasgow alcoholic hepatitis score 762, 763t
Glasgow criteria 1001, 1003t
Goodsall's rule 625f
Granulomatous gastritis 214
Grey Turner's sign 997f

H

Haemorrhoids
  classification of 584t
  degrees of internal 583f
  development of 582
  inflamed 587f
  position of 581f
  prolapsed 585f
  sclerotherapy of 590f
  second degree 584f
  third degree 585f
  treatment for 588
  types of 583f

Haggitt's classification 529f
Hamartomas 533
Hand-sewn technique 554
Hans Beger procedure 1021f
Hartmann's operation 692
Hartmann's pouch of gallbladder 954
Haustrations, loss of 492f
Head of pancreas, carcinoma of 1035f
Heart 772, 777
Heinecke–Mikulicz pyloroplasty 224f
Helicobacter pylori 209
Hemangioma 833, 834, 835
　of liver 836f
　of rectum 106f
Hematocrit 783
Hematologic diseases 45
Hemochromatosis 772
　types of 772
Hemoglobin for anemia 733
Hemolysis 76
Hemorrhage from appendicular stump 469
Hemorrhagic pancreatitis, acute 994
Hemorrhoidal mass 597f
Hemorrhoidectomy 602f
　closed 600f
　open
　　Milligan 597
　　Morgan 597
Hemorrhoids 580
Henley's operation 313f
Hepatectomy 856, 858, 859f
Hepatic abscess, aspiration of 817
Hepatic adenoma 837f, 838t
Hepatic artery anomalies 871
Hepatic encephalopathy 805
　grades of 807t
Hepatic failure, spider nevi of 731f
Hepatic functional status 857t
Hepatic resections 857
Hepatic venography 796
Hepatitis 748t
　A 745, 753
　　and B, passive immunoprophylaxis of 753t
　acute 743, 745
　　autoimmune 758
　B 746, 748, 750, 753
　　antiviral therapy in chronic 749t
　　virus 744
　C 746, 750, 751, 751t
　　treatment 755
　chronic 743, 745
　　autoimmune 758, 758t
　D 747, 750
　E 747
　virus antibodies 734
　virus antigen 734
　virus profile 811
Hepatoblastoma 840, 841f
Hepatocellular carcinoma 842, 843, 846f
　with ascites 846f

TNM classification of 844, 844t
types of 842
Hepatomegaly 737
causes of 739t
Hepatorenal syndrome 808
Hereditary hemochromatosis 773
Hereditary non-polyposis colon cancer 538, 550
Hernia 474
incisional 972
internal 343
mercedes repair of parastomal 714f
operative repair of parastomal 713f
paracolostomy 713f
paraesophageal 136f
parastomal 713
Herpes simplex virus 173
Hiatus hernia 134
types 134f
Hill repair
anesthesia 156
incision 156
modified 155, 155f
position 156
postoperative care 157
Hinchey's classification of diverticulitis 515f
Hirschsprung's disease 53, 572, 574f
Horseshoe abscess, drainage of 620f
Horsley's slit and oversewing of ulcer 286f
Hunt–Lawrence pouch 329f
Hydatid cyst of liver 828, 829f
Hyperplasia, focal nodular 833, 834, 835, 836f, 838t
Hyperplastic polyps 533
Hypertension, portal 793
complications 796
management 796, 802
Hypochondrial pain
left 8
right 7
Hypochondrium
left 20t
right 20t
Hypogastric pain 10t
Hypogastrium 20t

I

Ileal lipoma 402f
Ileal pouch–anal anastomosis 561
Ileocecal tuberculosis 368f
Ileoileal intussusception 359f, 360f, 362f
Ileoileal intussusception 361f
Ileorectal/ileoanal anastomosis 561
Ileosigmoid knotting 487
Ileostomy 683
mucosal slough of 708f
prolapse 712f
stenosis of 710f, 711f
Ileotransverse colostomy 558f
Ileum and ascending colon 559f

Iliac fossa
  left 20t
  right 20t
  with vomiting, pain in left 13
  with, pain in right 12
Immune modulators 748
Immune system disorders 45
Inflammatory disease of proximal colon, chronic 372f
Inflammatory polyps 533
Infrared coagulator 592f
Injury, type of 770
Insulin, secrete 986
Interferon and ribavirin therapy 752t
Intestinal atresia 353f
Intestinal diseases, small 351
  symptoms of 350
Intestinal obstruction 389, 476
  causes of 391t
Intestinal stomas 663
Intestinal tuberculosis 366, 368f
Intestine, large 477
  anatomy of 477
  injuries of 489
Intestine, small 347
  injuries of 357
  physiology 349
Intra-abdominal abscesses 302, 421, 421f
Intra-abdominal adhesions 424f
Intraductal short wave lithotripsy 975
Intragastric haemorrhage 283
  delayed 285

Iron 350
Irritable bowel syndrome 380
Ischemic colitis 502, 503t, 504f
Ischemic enteritis 386, 388f
Izbicki's procedure 1022f

J

Jaboulay pyloroplasty 226f
Janeway's gastrostomy 667, 668f
Jaundice 69, 726, 727, 727f
  classification of 84t
  mild 75
  obstructive 82, 86f, 1050
    causes 82
  postoperative 305
Jejunal diverticula 394f
Jejunal loop (efferent loop) herniation 300
Jejunogastric intussusception 345
Jejunojejunostomy with feeding jejunostomy 295f
Jejunostomy 672, 672f
Jejunum 273f
  internal herniation of 343f
Joints 772, 777

K

Kidney 777
Klebsiella species 814
Koch's continent ileostomy 684f
Kocher's maneuver 193
Kudo's classification 530f

L

Lactate dehydrogenase 734
Ladd's bands, division of 357*f*
Ladd's operation 357*f*
Large bowel, reconstructions of 552
Laser hemorrhoidectomy 600
Lay-open technique (fistulotomy) 626*f*, 628
Leger's procedure 1017*f*
Lilly technique 880
Limb pouch, triple 315*f*
Limb Roux-En-Y, triple 315*f*
Lithotripsy 975, 976
    complication 976
    mechanical 975
Liver 197, 720, 772, 777
    anatomy of 720
    calcified hydatid cyst of 830*f*
    injuries of 739
    laparoscopic 861
    mass in 846*f*
    multiloculated cyst of 826*f*
    multiple metastases of 850*f*
Liver abscess 814
    pyogenic 814
Liver biopsy 787
    and hepatic iron 774
Liver cyst 826*f*
    acquired 823
    congenital 822
    neoplastic 823, 832
        signs of 832
        symptoms of 832
    parasitic 823
Liver disease 726
    chronic 862
    drug-induced 768
    model for end-stage 762
    signs 729
    symptoms 727
    types of alcoholic 760
Liver dullness, obliteration of 7
Liver enzymes 811
Liver failure, signs of 730
Liver function tests 85, 733, 795
Liver injuries
    alcoholic 770*t*
    blood tests 742
    classification 740
    scale 741*t*
    signs of 741
    symptoms of 741
    types of 740*f*
    with hemoperitoneum 742*f*
Liver masses, focal 809
Liver parenchyma 860
Liver therapies, regional 851
Liver transplantation 771, 862, 863
    complications 866
    living donor and split 865
Liver tumors 834
    benign 833
Longmire operation, transverse 1020, 1021*f*
Loop ileostomy 712*f*

Loop obstruction, chronic afferent 340, 340f, 341
Loop ostomy 689
Los Angeles classification 143f
Lucey–Driscoll syndrome 82
Lumbar region 20t
Luminal nutrient deficiency 714
Lymph nodes of stomach 200f, 201f
Lymph nodes status 240t, 844, 939
Lymph nodes, classification of 198
Lymphatic drainage 436
Lymphatics 724
Lymphocytic gastritis 213
Lymphoid polyps 533
Lymphomas 402
   low-grade 249

M

Maddrey's discriminant function 762
Magnesium 350
Malabsorption and weight loss 321
Malignancies, types of 650
Mallory–Weiss tear of esophagus 181
   management 182
Mcburney's point 440f
Meckel's diverticulum 394f
Menetrier's disease 260
   management of 260
   signs of 260
   symptoms of 260
Mercadier procedure 1018f
Mesenteric artery, branch of superior 984
Mesenteric ischemia, classification of 388
Mesenteric vascular obstruction 386
Mesenteric vein, superior 853
Mesenteric vessels, division of 413f
Mesh rectopexy 656f
Mesoappendix
   clamping 463f
   division of 463f, 467f
Mesocolic vessels, division of 555f
Mesorectal excision 639, 640f
Mesosigmoidoplasty 483f
Metabolic liver diseases 772, 849, 862
Metastatic status 241t, 844, 939
Midgut volvulus 355f
Mirizzi's syndrome 896, 897f
   types of 897f
Mortensen's U-shaped colopexy 487f
Mucocele 895
   calcified 458f
Mucocutaneous infection 708
Mucocutaneous suturing 688f, 691f
Mucosa of ulcerative colitis 492f
Murphy's sign 892
Musshoff classification 248
Musshoff modification 404t
Myochosis 512f

N

Nasobiliary drainage/endobiliary stenting 911
Nausea 61, 62t
　acute 62t
　causes of 61, 62t
　chronic 62t
　management of 63
NDO plicator 160f
Necrosis,
　infection of 995
　percentage of 1000
Neoplastic polyps 524
Nerve supply 117, 436, 478, 870
Neuroanatomy 985
Nipple valve slippage complication 717
Nissen's fundoplication 151f
　anesthesia 153
　complications 154
　incision 153
　position 152
　postoperative care 154
Non-alcoholic steatohepatitis 767
Nonbleeding varices 798
Non-disposable bags 696
Non-drainable bags 698
Non-gallstone pancreatitis 1002
Non-neoplastic polyps 533
Nonspecific symptoms 75
Nutritional deficiencies 428, 428f
　management 429

O

Obesity, classification of 261t
Obstruction, nature of 83t
Obstructive calculus disease 908f
Obturator test 443f
Oddi dysfunction 933t
　sphincter of 932
Odor 705
　management 705
Ogilvie's syndrome 506, 507
　signs of 507
　symptoms of 507
Omental patch 222f
Oral nucleoside analogs 749
　of adenosine monophosphate 749
Oropharyngeal dysphagia 33
　propulsive causes of 34t
Orthotopic liver transplantation 864f
Osmotic watery diarrhea 44t
Ostomy
　complications of 707
　end loop 689
　postoperative management of 693
　separation of 708, 709f

P

Pain
　referred 5f
　site of 2t

Pancreas 197, 772, 983
- cell tumors of 1041
- divisum 984
- edematous 999f
- exocrine 985

Pancreatic calculi 1000f, 1013f
Pancreatic cystic tumors 1038t
Pancreatic disease 987
Pancreatic duct anatomy 983
Pancreatic enzymes 1012
- in body fluids 990

Pancreatic function tests 1010
Pancreatic head malignancy 1034f
Pancreatic leak 1048
Pancreatic left resection 1020
Pancreatic malignancy 1030, 1031
- TNM classification of 1031, 1032t

Pancreatic pseudocyst 1023, 1025f
- signs of 1024
- symptoms of 1024

Pancreatic resections 1043
Pancreatic secretions, leakage of 1048
Pancreatic surgery, complications of 1045
Pancreatitis 1009
Pancreatitis, acute 992, 999f, 1000, 1004t
- management of 1006f
- necrotizing 994
- severity of 1001

Pancreatitis, calcific 1013f
Pancreatitis, chronic 1008, 1009t, 1012t, 1014
Pancreatitis, postoperative 303
Pancreatoduodenectomy, surgical technique of 1044
Pancreatolauryl test 1011
Pancytopenia 795
Parabronchial pouch 132f
Paraesophageal hernia 136f
Paraileostomy fistula 715f
Paralytic ileus 385, 470
- causes of 385t
- step ladder pattern of 386f

Partington-Rochelle operation 1018, 1019f
Pedunculated colonic polyp 527f
Peg procedure 669
Peg tube, positioning of 671f
Pelvic and subcecal appendicitis 444t
Pelvic/paracolic abscess 472
Percutaneous endoscopic gastrostomy 669, 671f
- with jejunal extension 677, 677f

Percutaneous transhepatic cholangiogram 735
Periampullary carcinoma 1026, 1027, 1028f, 1029f
Perianal hematoma 611, 611f
- signs of 611
- symptoms of 611

Perihilar cholangiocarcinoma 945t
Perineal wound 644f
Peripheral antineutrophil cytoplasmic antibody 930
Peritoneal tuberculosis 365, 366

Pigment stones 883, 884f
Polycystic liver disease 824, 825, 827f, 828
Polypoid periampullary carcinoma 1029f
Polyposis syndromes 534, 535t
   management 536
Polyps
   anatomy of 523f
   multiple 528f
   type of 234t
Portal vein thrombosis 787-789
   causes of 788
   management 789
   signs 788
   symptoms 788
Portosystemic shunt 855f
   procedures 853
   types of 853t
Postappendicectomy 475f
Postesophagectomy complications 195
Posthepatic (post-sinusoidal) causes 794
Postoperative jaundice, management 306
Post-vagotomy diarrhea 320
Poth's operation 313f
Prehepatic (presinusoidal) causes 794
Prophylactic colectomy 536
Proteins 349
Proteus species 814

Prothrombin time 734, 783
Pseudocyst
   acute 1024
   chronic 1024
   types of 1024
Pseudomonas infection 912
Pseudopolyps 522f
Pseuodmembranous colitis 497
   management 499
   signs of 498
   symptoms of 498
Puborectalis muscle 50
Puestow-Gilesby operation 1017/1018f
Purse-string suture, application of 666f
Pus 895
Pyloric stenosis, congenital 251, 252f, 254f
Pyloromyotomy 254f
Pyloroplasty 266t, 268f
   laparoscopic 279f

Q

Quadrant pain, left
   lower 10t
   upper 3t
Quadrant pain, upper 3t
Quinolone 42

R

Radiation 4
Radiation colitis 500

Radiopaque gallstones 887f
   multiple 887f
   single 887f
Ranson criteria 1002f
Rectal examination 55, 732
Rectal malignancy 636
   management 638
Rectal polyps 635, 636f
   management 635
Rectal prolapse 653
   management 654
Rectal ulcer 661
Rectum and anal canal 569
Rectum
   injuries of 579
   physiology 571
   prolapse 654f
Red blood cells 777
Reflux esophagitis 137, 138f
Resection, low anterior 647f
Retching 61
Ripstein's procedure 656f
Rotor syndrome 72, 81, 81t, 330
Roux-En-Y gastric bypass 262
Roux-En-Y gastrojejunostomy, side-to-side 293f
Roux-En-Y reconstruction 302f
Rovsing's sign 441f
Rubber band ligation 593
Rumack-Mathew paracetamol nomogram 771f
Rumpf's operation 1019, 1020f
Rupture of stump 473

S

Savary–Miller classification 141, 142f
Schatzki's ring 129, 130f
Sclerosing cholangitis 929f, 930f
Sclerosing cholangitis, primary 928
   classification 933
   complications 930
   management 931, 934
Scopy-anastomotic ulcer 336f
Secretin pancreozymin test 1010
Secretory watery diarrhea 44t
Septic syndrome 994
Seromuscular suturing 273f
Serum albumin 783
Serum alkaline phosphatase 783
Serum alpha fetoprotein 811
Serum amylase, elevation of 996
Serum bilirubin 811
Serum iron 774
Short bowel syndrome 429, 430f
Shunt procedures 852
Sigmoid colon 641f
Sigmoid volvulus 480, 480f
Sigmoidoscopy, malignant growth 637f
Skin 772
   irritation 707
      management 707
   preparation of 699f
   problems of 706
   protection cream, application of 703f

Index

Sleeve gastrectomy, laparoscopic 261
Small bowel, diverticulitis of 393
Small bowel lymphoma 405f
   bleeding from 111f
   types of 404t
Solitary rectal ulcer 662f
Sphincterotomy, closed internal 616f
Sphincterotomy, open 616f
Spleen 197
Splenic artery, branch of 198
Splenic vein 853
Spyglass cholangiography 736
Squamous cell carcinoma 184
Stamm's gastrostomy 664, 666f
Stewart-way classification 919
   of bile duct injuries f 920
Stoma sites 682
Stoma, infection of 679
Stomach 273f
   acid secretion 202
   acidity in 215
   after GJ, removal of distal 279f
   and duodenum 197
   and jejunum, opening of 274f
   angiodysplasia of 111f
   anterior wall of 665f
   arterial supply to 197
   carcinoma 244f
   gastric hormones 203
   gastric mucosal barrier 203
   intrinsic factor 203
   lymphatic drainage of 198
   malignant growth 243f
   pepsinogen secretion 203
   physiology 202
   removal of 266t
   surgeries of 265, 267
   surgical anatomy 197
   with liver metastases, carcinoma 244f
Stomal obstruction 294
Stomas 663, 680
   diverting 685
Stone extraction 974
Stone in CBD, multiple 910f
Stools examination 84
Stress gastritis 212
Stretta procedure 161f
Strictures 383
Stricturoplasty, types of 384f
Submucosal plexus 117
Sutures
   application of 603f
   tightening 605f
Swallowing, physiology of 31
Synchronous lesions 540
Synergistic neurotoxins 806

T

Terrence Kennedy operation 316f
Thiersch operation 660f
Thoracic esophagus 116, 189f
Thrombosed and ulcerated pile masses 588f

Tissue diagnosis 757, 761, 774
Torsion of midgut 355f
Toxic injury to liver 781
Toxic megacolon 492f
Toxic-metabolic pancreatitis 1009
Tracheoesophageal fistula 122f
Transaminases and bilirubin 816
Transduodenal sphincterotomy 978
Transhiatal esophagectomy 193
Transjugular intrahepatic
portosystemic shunt 180,
789, 789f, 797
Transthoracic Nissen fundoplication 151
Transthoracic procedure 147
Trauma 706
management 707
Traveler's diarrhea 42, 44
Trichobezoar 257f
by laparotomy, removal of 258f
Tuberculosis, of mesenteric lymph nodes 365, 366
Tumor
benign 182, 401
diagnosis 183
management 183, 401
signs 183
symptoms 183
carcinoid 453
malignant 402, 406
management 406, 407
mucinous 456
Tumor of liver, rare benign 834
Tumor status 240t

U

Ulcer, anastomotic 335
diagnosis 335
management 336
Ulcer
excision of 266t
location of 217t
recurrent 336
Ulcerations, marginal 1049
Ulcerative colitis 375t, 490, 493f
malignant growth with 545f
Ulcerative type 365, 366
Umbilical region 20t
Uncut Roux operation 333f
Unresectable tumors 851
Ureter
left 642f
right 642f
Ureteric colic 450t
Urine 1011
examination 84

V

Vaccine, type of 753
van De Kamer test 1011
Varicella zoster virus 173
Vasoactive inhibitory peptide 311
Vasotopic drugs 589
Vein, portal 853
Venous diseases 387
Venous drainage 117, 198, 478, 722, 870
Ventral hernia 475f

Vermiform appendix 435
Viral hepatitis 76, 734, 743
    complications 747
    management 747
    signs of 745
    symptoms of 745
Vitamin B_{12} 681
Vitamin K 350
Volvulus 479
    of midgut 354
    of reservoir 719
Vomiting 61, 62t
    acute 62t
    causes of 61, 62t
    chronic 62t
    management of 63

W

Water-soluble vitamins 350
WBC and platelet counts 783
Weight loss pathogenesis 322f

Wells Ivalon sponge rectopexy 656f
Whipple operation 1021f
Whipple's disease 377, 378
Whipple's operation 1029
Wilson's disease 776, 783
    complications 777
    management 777
    signs of 776
    symptoms of 776
Witzel's gastrostomy 667, 667f
Witzel's open surgical jejunostomy 673f
Wound infection 471f
    after appendicectomy 471
    after colonic surgery 563
Wound, perineal 644f

Z

Zenker's diverticulum 132f
Zollinger-Ellison syndrome 228